ACCESS TO
Health
Risk
Behavior
in the United States

ACCESS TO

Health
Risk
Behavior

in the United States

A State-by-State Look
at Teens and Adults

*BY THE EDITORS OF
NEW STRATEGIST
PUBLICATIONS*

New Strategist Publications, Inc.
Ithaca, New York

New Strategist Publications, Inc.
P.O. Box 242, Ithaca, New York 14851
800/848-0842; 607/273-0913
www.newstrategist.com

ISBN 1-885070-59-4

Printed in the United States of America

Contents

Tables

Part One: Adults

Part Two: Youth

Results from the 2001 Youth Risk Behavior Surveillance System

Trends from the Youth Risk Behavior Surveillance System

Foreword

We live in a time when the relationships between human behavior and health conditions are better understood, and both public policy makers and businesses are struggling with concerns such as access to and the high cost of health insurance, the rapidly rising price of prescription drugs, and the growing prevalence of obesity in the American population. We also live in a time of increasing reliance by policy makers and business leaders on a broad range of data to make informed decisions. Frequently, these data are not easily accessible in the form needed or for the geographic units wanted.

New Strategist Publications recognizes the growing importance of providing easy access to data on youth and adult health behavior and has created a book that will be a valuable addition to audiences needing both general and detailed health behavior information. Using data from the Behavioral Risk Factor Surveillance System (BRFSS) and the Youth Risk Behavior Surveillance System (YRBSS), the two best data sources on health behavior in the United States, New Strategist's editors have generated a compendium of more than 200 tables containing a wide range of health behavior information for the United States and individual states, easing the process of making cross-state comparisons. In addition, the youth data presented are for two time periods, making valuable trend analysis possible.

The tables contain important health behavior factors cross-tabulated by demographic factors that are known to be related to health risk behavior such as age, education, sex, and household income. The detailed data make it feasible to examine factors related to health risk behavior in depth, and to observe if these relationships vary or are the same across states. Adding data for two time periods is quite useful in understanding the effects of the addition or elimination of new public and private programs and policies designed to influence health behavior. While the BRFSS and YRFSS websites allow the user to create custom tables, it is not possible to generate many of the tables found in the book without spending hours at the task.

Through its reference books, New Strategist brings demographic information to a broad range of audiences, including those in health care. With this volume, New Strategist reveals its strong commitment to advancing the discussion of important public policy issues by providing improved access to the data needed to better understand them.

Louis G. Pol
Dean, College of Business Administration
University of Nebraska at Omaha
October 6, 2003

A Message from New Strategist Publications

New Strategist Publications specializes in providing easy access to increasingly inaccessible government data. Providing such access is becoming ever more important as the Internet and electronic publishing replace paper products in the reference book industry.

The rise of the Internet has changed the way the federal government disseminates information. Many government agencies have stopped producing paper reports, while others publish paper editions only of summary data and not the details. To get at the details, government web sites often require users to navigate huge spreadsheets—some literally hundreds of pages long. Others allow users to create customized tables from their databases, but only one variable at a time. Like blind people describing an elephant, often we see only the parts—the trunk, a leg, the tail—and not the whole.

Until now. With the publication of the ACCESS TO series, New Strategist Publications, the leader in demographic reference book publishing, is putting government data back into the hands of the American public. *ACCESS TO: Health Risk Behavior in the United States: A State-by-State Look at Teens and Adults* reveals the findings of two important government health surveys in one volume. The first, the Behavioral Risk Factor Surveillance System (BRFSS), is a state-by-state examination of the health and health-risk behaviors of adults aged 18 or older. The second, the Youth Risk Behavior Surveillance System (YRBSS), is a state (and sometimes local) level examination of the health and health risk behavior of students in grades 9 through 12. The results of both surveys are available piecemeal online. This book presents them in their entirety for a comprehensive look at Americans' health at the state level.

ACCESS TO: Health Risk Behavior in the United States: A State-by-State Look at Teens and Adults presents data from the 2001 BRFSS survey. Data for earlier years are shown for questions not asked in 2001. In those cases, data for the latest year available are presented. Not every state fielded every question, so if a state is missing from the list, it means it did not include the question in its survey. For most questions, state-level data are shown by age, education, household income, and sex. While race and Hispanic origin data are available from BRFSS, they are not included in this book. In many states, sample sizes are too small to make reliable estimates for racial subgroups. Those interested in exploring answers to BRFSS health questions by state and race should visit the BRFSS web site (http://www.cdc.gov/brfss/) where such data can be explored state-by-state and question-by-question. Be sure to check the size of the standard errors on any results before depending on the data, however.

ACCESS TO: Health Risk Behavior in the United States: A State-by-State Look at Teens and Adults also includes the data from the 2001 YRBSS. Answers to questions asked of the nation's high school students are shown by state and for some local areas. Demographic breaks (sex, race, Hispanic origin, and grade) are shown at the national level only. Also included is the

Center for Disease Control's analysis of the 2001 data that appeared in *Morbidity and Mortality Weekly Report*. In addition, the book includes trend data for participating states.

ACCESS TO: Health Risk Behavior in the United States: A State-by-State Look at Teens and Adults gives readers handy access to important state-level health data not comprehensively available elsewhere. With the data in hand, researchers, health providers, and businesses can become better informed about the health status and behavior of the American population.

New Strategist Publications, Inc.

P.O. Box 242, Ithaca, NY 14851

phone: 607 / 273-0913; toll free 800 / 848-0842

fax: 607 / 277-0481

e-mail: demographics@newstrategist.com

website: www.newstrategist.com

Part One: Adults

Behavioral Risk Factor Surveillance System

Behavioral Risk Factor Surveillance System

Centers for Disease Control and Prevention (CDC)
U.S. Department of Health and Human Services

(The following descriptions of the Behavioral Risk Factor Surveillance System appear on the BRFSS web site.)

Nearly 40 percent of deaths in America can be attributed to smoking, physical inactivity, poor diet, or alcohol misuse—behaviors practiced by many people every day for much of their lives. For 18 years, the Centers for Disease Control and Prevention (CDC) has helped states survey U.S. adults to learn more about a wide range of behaviors that affect their health. A strong focus has been on the following behaviors, which are linked with heart disease, stroke, cancer, and diabetes—the nation's leading killers:

- Not getting enough physical activity
- Eating a high-fat, low-fiber diet
- Using tobacco and alcohol
- Not getting medical care that is known to save lives (for example, mammograms, Pap smears, colorectal cancer screening, and flu shots)

The surveys have given us a wealth of knowledge about these and other harmful behaviors—how common they are, whether they are increasing over time, and which people might be most at risk. Such information is essential to public health agencies at the national, state, and local levels.

We must continue to monitor health behaviors to ensure our programs are on track, because chronic diseases are a growing public health threat. Heart disease is the leading cause of death in this country, accounting for more than 30 percent of all deaths. Cancer is the second leading cause, accounting for about 25 percent of all deaths.

About the BRFSS

The Behavioral Risk Factor Surveillance System (BRFSS) is a collaborative project of the Centers for Disease Control and Prevention (CDC) and U.S. states and territories. The BRFSS, administered and supported by CDC's Behavioral Surveillance Branch, is an ongoing data collection program designed to measure behavioral risk factors in the adult population 18 years of age or older living in households. The BRFSS was initiated in 1984, with 15 states collecting surveillance data on risk behavior. Today, all 50 states, three territories, and the District of Columbia take part in the survey. The BRFSS is the primary source of information on health-related behaviors of Americans.

The objective of the BRFSS is to collect uniform, state-specific data on preventive health practices and risk behaviors that are linked to chronic diseases, injuries, and preventable infectious diseases in the adult population. Factors assessed by the BRFSS include tobacco use, health care coverage, HIV / AIDS knowledge or prevention, physical activity, and fruit and vegetable consumption. Data are collected from a random sample of adults (one per household) through a telephone survey.

State and local health departments rely heavily on data from the BRFSS to determine priority health issues and identify populations at highest risk for illness, disability, and death. States use the data in a variety of ways:

- To develop strategic plans and target prevention programs
- To monitor the effectiveness of interventions and progress in meeting prevention goals
- To educate the public, the health community, and policy makers about disease prevention
- To support community policies that promote health and prevent disease

The BRFSS field operations are managed by state health departments with guidelines provided by the CDC. These health departments participate in developing the survey instrument and conduct the interviews either in-house or through use of contractors. The data are transmitted to the CDC's National Center for Chronic Disease Prevention and Health Promotion's Behavioral Surveillance Branch for editing, processing, weighting, and analysis. An edited and weighted data file is provided to each participating health department for each year of data collection, and summary reports of state specific data are prepared by CDC. Health departments use the data for a variety of purposes, including identifying demographic variations in health related behaviors, targeting services, addressing emergent and critical health issues, proposing legislation for health initiatives and measuring progress toward state and national health objectives.

BRFSS data also help public health professionals monitor progress in meeting the nation's health objectives outlined in Healthy People 2010. BRFSS information is used by researchers, voluntary and professional organizations, and managed care organizations to target prevention efforts. Recognizing the value of the BRFSS, Canada, Australia, Russia, and other countries have asked CDC to help them establish similar surveillance systems for their own populations.

Uses of the BRFSS

CDC's Behavioral Risk Factor Surveillance System benefits states in many ways. The BRFSS data can be analyzed according to age, sex, education, income, race, ethnicity, and other variables. This allows states to find groups at highest risk for health problems and make better use of scarce resources to prevent these problems.

The BRFSS is designed to examine trends over time. For example, state-based data from the BRFSS have revealed a national epidemic of obesity.

States can readily address urgent and emerging health issues. Questions may be added for a wide range of important health issues, such as diabetes, arthritis, tobacco use, folic acid consumption, health care coverage, and even terrorism. For example, following the bomb explosion at the Alfred P. Murrah Federal Building in Oklahoma City, the Oklahoma BRFSS included questions on such issues as stress, nightmares, and feelings of hopelessness so that health department personnel could better address the psychological impact of the disaster. New York State was able to use the survey to collect data in response to the terrorist attacks on the World Trade Center.

States can use the BRFSS to find out if their programs are working and keep them on track. In Arkansas, for example, health officials are using the BRFSS to determine if the state's breast care program is boosting the percentage of women over 40 who have mammograms. The state also uses

BRFSS data to improve and refine the program, which provides breast cancer education, screening, and treatment to women with limited resources.

The BRFSS is flexible in that it allows states to add timely questions specific to their needs. Yet standard core questions enable health professionals to make comparisons among states and reach national conclusions. BRFSS data have highlighted wide state-to-state differences in key health issues. In 2000, for example, the percentage of adults who smoked ranged from a low of 13 percent in Utah to a high of 30 percent in Kentucky.

Oregon is one state that has used BRFSS findings to inform public policy. The fight to pass workplace smoking bans had been tough in Oregon. Supporters of workplace smoking bans were called health fanatics who were out of step with the wishes of ordinary citizens. The BRFSS produced powerful evidence that proved otherwise. The surveys revealed that about 9 in 10 Oregonians thought breathing secondhand smoke was harmful to health and that people should be protected. As a result, workplace smoking bans have been passed in communities across the state. About 30 percent of Oregonians now live in localities where smoking is banned in all or nearly all workplaces.

Flu and pneumonia are common causes of death for older Americans, but not all seniors get flu shots or pneumonia vaccinations. New York health officials used the BRFSS to identify populations with the greatest needs. They found that older adults living in New York City were far less likely to be vaccinated against flu or pneumonia than elders elsewhere in the state. Vaccination rates were also low among African Americans and Hispanics across the state. The BRFSS revealed good news as well: flu and pneumonia vaccination rates have increased dramatically statewide, particularly in areas where vaccination campaigns have been launched. Now, about half of all state residents over age 65 are vaccinated.

With the help of state health officials, Kansas City employers used BRFSS survey methods to identify serious health problems and risks affecting employees and their families. By improving the health of employees and dependents, the companies hope to cut health care costs and absenteeism. Two serious health conditions—diabetes and depression—were identified and are now being targeted. The employers concluded that community approaches, rather than just workplace programs, are the answer, and strong community partnerships are essential.

The BRFSS faces many challenges. As more people become aware of the system's usefulness, more questions are being added to the surveys. The challenge is keeping the phone interviews to a reasonable length. In addition, caller ID, cell phones, and competition from telemarketers are making it difficult for interviewers to contact and survey people by phone. Yet another challenge is how to continually increase the number of adults interviewed to meet the rising demand for data at the state, city, county, district, and subpopulation levels. These challenges might dictate future changes in the BRFSS. For example, we might need to establish several different surveillance systems or change the way we collect data. Whatever direction the BRFSS takes, CDC must work closely with state and federal partners to continue providing data useful for good public health research and practice.

History of the BRFSS

By the early 1980s, scientific research clearly showed that personal health behaviors played a major role in premature morbidity and mortality. Although national estimates of health risk behaviors among U.S. adult populations had been periodically obtained through surveys conducted by the National Center for Health Statistics (NCHS), these data were not available on a state-specific basis. This deficiency was viewed as critical for state health agencies that have the primary role of targeting resources to reduce behavioral risks and their consequent illnesses. National data may not be appropriate for any given state; however, state and local agency participation was critical to achieve national health goals.

About the same time as personal health behaviors received wider recognition in relation to chronic disease morbidity and mortality, telephone surveys emerged as an acceptable method for determining the prevalence of many health risk behaviors among populations. In addition to their cost advantages, telephone surveys were especially desirable at the state and local level, where the necessary expertise and resources for conducting area probability sampling for in-person household interviews were not likely to be available.

As a result, surveys were developed and conducted to monitor state-level prevalence of the major behavioral risks among adults associated with premature morbidity and mortality. The basic philosophy was to collect data on actual behaviors, rather than on attitudes or knowledge, that would be especially useful for planning, initiating, supporting, and evaluating health promotion and disease prevention programs.

To determine feasibility of behavioral surveillance, initial point-in-time state surveys were conducted in 29 states from 1981 to 1983. In 1984, The Centers for Disease Control and Prevention established the Behavioral Risk Factor Surveillance System, and 15 states participated in monthly data collection. Although the BRFSS was designed to collect state-level data, a number of states from the outset stratified their samples to allow them to estimate prevalence for regions within their respective states.

CDC developed a standard core questionnaire for states to use to provide data that could be compared across states. The BRFSS, administered and supported by the Division of Adult and Community Health, National Center for Chronic Disease Prevention and Health Promotion, CDC, is an on-going data collection program. By 1994, all states, the District of Columbia, and three territories were participating in the BRFSS.

Methodology of the BRFSS

The health characteristics estimated from the BRFSS pertain only to the adult population aged 18 years and older living in households. Respondents are identified through telephone-based methods. Although approximately 95 percent of U.S. households have telephones, coverage ranges from 87 to 98 percent across states and varies for subgroups as well. For example, persons living in the South, minorities, and those in lower socioeconomic groups typically have lower telephone coverage. No direct method of compensating for nontelephone coverage is employed by the BRFSS; however, poststratification weights are used, and may partially correct for any bias caused by nontelephone coverage. These weights adjust for differences in probability of selection and nonresponse, as well as noncoverage, and must be used for deriving representative population based estimates of risk behavior prevalence.

The BRFSS questionnaire. The questionnaire has three parts: (1) the core component; (2) optional modules; and (3) state-added questions.

The *core* is a standard set of questions asked by all states. It includes queries about current health-related perceptions, conditions, and behaviors (e.g., health status, health insurance, diabetes, tobacco use, selected cancer screening procedures, and HIV/AIDS risks) and questions on demographic characteristics. *Optional CDC modules* are sets of questions on specific topics (e.g., cardiovascular disease, oral health) that states elect to use on their questionnaires. In 2001, 14 modules were supported by CDC. *State-added questions* are developed or acquired by participating states and added to their questionnaires. State-added questions are not edited or evaluated by CDC.

Each year, the states and CDC agree on the content of the core component and optional modules. For comparability, many questions are taken from established national surveys, such as the National Health Interview Survey or the National Health and Nutrition Examination Survey. This practice allows the BRFSS to take advantage of questions that may have been tested and allows states to compare their data with those from other surveys. Any new questions proposed as additions to the BRFSS must go through cognitive testing and field testing prior to their inclusion on the survey. BRFSS protocol specifies that all states ask the core component questions without modification; they may choose to add any, all, or none of the optional modules; and states may add questions of their choosing at the end of the questionnaire.

Although CDC supported 14 modules in 2001, it is not feasible for a state to use them all. States are selective with their choices of modules and state-specific questions to keep the questionnaire at a reasonable length (though there is wide variation across states in the total number of questions for a given year, ranging from a low of about 90 to 150 or more). New questionnaires are implemented in January, and usually remain unchanged throughout the year. However, the flexibility of state-added questions does permit additions, changes, and deletions at any time during the year.

Before the beginning of the calendar year, CDC provides states with the text of the core component and the optional modules that will be supported for the coming year. States select their optional modules and choose any state-added question(s). Each state then constructs its questionnaire. The core component is asked first, optional modules are asked next, and state-added questions last. This ordering ensures comparability across states and follows CDC protocol. Generally, the only changes allowed are the limited insertion of state-added questions on topics related to core questions. Such exceptions are to be agreed upon in consultation with CDC. However, even with these exceptions, the policy has not been followed in every instance.

Once the content (core, modules, and state-added) of the questionnaire is determined by a state, it is used without changes for one calendar year. If a significant portion of the state population does not speak English, states have the option of translating the questionnaire into other languages. At the present time, CDC provides only a Spanish version of the core questionnaire and optional modules.

Data collection and processing. Data for a state may be collected directly by the state health department or through a contractor. In 2001, 14 state health departments collected their data in-house; 40 contracted data collection to university survey research centers or commercial firms.

Interviews are conducted through computer-assisted telephone interviewing (CATI). Following specifications provided by CDC, state health personnel or contractors conduct the interviews. The core portion of the questionnaire lasts an average of 10 minutes. Interview time for modules and state-added questions is dependent upon the number of questions used, but generally extend the interview period by an additional 5 to 10 minutes. Telephone interviewing is conducted during each calendar month, and calls are made seven days per week, during both day and evening hours.

CDC begins to process data for the survey year as soon as states or their contractors begin submitting data, and it continues processing data throughout the survey year. Once the entire year of data for a state has been received and validated, several year-end programs are run on the data. These programs perform some additional, limited data cleanup and fixes specific to the state and data year, and they produce reports that identify potential analytic problems with the data set. Once these programs are complete, the data are ready for assigning weights and adding new variables.

Not all of the variables that appear on the public use data set are taken directly from the state files. CDC prepares a set of SAS programs that prepare the data for analysis and add weighting and risk factor calculations as variables to the data file. To create the risk factor calculations, several variables from the data file are combined. Creation of the variables varies in complexity; some only combine codes, while others require sorting and combining selected codes from multiple variables.

Limitations of BRFSS data. BRFSS data vary somewhat by state with respect to data collection, sampling design, and sample size. In a few states, a portion of sample records intended for use during one month may have been completed in another month. Several states do not collect data all 12 months of the year. Although almost all states collect data monthly, the annual number of interviews ranges from 871 in Guam to 8,628 in Massachusetts. Estimates for some states are therefore based upon smaller sample sizes, and for rare events, may yield unstable estimates. Some items such as immunizations are affected by seasonality, and estimates for these items may be biased for subpopulations.

All data collection systems are subject to error, and records may be incomplete or contain inaccurate information. Respondents may not remember essential information, a question may not mean the same thing to different respondents, and some individuals may not respond at all. It is not always possible to measure the magnitude of these errors or their impact on the data. The data user must make his or her own evaluation of the data. Overall estimates generally have relatively small sampling errors, but estimates for certain population subgroups may be based on small numbers and have relatively large sampling errors. When the number of events is small and the probability of such an event is small, considerable caution must be observed in interpreting the estimates or differences among groups and areas.

For more information

To learn more about BRFSS or to examine additional survey results, visit the BRFSS web site at http://www.cdc.gov/brfss/.

1.1 Alcohol Consumption by Age, 1999

"During the past month, have you had at least
one drink of any alcoholic beverage?"

(percent of people aged 18 or older responding "yes," by state and age, 1999)

	total	18 to 24	25 to 34	35 to 44	45 to 54	55 to 64	65 or older
U.S. total	**54.2%**	**61.1%**	**62.1%**	**58.2%**	**56.0%**	**47.2%**	**36.1%**
Alabama	39.6	52.3	55.2	40.4	35.4	31.7	23.1
Alaska	56.9	65.6	58.5	57.0	59.9	50.9	38.2
Arizona	34.5	28.2	33.8	31.7	40.6	31.5	39.4
Arkansas	38.3	49.5	49.5	43.1	36.3	29.4	24.9
California	60.4	64.8	67.7	60.1	59.8	55.0	51.8
Colorado	64.2	67.9	70.8	70.6	64.7	60.1	44.3
Connecticut	59.4	69.9	63.6	62.7	59.5	52.4	49.1
Delaware	60.0	61.3	68.6	66.2	63.6	50.5	46.3
District of Columbia	50.3	59.4	57.2	56.3	50.0	46.9	30.5
Florida	55.2	56.3	61.2	59.4	61.0	47.5	46.5
Georgia	47.7	51.6	61.4	51.3	46.7	38.7	27.1
Hawaii	48.6	58.5	52.9	50.8	51.8	45.5	33.1
Idaho	48.9	52.8	55.6	54.0	51.2	42.9	35.5
Illinois	57.3	74.8	67.0	62.6	62.6	46.1	35.6
Indiana	54.3	67.6	61.8	62.7	53.3	52.4	30.4
Iowa	55.0	67.9	63.9	60.9	59.4	48.9	34.5
Kansas	46.8	60.2	55.7	53.5	48.9	39.4	24.9
Kentucky	34.9	44.7	46.1	42.8	35.3	21.1	16.7
Louisiana	45.4	54.0	54.8	52.1	49.8	36.1	22.2
Maine	59.8	65.8	68.1	65.9	61.1	60.1	40.0
Maryland	57.8	65.8	62.4	63.0	61.0	52.4	38.9
Massachusetts	61.5	64.0	69.6	67.0	64.0	55.9	47.2
Michigan	59.2	71.9	66.0	64.4	59.4	50.7	41.7
Minnesota	51.1	54.7	57.6	49.0	57.1	46.0	41.0
Mississippi	38.6	45.8	53.6	42.1	37.8	31.2	18.8
Missouri	53.4	65.3	62.9	58.3	53.8	47.2	35.0
Montana	56.9	66.8	65.5	66.5	56.4	45.3	40.8
Nebraska	52.2	59.5	62.0	57.9	56.6	46.0	32.6
Nevada	63.1	73.8	63.1	66.3	62.2	60.8	54.4
New Hampshire	64.2	73.1	70.1	67.9	66.3	54.9	49.1
New Jersey	54.0	61.6	63.2	55.4	55.2	51.0	40.4
New Mexico	54.1	57.5	65.6	60.1	52.6	50.3	34.3
New York	52.6	62.6	54.1	56.0	52.5	50.3	42.6
North Carolina	41.7	55.7	49.1	47.9	40.4	33.7	22.1
North Dakota	55.4	69.5	67.6	62.3	56.1	44.2	33.4
Ohio	43.8	63.1	52.1	50.9	40.8	36.9	22.6
Oklahoma	28.6	39.7	38.4	30.6	31.1	23.3	11.1
Oregon	60.9	63.3	67.4	69.2	61.1	49.9	50.2
Pennsylvania	51.5	61.0	62.6	58.1	50.3	42.5	36.9
Rhode Island	58.3	58.4	67.9	64.8	63.1	52.8	42.7
South Carolina	42.0	47.4	50.4	49.1	43.0	34.5	23.6
South Dakota	58.6	68.6	67.6	65.1	60.8	50.2	40.9
Tennessee	29.7	35.7	38.6	38.4	28.3	19.4	14.4
Texas	54.8	60.3	62.2	59.1	56.4	47.3	36.7
Utah	29.7	35.2	30.0	37.4	29.3	22.3	17.6
Vermont	60.5	69.5	69.2	64.3	62.5	56.1	40.8
Virginia	54.3	58.7	59.7	59.6	59.0	49.9	29.2
Washington	60.7	63.0	71.9	63.9	58.7	59.3	45.5
West Virginia	32.6	47.4	43.0	40.9	30.4	19.5	17.9
Wisconsin	71.1	77.2	77.5	77.7	72.1	69.2	54.6
Wyoming	56.1	61.8	65.5	58.2	56.0	52.0	41.8

Source: Compiled by New Strategist based on the Centers for Disease Control and Prevention Behavioral Risk Factor Surveillance System Survey, Internet site http://www.cdc.gov/brfss/index.htm

1.2 Alcohol Consumption by Education, 1999

*"During the past month, have you had at least
one drink of any alcoholic beverage?"*

(percent of people aged 18 or older responding "yes," by state and educational attainment, 1999)

	total	less than high school	high school graduate	some college	college graduate
U.S. total	**54.2%**	**34.2%**	**49.6%**	**57.9%**	**64.3%**
Alabama	39.6	24.4	33.0	45.7	57.3
Alaska	56.9	36.6	51.6	61.0	65.5
Arizona	34.5	15.6	32.3	36.8	44.7
Arkansas	38.3	24.5	36.9	43.6	45.2
California	60.4	45.7	56.2	63.8	70.8
Colorado	64.2	46.1	58.7	64.4	74.0
Connecticut	59.4	36.4	52.0	64.0	69.6
Delaware	60.0	39.0	54.9	58.3	72.7
District of Columbia	50.3	34.4	40.8	47.8	62.6
Florida	55.2	36.0	51.5	57.0	66.6
Georgia	47.7	29.9	40.7	51.6	61.3
Hawaii	48.6	27.5	45.2	50.6	54.8
Idaho	48.9	37.7	48.3	47.9	56.2
Illinois	57.3	29.4	54.6	61.3	68.4
Indiana	54.3	35.6	52.3	52.5	69.2
Iowa	55.0	33.4	51.0	58.7	65.7
Kansas	46.8	33.2	39.4	51.6	56.6
Kentucky	34.9	17.0	33.9	42.3	47.6
Louisiana	45.4	25.9	45.7	52.5	52.5
Maine	59.8	45.5	52.5	64.1	72.3
Maryland	57.8	37.0	52.0	59.3	68.4
Massachusetts	61.5	35.6	55.3	62.5	72.4
Michigan	59.2	40.5	55.9	61.4	67.7
Minnesota	51.1	35.4	47.7	50.7	59.2
Mississippi	38.6	24.5	33.1	44.5	52.9
Missouri	53.4	36.3	47.7	58.2	67.5
Montana	56.9	41.8	53.7	60.4	63.3
Nebraska	52.2	33.4	48.5	54.0	62.2
Nevada	63.1	57.2	61.6	64.3	66.9
New Hampshire	64.2	32.9	51.2	69.4	78.5
New Jersey	54.0	22.6	46.9	60.8	68.3
New Mexico	54.1	35.7	50.8	58.3	65.0
New York	52.6	30.3	45.9	59.2	64.9
North Carolina	41.7	21.1	35.7	46.7	59.2
North Dakota	55.4	35.3	56.0	58.0	62.1
Ohio	43.8	19.8	42.0	48.1	57.9
Oklahoma	28.6	17.4	25.6	31.4	38.0
Oregon	60.9	46.5	54.4	63.9	69.8
Pennsylvania	51.5	34.6	45.8	57.8	62.4
Rhode Island	58.3	33.7	51.0	63.2	72.2
South Carolina	42.0	23.2	38.7	46.6	54.6
South Dakota	58.6	42.6	55.4	61.4	65.8
Tennessee	29.7	18.1	25.2	33.5	42.0
Texas	54.8	40.5	53.8	57.4	63.8
Utah	29.7	29.4	36.7	24.0	29.3
Vermont	60.5	39.4	55.2	62.7	72.3
Virginia	54.3	30.9	43.0	58.7	67.9
Washington	60.7	44.2	54.8	60.7	70.6
West Virginia	32.6	15.3	30.3	39.7	49.9
Wisconsin	71.1	53.2	69.1	73.0	78.0
Wyoming	56.1	34.1	56.3	55.5	62.6

Source: Compiled by New Strategist based on the Centers for Disease Control and Prevention Behavioral Risk Factor Surveillance System Survey, Internet site http://www.cdc.gov/brfss/index.htm

1.3 Alcohol Consumption by Household Income, 1999

"During the past month, have you had at least one drink of any alcoholic beverage?"

(percent of people aged 18 or older responding "yes," by state and household income, 1999)

	total	less than $15,000	$15,000 to $24,999	$25,000 to $34,999	$35,000 to $49,999	$50,000 or more
U.S. total	**54.2%**	**40.2%**	**45.7%**	**53.3%**	**59.9%**	**67.5%**
Alabama	39.6	25.2	36.9	45.2	44.0	52.4
Alaska	56.9	45.4	50.4	53.1	57.3	64.0
Arizona	34.5	31.1	25.2	32.6	44.4	52.1
Arkansas	38.3	23.8	34.7	40.0	40.9	51.8
California	60.4	49.1	50.8	60.7	63.9	71.6
Colorado	64.2	43.3	56.3	62.2	62.1	78.5
Connecticut	59.4	47.9	48.2	56.7	64.7	71.2
Delaware	60.0	34.8	46.9	55.3	66.2	73.0
District of Columbia	50.3	41.5	40.8	44.3	64.7	67.4
Florida	55.2	33.6	46.8	52.6	60.8	72.0
Georgia	47.7	30.5	42.0	44.1	52.6	61.4
Hawaii	48.6	51.7	44.9	48.1	49.0	54.5
Idaho	48.9	38.2	46.4	46.5	49.4	61.1
Illinois	57.3	39.2	40.2	54.3	62.7	73.9
Indiana	54.3	28.2	42.4	57.6	61.9	70.9
Iowa	55.0	40.3	43.6	54.0	60.9	67.1
Kansas	46.8	36.6	40.3	42.2	47.2	63.8
Kentucky	34.9	19.8	28.2	35.1	43.7	49.0
Louisiana	45.4	33.9	42.9	44.6	52.1	58.6
Maine	59.8	40.1	58.0	59.7	68.1	72.5
Maryland	57.8	41.8	48.7	53.5	58.5	68.3
Massachusetts	61.5	44.7	46.5	62.2	71.1	75.4
Michigan	59.2	41.7	56.6	55.1	61.5	69.3
Minnesota	51.1	40.8	42.7	50.8	44.2	59.9
Mississippi	38.6	26.0	32.6	43.1	42.0	58.2
Missouri	53.4	34.0	42.3	54.8	59.6	71.4
Montana	56.9	49.4	49.0	57.1	62.4	68.8
Nebraska	52.2	41.5	45.6	55.8	61.7	63.1
Nevada	63.1	52.2	62.0	61.1	61.6	71.2
New Hampshire	64.2	44.9	50.0	61.5	68.8	76.1
New Jersey	54.0	35.4	37.8	46.2	60.2	70.7
New Mexico	54.1	40.3	52.9	51.8	61.5	69.3
New York	52.6	42.0	46.7	48.4	65.5	70.8
North Carolina	41.7	23.6	32.7	40.0	47.0	58.8
North Dakota	55.4	44.7	50.9	56.8	59.2	69.5
Ohio	43.8	32.1	37.9	35.5	48.9	57.4
Oklahoma	28.6	29.0	28.6	29.8	35.2	52.3
Oregon	60.9	49.3	52.7	59.3	63.8	71.0
Pennsylvania	51.5	37.1	45.8	55.6	53.6	66.4
Rhode Island	58.3	46.0	47.7	63.7	65.4	73.5
South Carolina	42.0	30.0	36.9	40.1	45.5	61.3
South Dakota	58.6	53.0	52.7	60.4	65.6	72.2
Tennessee	29.7	23.2	30.5	30.7	41.8	42.8
Texas	54.8	42.8	49.4	56.3	58.7	67.2
Utah	29.7	26.2	30.0	26.4	30.7	35.0
Vermont	60.5	47.0	54.9	63.9	63.6	76.8
Virginia	54.3	32.7	38.2	52.5	51.6	67.6
Washington	60.7	52.2	52.8	58.1	63.5	71.1
West Virginia	32.6	19.1	24.4	31.9	42.7	52.5
Wisconsin	71.1	59.6	59.6	71.3	75.4	83.1
Wyoming	56.1	42.7	51.7	56.8	61.6	66.3

Source: Compiled by New Strategist based on the Centers for Disease Control and Prevention Behavioral Risk Factor Surveillance System Survey, Internet site http://www.cdc.gov/brfss/index.htm

1.4 Alcohol Consumption by Sex, 1999

"During the past month, have you had at least one drink of any alcoholic beverage?"

(percent of people aged 18 or older responding "yes," by state and sex, 1999)

	total	men	women
U.S. total	**54.2%**	**62.4%**	**45.9%**
Alabama	39.6	49.8	30.6
Alaska	56.9	62.8	50.4
Arizona	34.5	43.4	26.1
Arkansas	38.3	46.7	30.8
California	60.4	68.4	52.5
Colorado	64.2	72.3	56.3
Connecticut	59.4	66.3	53.2
Delaware	60.0	70.4	50.6
District of Columbia	50.3	53.5	47.6
Florida	55.2	62.7	48.3
Georgia	47.7	59.0	37.4
Hawaii	48.6	59.3	37.8
Idaho	48.9	55.1	43.0
Illinois	57.3	67.4	47.3
Indiana	54.3	62.5	46.8
Iowa	55.0	65.2	45.8
Kansas	46.8	56.8	37.5
Kentucky	34.9	43.5	27.1
Louisiana	45.4	56.1	35.9
Maine	59.8	68.4	51.9
Maryland	57.8	66.1	50.2
Massachusetts	61.5	66.4	57.1
Michigan	59.2	68.0	51.1
Minnesota	51.1	55.5	46.9
Mississippi	38.6	50.0	28.6
Missouri	53.4	62.3	45.3
Montana	56.9	64.3	49.9
Nebraska	52.2	61.9	43.2
Nevada	63.1	68.9	57.2
New Hampshire	64.2	71.3	57.6
New Jersey	54.0	59.3	49.2
New Mexico	54.1	62.9	45.8
New York	52.6	60.3	45.7
North Carolina	41.7	52.2	32.2
North Dakota	55.4	65.2	45.9
Ohio	43.8	52.9	35.7
Oklahoma	28.6	35.7	22.2
Oregon	60.9	65.7	56.3
Pennsylvania	51.5	60.5	43.4
Rhode Island	58.3	65.3	52.1
South Carolina	42.0	52.0	32.9
South Dakota	58.6	68.1	49.6
Tennessee	29.7	38.9	21.5
Texas	54.8	65.8	44.4
Utah	29.7	36.1	23.7
Vermont	60.5	66.8	54.8
Virginia	54.3	61.8	47.3
Washington	60.7	66.6	55.0
West Virginia	32.6	42.1	24.2
Wisconsin	71.1	80.6	62.3
Wyoming	56.1	66.4	46.0

Source: Compiled by New Strategist based on the Centers for Disease Control and Prevention Behavioral Risk Factor Surveillance System Survey, Internet site http://www.cdc.gov/brfss/index.htm

1.5 Alcohol Consumption: Binge Drinking by Age, 2001

"How many times during the past month did you
have five or more drinks on an occasion?"

(percent of people aged 18 or older responding "one or more," by state and age, 2001)

	total	18 to 24	25 to 34	35 to 44	45 to 54	55 to 64	65 or older
U.S. total	**27.0%**	**48.3%**	**35.4%**	**27.3%**	**19.6%**	**13.2%**	**7.1%**
Alabama	27.8	40.2	32.6	29.4	22.1	18.2	10.5
Alaska	29.6	45.5	37.5	33.6	18.0	10.7	16.1
Arizona	30.0	60.0	43.5	33.0	15.3	17.7	7.9
Arkansas	29.1	42.9	36.3	31.2	27.8	14.2	7.3
California	26.8	52.2	34.6	27.0	19.0	17.6	5.0
Colorado	25.5	49.8	37.0	27.0	16.3	11.4	2.3
Connecticut	21.9	48.0	33.2	23.3	14.4	10.9	5.6
Delaware	26.8	50.6	38.8	25.2	21.1	11.1	6.6
District of Columbia	24.6	52.9	35.4	19.2	13.7	11.9	6.8
Florida	22.5	43.4	28.9	26.6	23.1	13.8	6.4
Georgia	24.7	41.6	27.0	27.1	19.6	13.6	5.0
Hawaii	23.0	38.5	29.1	54.5	14.3	16.9	7.0
Idaho	26.3	48.7	33.9	24.4	24.7	12.2	6.9
Illinois	30.0	53.2	42.1	27.7	22.1	16.1	10.0
Indiana	27.7	50.5	30.6	27.7	21.5	15.6	6.8
Iowa	28.1	54.6	37.5	29.1	19.6	15.7	4.4
Kansas	28.9	52.2	36.7	28.6	18.0	14.6	5.5
Kentucky	26.4	42.0	29.3	29.0	19.5	13.6	8.8
Louisiana	31.3	46.0	34.5	34.5	25.1	20.2	12.4
Maine	28.1	55.8	36.9	25.3	23.8	14.4	6.0
Maryland	21.5	40.8	32.8	20.8	14.9	8.8	7.6
Massachusetts	27.6	57.9	40.2	27.5	17.9	12.8	7.0
Michigan	31.3	51.1	43.1	29.5	24.5	18.1	11.6
Minnesota	29.4	64.4	37.1	28.9	21.2	15.7	6.7
Mississippi	30.4	41.6	35.2	30.4	27.1	13.3	12.3
Missouri	28.6	56.3	31.9	29.2	21.2	13.1	7.7
Montana	29.8	51.9	40.4	31.1	24.0	17.1	6.0
Nebraska	28.9	53.2	37.3	28.6	20.4	12.9	8.8
Nevada	27.6	45.8	42.8	29.7	20.2	15.9	9.6
New Hampshire	24.1	50.0	31.2	26.7	15.9	13.6	4.9
New Jersey	23.2	48.3	33.4	25.0	16.3	8.2	7.0
New Mexico	28.8	46.9	36.3	34.4	20.1	18.5	8.3
New York	25.0	51.5	31.8	24.0	18.0	12.7	9.9
North Carolina	23.8	37.6	33.1	22.7	19.1	7.2	6.2
North Dakota	34.7	59.5	44.9	34.4	27.3	15.7	7.5
Ohio	29.7	52.6	40.2	32.3	20.8	13.7	7.7
Oklahoma	27.7	44.0	35.5	23.6	24.5	8.4	11.9
Oregon	25.2	50.0	36.4	23.6	18.2	13.4	6.6
Pennsylvania	27.4	47.8	38.9	29.1	23.0	10.2	6.4
Rhode Island	23.8	50.9	30.4	27.2	15.0	14.0	6.1
South Carolina	26.5	48.3	33.4	24.5	22.0	12.7	5.8
South Dakota	30.3	54.8	43.5	32.6	20.0	9.0	5.7
Tennessee	25.3	47.5	28.7	19.6	23.0	9.9	11.8
Texas	29.4	53.2	33.8	29.1	25.7	13.1	7.9
Utah	32.5	48.1	39.0	30.9	27.9	29.9	7.4
Vermont	24.6	53.0	32.5	25.2	13.5	10.7	7.0
Virginia	26.2	49.6	35.6	26.7	15.3	9.5	9.5
Washington	24.1	44.9	32.5	22.4	21.7	12.0	7.7
West Virginia	29.0	63.3	34.5	24.2	17.7	13.8	6.1
Wisconsin	36.4	64.9	50.3	41.2	28.4	21.4	8.5
Wyoming	29.1	48.6	38.4	29.1	23.2	14.4	12.6

Source: Compiled by New Strategist based on the Centers for Disease Control and Prevention Behavioral Risk Factor Surveillance System Survey, Internet site http://www.cdc.gov/brfss/index.htm

1.6 Alcohol Consumption: Binge Drinking by Education, 2001

*"How many times during the past month did you
have five or more drinks on an occasion?"*

(percent of people aged 18 or older responding "one or more," by state and educational attainment, 2001)

	total	less than high school	high school graduate	some college	college graduate
U.S. total	**27.0%**	**35.5%**	**30.2%**	**28.7%**	**20.5%**
Alabama	27.8	35.6	28.7	30.6	22.2
Alaska	29.6	40.8	34.8	31.6	21.4
Arizona	30.0	37.1	34.1	33.0	21.8
Arkansas	29.1	39.2	35.3	30.1	18.7
California	26.8	45.0	34.1	26.6	17.0
Colorado	25.5	41.3	29.5	29.1	17.8
Connecticut	21.9	29.1	24.4	23.1	19.3
Delaware	26.8	36.9	27.4	31.8	21.4
District of Columbia	24.6	26.6	36.7	19.9	22.1
Florida	22.5	32.6	24.9	22.9	17.6
Georgia	24.7	46.7	30.3	25.4	16.6
Hawaii	23.0	30.1	33.1	24.3	12.2
Idaho	26.3	26.8	31.5	27.4	20.1
Illinois	30.0	35.2	29.8	32.8	26.6
Indiana	27.7	41.5	30.6	29.5	19.5
Iowa	28.1	43.2	30.0	31.2	20.4
Kansas	28.9	42.3	32.7	30.2	23.2
Kentucky	26.4	31.7	30.2	28.3	18.2
Louisiana	31.3	36.4	38.9	29.9	22.9
Maine	28.1	45.9	31.3	31.0	19.8
Maryland	21.5	21.2	25.4	28.6	15.9
Massachusetts	27.6	43.3	34.4	28.2	22.8
Michigan	31.3	44.0	34.9	34.0	22.0
Minnesota	29.4	40.7	32.8	30.4	24.3
Mississippi	30.4	39.0	34.8	31.9	21.1
Missouri	28.6	33.9	32.3	29.8	22.5
Montana	29.8	42.4	29.2	34.3	23.1
Nebraska	28.9	34.4	32.6	30.3	22.5
Nevada	27.6	38.7	27.6	27.4	25.0
New Hampshire	24.1	36.3	30.4	25.3	17.8
New Jersey	23.2	29.5	27.0	26.6	18.1
New Mexico	28.8	37.6	38.9	30.0	16.4
New York	25.0	28.2	23.8	29.5	22.0
North Carolina	23.8	27.2	24.8	27.5	19.3
North Dakota	34.7	28.5	38.8	35.3	31.5
Ohio	29.7	46.2	33.9	28.1	22.6
Oklahoma	27.7	40.0	29.4	25.5	24.0
Oregon	25.2	38.8	28.8	24.7	18.7
Pennsylvania	27.4	34.7	30.6	28.6	21.6
Rhode Island	23.8	31.8	25.4	28.3	17.5
South Carolina	26.5	39.8	33.8	25.6	18.5
South Dakota	30.3	22.1	32.8	33.5	26.0
Tennessee	25.3	37.1	28.2	29.8	12.8
Texas	29.4	42.6	35.6	29.2	19.7
Utah	32.5	52.8	38.7	28.0	23.8
Vermont	24.6	40.2	29.5	27.3	17.5
Virginia	26.2	33.6	32.4	25.9	21.9
Washington	24.1	37.3	29.7	23.3	19.1
West Virginia	29.0	33.2	33.8	29.8	18.5
Wisconsin	36.4	34.2	41.9	39.0	28.0
Wyoming	29.1	40.5	33.2	29.6	22.0

Source: Compiled by New Strategist based on the Centers for Disease Control and Prevention Behavioral Risk Factor Surveillance System Survey, Internet site http://www.cdc.gov/brfss/index.htm

1.7 Alcohol Consumption: Binge Drinking by Household Income, 2001

"How many times during the past month did you
have five or more drinks on an occasion?"

(percent of people aged 18 or older responding "one or more," by state and household income, 2001)

	total	less than $15,000	$15,000 to $24,999	$25,000 to $34,999	$35,000 to $49,999	$50,000 or more
U.S. total	**27.0%**	**35.4%**	**30.9%**	**29.2%**	**27.4%**	**23.4%**
Alabama	27.8	36.3	38.6	30.6	25.8	20.8
Alaska	29.6	35.2	36.5	36.0	24.0	30.4
Arizona	30.0	39.2	41.1	32.2	29.4	26.3
Arkansas	29.1	30.2	38.4	24.9	27.4	25.1
California	26.8	31.9	33.2	29.1	29.6	23.2
Colorado	25.5	44.3	38.1	25.7	27.6	21.1
Connecticut	21.9	34.2	25.7	28.1	22.1	20.5
Delaware	26.8	33.7	33.2	34.7	32.8	23.1
District of Columbia	24.6	52.7	27.6	24.1	30.5	18.3
Florida	22.5	21.9	25.8	25.7	27.6	21.3
Georgia	24.7	36.7	30.2	27.3	22.4	22.2
Hawaii	23.0	29.4	27.8	29.8	23.2	17.2
Idaho	26.3	30.9	31.2	32.5	23.8	20.7
Illinois	30.0	48.7	27.1	28.0	28.9	32.3
Indiana	27.7	41.3	35.0	33.7	26.8	22.3
Iowa	28.1	37.6	32.7	28.8	28.4	26.2
Kansas	28.9	36.2	35.9	32.4	31.1	24.4
Kentucky	26.4	21.9	33.0	25.7	29.2	24.3
Louisiana	31.3	32.4	35.5	32.2	35.3	27.5
Maine	28.1	36.0	34.3	31.6	28.5	24.7
Maryland	21.5	41.1	26.3	27.2	24.8	19.5
Massachusetts	27.6	38.6	32.3	30.9	28.4	27.3
Michigan	31.3	48.1	33.7	34.9	32.8	28.3
Minnesota	29.4	42.0	28.5	39.3	29.4	27.5
Mississippi	30.4	34.2	27.3	29.9	38.0	24.9
Missouri	28.6	35.2	32.3	34.5	27.4	25.4
Montana	29.8	41.5	38.8	32.3	24.2	22.0
Nebraska	28.9	40.3	35.9	27.8	30.1	26.1
Nevada	27.6	32.5	26.9	25.9	28.2	27.4
New Hampshire	24.1	27.1	30.3	26.6	22.0	22.8
New Jersey	23.2	45.7	28.1	21.6	24.1	22.5
New Mexico	28.8	30.5	37.6	34.6	30.0	21.2
New York	25.0	28.0	24.6	23.3	25.8	24.7
North Carolina	23.8	29.6	31.7	27.5	25.4	19.1
North Dakota	34.7	48.7	41.7	31.8	27.7	34.4
Ohio	29.7	39.2	31.4	34.8	31.9	27.3
Oklahoma	27.7	41.7	35.8	27.3	26.9	19.4
Oregon	25.2	36.5	30.3	30.0	24.6	20.9
Pennsylvania	27.4	40.4	30.2	29.4	29.5	23.7
Rhode Island	23.8	36.7	26.2	29.3	28.7	20.5
South Carolina	26.5	44.6	32.3	29.5	25.7	21.1
South Dakota	30.3	43.5	33.3	31.9	28.3	29.5
Tennessee	25.3	28.4	31.8	22.7	29.8	16.3
Texas	29.4	38.8	37.9	35.2	30.9	25.0
Utah	32.5	43.1	37.7	43.7	33.2	26.3
Vermont	24.6	38.9	28.7	29.4	27.1	19.9
Virginia	26.2	39.8	33.0	39.2	23.3	22.6
Washington	24.1	26.4	28.2	29.3	24.1	22.4
West Virginia	29.0	31.5	40.1	31.7	21.3	21.8
Wisconsin	36.4	46.7	37.1	36.2	36.6	38.5
Wyoming	29.1	42.9	35.1	28.6	26.2	25.7

Source: Compiled by New Strategist based on the Centers for Disease Control and Prevention Behavioral Risk Factor Surveillance System Survey, Internet site http://www.cdc.gov/brfss/index.htm

1.8 Alcohol Consumption: Binge Drinking by Sex, 2001

"How many times during the past month did you have five or more drinks on an occasion?"

(percent of people aged 18 or older responding "one or more," by state and sex, 2001)

	total	men	women
U.S. total	**27.0%**	**36.5%**	**15.5%**
Alabama	27.8	39.0	12.5
Alaska	29.6	38.6	19.5
Arizona	30.0	39.3	18.3
Arkansas	29.1	38.5	15.7
California	26.8	36.4	14.0
Colorado	25.5	35.6	12.8
Connecticut	21.9	30.1	12.7
Delaware	26.8	37.0	13.7
District of Columbia	24.6	32.6	16.3
Florida	22.5	29.8	13.9
Georgia	24.7	32.0	14.7
Hawaii	23.0	30.0	11.4
Idaho	26.3	35.0	14.5
Illinois	30.0	37.4	20.8
Indiana	27.7	37.2	15.0
Iowa	28.1	37.3	17.2
Kansas	28.9	39.1	16.0
Kentucky	26.4	35.9	12.6
Louisiana	31.3	42.7	16.7
Maine	28.1	39.2	14.2
Maryland	21.5	30.0	11.6
Massachusetts	27.6	37.6	17.0
Michigan	31.3	41.1	19.8
Minnesota	29.4	40.8	16.4
Mississippi	30.4	40.0	16.7
Missouri	28.6	38.7	16.2
Montana	29.8	39.4	17.2
Nebraska	28.9	37.8	17.8
Nevada	27.6	38.7	14.3
New Hampshire	24.1	33.3	14.1
New Jersey	23.2	31.1	14.3
New Mexico	28.8	40.9	12.7
New York	25.0	32.6	16.2
North Carolina	23.8	30.5	13.9
North Dakota	34.7	46.7	19.6
Ohio	29.7	39.2	18.5
Oklahoma	27.7	37.8	13.5
Oregon	25.2	33.6	14.1
Pennsylvania	27.4	38.7	14.1
Rhode Island	23.8	31.1	16.2
South Carolina	26.5	34.6	15.6
South Dakota	30.3	38.7	19.3
Tennessee	25.3	34.2	11.1
Texas	29.4	38.9	16.9
Utah	32.5	41.8	19.0
Vermont	24.6	32.4	15.7
Virginia	26.2	34.0	16.9
Washington	24.1	33.7	12.8
West Virginia	29.0	35.2	18.9
Wisconsin	36.4	48.0	23.5
Wyoming	29.1	39.3	17.0

Source: Compiled by New Strategist based on the Centers for Disease Control and Prevention Behavioral Risk Factor Surveillance System Survey, Internet site http://www.cdc.gov/brfss/index.htm

1.9 Asthma by Age, 2001

"Has a doctor ever told you that you have asthma?"

(percent of people aged 18 or older responding "yes," by state and age, 2001)

	total	18 to 24	25 to 34	35 to 44	45 to 54	55 to 64	65 or older
U.S. total	**11.2%**	**14.9%**	**11.5%**	**10.2%**	**10.3%**	**10.3%**	**8.8%**
Alabama	9.7	10.4	10.5	8.6	9.6	10.9	8.8
Alaska	11.5	12.4	9.2	12.9	13.8	8.0	11.3
Arizona	12.4	15.8	7.5	11.4	10.3	9.5	10.4
Arkansas	10.6	15.7	10.4	14.1	10.2	11.7	13.3
California	12.4	10.9	12.3	11.3	15.2	11.2	12.8
Colorado	12.1	18.7	12.4	10.0	13.8	9.6	10.5
Connecticut	12.3	18.4	14.0	13.0	12.3	10.3	8.5
Delaware	12.0	24.8	10.9	10.8	10.0	10.3	7.9
District of Columbia	12.0	13.8	14.7	11.9	12.8	9.8	8.3
Florida	9.9	13.8	11.4	9.6	9.3	10.3	7.3
Georgia	11.0	14.3	10.6	10.5	10.0	11.3	10.1
Hawaii	12.2	19.4	9.0	13.8	15.8	10.4	6.8
Idaho	11.7	12.9	13.3	12.1	8.9	12.7	11.1
Illinois	11.3	19.1	13.6	9.8	8.7	11.0	7.9
Indiana	11.3	15.0	13.2	11.5	10.8	8.5	9.3
Iowa	9.7	16.0	11.5	9.5	9.0	5.5	7.6
Kansas	11.7	19.1	11.3	10.3	10.6	11.0	10.2
Kentucky	10.9	14.5	9.3	9.4	10.0	12.4	11.7
Louisiana	9.1	10.3	10.0	9.2	9.1	7.2	8.9
Maine	12.6	20.4	13.9	10.5	10.3	12.9	10.9
Maryland	11.1	15.9	12.6	9.6	10.5	13.1	7.5
Massachusetts	13.1	17.5	15.3	13.7	11.5	11.7	9.6
Michigan	12.4	21.2	13.6	10.7	10.5	12.5	8.6
Minnesota	10.1	14.6	11.3	8.3	9.2	12.3	7.2
Mississippi	9.2	11.4	8.1	9.1	8.5	10.3	7.9
Missouri	12.0	18.8	11.3	14.4	13.6	7.5	7.4
Montana	11.8	13.3	14.0	12.1	10.4	8.0	12.3
Nebraska	8.4	16.0	7.3	7.5	6.9	7.4	7.5
Nevada	13.3	15.7	17.3	9.6	14.0	15.7	9.6
New Hampshire	12.5	17.7	17.2	10.4	9.5	14.0	8.0
New Jersey	9.4	18.0	11.0	8.1	8.2	9.2	5.8
New Mexico	10.8	13.9	10.0	10.2	11.4	9.5	10.0
New York	11.1	13.5	11.8	9.6	12.8	9.9	9.7
North Carolina	10.1	14.8	10.1	8.8	8.7	11.8	8.1
North Dakota	9.1	13.1	11.7	7.7	7.6	8.0	7.4
Ohio	9.8	10.2	10.1	11.6	8.1	9.7	9.0
Oklahoma	10.1	11.6	12.3	7.9	10.7	10.6	8.4
Oregon	13.0	14.5	13.3	11.7	12.7	16.2	10.9
Pennsylvania	10.7	18.9	11.6	10.1	11.4	7.8	6.9
Rhode Island	12.1	16.4	15.9	12.4	11.3	12.0	7.1
South Carolina	10.8	13.0	10.1	10.0	10.4	10.4	11.4
South Dakota	7.7	9.5	7.6	6.2	7.2	10.2	7.2
Tennessee	9.3	9.3	9.7	8.8	7.7	11.0	10.1
Texas	9.6	12.7	9.2	8.8	9.5	9.8	8.6
Utah	10.7	10.6	11.7	9.4	11.0	12.4	10.0
Vermont	12.1	17.1	12.5	12.8	10.1	11.0	9.7
Virginia	11.4	17.4	9.7	11.5	10.2	9.2	11.4
Washington	12.0	14.8	12.6	10.9	10.2	14.8	10.0
West Virginia	12.5	18.9	11.6	11.7	12.9	10.3	11.2
Wisconsin	10.9	15.8	15.0	8.6	10.4	8.3	8.1
Wyoming	11.6	16.6	13.8	11.8	8.7	12.3	8.4

Source: Compiled by New Strategist based on the Centers for Disease Control and Prevention Behavioral Risk Factor Surveillance System Survey. Internet site http://www.cdc.gov/brfss/index.htm

1.10 Asthma by Education, 2001

"Has a doctor ever told you that you have asthma?"

(percent of people aged 18 or older responding "yes," by state and educational attainment, 2001)

	total	less than high school	high school graduate	some college	college graduate
U.S. total	**11.2%**	**12.9%**	**10.2%**	**12.0%**	**10.0%**
Alabama	9.7	14.6	7.7	9.4	9.7
Alaska	11.5	17.6	10.2	10.8	12.1
Arizona	12.4	13.2	11.2	15.0	10.4
Arkansas	10.6	15.1	8.7	11.6	9.5
California	12.4	8.7	15.0	13.4	11.8
Colorado	12.1	7.8	13.3	12.5	12.4
Connecticut	12.3	14.2	11.2	14.1	11.5
Delaware	12.0	16.2	12.4	12.8	9.9
District of Columbia	12.0	10.6	14.6	11.0	11.4
Florida	9.9	9.9	9.9	10.3	9.3
Georgia	11.0	15.1	10.3	11.4	9.3
Hawaii	12.2	10.9	14.3	12.5	9.7
Idaho	11.7	13.1	12.7	11.6	10.2
Illinois	11.3	14.8	9.7	13.0	10.1
Indiana	11.3	15.1	9.2	13.9	10.6
Iowa	9.7	12.1	8.6	11.7	8.2
Kansas	11.7	16.0	10.0	12.7	11.4
Kentucky	10.9	14.8	10.3	11.0	8.3
Louisiana	9.1	10.7	8.8	10.6	7.0
Maine	12.6	12.7	12.6	13.7	11.8
Maryland	11.1	18.4	12.1	11.4	8.5
Massachusetts	13.1	17.8	12.5	13.1	12.5
Michigan	12.4	14.5	12.0	14.1	10.0
Minnesota	10.1	12.9	9.5	10.5	9.6
Mississippi	9.2	12.5	7.8	8.2	9.6
Missouri	12.0	15.4	9.6	14.1	10.9
Montana	11.8	11.9	11.3	12.0	12.3
Nebraska	8.4	8.3	6.9	10.9	7.8
Nevada	13.3	11.7	13.4	12.4	14.9
New Hampshire	12.5	13.7	11.1	13.8	12.5
New Jersey	9.4	10.0	8.0	12.0	8.6
New Mexico	10.8	9.6	8.2	15.5	9.8
New York	11.1	13.0	8.9	13.2	10.2
North Carolina	10.1	10.5	12.5	8.1	8.4
North Dakota	9.1	12.4	9.5	8.9	7.9
Ohio	9.8	14.7	9.0	10.5	8.1
Oklahoma	10.1	10.4	9.6	12.0	8.4
Oregon	13.0	12.3	14.1	12.6	12.5
Pennsylvania	10.7	10.3	9.2	13.8	10.3
Rhode Island	12.1	11.8	11.9	12.7	12.1
South Carolina	10.8	14.9	9.3	12.0	9.0
South Dakota	7.7	8.2	6.9	8.1	8.0
Tennessee	9.3	13.6	8.9	10.3	5.8
Texas	9.6	7.2	8.8	11.9	10.0
Utah	10.7	11.5	10.0	12.4	9.4
Vermont	12.1	16.5	11.2	11.2	12.7
Virginia	11.4	14.8	10.5	12.2	10.5
Washington	12.0	15.1	12.4	12.4	10.4
West Virginia	12.5	15.5	12.6	12.0	9.5
Wisconsin	10.9	15.1	11.0	12.0	8.2
Wyoming	11.6	9.3	10.3	13.7	11.5

Source: Compiled by New Strategist based on the Centers for Disease Control and Prevention Behavioral Risk Factor Surveillance System Survey, Internet site http://www.cdc.gov/brfss/index.htm

1.11 Asthma by Household Income, 2001

"Has a doctor ever told you that you have asthma?"

(percent of people aged 18 or older responding "yes," by state and household income, 2001)

	total	less than $15,000	$15,000 to $24,999	$25,000 to $34,999	$35,000 to $49,999	$50,000 or more
U.S. total	**11.2%**	**15.4%**	**12.3%**	**10.7%**	**10.5%**	**10.0%**
Alabama	9.7	13.8	9.5	10.2	8.9	7.0
Alaska	11.5	17.0	12.0	14.0	10.2	10.2
Arizona	12.4	13.5	13.9	11.7	12.3	11.9
Arkansas	10.6	17.0	12.4	6.7	11.0	8.7
California	12.4	11.3	14.1	10.2	15.1	12.3
Colorado	12.1	14.6	11.0	11.7	11.3	13.1
Connecticut	12.3	19.9	14.2	13.3	10.4	11.9
Delaware	12.0	14.2	12.6	11.7	11.3	9.9
District of Columbia	12.0	11.1	13.0	11.0	12.5	11.4
Florida	9.9	15.4	10.6	8.5	8.8	10.0
Georgia	11.0	16.4	12.3	12.6	7.8	10.5
Hawaii	12.2	12.8	13.0	8.7	15.7	9.7
Idaho	11.7	17.9	14.1	9.3	10.4	9.6
Illinois	11.3	13.6	13.4	9.0	11.9	11.5
Indiana	11.3	16.3	13.9	13.7	8.5	9.2
Iowa	9.7	11.3	10.7	11.2	9.3	7.6
Kansas	11.7	16.1	16.0	14.1	8.3	9.7
Kentucky	10.9	20.0	11.2	11.4	8.7	6.3
Louisiana	9.1	12.8	9.3	10.0	8.5	6.6
Maine	12.6	21.7	13.3	13.0	8.6	11.4
Maryland	11.1	9.9	16.6	10.7	10.5	9.2
Massachusetts	13.1	18.8	15.3	14.4	12.1	11.9
Michigan	12.4	18.8	13.1	13.9	12.7	10.1
Minnesota	10.1	14.9	12.8	7.3	9.7	10.1
Mississippi	9.2	12.1	11.1	6.4	6.9	8.0
Missouri	12.0	15.5	14.1	13.9	9.8	11.4
Montana	11.8	14.9	13.7	9.8	12.9	9.0
Nebraska	8.4	15.7	9.7	7.0	7.7	7.8
Nevada	13.3	15.0	10.0	18.2	14.5	12.9
New Hampshire	12.5	14.9	12.7	9.6	11.3	13.7
New Jersey	9.4	9.9	9.3	8.9	9.3	10.0
New Mexico	10.8	13.3	10.1	9.0	11.6	11.1
New York	11.1	15.8	10.1	9.8	12.5	10.3
North Carolina	10.1	11.6	12.7	7.6	9.9	8.7
North Dakota	9.1	13.2	10.4	8.5	8.5	7.5
Ohio	9.8	16.2	13.1	12.0	7.4	7.0
Oklahoma	10.1	15.7	11.2	8.1	12.4	7.2
Oregon	13.0	19.6	11.3	15.7	12.6	11.4
Pennsylvania	10.7	18.2	11.6	9.7	10.4	8.8
Rhode Island	12.1	14.4	13.9	10.5	11.8	10.9
South Carolina	10.8	15.7	9.6	10.9	9.4	9.9
South Dakota	7.7	11.2	8.6	6.5	7.4	7.1
Tennessee	9.3	19.7	11.5	7.3	8.3	7.0
Texas	9.6	10.4	8.2	10.4	9.9	10.4
Utah	10.7	18.4	12.9	12.4	8.4	10.9
Vermont	12.1	18.8	14.6	10.8	10.5	10.7
Virginia	11.4	17.6	11.5	12.4	10.4	10.0
Washington	12.0	19.5	13.1	12.7	11.7	9.9
West Virginia	12.5	17.6	14.8	11.9	8.9	8.3
Wisconsin	10.9	10.8	11.7	10.9	11.3	9.1
Wyoming	11.6	15.5	12.2	10.6	11.8	10.4

Source: Compiled by New Strategist based on the Centers for Disease Control and Prevention Behavioral Risk Factor Surveillance System Survey, Internet site http://www.cdc.gov/brfss/index.htm

1.12 Asthma by Sex, 2001

"Has a doctor ever told you that you have asthma?"

(percent of people aged 18 or older responding "yes," by state and sex, 2001)

	total	men	women
U.S. total	**11.2%**	**9.5%**	**12.7%**
Alabama	9.7	7.8	11.4
Alaska	11.5	8.8	14.4
Arizona	12.4	10.5	14.2
Arkansas	10.6	9.0	12.0
California	12.4	9.7	15.1
Colorado	12.1	7.7	16.4
Connecticut	12.3	11.1	13.4
Delaware	12.0	9.9	13.9
District of Columbia	12.0	9.2	14.4
Florida	9.9	10.3	11.6
Georgia	11.0	10.3	11.6
Hawaii	12.2	11.0	13.3
Idaho	11.7	10.6	12.7
Illinois	11.3	8.9	13.5
Indiana	11.3	9.0	13.4
Iowa	9.7	8.2	11.1
Kansas	11.7	9.9	13.3
Kentucky	10.9	8.6	13.0
Louisiana	9.1	8.3	9.9
Maine	12.6	10.7	14.5
Maryland	11.1	9.2	12.8
Massachusetts	13.1	11.0	14.9
Michigan	12.4	10.6	14.0
Minnesota	10.1	9.8	10.4
Mississippi	9.2	8.7	9.5
Missouri	12.0	11.3	12.5
Montana	11.8	10.6	13.0
Nebraska	8.4	7.9	8.9
Nevada	13.3	12.4	14.2
New Hampshire	12.5	11.6	13.3
New Jersey	9.4	6.9	11.7
New Mexico	10.8	8.7	12.7
New York	11.1	9.4	12.6
North Carolina	10.1	8.5	11.4
North Dakota	9.1	7.7	10.4
Ohio	9.8	8.3	11.1
Oklahoma	10.1	8.5	11.5
Oregon	13.0	10.5	15.3
Pennsylvania	10.7	9.6	11.7
Rhode Island	12.1	9.9	14.1
South Carolina	10.8	9.8	11.6
South Dakota	7.7	7.5	7.9
Tennessee	9.3	7.2	11.3
Texas	9.6	8.2	10.9
Utah	10.7	10.4	11.0
Vermont	12.1	9.9	14.1
Virginia	11.4	9.5	13.1
Washington	12.0	9.8	14.1
West Virginia	12.5	10.8	13.9
Wisconsin	10.9	9.7	12.0
Wyoming	11.6	12.0	11.3

Source: Compiled by New Strategist based on the Centers for Disease Control and Prevention Behavioral Risk Factor Surveillance System Survey, Internet site http://www.cdc.gov/brfss/index.htm

1.13 Bicycle Helmet Use by Children, 1999

"During the past year, how often has the child (5 to 15 years old)
worn a bicycle helmet when riding a bicycle?"

(percent of people aged 18 or older living in households with children aged 5 to 15 responding "always," by state, 1999)

	child always wears bicycle helmet
U.S. total	**33.1%**
Alabama	31.9
Alaska	42.6
Arizona	35.4
Arkansas	14.0
California	52.4
Colorado	40.1
Connecticut	64.5
Delaware	57.3
District of Columbia	36.7
Florida	53.2
Georgia	39.9
Hawaii	43.6
Idaho	29.4
Illinois	25.5
Indiana	16.3
Iowa	20.8
Kansas	28.1
Kentucky	26.1
Louisiana	14.4
Maine	57.2
Maryland	46.1
Massachusetts	58.2
Michigan	26.8
Minnesota	27.8
Mississippi	17.1
Missouri	27.1
Montana	34.4
Nebraska	23.6
Nevada	29.2
New Hampshire	64.2
New Jersey	58.0
New Mexico	28.3
New York	56.2
North Carolina	30.9
North Dakota	17.4
Ohio	38.8
Oklahoma	30.6
Oregon	61.9
Pennsylvania	56.5
Rhode Island	52.8
South Carolina	24.7
South Dakota	13.6
Tennessee	42.0
Texas	28.9
Utah	25.8
Vermont	63.9
Virginia	44.2
Washington	55.1
West Virginia	60.3
Wisconsin	26.6
Wyoming	29.2

Source: Compiled by New Strategist based on the Centers for Disease Control and Prevention Behavioral Risk Factor Surveillance System Survey, Internet site http://www.cdc.gov/brfss/index.htm

1.14 Cholesterol Ever Checked by Age, 2001

"Have you ever had your blood cholesterol checked?"

(percent of people aged 18 or older responding "yes," by state and age, 2001)

	total	18 to 24	25 to 34	35 to 44	45 to 54	55 to 64	65 or older
U.S. total	**77.0%**	**46.5%**	**63.2%**	**76.7%**	**87.6%**	**92.8%**	**93.7%**
Alabama	76.8	46.3	64.3	75.5	89.0	91.1	91.3
Alaska	74.3	42.1	63.5	75.5	85.9	89.0	93.4
Arizona	76.4	44.2	60.7	70.6	88.2	93.1	97.0
Arkansas	75.5	49.9	60.7	71.0	82.5	86.4	94.4
California	74.7	45.9	60.4	72.1	87.4	89.5	94.0
Colorado	77.0	42.8	63.2	75.1	90.3	93.6	92.3
Connecticut	83.4	55.2	70.3	86.1	89.5	95.7	94.3
Delaware	81.5	58.6	65.3	80.7	90.7	94.8	96.1
District of Columbia	83.3	59.1	71.0	88.7	92.6	91.8	92.0
Florida	81.1	51.0	69.9	77.6	85.7	93.4	93.5
Georgia	78.9	57.0	63.3	82.6	86.9	90.3	94.0
Hawaii	78.3	49.5	63.4	76.3	87.5	94.0	94.0
Idaho	73.0	36.2	56.9	70.3	84.9	91.1	91.0
Illinois	74.3	46.6	58.9	75.6	84.5	92.7	88.3
Indiana	77.1	46.5	59.5	77.7	86.0	94.2	94.5
Iowa	77.0	46.1	59.7	76.5	89.5	90.6	92.3
Kansas	76.7	45.6	59.5	74.5	88.8 ·	95.2	92.4
Kentucky	75.2	49.7	61.6	74.2	81.4	89.9	91.0
Louisiana	75.9	51.4	64.3	72.1	86.0	91.0	92.2
Maine	81.4	47.6	67.3	82.3	91.0	94.5	94.3
Maryland	83.5	56.7	71.2	84.4	91.9	94.6	96.1
Massachusetts	84.7	57.7	75.6	85.8	92.1	95.2	95.6
Michigan	79.2	45.0	64.9	80.0	90.1	92.0	95.9
Minnesota	81.3	46.9	68.1	82.6	91.8	95.8	94.4
Mississippi	73.7	44.7	63.7	71.9	82.6	90.5	90.1
Missouri	76.7	44.3	59.4	75.7	86.8	93.2	92.0
Montana	75.3	49.9	53.2	71.3	84.1	92.2	93.8
Nebraska	69.7	38.2	49.3	66.5	84.6	87.6	89.1
Nevada	77.6	45.5	60.1	75.4	88.3	94.4	94.1
New Hampshire	81.4	49.1	68.3	82.9	93.7	95.2	93.0
New Jersey	82.5	56.5	71.7	81.8	88.2	93.3	95.4
New Mexico	72.1	38.7	52.3	71.3	85.8	90.8	92.2
New York	80.4	58.5	66.3	80.6	86.9	95.2	90.9
North Carolina	79.0	54.9	61.8	82.0	86.7	95.3	93.2
North Dakota	76.1	45.7	59.7	74.2	87.3	92.4	94.4
Ohio	76.1	44.7	57.7	77.1	86.3	92.4	92.0
Oklahoma	76.0	47.5	64.1	78.0	88.8	93.0	94.2
Oregon	76.5	54.0	75.9	84.2	91.1	93.5	94.6
Pennsylvania	79.4	44.2	63.9	77.0	82.2	90.0	92.2
Rhode Island	83.4	36.1	61.2	73.6	85.5	94.6	96.8
South Carolina	80.7	54.4	70.9	80.8	89.1	94.1	93.7
South Dakota	74.4	45.5	63.2	70.5	84.0	84.6	83.6
Tennessee	72.8	45.5	63.2	70.5	84.0	84.6	83.6
Texas	73.8	42.7	57.3	74.9	86.7	90.4	93.1
Utah	74.6	40.6	60.6	78.8	87.8	91.8	92.1
Vermont	80.9	54.1	67.1	83.6	89.2	93.1	93.9
Virginia	80.6	53.9	65.3	81.9	89.5	95.2	95.1
Washington	78.1	35.7	61.1	80.6	90.2	95.3	94.2
West Virginia	79.4	52.9	60.3	77.1	89.9	93.3	93.0
Wisconsin	77.2	40.0	61.9	75.9	87.9	95.9	94.5
Wyoming	76.3	39.8	57.7	76.3	88.3	92.3	95.9

Source: Compiled by New Strategist based on the Centers for Disease Control and Prevention Behavioral Risk Factor Surveillance System Survey. Internet site http://www.cdc.gov/brfss/index.htm

1.15 Cholesterol Ever Checked by Education, 2001

"Have you ever had your blood cholesterol checked?"

(percent of people aged 18 or older responding "yes," by state and educational attainment, 2001)

	total	less than high school	high school graduate	some college	college graduate
U.S. total	**77.0%**	**70.7%**	**73.1%**	**77.2%**	**85.1%**
Alabama	76.8	74.4	72.8	77.5	84.1
Alaska	74.3	61.9	64.3	77.8	83.7
Arizona	76.4	63.2	73.3	74.4	87.4
Arkansas	75.5	73.8	71.3	75.1	83.2
California	74.7	58.9	70.0	76.5	85.1
Colorado	77.0	56.8	73.1	76.1	86.8
Connecticut	83.4	72.5	80.5	81.8	89.0
Delaware	81.5	71.9	81.1	79.7	85.8
District of Columbia	83.3	80.5	76.3	79.2	89.5
Florida	81.1	66.1	76.8	83.2	90.4
Georgia	78.9	73.8	73.8	80.0	85.2
Hawaii	78.3	75.9	71.8	79.5	84.7
Idaho	73.0	62.2	67.9	74.7	80.5
Illinois	74.3	61.0	69.3	74.4	82.8
Indiana	77.1	67.5	73.1	79.0	85.1
Iowa	77.0	71.1	75.2	75.1	84.0
Kansas	76.7	65.2	73.2	76.2	83.1
Kentucky	75.2	71.3	74.0	74.9	81.6
Louisiana	75.9	73.1	72.3	74.4	84.9
Maine	81.4	82.1	74.7	82.4	89.1
Maryland	83.5	74.7	82.5	80.5	88.1
Massachusetts	84.7	76.8	80.8	84.1	89.3
Michigan	79.2	75.6	73.9	80.6	85.7
Minnesota	81.3	70.5	77.5	81.6	86.7
Mississippi	73.7	69.9	69.9	73.7	82.7
Missouri	76.7	73.0	74.4	74.8	83.3
Montana	75.3	66.1	68.9	77.8	84.3
Nebraska	69.7	68.2	62.0	70.5	81.3
Nevada	77.6	72.3	72.0	76.7	86.4
New Hampshire	81.4	66.7	76.7	81.8	88.6
New Jersey	82.5	70.2	79.6	84.2	87.0
New Mexico	72.1	60.7	65.8	75.7	83.2
New York	80.4	68.6	77.0	81.3	88.0
North Carolina	79.0	76.0	75.2	78.3	85.9
North Dakota	76.1	80.7	73.0	73.3	81.0
Ohio	76.1	70.2	70.9	76.8	86.2
Oklahoma	76.0	68.6	73.0	77.0	83.5
Oregon	76.5	56.9	70.3	78.5	88.8
Pennsylvania	79.4	71.7	78.5	79.3	83.8
Rhode Island	83.4	73.8	77.7	85.1	91.9
South Carolina	80.7	70.6	78.8	81.1	88.2
South Dakota	74.4	74.7	69.5	72.1	82.5
Tennessee	72.8	69.6	68.9	74.7	79.0
Texas	73.8	54.9	71.8	78.2	85.0
Utah	74.6	53.7	67.2	75.4	85.6
Vermont	80.9	78.9	77.0	80.6	85.5
Virginia	80.6	76.7	78.0	76.7	86.9
Washington	78.1	55.0	74.6	79.3	85.0
West Virginia	79.4	77.6	77.8	80.7	83.4
Wisconsin	77.2	70.8	73.8	76.5	84.3
Wyoming	76.3	63.4	71.4	75.3	87.0

Source: Compiled by New Strategist based on the Centers for Disease Control and Prevention Behavioral Risk Factor Surveillance System Survey. Internet site http://www.cdc.gov/brfss/index.htm

1.16 Cholesterol Ever Checked by Household Income, 2001

"Have you ever had your blood cholesterol checked?"

(percent of people aged 18 or older responding "yes," by state and household income, 2001)

	total	less than $15,000	$15,000 to $24,999	$25,000 to $34,999	$35,000 to $49,999	$50,000 or more
U.S. total	**77.0%**	**70.1%**	**71.6%**	**72.8%**	**78.3%**	**84.9%**
Alabama	76.8	69.0	74.6	71.8	78.1	83.8
Alaska	74.3	59.6	64.3	67.9	75.1	82.9
Arizona	76.4	65.8	61.4	71.1	81.2	84.9
Arkansas	75.5	68.7	70.8	70.0	74.2	82.9
California	74.7	63.6	61.4	70.7	73.7	84.2
Colorado	77.0	65.6	66.4	67.1	77.9	84.9
Connecticut	83.4	76.6	74.2	76.7	84.6	88.8
Delaware	81.5	78.7	74.8	72.7	77.6	85.6
District of Columbia	83.3	82.9	74.7	73.5	78.7	93.3
Florida	81.1	74.8	73.9	82.2	82.1	86.7
Georgia	78.9	72.7	73.5	75.6	78.8	84.7
Hawaii	78.3	65.4	75.1	75.4	80.6	86.9
Idaho	73.0	66.6	65.3	67.6	73.9	83.1
Illinois	74.3	72.7	65.0	71.7	70.9	79.8
Indiana	77.1	76.0	71.9	71.7	74.0	82.8
Iowa	77.0	68.5	76.1	73.4	75.1	84.2
Kansas	76.7	70.0	72.1	70.9	77.4	82.9
Kentucky	75.2	71.9	68.6	73.8	75.4	82.2
Louisiana	75.9	70.5	68.7	72.1	80.1	84.6
Maine	81.4	84.3	77.8	76.1	83.7	85.2
Maryland	83.5	74.0	75.7	79.5	83.8	87.8
Massachusetts	84.7	79.1	78.3	81.0	82.8	89.2
Michigan	79.2	64.8	73.3	76.9	78.8	85.4
Minnesota	81.3	77.0	78.2	74.4	79.3	85.7
Mississippi	73.7	63.6	71.4	76.5	80.5	80.2
Missouri	76.7	75.2	67.4	74.5	76.9	81.5
Montana	75.3	68.7	66.7	70.4	78.3	83.3
Nebraska	69.7	59.2	70.1	66.7	68.2	79.2
Nevada	77.6	72.5	66.0	74.8	77.1	82.8
New Hampshire	81.4	76.5	73.8	72.8	81.5	87.4
New Jersey	82.5	68.7	75.6	78.5	82.8	86.8
New Mexico	72.1	61.8	62.9	68.5	72.1	85.2
New York	80.4	74.4	69.2	81.5	77.0	87.8
North Carolina	79.0	72.0	72.9	75.5	80.1	87.2
North Dakota	76.1	66.6	69.2	71.8	76.8	83.9
Ohio	76.1	68.0	72.8	70.5	76.7	81.8
Oklahoma	76.0	72.9	68.4	68.6	78.3	86.3
Oregon	76.5	63.0	66.3	72.9	75.8	88.1
Pennsylvania	79.4	70.2	79.1	74.7	80.6	83.7
Rhode Island	83.4	70.7	81.9	80.6	85.1	90.0
South Carolina	80.7	71.7	75.5	78.3	81.7	87.5
South Dakota	74.4	69.7	69.8	68.1	75.1	81.6
Tennessee	72.8	65.4	70.6	73.3	69.4	80.5
Texas	73.8	60.2	62.8	72.1	76.1	84.9
Utah	74.6	64.3	63.9	67.7	76.2	83.0
Vermont	80.9	77.6	76.9	76.0	81.9	86.5
Virginia	80.6	72.0	77.0	70.8	79.1	87.8
Washington	78.1	69.0	69.0	71.2	75.8	85.8
West Virginia	79.4	80.0	73.4	78.3	81.9	86.9
Wisconsin	77.2	65.2	72.1	75.0	76.6	82.5
Wyoming	76.3	71.6	67.0	70.8	79.1	82.5

Source: Compiled by New Strategist based on the Centers for Disease Control and Prevention Behavioral Risk Factor Surveillance System Survey, Internet site http://www.cdc.gov/brfss/index.htm

1.17 Cholesterol Ever Checked by Sex, 2001

"Have you ever had your blood cholesterol checked?"

(percent of people aged 18 or older responding "yes," by state and sex, 2001)

	total	men	women
U.S. total	**77.0%**	**74.9%**	**79.5%**
Alabama	76.8	76.4	77.3
Alaska	74.3	74.7	73.8
Arizona	76.4	74.9	77.8
Arkansas	75.5	73.9	76.9
California	74.7	71.2	78.2
Colorado	77.0	74.2	79.6
Connecticut	83.4	81.3	85.4
Delaware	81.5	79.2	83.7
District of Columbia	83.3	80.2	85.9
Florida	81.1	78.4	83.6
Georgia	78.9	77.4	80.3
Hawaii	78.3	77.1	79.5
Idaho	73.0	70.9	75.0
Illinois	74.3	72.2	76.2
Indiana	77.1	75.3	78.8
Iowa	77.0	73.6	80.1
Kansas	76.7	75.1	78.3
Kentucky	75.2	73.0	77.2
Louisiana	75.9	74.2	77.5
Maine	81.4	78.0	84.5
Maryland	83.5	81.8	85.1
Massachusetts	84.7	83.0	86.2
Michigan	79.2	75.6	82.4
Minnesota	81.3	75.8	86.5
Mississippi	73.7	72.7	74.7
Missouri	76.7	75.0	78.2
Montana	75.3	72.9	77.7
Nebraska	69.7	66.5	72.6
Nevada	77.6	75.0	80.2
New Hampshire	81.4	79.3	83.3
New Jersey	82.5	81.6	83.3
New Mexico	72.1	68.8	75.3
New York	80.4	78.5	82.1
North Carolina	79.0	76.6	81.3
North Dakota	76.1	73.5	78.6
Ohio	76.1	74.0	77.9
Oklahoma	76.0	74.2	77.7
Oregon	76.5	74.5	78.5
Pennsylvania	79.4	79.2	79.5
Rhode Island	83.4	80.9	85.7
South Carolina	80.7	79.9	81.5
South Dakota	74.4	71.4	77.2
Tennessee	72.8	70.9	74.5
Texas	73.8	70.4	77.0
Utah	74.6	72.8	76.3
Vermont	80.9	78.2	83.3
Virginia	80.6	78.8	82.3
Washington	78.1	75.0	81.0
West Virginia	79.4	78.4	80.3
Wisconsin	77.2	73.6	80.5
Wyoming	76.3	72.6	79.9

Source: Compiled by New Strategist based on the Centers for Disease Control and Prevention Behavioral Risk Factor Surveillance System Survey, Internet site http://www.cdc.gov/brfss/index.htm

1.18 Cholesterol: Last Time Checked by Age, 2001

"About how long has it been since you last had your blood cholesterol checked?"

(percent of people aged 18 or older responding "past year," by state and age, 2001)

	total	18 to 24	25 to 34	35 to 44	45 to 54	55 to 64	65 or older
U.S. total	**71.7%**	**66.1%**	**60.9%**	**61.7%**	**70.9%**	**80.0%**	**85.5%**
Alabama	71.9	68.0	65.7	61.6	68.4	78.5	85.4
Alaska	63.0	62.1	57.5	57.2	59.5	69.9	82.6
Arizona	71.7	73.2	55.4	67.2	71.4	72.5	85.6
Arkansas	70.4	69.4	62.8	60.6	67.8	72.8	83.2
California	68.7	67.9	58.3	59.5	67.5	79.3	82.6
Colorado	63.6	59.5	49.1	52.6	62.7	75.7	82.2
Connecticut	73.6	72.1	59.8	64.2	73.1	84.0	86.7
Delaware	73.5	72.4	68.0	59.9	70.7	82.9	86.4
District of Columbia	76.9	61.5	65.6	72.4	78.7	84.2	92.9
Florida	80.3	69.8	69.1	71.1	79.0	86.3	91.2
Georgia	71.9	67.0	69.2	66.6	73.7	79.9	81.2
Hawaii	76.5	71.5	64.9	68.6	72.8	83.9	92.2
Idaho	60.0	59.9	45.9	44.3	59.2	69.3	77.2
Illinois	70.1	72.2	60.8	55.4	69.2	82.1	83.8
Indiana	69.6	61.2	58.5	60.4	68.3	76.6	84.6
Iowa	70.0	65.1	57.0	57.7	69.5	79.1	82.5
Kansas	67.3	61.6	55.5	54.0	64.5	77.8	83.2
Kentucky	74.1	70.7	64.6	61.9	75.9	81.2	86.4
Louisiana	78.6	75.5	67.6	73.3	78.2	84.9	89.3
Maine	71.7	61.6	61.1	59.8	71.6	80.2	87.9
Maryland	74.2	73.6	63.6	65.2	72.8	82.6	89.9
Massachusetts	73.3	66.3	64.5	63.6	71.2	80.9	89.2
Michigan	72.4	61.9	55.4	65.1	73.5	81.0	87.6
Minnesota	68.4	65.9	56.4	61.1	66.3	79.0	81.2
Mississippi	71.7	66.0	61.2	66.6	69.1	82.5	81.2
Missouri	73.1	68.2	58.0	63.6	74.3	83.4	83.2
Montana	64.9	54.7	51.9	52.8	65.2	71.4	80.0
Nebraska	71.1	65.9	62.0	62.0	69.2	78.8	80.6
Nevada	69.9	63.1	56.2	59.1	68.7	82.3	84.9
New Hampshire	69.4	60.8	53.6	60.0	69.8	82.8	85.1
New Jersey	77.1	68.8	66.9	70.0	78.9	84.4	88.2
New Mexico	70.1	63.8	60.5	64.1	66.7	76.4	83.8
New York	76.8	73.8	68.1	68.4	78.5	81.5	88.5
North Carolina	77.6	74.0	68.7	70.1	76.5	87.4	86.4
North Dakota	68.1	62.5	51.4	58.0	65.2	75.4	86.1
Ohio	71.7	71.7	60.1	59.7	71.0	78.5	85.4
Oklahoma	72.7	71.7	62.6	66.8	71.2	74.7	84.7
Oregon	62.5	51.7	46.9	53.1	60.2	70.6	78.6
Pennsylvania	71.6	62.7	55.0	61.4	70.9	78.5	87.5
Rhode Island	78.7	75.5	66.2	71.6	77.9	85.9	91.5
South Carolina	77.1	75.8	67.7	69.7	78.4	82.5	88.6
South Dakota	69.9	62.8	57.0	60.8	66.3	78.3	84.1
Tennessee	77.0	65.0	72.1	67.5	77.8	87.7	85.7
Texas	72.7	70.8	65.2	63.8	72.1	78.1	85.7
Utah	61.7	54.1	47.3	50.8	62.4	72.5	81.4
Vermont	66.7	57.0	52.5	56.9	66.0	78.7	85.3
Virginia	70.0	65.2	54.9	61.2	72.3	77.8	86.6
Washington	63.1	60.3	51.0	50.1	60.4	73.9	80.9
West Virginia	79.4	76.8	67.8	72.0	78.7	82.9	90.1
Wisconsin	64.4	58.1	43.0	52.5	63.5	77.9	81.4
Wyoming	71.3	69.4	61.6	58.5	68.1	80.5	88.6

Source: Compiled by New Strategist based on the Centers for Disease Control and Prevention Behavioral Risk Factor Surveillance System Survey, Internet site http://www.cdc.gov/brfss/index.htm

1.19 Cholesterol: Last Time Checked by Education, 2001

"About how long has it been since you last had your blood cholesterol checked?"

(percent of people aged 18 or older responding "past year," by state and educational attainment, 2001)

	total	less than high school	high school graduate	some college	college graduate
U.S. total	**71.7%**	**79.0%**	**74.3%**	**70.7%**	**68.6%**
Alabama	71.9	78.1	70.5	70.0	72.0
Alaska	63.0	70.3	61.7	62.9	62.8
Arizona	71.7	81.3	76.9	68.8	67.0
Arkansas	70.4	76.0	72.7	64.5	70.0
California	68.7	67.5	70.6	69.6	67.1
Colorado	63.6	67.6	66.2	62.9	61.6
Connecticut	73.6	84.6	77.4	73.2	69.3
Delaware	73.5	84.2	74.8	74.0	69.7
District of Columbia	76.9	83.9	84.1	82.7	69.8
Florida	80.3	82.3	80.4	80.7	79.0
Georgia	71.9	75.8	71.5	73.0	69.5
Hawaii	76.5	91.0	76.7	74.5	75.2
Idaho	60.0	66.0	61.6	60.0	56.9
Illinois	70.1	71.8	72.7	72.3	65.8
Indiana	69.6	76.1	71.0	67.7	67.5
Iowa	70.0	80.8	69.9	70.2	66.7
Kansas	67.3	79.9	68.9	65.3	65.3
Kentucky	74.1	78.9	75.4	70.3	72.2
Louisiana	78.6	85.6	79.2	75.2	76.2
Maine	71.7	82.1	74.6	69.0	67.9
Maryland	74.2	82.7	75.9	74.4	71.2
Massachusetts	73.3	82.7	77.8	73.7	68.8
Michigan	72.4	80.1	75.5	70.8	67.9
Minnesota	68.4	81.0	71.3	68.4	63.9
Mississippi	71.7	70.3	74.4	71.9	68.8
Missouri	73.1	75.9	75.1	74.0	68.5
Montana	64.9	67.2	65.7	64.6	63.7
Nebraska	71.1	77.8	76.5	70.3	63.2
Nevada	69.9	73.1	71.3	67.3	70.6
New Hampshire	69.4	75.5	69.8	70.0	67.7
New Jersey	77.1	90.0	82.0	73.5	72.9
New Mexico	70.1	71.3	75.3	67.3	67.7
New York	76.8	84.7	79.9	76.0	72.6
North Carolina	77.6	82.4	80.8	78.3	71.4
North Dakota	68.1	78.6	72.0	64.4	64.8
Ohio	71.7	74.6	74.5	71.9	66.7
Oklahoma	72.7	77.9	74.2	70.5	70.9
Oregon	62.5	66.5	66.9	63.4	57.1
Pennsylvania	71.6	81.3	76.0	71.4	62.2
Rhode Island	78.7	84.0	83.2	76.0	75.6
South Carolina	77.1	82.7	79.5	75.4	73.5
South Dakota	69.9	79.0	70.2	70.6	66.1
Tennessee	77.0	85.5	77.9	76.2	71.6
Texas	72.7	78.0	73.2	72.9	69.5
Utah	61.7	68.0	64.8	59.9	60.2
Vermont	66.7	77.1	71.8	67.1	59.6
Virginia	70.0	80.2	72.6	69.4	65.9
Washington	63.1	64.9	66.8	64.2	59.1
West Virginia	79.4	85.9	77.1	80.4	76.8
Wisconsin	64.4	73.2	66.5	64.4	59.5
Wyoming	71.3	79.1	69.3	72.9	70.1

Source: Compiled by New Strategist based on the Centers for Disease Control and Prevention Behavioral Risk Factor Surveillance System Survey, Internet site http://www.cdc.gov/brfss/index.htm

1.20 Cholesterol: Last Time Checked by Household Income, 2001

"About how long has it been since you last had your blood cholesterol checked?"

(percent of people aged 18 or older responding "past year," by state and household income, 2001)

	total	less than $15,000	$15,000 to $24,999	$25,000 to $34,999	$35,000 to $49,999	$50,000 or more
U.S. total	**71.7%**	**76.0%**	**74.6%**	**72.0%**	**69.6%**	**69.3%**
Alabama	71.9	74.3	74.5	71.8	66.9	69.2
Alaska	63.0	64.0	54.3	58.2	63.1	64.4
Arizona	71.7	85.0	69.9	72.0	75.0	66.2
Arkansas	70.4	69.6	73.9	70.7	66.1	68.9
California	68.7	69.1	72.5	68.1	70.1	65.9
Colorado	63.6	61.4	63.3	65.5	66.2	58.5
Connecticut	73.6	80.0	78.0	77.9	76.0	69.8
Delaware	73.5	78.2	78.8	71.1	70.7	69.6
District of Columbia	76.9	81.0	79.2	81.6	71.5	73.0
Florida	80.3	75.0	81.3	79.7	79.2	78.5
Georgia	71.9	77.4	72.7	72.6	71.2	69.8
Hawaii	76.5	76.4	77.8	70.1	77.5	74.1
Idaho	60.0	65.5	60.4	58.5	61.9	56.2
Illinois	70.1	68.5	72.7	74.0	71.8	66.4
Indiana	69.6	74.5	71.0	68.4	69.1	67.8
Iowa	70.0	70.6	71.3	70.2	66.3	70.4
Kansas	67.3	73.5	71.7	65.1	62.0	65.4
Kentucky	74.1	74.6	74.7	75.6	74.3	69.8
Louisiana	78.6	81.4	79.9	79.8	76.6	75.0
Maine	71.7	77.0	76.3	73.3	64.1	67.4
Maryland	74.2	72.8	80.6	78.5	74.1	69.6
Massachusetts	73.3	76.1	79.5	75.6	72.1	70.0
Michigan	72.4	76.0	75.3	68.4	73.4	69.4
Minnesota	68.4	75.7	72.4	68.4	67.6	66.4
Mississippi	71.7	76.5	69.1	70.7	74.7	70.8
Missouri	73.1	77.6	77.0	72.4	69.5	70.4
Montana	64.9	59.6	63.7	64.5	61.3	69.2
Nebraska	71.1	77.4	73.3	73.5	69.1	65.7
Nevada	69.9	80.8	77.6	72.1	64.1	66.3
New Hampshire	69.4	73.2	77.8	74.2	67.4	65.8
New Jersey	77.1	82.9	83.6	77.5	80.0	73.0
New Mexico	70.1	73.8	72.2	69.2	67.5	66.9
New York	76.8	78.9	81.1	80.8	75.2	72.8
North Carolina	77.6	81.5	83.9	77.3	70.7	75.7
North Dakota	68.1	73.9	72.0	65.5	63.7	66.0
Ohio	71.7	76.2	75.3	70.8	70.7	69.5
Oklahoma	72.7	73.4	74.3	71.9	72.6	68.3
Oregon	62.5	61.0	64.8	63.4	64.1	59.1
Pennsylvania	71.6	79.1	77.4	73.3	68.8	65.1
Rhode Island	78.7	81.8	81.5	82.8	76.9	75.4
South Carolina	77.1	78.3	77.2	78.7	75.5	75.9
South Dakota	69.9	76.6	70.2	71.6	66.8	66.6
Tennessee	77.0	79.3	77.7	78.7	67.9	75.1
Texas	72.7	75.8	73.6	75.1	69.8	69.8
Utah	61.7	61.2	63.3	67.9	54.8	60.9
Vermont	66.7	72.8	70.2	66.6	64.4	62.4
Virginia	70.0	80.1	74.8	72.3	68.1	66.4
Washington	63.1	72.0	65.6	64.2	64.2	59.6
West Virginia	79.4	80.3	82.3	77.5	76.4	78.1
Wisconsin	64.4	67.1	70.1	66.4	61.1	59.0
Wyoming	71.3	73.1	71.6	71.3	65.3	72.7

Source: Compiled by New Strategist based on the Centers for Disease Control and Prevention Behavioral Risk Factor Surveillance System Survey, Internet site http://www.cdc.gov/brfss/index.htm

1.21 Cholesterol: Last Time Checked by Sex, 2001

"About how long has it been since you last had your blood cholesterol checked?"

(percent of people aged 18 or older responding "past year," by state and sex, 2001)

	total	men	women
U.S. total	**71.7%**	**71.0%**	**72.3%**
Alabama	71.9	71.7	72.0
Alaska	63.0	64.7	61.1
Arizona	71.7	68.8	74.4
Arkansas	70.4	71.0	70.0
California	68.7	67.9	69.5
Colorado	63.6	62.6	64.4
Connecticut	73.6	73.5	73.6
Delaware	73.5	75.4	72.0
District of Columbia	76.9	73.3	79.7
Florida	80.3	79.3	81.1
Georgia	71.9	71.0	72.6
Hawaii	76.5	74.2	78.7
Idaho	60.0	59.0	60.9
Illinois	70.1	69.2	70.8
Indiana	69.6	69.1	70.0
Iowa	70.0	71.3	68.9
Kansas	67.3	67.5	67.1
Kentucky	74.1	73.2	74.9
Louisiana	78.6	77.2	79.8
Maine	71.7	70.6	72.7
Maryland	74.2	73.1	75.1
Massachusetts	73.3	73.2	73.4
Michigan	72.4	71.8	72.9
Minnesota	68.4	66.2	70.3
Mississippi	71.7	69.8	73.4
Missouri	73.1	73.6	72.7
Montana	64.9	63.6	66.1
Nebraska	71.1	70.9	71.3
Nevada	69.9	67.4	72.4
New Hampshire	69.4	69.2	69.6
New Jersey	77.1	74.7	79.2
New Mexico	70.1	67.6	72.2
New York	76.8	76.3	77.3
North Carolina	77.6	74.6	80.1
North Dakota	68.1	66.4	69.7
Ohio	71.7	71.8	71.6
Oklahoma	72.7	72.6	72.8
Oregon	62.5	59.7	65.0
Pennsylvania	71.6	71.3	72.0
Rhode Island	78.7	77.6	79.6
South Carolina	77.1	77.7	76.5
South Dakota	69.9	68.5	71.1
Tennessee	77.0	75.4	78.3
Texas	72.7	70.4	74.6
Utah	61.7	59.5	63.8
Vermont	66.7	65.5	67.8
Virginia	70.0	70.4	69.7
Washington	63.1	61.1	64.9
West Virginia	79.4	78.7	80.1
Wisconsin	64.4	63.9	64.8
Wyoming	71.3	78.7	80.1

Source: Compiled by New Strategist based on the Centers for Disease Control and Prevention Behavioral Risk Factor Surveillance System Survey, Internet site http://www.cdc.gov/brfss/index.htm

1.22 High Cholesterol by Age, 2001

"Have you ever been told by a doctor or other health professional that your blood cholesterol is high?"

(percent of people aged 18 or older responding "yes," by state and age, 2001)

	total	18 to 24	25 to 34	35 to 44	45 to 54	55 to 64	65 or older
U.S. total	**30.2%**	**8.1%**	**14.2%**	**23.1%**	**33.4%**	**43.9%**	**43.9%**
Alabama	32.9	12.1	13.9	22.3	34.4	48.0	51.8
Alaska	28.7	6.6	11.0	24.7	37.5	47.7	41.0
Arizona	30.3	4.6	11.5	31.4	28.2	39.1	45.7
Arkansas	29.9	8.2	11.5	23.2	30.0	44.0	44.0
California	31.7	8.5	18.6	24.2	36.4	43.1	46.9
Colorado	29.4	9.8	14.7	22.1	26.4	45.7	48.4
Connecticut	29.8	9.3	16.3	22.6	30.7	42.8	43.5
Delaware	30.5	6.6	14.5	24.8	30.0	47.1	46.3
District of Columbia	29.0	18.5	14.7	21.0	29.6	41.8	46.6
Florida	31.0	7.9	13.5	20.4	30.9	44.7	44.4
Georgia	31.9	11.9	15.1	25.2	37.5	47.2	48.5
Hawaii	25.1	5.0	14.5	20.4	29.7	36.8	31.8
Idaho	30.3	6.1	11.5	22.4	35.4	41.6	43.5
Illinois	29.4	8.1	14.7	21.4	35.2	45.0	40.6
Indiana	30.1	7.3	11.3	25.5	33.2	43.5	41.9
Iowa	30.4	5.6	13.5	22.2	33.8	39.6	45.3
Kansas	29.2	9.0	14.2	21.7	33.4	40.6	40.8
Kentucky	31.1	9.6	13.8	26.5	35.9	45.2	41.2
Louisiana	27.6	7.0	13.9	23.1	31.7	43.2	38.5
Maine	30.3	5.2	16.5	26.6	30.6	41.1	43.1
Maryland	31.1	9.9	14.9	23.8	35.7	46.3	46.7
Massachusetts	29.7	10.1	15.7	23.0	32.7	42.2	44.6
Michigan	33.6	9.6	17.0	27.9	38.3	44.9	46.9
Minnesota	30.2	9.6	13.2	22.3	31.7	48.1	43.9
Mississippi	31.0	2.6	15.3	22.0	35.9	47.8	46.4
Missouri	31.3	7.2	14.6	24.8	33.8	44.8	41.8
Montana	29.0	6.2	12.1	21.0	30.0	42.8	40.8
Nebraska	27.8	8.3	12.9	18.7	29.1	38.9	39.2
Nevada	36.5	4.3	22.6	28.3	44.9	42.8	50.2
New Hampshire	31.0	8.2	20.3	22.6	32.9	47.8	43.9
New Jersey	30.2	10.3	13.3	21.4	33.7	42.5	45.9
New Mexico	24.8	2.3	8.4	22.1	24.9	34.2	39.0
New York	30.1	11.8	17.3	22.9	32.9	39.1	45.4
North Carolina	28.9	6.7	14.0	24.4	30.7	39.9	44.6
North Dakota	29.6	6.1	12.3	23.5	34.9	40.8	41.5
Ohio	32.8	4.2	17.5	25.4	33.7	49.9	46.3
Oklahoma	29.6	10.6	12.9	21.1	31.6	48.1	41.3
Oregon	32.1	2.4	14.6	26.2	35.7	43.9	42.9
Pennsylvania	32.5	10.4	15.6	23.1	33.1	45.6	46.7
Rhode Island	33.1	18.7	17.0	25.3	36.8	52.0	43.2
South Carolina	27.8	5.5	9.2	23.9	33.0	41.4	43.0
South Dakota	29.5	3.4	13.0	22.1	31.4	43.8	41.8
Tennessee	33.2	9.3	18.6	24.5	41.7	44.9	44.1
Texas	31.8	8.4	14.8	25.2	34.6	49.2	46.5
Utah	29.0	7.1	11.9	21.7	38.3	44.9	40.6
Vermont	29.5	6.4	14.4	20.3	33.6	45.1	45.4
Virginia	30.7	10.1	15.2	20.8	33.4	47.6	48.4
Washington	29.2	5.9	16.4	24.2	29.3	40.5	41.2
West Virginia	37.7	12.0	14.2	25.7	46.4	50.6	50.8
Wisconsin	29.7	5.4	12.3	21.3	30.6	43.3	44.8
Wyoming	30.5	9.6	13.2	25.6	32.9	43.9	40.9

Source: Compiled by New Strategist based on the Centers for Disease Control and Prevention Behavioral Risk Factor Surveillance System Survey, Internet site http://www.cdc.gov/brfss/index.htm

1.23 High Cholesterol by Education, 2001

"Have you ever been told by a doctor or other health professional
that your blood cholesterol is high?"

(percent of people aged 18 or older responding "yes." by state and educational attainment, 2001)

	total	less than high school	high school graduate	some college	college graduate
U.S. total	**30.2%**	**36.0%**	**31.7%**	**29.3%**	**27.0%**
Alabama	32.9	43.0	32.5	27.5	33.0
Alaska	28.7	27.9	27.3	29.3	29.0
Arizona	30.3	32.0	32.3	33.6	24.9
Arkansas	29.9	40.8	31.8	24.8	26.0
California	31.7	36.7	30.7	31.7	30.3
Colorado	29.4	31.6	29.9	31.0	27.5
Connecticut	29.8	35.1	32.1	32.0	26.1
Delaware	30.5	36.0	31.0	31.4	28.0
District of Columbia	29.0	44.0	27.9	29.4	25.9
Florida	31.0	35.9	31.6	31.3	28.5
Georgia	31.9	38.0	36.7	31.5	25.8
Hawaii	25.1	29.3	25.2	25.1	24.3
Idaho	30.3	34.0	31.5	30.2	28.3
Illinois	29.4	31.0	29.8	32.2	26.4
Indiana	30.1	34.6	33.3	29.7	24.9
Iowa	30.4	40.3	32.5	28.7	25.8
Kansas	29.2	37.3	31.2	28.9	26.2
Kentucky	31.1	41.2	32.0	25.9	27.3
Louisiana	27.6	34.1	27.8	24.6	25.7
Maine	30.3	40.3	31.2	28.2	28.5
Maryland	31.1	38.7	30.3	31.8	29.6
Massachusetts	29.7	34.5	33.5	30.5	26.2
Michigan	33.6	34.5	33.5	30.5	26.2
Minnesota	30.2	37.9	37.7	32.7	28.6
Mississippi	31.0	36.4	37.1	27.6	26.0
Missouri	31.3	38.2	33.0	27.8	26.9
Montana	29.0	30.3	31.5	27.0	27.9
Nebraska	27.8	26.7	32.4	26.9	23.6
Nevada	36.5	41.4	31.0	39.6	36.3
New Hampshire	31.0	32.3	31.8	31.6	29.9
New Jersey	30.2	32.6	34.7	29.2	26.8
New Mexico	24.8	22.2	25.0	25.5	25.6
New York	30.1	37.4	31.2	28.5	28.2
North Carolina	28.9	33.7	29.3	31.3	24.4
North Dakota	29.6	36.0	31.2	27.3	28.5
Ohio	32.8	34.7	36.9	27.9	31.2
Oklahoma	29.6	36.0	30.5	29.7	24.7
Oregon	32.1	39.1	36.3	30.8	27.9
Pennsylvania	32.5	43.0	35.3	30.3	26.6
Rhode Island	33.1	39.5	37.3	30.8	29.6
South Carolina	27.8	38.4	26.1	28.4	24.4
South Dakota	29.5	33.9	32.8	28.3	26.1
Tennessee	33.2	39.1	34.9	33.4	27.3
Texas	31.8	31.9	30.0	34.1	31.3
Utah	29.0	31.2	27.5	30.3	28.5
Vermont	29.5	43.5	32.7	28.1	24.4
Virginia	30.7	41.8	30.8	29.9	28.3
Washington	29.2	31.5	32.2	28.9	27.1
West Virginia	37.7	50.4	37.3	34.2	30.6
Wisconsin	29.7	35.6	33.6	26.7	26.4
Wyoming	30.5	31.2	31.6	31.3	28.4

Source: Compiled by New Strategist based on the Centers for Disease Control and Prevention Behavioral Risk Factor Surveillance System Survey, Internet site http://www.cdc.gov/brfss/index.htm

1.24 High Cholesterol by Household Income, 2001

"Have you ever been told by a doctor or other health professional
that your blood cholesterol is high?"

(percent of people aged 18 or older responding "yes," by state and household income, 2001)

	total	less than $15,000	$15,000 to $24,999	$25,000 to $34,999	$35,000 to $49,999	$50,000 or more
U.S. total	30.2%	36.1%	32.3%	30.1%	28.9%	28.1%
Alabama	32.9	40.6	32.3	26.9	31.3	31.7
Alaska	28.7	36.1	27.1	21.5	30.3	28.1
Arizona	30.3	38.1	29.8	30.4	30.1	28.8
Arkansas	29.9	34.3	32.6	28.7	31.5	24.0
California	31.7	33.0	34.0	33.3	32.7	29.0
Colorado	29.4	38.6	30.8	32.6	28.3	26.7
Connecticut	29.8	34.1	31.5	30.0	28.5	29.2
Delaware	30.5	31.4	39.0	30.6	27.9	26.3
District of Columbia	29.0	37.1	31.6	27.1	25.8	26.3
Florida	31.0	34.7	35.2	27.9	26.7	28.7
Georgia	31.9	37.2	34.8	29.2	26.8	30.7
Hawaii	25.1	34.2	16.2	26.2	29.5	25.4
Idaho	30.3	36.5	29.0	27.7	30.6	28.4
Illinois	29.4	44.7	34.5	31.2	24.3	28.1
Indiana	30.1	35.3	30.6	31.0	32.5	26.9
Iowa	30.4	32.9	34.3	32.2	32.3	24.2
Kansas	29.2	37.0	31.8	24.1	30.6	27.1
Kentucky	31.1	39.3	34.7	33.2	30.0	24.8
Louisiana	27.6	35.2	26.4	23.7	27.5	26.5
Maine	30.3	35.3	33.1	30.8	29.0	26.6
Maryland	31.1	31.4	32.9	35.1	26.5	31.0
Massachusetts	29.7	32.0	34.9	33.1	29.4	28.2
Michigan	33.6	42.8	38.0	33.7	32.7	28.6
Minnesota	30.2	37.8	34.3	32.1	31.8	26.6
Mississippi	31.0	39.2	31.9	28.3	28.4	28.1
Missouri	31.3	36.3	32.7	29.4	29.2	28.7
Montana	29.0	28.0	26.8	31.6	24.2	29.4
Nebraska	27.8	31.8	26.7	29.1	28.9	24.8
Nevada	36.5	52.8	37.7	30.2	32.2	36.8
New Hampshire	31.0	40.2	34.8	32.8	27.1	30.1
New Jersey	30.2	37.3	33.7	29.8	29.0	27.2
New Mexico	24.8	30.6	23.8	23.4	24.1	24.2
New York	30.1	31.8	35.8	37.9	25.6	27.0
North Carolina	28.9	34.8	33.7	26.7	29.4	25.0
North Dakota	29.6	28.3	31.6	30.8	24.3	30.4
Ohio	32.8	39.9	39.0	32.6	28.1	30.8
Oklahoma	29.6	39.0	31.1	26.5	30.2	25.7
Oregon	32.1	37.6	29.9	34.4	31.7	30.4
Pennsylvania	32.5	36.2	37.9	33.4	28.9	29.6
Rhode Island	33.1	40.4	28.4	33.1	38.3	30.9
South Carolina	27.8	42.2	27.1	27.6	25.4	27.5
South Dakota	29.5	33.2	31.1	28.8	27.2	26.9
Tennessee	33.2	49.3	42.0	28.1	29.1	27.7
Texas	31.8	34.0	31.0	33.1	27.0	32.8
Utah	29.0	36.0	25.7	29.3	29.6	28.3
Vermont	29.5	34.6	32.3	28.3	30.8	25.8
Virginia	30.7	44.5	32.2	32.5	26.4	28.5
Washington	29.2	30.5	34.3	35.2	26.1	26.2
West Virginia	37.7	46.8	39.7	39.3	35.2	32.1
Wisconsin	29.7	34.5	36.9	28.5	32.2	23.1
Wyoming	30.5	31.2	28.3	31.8	28.1	29.5

Source: Compiled by New Strategist based on the Centers for Disease Control and Prevention Behavioral Risk Factor Surveillance System Survey, Internet site http://www.cdc.gov/brfss/index.htm

1.25 High Cholesterol by Sex, 2001

"Have you ever been told by a doctor or other health professional that your blood cholesterol is high?"

(percent of people aged 18 or older responding "yes," by state and sex, 2001)

	total	men	women
U.S. total	**30.2%**	**31.1%**	**29.7%**
Alabama	32.9	34.1	31.7
Alaska	28.7	28.2	29.4
Arizona	30.3	30.0	30.7
Arkansas	29.9	30.0	29.7
California	31.7	34.8	28.9
Colorado	29.4	33.0	26.2
Connecticut	29.8	30.7	29.0
Delaware	30.5	31.0	30.1
District of Columbia	29.0	28.0	29.9
Florida	31.0	30.2	31.7
Georgia	31.9	32.8	31.1
Hawaii	25.1	25.7	24.5
Idaho	30.3	31.1	29.6
Illinois	29.4	30.0	28.8
Indiana	30.1	30.4	29.8
Iowa	30.4	33.4	27.8
Kansas	29.2	28.9	29.6
Kentucky	31.1	31.5	30.9
Louisiana	27.6	27.7	27.6
Maine	30.3	31.4	29.4
Maryland	31.1	34.1	28.4
Massachusetts	29.7	31.5	28.2
Michigan	33.6	36.0	31.5
Minnesota	30.2	31.6	29.0
Mississippi	31.0	30.3	31.6
Missouri	31.3	31.5	31.1
Montana	29.0	29.4	28.6
Nebraska	27.8	29.1	26.6
Nevada	36.5	35.7	37.2
New Hampshire	31.0	34.6	27.9
New Jersey	30.2	29.7	30.7
New Mexico	24.8	26.8	23.2
New York	30.1	33.1	27.6
North Carolina	28.9	27.1	30.5
North Dakota	29.6	28.4	30.7
Ohio	32.8	35.9	30.1
Oklahoma	29.6	29.2	30.0
Oregon	32.1	34.1	30.3
Pennsylvania	32.5	33.9	31.2
Rhode Island	33.1	35.2	31.4
South Carolina	27.8	28.4	27.3
South Dakota	29.5	28.1	30.8
Tennessee	33.2	35.6	31.1
Texas	31.8	32.2	31.4
Utah	29.0	31.1	26.9
Vermont	29.5	31.3	27.9
Virginia	30.7	31.7	29.7
Washington	29.2	30.8	27.7
West Virginia	37.7	36.6	38.6
Wisconsin	29.7	33.1	26.7
Wyoming	30.5	31.2	29.9

Source: Compiled by New Strategist based on the Centers for Disease Control and Prevention Behavioral Risk Factor Surveillance System Survey, Internet site http://www.cdc.gov/brfss/index.htm

1.26 Colorectal Cancer Screening: Ever Had a Colonoscopy Exam by Age, 1999

"Have you ever had a sigmoidoscopy or colonoscopy exam?"

(percent of people aged 18 or older responding "yes," by state and age, 1999)

	total	40 to 49	50 to 59	60 to 64	65 or older
U.S. total	**33.7%**	**15.7%**	**33.0%**	**45.4%**	**51.5%**
Alabama	34.9	20.6	31.0	42.9	49.1
Alaska	35.4	19.6	35.2	68.5	67.7
Arizona	30.8	19.8	26.7	33.4	44.5
Arkansas	34.4	18.3	34.7	41.4	47.4
California	35.1	13.0	38.5	47.8	57.5
Colorado	32.4	13.9	29.8	50.0	55.4
Connecticut	36.8	14.9	40.1	50.2	55.6
Delaware	43.9	22.3	46.9	51.8	64.6
District of Columbia	37.1	14.1	34.2	53.6	58.5
Florida	36.2	14.7	32.0	47.5	52.9
Georgia	36.7	18.8	38.3	55.1	53.9
Hawaii	31.9	9.4	27.3	61.8	54.1
Idaho	32.2	15.1	30.8	45.9	49.1
Illinois	34.4	15.3	35.4	48.3	49.2
Indiana	36.1	22.8	35.4	41.0	50.4
Iowa	36.2	14.9	35.3	50.8	52.9
Kansas	30.2	13.7	27.5	39.9	46.6
Kentucky	28.2	15.8	27.3	36.6	40.3
Louisiana	29.3	15.6	25.5	36.1	46.2
Maine	33.7	15.6	32.8	50.9	48.5
Maryland	39.3	19.3	41.0	59.4	57.8
Massachusetts	33.8	14.5	37.4	41.4	49.7
Michigan	40.1	22.0	40.2	54.5	56.1
Minnesota	37.2	17.1	37.9	44.6	56.3
Mississippi	30.8	18.5	27.9	35.1	45.5
Missouri	30.1	13.7	29.2	37.5	44.8
Montana	33.3	14.5	28.0	53.8	52.9
Nebraska	26.9	14.1	26.7	31.1	39.1
Nevada	33.4	16.2	29.2	49.9	54.7
New Hampshire	34.4	16.7	37.6	47.1	54.3
New Jersey	34.4	14.9	36.9	45.2	49.6
New Mexico	32.0	13.3	32.8	45.0	51.2
New York	32.2	12.5	31.7	39.8	51.8
North Carolina	32.0	18.0	28.7	38.1	48.9
North Dakota	33.5	16.9	30.8	39.9	50.3
Ohio	34.5	21.4	29.9	45.5	48.2
Oklahoma	30.2	14.2	28.1	39.4	44.8
Oregon	36.5	16.3	35.4	58.7	53.7
Pennsylvania	32.4	16.6	31.8	38.7	45.3
Rhode Island	37.3	14.2	39.2	46.9	55.6
South Carolina	32.9	16.1	33.5	38.4	50.5
South Dakota	35.1	14.0	33.3	47.5	52.2
Tennessee	31.9	17.3	28.5	44.3	46.7
Texas	34.1	16.0	34.3	46.3	52.9
Utah	32.3	13.6	32.2	43.8	55.4
Vermont	31.5	13.5	33.5	38.9	51.1
Virginia	34.2	19.1	36.8	45.4	54.2
Washington	38.7	17.5	39.2	65.4	55.8
West Virginia	30.1	19.5	29.0	31.5	40.1
Wisconsin	41.2	19.9	44.6	50.5	58.8
Wyoming	33.2	13.1	36.6	49.6	53.7

Source: Compiled by New Strategist based on the Centers for Disease Control and Prevention Behavioral Risk Factor Surveillance System Survey, Internet site http://www.cdc.gov/brfss/index.htm

1.27 Colorectal Cancer Screening: Ever Had a Colonoscopy Exam by Education, 1999

"Have you ever had a sigmoidoscopy or colonoscopy exam?"

(percent of people aged 18 or older responding "yes," by state and educational attainment, 1999)

	total	less than high school	high school graduate	some college	college graduate
U.S. total	**33.7%**	**34.4%**	**31.8%**	**32.6%**	**35.9%**
Alabama	34.9	35.9	34.9	33.7	34.7
Alaska	35.4	31.0	31.0	41.4	35.8
Arizona	30.8	28.4	24.9	32.8	38.0
Arkansas	34.4	36.6	32.0	33.3	36.9
California	35.1	28.3	31.6	39.6	38.0
Colorado	32.4	17.0	33.0	32.5	36.0
Connecticut	36.8	43.5	39.8	33.2	34.4
Delaware	43.9	38.6	38.0	41.9	52.7
District of Columbia	37.1	43.7	35.7	32.0	37.3
Florida	36.2	33.5	34.8	35.4	39.9
Georgia	36.7	39.8	28.9	40.2	41.5
Hawaii	31.9	39.9	33.9	32.1	28.3
Idaho	32.2	33.6	32.2	31.1	32.8
Illinois	34.4	32.6	34.5	39.0	30.9
Indiana	36.1	36.9	34.9	41.4	33.5
Iowa	36.2	43.5	37.8	31.3	34.5
Kansas	30.2	36.6	29.4	27.9	31.4
Kentucky	28.2	30.4	26.2	31.1	25.1
Louisiana	29.3	30.1	27.3	33.2	27.5
Maine	33.7	37.0	35.8	30.4	32.9
Maryland	39.3	35.2	35.9	41.0	42.9
Massachusetts	33.8	28.4	32.3	34.0	36.6
Michigan	40.1	42.0	34.7	43.8	42.6
Minnesota	37.2	48.8	35.4	36.1	36.2
Mississippi	30.8	29.5	27.0	32.7	35.8
Missouri	30.1	30.0	28.3	33.9	29.6
Montana	33.3	49.7	31.7	29.9	32.5
Nebraska	26.9	39.1	26.6	25.3	28.3
Nevada	33.4	44.7	30.0	32.4	33.9
New Hampshire	34.4	36.6	37.8	26.9	37.1
New Jersey	34.4	25.6	32.2	30.2	42.5
New Mexico	32.0	32.8	26.6	32.7	35.4
New York	32.2	25.9	31.4	31.0	37.1
North Carolina	32.0	30.7	28.8	29.4	39.9
North Dakota	33.5	41.3	31.8	28.8	35.5
Ohio	34.5	42.9	31.8	34.6	33.3
Oklahoma	30.2	31.1	27.7	30.0	34.1
Oregon	36.5	29.2	37.0	36.3	38.4
Pennsylvania	32.4	31.3	32.2	29.7	35.3
Rhode Island	37.3	36.8	37.9	35.2	38.4
South Carolina	32.9	30.4	29.1	35.5	38.1
South Dakota	35.1	39.4	36.4	32.0	34.3
Tennessee	31.9	30.5	30.8	32.0	34.9
Texas	34.1	25.6	31.7	36.9	39.2
Utah	32.3	40.2	27.7	31.1	36.7
Vermont	31.5	31.2	28.2	32.2	34.3
Virginia	34.2	39.7	31.3	29.6	37.9
Washington	38.7	37.9	39.0	38.1	39.4
West Virginia	30.1	32.5	27.8	25.9	36.7
Wisconsin	41.2	46.3	37.0	45.6	40.9
Wyoming	33.2	41.6	30.4	31.7	36.1

Source: Compiled by New Strategist based on the Centers for Disease Control and Prevention Behavioral Risk Factor Surveillance System Survey, Internet site http://www.cdc.gov/brfss/index.htm

1.28 Colorectal Cancer Screening: Ever Had a Colonoscopy Exam by Household Income, 1999

"Have you ever had a sigmoidoscopy or colonoscopy exam?"

(percent of people aged 18 or older responding "yes," by state and household income, 1999)

	total	less than $15,000	$15,000 to $24,999	$25,000 to $34,999	$35,000 to $49,999	$50,000 or more
U.S. total	**33.7%**	**35.2%**	**35.3%**	**33.4%**	**30.8%**	**31.6%**
Alabama	34.9	37.8	36.4	30.3	34.3	29.7
Alaska	35.4	35.1	51.3	19.0	42.3	32.5
Arizona	30.8	45.7	38.9	33.1	29.0	21.8
Arkansas	34.4	34.4	32.9	34.6	30.6	36.5
California	35.1	28.8	37.7	36.1	36.8	35.2
Colorado	32.4	39.7	29.5	43.8	27.7	29.3
Connecticut	36.8	40.6	37.6	40.7	30.9	37.2
Delaware	43.9	46.5	38.5	44.2	41.3	44.2
District of Columbia	37.1	53.0	35.3	43.3	30.4	41.8
Florida	36.2	33.9	35.1	34.2	33.1	35.0
Georgia	36.7	33.6	37.5	42.7	36.0	37.1
Hawaii	31.9	29.5	36.7	31.5	36.6	26.6
Idaho	32.2	31.5	35.3	33.2	27.7	30.9
Illinois	34.4	48.0	35.3	25.3	33.3	30.4
Indiana	36.1	35.8	33.2	37.9	31.0	33.7
Iowa	36.2	40.6	43.5	39.8	29.5	30.8
Kansas	30.2	31.4	29.5	35.2	25.0	26.1
Kentucky	28.2	29.7	29.6	23.5	24.0	26.3
Louisiana	29.3	31.0	35.2	31.6	19.7	28.3
Maine	33.7	33.3	30.2	32.8	31.5	31.3
Maryland	39.3	33.6	37.6	43.7	34.8	37.6
Massachusetts	33.8	40.2	35.8	32.8	33.1	29.3
Michigan	40.1	41.7	45.9	48.9	38.9	33.7
Minnesota	37.2	50.4	41.6	39.1	31.1	33.7
Mississippi	30.8	27.2	32.7	31.9	28.6	32.1
Missouri	30.1	32.7	32.7	28.8	24.9	26.2
Montana	33.3	41.6	33.9	30.2	36.0	25.7
Nebraska	26.9	34.5	31.9	27.4	23.8	22.8
Nevada	33.4	41.8	43.2	29.7	28.3	29.5
New Hampshire	34.4	35.2	46.6	38.3	30.9	29.3
New Jersey	34.4	45.4	36.3	26.6	32.2	37.4
New Mexico	32.0	34.0	26.4	36.9	30.0	33.5
New York	32.2	32.3	29.5	31.8	33.4	35.7
North Carolina	32.0	27.9	36.5	31.0	25.2	33.6
North Dakota	33.5	36.5	36.7	33.7	28.1	31.4
Ohio	34.5	40.2	42.5	32.8	27.2	27.4
Oklahoma	30.2	30.6	28.0	36.3	20.8	33.4
Oregon	36.5	33.6	45.0	33.4	30.6	36.6
Pennsylvania	32.4	35.5	34.6	32.1	31.9	27.6
Rhode Island	37.3	47.6	41.0	33.4	36.8	31.5
South Carolina	32.9	35.3	29.0	31.6	31.6	31.6
South Dakota	35.1	40.6	42.2	33.8	28.2	30.2
Tennessee	31.9	33.8	34.4	37.0	25.8	28.6
Texas	34.1	30.2	31.5	36.4	34.5	36.8
Utah	32.3	39.0	32.7	33.6	28.9	28.8
Vermont	31.5	35.9	30.6	24.8	28.7	33.1
Virginia	34.2	35.9	33.5	32.0	32.3	33.7
Washington	38.7	41.4	44.1	39.6	40.1	33.1
West Virginia	30.1	28.2	29.7	29.7	30.7	31.7
Wisconsin	41.2	51.4	40.7	45.5	36.0	38.0
Wyoming	33.2	32.3	34.8	34.6	29.4	32.5

Source: Compiled by New Strategist based on the Centers for Disease Control and Prevention Behavioral Risk Factor Surveillance System Survey, Internet site http://www.cdc.gov/brfss/index.htm

1.29 Colorectal Cancer Screening: Ever Had a Colonoscopy Exam by Sex, 1999

"Have you ever had a sigmoidoscopy or colonoscopy exam?"

(percent of people aged 18 or older responding "yes," by state and sex, 1999)

	total	men	women
U.S. total	**33.7%**	**33.9%**	**32.6%**
Alabama	34.9	34.0	35.6
Alaska	35.4	38.9	31.8
Arizona	30.8	29.5	32.0
Arkansas	34.4	33.1	35.4
California	35.1	37.8	32.7
Colorado	32.4	34.7	30.4
Connecticut	36.8	37.6	36.1
Delaware	43.9	45.6	42.5
District of Columbia	37.1	40.7	34.2
Florida	36.2	37.0	35.6
Georgia	36.7	37.9	35.8
Hawaii	31.9	33.6	30.4
Idaho	32.2	31.9	32.5
Illinois	34.4	31.7	36.9
Indiana	36.1	38.2	34.3
Iowa	36.2	33.7	38.2
Kansas	30.2	30.0	30.3
Kentucky	28.2	36.7	29.4
Louisiana	29.3	31.4	27.5
Maine	33.7	30.2	36.7
Maryland	39.3	42.5	36.4
Massachusetts	33.8	35.9	32.0
Michigan	40.1	45.4	35.8
Minnesota	37.2	36.7	37.6
Mississippi	30.8	30.0	31.4
Missouri	30.1	28.2	31.6
Montana	33.3	33.1	33.5
Nebraska	26.9	26.2	27.5
Nevada	33.4	31.0	35.6
New Hampshire	34.4	37.9	31.2
New Jersey	34.4	37.2	32.0
New Mexico	32.0	32.1	32.0
New York	32.2	34.5	30.3
North Carolina	32.0	31.0	32.9
North Dakota	33.5	35.9	31.3
Ohio	34.5	35.0	34.1
Oklahoma	30.2	31.8	28.8
Oregon	36.5	36.8	36.1
Pennsylvania	32.4	33.9	31.2
Rhode Island	37.3	37.4	37.2
South Carolina	32.9	32.7	33.0
South Dakota	35.1	32.8	37.1
Tennessee	31.9	31.4	32.2
Texas	34.1	35.7	32.7
Utah	32.3	33.1	31.6
Vermont	31.5	31.0	31.9
Virginia	34.2	37.2	31.7
Washington	38.7	39.4	38.0
West Virginia	30.1	29.9	30.2
Wisconsin	41.2	42.2	40.3
Wyoming	33.2	36.8	29.9

Source: Compiled by New Strategist based on the Centers for Disease Control and Prevention Behavioral Risk Factor Surveillance System Survey, Internet site http://www.cdc.gov/brfss/index.htm

1.30 Colorectal Cancer Screening: Last Colonoscopy Exam by Age, 1999

"When did you have your last sigmoidoscopy or colonoscopy exam?"

(percent of people aged 18 or older responding "past year," by state and age, 1999)

	total	40 to 49	50 to 59	60 to 64	65 or older
U.S. total	**32.8%**	**26.9%**	**33.1%**	**31.8%**	**34.5%**
Alabama	29.3	21.9	26.5	41.3	30.1
Alaska	33.6	40.4	36.6	19.9	33.3
Arizona	43.3	53.4	47.2	39.2	37.8
Arkansas	29.3	24.7	31.3	26.1	30.8
California	31.7	26.3	34.0	25.6	33.5
Colorado	21.5	19.0	20.4	22.0	22.8
Connecticut	37.7	21.1	44.4	26.2	41.4
Delaware	36.0	25.3	44.0	36.8	35.2
District of Columbia	48.3	44.6	39.8	54.9	51.2
Florida	34.0	32.2	31.5	34.4	35.2
Georgia	31.0	23.3	26.9	28.1	38.7
Hawaii	25.2	21.7	22.6	24.9	27.3
Idaho	29.4	26.5	31.0	28.4	29.8
Illinois	34.0	16.5	33.4	41.7	37.7
Indiana	30.8	16.6	35.6	26.5	36.7
Iowa	27.5	29.3	27.8	29.1	26.5
Kansas	32.8	28.3	37.6	28.0	33.3
Kentucky	31.1	26.0	32.6	37.1	30.8
Louisiana	38.0	30.3	38.6	51.9	37.3
Maine	32.7	25.1	34.3	29.2	35.3
Maryland	34.6	34.5	32.4	39.7	34.6
Massachusetts	38.2	33.7	43.8	38.1	36.4
Michigan	32.8	29.7	37.5	22.7	34.2
Minnesota	35.7	31.9	41.2	40.1	32.9
Mississippi	33.9	26.9	32.1	35.0	37.8
Missouri	29.3	20.2	28.9	29.7	32.2
Montana	27.7	27.0	19.3	25.0	32.4
Nebraska	26.2	12.7	17.8	32.3	33.8
Nevada	25.5	23.0	33.1	10.6	27.0
New Hampshire	32.3	27.2	36.1	18.0	36.6
New Jersey	40.0	37.2	40.7	39.2	40.6
New Mexico	30.3	21.9	35.9	25.5	31.5
New York	40.7	29.3	40.8	46.8	42.4
North Carolina	39.1	32.3	48.5	38.3	37.1
North Dakota	28.3	15.5	31.1	34.0	30.4
Ohio	31.9	23.5	26.5	47.0	34.7
Oklahoma	36.1	46.9	32.3	34.1	35.2
Oregon	30.4	35.0	27.1	27.4	31.7
Pennsylvania	35.1	29.4	34.7	29.4	38.5
Rhode Island	41.8	37.9	35.2	43.4	45.7
South Carolina	40.1	39.5	38.5	35.5	42.4
South Dakota	31.2	25.0	38.7	31.4	29.9
Tennessee	35.6	35.8	36.1	37.9	34.4
Texas	33.6	35.7	33.2	34.1	33.0
Utah	34.3	32.7	32.8	29.9	36.9
Vermont	33.2	23.4	32.3	28.1	38.4
Virginia	31.4	25.5	39.0	28.3	29.3
Washington	26.4	18.7	32.4	24.7	26.5
West Virginia	32.9	23.6	28.7	35.5	38.6
Wisconsin	31.7	29.1	27.9	43.9	31.6
Wyoming	27.8	22.3	30.3	21.8	30.3

Source: Compiled by New Strategist based on the Centers for Disease Control and Prevention Behavioral Risk Factor Surveillance System Survey, Internet site http://www.cdc.gov/brfss/index.htm

1.31 Colorectal Cancer Screening: Last Colonoscopy Exam by Education, 1999

"When did you have your last sigmoidoscopy or colonoscopy exam?"

(percent of people aged 18 or older responding "past year," by state and educational attainment, 1999)

	total	less than high school	high school graduate	some college	college graduate
U.S. total	**32.8%**	**37.9%**	**33.9%**	**32.0%**	**30.4%**
Alabama	29.3	29.4	25.8	33.4	31.2
Alaska	33.6	41.1	26.4	31.7	40.1
Arizona	43.3	54.1	47.6	39.2	40.2
Arkansas	29.3	29.4	29.6	26.2	32.0
California	31.7	33.7	31.1	33.4	29.4
Colorado	21.5	41.7	22.5	20.9	18.7
Connecticut	37.7	44.3	38.2	35.8	35.2
Delaware	36.0	48.6	36.5	32.1	34.9
District of Columbia	48.3	58.0	50.7	52.2	41.2
Florida	34.0	41.9	34.9	33.3	30.5
Georgia	31.0	40.9	31.8	22.3	31.0
Hawaii	25.2	32.2	27.6	20.2	24.8
Idaho	29.4	33.6	32.2	25.4	28.9
Illinois	34.0	32.9	41.0	34.8	24.5
Indiana	30.8	41.1	25.2	29.1	36.9
Iowa	27.5	35.7	27.3	24.3	26.0
Kansas	32.8	29.1	35.9	28.3	35.2
Kentucky	31.1	34.7	29.0	33.3	26.5
Louisiana	38.0	47.9	39.6	29.5	37.4
Maine	32.7	46.6	35.7	30.3	24.0
Maryland	34.6	40.9	41.0	30.1	29.8
Massachusetts	38.2	48.5	32.4	36.1	42.1
Michigan	32.8	36.9	33.6	33.6	29.3
Minnesota	35.7	32.0	38.1	36.1	33.5
Mississippi	33.9	38.0	29.1	34.5	35.0
Missouri	29.3	37.9	26.4	31.1	25.5
Montana	27.7	33.4	29.7	32.0	19.2
Nebraska	26.2	34.7	26.8	21.8	25.4
Nevada	25.5	13.0	26.2	30.1	26.4
New Hampshire	32.3	40.0	35.8	28.0	29.9
New Jersey	40.0	50.6	40.3	40.1	37.8
New Mexico	30.3	38.1	25.2	30.4	29.5
New York	40.7	55.5	37.9	39.4	40.1
North Carolina	39.1	33.9	37.7	42.5	42.2
North Dakota	28.3	27.9	23.9	29.2	33.9
Ohio	31.9	38.1	31.6	32.5	24.1
Oklahoma	36.1	34.5	36.0	35.4	37.6
Oregon	30.4	31.2	28.7	32.2	30.3
Pennsylvania	35.1	39.1	34.7	39.7	30.6
Rhode Island	41.8	50.8	44.9	36.9	37.0
South Carolina	40.1	46.3	41.7	32.8	40.2
South Dakota	31.2	37.8	34.5	28.1	25.4
Tennessee	35.6	35.3	34.3	38.5	34.1
Texas	33.6	44.8	34.5	29.4	31.8
Utah	34.3	42.8	40.2	38.6	24.9
Vermont	33.2	19.5	36.6	32.8	34.0
Virginia	31.4	37.5	29.9	34.0	27.4
Washington	26.4	47.7	25.2	24.7	24.3
West Virginia	32.9	33.9	36.0	29.9	28.0
Wisconsin	31.7	40.6	31.6	31.3	27.3
Wyoming	27.8	35.3	23.3	27.9	30.4

Source: Compiled by New Strategist based on the Centers for Disease Control and Prevention Behavioral Risk Factor Surveillance System Survey, Internet site http://www.cdc.gov/brfss/index.htm

1.32 Colorectal Cancer Screening: Last Colonoscopy Exam by Household Income, 1999

"When did you have your last sigmoidoscopy or colonoscopy exam?"

(percent of people aged 18 or older responding "past year," by state and household income, 1999)

	total	less than $15,000	$15,000 to $24,999	$25,000 to $34,999	$35,000 to $49,999	$50,000 or more
U.S. total	**32.8%**	**32.8%**	**33.5%**	**33.3%**	**32.3%**	**31.3%**
Alabama	29.3	34.9	26.7	33.7	32.3	30.9
Alaska	33.6	40.8	32.1	36.8	28.0	41.3
Arizona	43.3	42.2	45.9	48.6	53.3	42.6
Arkansas	29.3	34.9	23.7	31.7	26.3	29.4
California	31.7	37.9	26.6	44.9	28.6	29.7
Colorado	21.5	24.3	16.6	21.8	25.5	18.9
Connecticut	37.7	42.4	52.9	39.3	35.2	34.9
Delaware	36.0	32.3	38.0	45.2	36.6	35.8
District of Columbia	48.3	36.1	68.7	62.3	43.6	39.6
Florida	34.0	38.9	34.3	33.4	36.0	30.8
Georgia	31.0	39.4	23.2	35.9	34.2	25.5
Hawaii	25.2	42.8	23.2	21.2	25.0	22.6
Idaho	29.4	32.1	29.3	33.2	20.6	32.6
Illinois	34.0	42.4	50.6	44.5	33.9	23.5
Indiana	30.8	18.3	28.4	25.6	23.8	32.0
Iowa	27.5	32.5	29.6	26.5	27.5	27.4
Kansas	32.8	30.1	33.3	35.3	30.9	33.7
Kentucky	31.1	28.1	30.8	36.8	38.9	24.0
Louisiana	38.0	46.3	48.3	37.0	21.4	33.9
Maine	32.7	34.9	43.7	25.5	40.5	24.3
Maryland	34.6	32.7	49.3	35.8	37.7	28.0
Massachusetts	38.2	29.4	44.3	35.4	26.5	36.9
Michigan	32.8	27.5	38.1	37.1	32.7	31.6
Minnesota	35.7	29.4	41.5	31.2	37.5	36.0
Mississippi	33.9	43.3	39.1	20.8	35.5	32.3
Missouri	29.3	32.7	32.0	21.3	22.2	29.1
Montana	27.7	26.6	29.0	31.2	28.3	24.2
Nebraska	26.2	30.7	26.8	24.3	17.7	22.4
Nevada	25.5	17.0	25.5	15.4	34.6	26.3
New Hampshire	32.3	61.1	33.7	29.3	28.4	29.6
New Jersey	40.0	29.6	47.7	29.4	37.0	41.2
New Mexico	30.3	33.3	29.4	25.5	24.5	34.1
New York	40.7	47.7	50.7	30.5	29.1	41.9
North Carolina	39.1	33.9	42.2	38.6	42.5	34.3
North Dakota	28.3	31.5	22.6	28.7	34.6	31.9
Ohio	31.9	29.5	35.2	32.1	41.9	27.4
Oklahoma	36.1	36.3	42.7	44.0	30.7	34.3
Oregon	30.4	33.8	34.2	15.3	37.5	31.1
Pennsylvania	35.1	38.1	39.1	40.1	31.5	30.7
Rhode Island	41.8	48.0	40.3	40.6	36.9	36.4
South Carolina	40.1	42.8	42.8	27.8	42.4	40.9
South Dakota	31.2	32.2	29.5	26.1	29.6	32.5
Tennessee	35.6	32.3	40.3	40.6	30.7	35.8
Texas	33.6	39.0	36.0	38.5	32.3	31.8
Utah	34.3	48.5	31.1	41.1	33.5	28.9
Vermont	33.2	28.2	27.1	41.4	29.8	35.2
Virginia	31.4	32.6	36.0	31.2	34.0	27.0
Washington	26.4	32.4	26.2	31.9	24.2	24.8
West Virginia	32.9	29.5	31.9	29.9	39.2	26.2
Wisconsin	31.7	27.8	32.0	39.2	30.2	31.8
Wyoming	27.8	28.8	16.5	34.5	31.7	29.4

Source: Compiled by New Strategist based on the Centers for Disease Control and Prevention Behavioral Risk Factor Surveillance System Survey, Internet site http://www.cdc.gov/brfss/index.htm

1.33 Colorectal Cancer Screening: Last Colonoscopy Exam by Sex, 1999

"When did you have your last sigmoidoscopy or colonoscopy exam?"

(percent of people aged 18 or older responding "past year," by state and sex, 1999)

	total	men	women
U.S. total	**32.8%**	**35.5%**	**31.1%**
Alabama	29.3	35.1	24.7
Alaska	33.6	37.0	29.2
Arizona	43.3	44.8	42.1
Arkansas	29.3	36.1	23.8
California	31.7	34.8	28.5
Colorado	21.5	20.5	22.5
Connecticut	37.7	38.6	36.8
Delaware	36.0	39.3	32.9
District of Columbia	48.3	48.3	48.3
Florida	34.0	35.6	32.5
Georgia	31.0	32.4	29.6
Hawaii	25.2	24.5	26.0
Idaho	29.4	31.0	28.0
Illinois	34.0	36.5	31.9
Indiana	30.8	38.4	23.8
Iowa	27.5	28.7	26.7
Kansas	32.8	34.4	31.4
Kentucky	31.1	34.8	28.3
Louisiana	38.0	43.7	32.6
Maine	32.7	38.7	28.5
Maryland	34.6	34.7	34.5
Massachusetts	38.2	36.9	39.4
Michigan	32.8	34.7	30.8
Minnesota	35.7	36.2	35.2
Mississippi	33.9	32.5	35.1
Missouri	29.3	25.9	31.9
Montana	27.7	29.9	25.7
Nebraska	26.2	27.0	25.6
Nevada	25.5	27.5	23.8
New Hampshire	32.3	36.5	27.6
New Jersey	40.0	44.2	35.7
New Mexico	30.3	31.7	29.1
New York	40.7	40.4	41.0
North Carolina	39.1	39.9	38.6
North Dakota	28.3	26.1	30.7
Ohio	31.9	38.1	26.4
Oklahoma	36.1	36.4	35.8
Oregon	30.4	32.6	28.4
Pennsylvania	35.1	37.6	32.8
Rhode Island	41.8	43.6	40.2
South Carolina	40.1	43.8	37.0
South Dakota	31.2	35.1	28.2
Tennessee	35.6	35.5	35.7
Texas	33.6	35.7	31.6
Utah	34.3	34.1	34.6
Vermont	33.2	36.4	30.3
Virginia	31.4	31.5	31.4
Washington	26.4	28.9	24.0
West Virginia	32.9	33.8	32.1
Wisconsin	31.7	39.0	24.8
Wyoming	27.8	33.5	21.4

Source: Compiled by New Strategist based on the Centers for Disease Control and Prevention Behavioral Risk Factor Surveillance System Survey, Internet site http://www.cdc.gov/brfss/index.htm

1.34 Colorectal Cancer Screening: Use of Home Blood Stool Test Kit by Age, 1999

"Have you ever used a home blood stool test kit to determine whether your stool contained blood?"

(percent of people aged 18 or older responding "yes," by state and age, 1999)

	total	40 to 49	50 to 59	60 to 64	65 or older
U.S. total	**31.1%**	**13.8%**	**30.5%**	**40.5%**	**46.3%**
Alabama	26.7	12.4	22.6	35.2	40.6
Alaska	21.5	12.7	28.4	23.1	36.8
Arizona	45.7	26.0	43.5	56.9	64.7
Arkansas	30.0	14.2	28.8	33.1	44.6
California	26.0	11.7	27.2	35.8	41.0
Colorado	33.6	14.4	32.9	48.6	56.5
Connecticut	34.6	14.8	40.3	46.8	49.3
Delaware	33.5	20.3	31.9	39.9	48.9
District of Columbia	42.5	23.8	39.9	49.5	62.3
Florida	34.7	13.3	30.0	44.5	52.1
Georgia	30.2	20.9	30.6	36.1	40.5
Hawaii	32.0	15.1	33.2	43.7	47.6
Idaho	30.1	13.4	30.9	42.5	45.0
Illinois	27.6	11.6	24.4	50.8	39.8
Indiana	27.1	13.9	29.9	32.9	37.9
Iowa	39.5	19.2	38.2	48.9	56.8
Kansas	28.7	12.0	32.7	41.1	39.9
Kentucky	30.8	18.9	30.1	38.5	42.2
Louisiana	29.4	17.1	25.6	36.5	44.4
Maine	36.0	12.4	37.1	50.3	55.3
Maryland	40.0	21.8	43.6	59.7	54.5
Massachusetts	33.1	12.6	38.5	43.0	48.4
Michigan	39.0	17.2	42.6	51.6	56.3
Minnesota	32.8	14.9	32.0	42.5	50.3
Mississippi	21.5	10.4	17.6	32.6	33.7
Missouri	30.2	11.8	29.9	39.6	45.8
Montana	30.8	12.1	29.6	56.1	45.5
Nebraska	31.2	12.9	33.5	34.2	47.9
Nevada	25.5	8.7	27.7	35.1	41.8
New Hampshire	34.7	14.3	43.9	41.2	55.4
New Jersey	33.6	11.8	35.3	49.7	50.7
New Mexico	29.1	13.7	29.3	36.0	46.4
New York	31.0	15.4	29.2	39.2	47.1
North Carolina	44.3	28.5	43.6	55.3	59.5
North Dakota	29.9	12.4	28.5	35.6	46.6
Ohio	32.8	14.7	34.4	46.9	45.7
Oklahoma	28.1	13.0	26.6	35.7	41.7
Oregon	40.4	17.5	41.0	55.3	61.0
Pennsylvania	32.5	13.8	30.0	42.4	48.3
Rhode Island	31.1	14.1	30.5	38.6	46.0
South Carolina	31.7	16.2	34.1	36.7	46.3
South Dakota	32.3	12.6	33.9	33.6	49.6
Tennessee	27.2	13.4	24.8	37.8	41.0
Texas	26.9	13.1	24.8	33.8	43.9
Utah	25.7	11.6	27.5	34.7	41.2
Vermont	36.6	16.3	41.1	51.4	54.9
Virginia	31.6	21.0	34.8	46.0	40.5
Washington	41.3	19.0	40.9	62.4	61.9
West Virginia	24.9	11.0	24.2	37.0	34.4
Wisconsin	31.6	14.4	29.2	50.3	46.3
Wyoming	23.7	12.6	26.0	30.7	35.4

Source: Compiled by New Strategist based on the Centers for Disease Control and Prevention Behavioral Risk Factor Surveillance System Survey, Internet site http://www.cdc.gov/brfss/index.htm

1.35 Colorectal Cancer Screening: Use of Home Blood Stool Test Kit by Education, 1999

"Have you ever used a home blood stool test kit to determine
whether your stool contained blood?"

(percent of people aged 18 or older responding "yes," by state and educational attainment, 1999)

	total	less than high school	high school graduate	some college	college graduate
U.S. total	**31.1%**	**29.2%**	**30.2%**	**32.3%**	**34.0%**
Alabama	26.7	19.7	28.4	28.7	30.5
Alaska	21.5	18.5	19.8	28.3	17.5
Arizona	45.7	12.5	48.2	49.2	51.6
Arkansas	30.0	24.6	27.1	32.3	36.4
California	26.0	13.1	24.8	31.6	29.4
Colorado	33.6	29.3	32.2	31.0	37.8
Connecticut	34.6	43.2	33.8	30.7	35.2
Delaware	33.5	32.0	28.7	36.5	37.0
District of Columbia	42.5	38.1	38.4	47.9	45.2
Florida	34.7	26.9	34.8	32.6	40.4
Georgia	30.2	26.1	25.4	35.0	34.3
Hawaii	32.0	37.1	30.6	31.0	32.8
Idaho	30.1	30.1	28.7	27.8	34.2
Illinois	27.6	24.8	29.3	25.3	28.8
Indiana	27.1	15.7	28.9	33.3	25.4
Iowa	39.5	39.9	40.4	37.4	39.8
Kansas	28.7	21.7	26.8	32.5	30.5
Kentucky	30.8	30.5	28.7	32.7	33.1
Louisiana	29.4	27.4	26.9	36.9	27.6
Maine	36.0	34.1	35.9	34.8	37.9
Maryland	40.0	35.3	36.7	45.5	41.8
Massachusetts	33.1	28.0	33.8	32.3	34.4
Michigan	39.0	37.9	33.1	43.5	43.2
Minnesota	32.8	38.6	31.5	32.3	32.9
Mississippi	21.5	18.9	20.2	23.8	24.2
Missouri	30.2	32.1	26.2	28.7	36.6
Montana	30.8	34.5	30.6	28.4	31.8
Nebraska	31.2	31.8	30.0	32.5	31.8
Nevada	25.5	22.2	23.4	24.9	30.5
New Hampshire	34.7	29.1	32.4	35.9	37.4
New Jersey	33.6	29.1	32.1	34.0	36.8
New Mexico	29.1	21.0	27.5	27.3	36.3
New York	31.0	28.2	30.3	35.3	29.8
North Carolina	44.3	40.0	42.8	44.3	50.8
North Dakota	29.9	30.6	30.2	26.5	33.3
Ohio	32.8	30.3	30.8	34.8	37.5
Oklahoma	28.1	25.7	27.6	28.9	29.9
Oregon	40.4	33.9	39.2	41.4	42.5
Pennsylvania	32.5	34.9	33.8	29.5	31.6
Rhode Island	31.1	29.3	32.1	28.9	32.4
South Carolina	31.7	26.2	30.3	33.9	36.7
South Dakota	32.3	33.8	31.0	31.8	34.3
Tennessee	27.2	28.0	23.5	31.2	27.4
Texas	26.9	16.9	25.4	27.0	33.9
Utah	25.7	23.7	20.6	25.5	31.1
Vermont	36.6	40.4	34.1	36.9	37.8
Virginia	31.6	32.0	26.8	27.7	39.0
Washington	41.3	34.6	42.9	39.5	43.3
West Virginia	24.9	23.2	23.4	26.6	29.5
Wisconsin	31.6	33.1	31.3	32.7	30.8
Wyoming	23.7	24.1	21.0	22.4	28.5

Source: Compiled by New Strategist based on the Centers for Disease Control and Prevention Behavioral Risk Factor Surveillance System Survey, Internet site http://www.cdc.gov/brfss/index.htm

1.36 Colorectal Cancer Screening: Use of Home Blood Stool Test Kit by Household Income, 1999

"Have you ever used a home blood stool test kit to determine whether your stool contained blood?"

(percent of people aged 18 or older responding "yes," by state and household income, 1999)

	total	less than $15,000	$15,000 to $24,999	$25,000 to $34,999	$35,000 to $49,999	$50,000 or more
U.S. total	**31.1%**	**31.5%**	**32.7%**	**30.6%**	**28.0%**	**30.2%**
Alabama	26.7	22.6	25.5	27.7	23.0	27.4
Alaska	21.5	18.5	16.1	29.5	29.5	19.7
Arizona	45.7	41.6	42.0	48.7	62.6	54.6
Arkansas	30.0	28.9	26.1	31.9	28.3	31.5
California	26.0	17.5	25.2	31.2	25.2	28.1
Colorado	33.6	27.3	33.7	37.9	29.9	31.2
Connecticut	34.6	39.6	32.5	35.7	28.6	32.8
Delaware	33.5	44.8	31.6	36.3	29.2	31.1
District of Columbia	42.5	44.4	35.0	46.9	41.8	49.8
Florida	34.7	28.9	33.1	35.1	35.7	34.7
Georgia	30.2	21.2	25.8	32.7	19.9	32.9
Hawaii	32.0	31.5	40.1	34.9	29.3	28.7
Idaho	30.1	28.5	37.5	29.0	25.6	29.2
Illinois	27.6	30.7	33.6	25.6	27.4	22.8
Indiana	27.1	25.2	26.9	27.3	19.4	27.7
Iowa	39.5	42.8	44.2	39.4	36.6	36.5
Kansas	28.7	25.6	29.0	27.8	27.5	27.1
Kentucky	30.8	30.1	31.7	30.3	27.8	31.0
Louisiana	29.4	31.5	30.9	26.2	29.5	25.1
Maine	36.0	45.0	36.4	33.0	32.9	27.5
Maryland	40.0	35.4	38.4	40.1	35.1	41.9
Massachusetts	33.1	35.4	33.0	38.5	26.2	28.8
Michigan	39.0	34.3	43.6	48.1	31.9	36.9
Minnesota	32.8	45.8	39.6	35.4	25.9	28.4
Mississippi	21.5	17.6	20.8	20.0	16.8	24.9
Missouri	30.2	29.5	30.4	21.6	29.4	28.1
Montana	30.8	36.1	30.7	27.3	29.8	26.5
Nebraska	31.2	33.8	34.7	31.6	27.0	27.6
Nevada	25.5	34.2	32.2	20.3	20.2	21.7
New Hampshire	34.7	35.5	31.4	40.9	35.8	30.6
New Jersey	33.6	32.6	36.6	26.6	24.6	35.0
New Mexico	29.1	24.2	24.8	26.4	27.7	34.5
New York	31.0	35.0	34.1	31.9	26.0	31.8
North Carolina	44.3	38.2	49.5	40.4	35.5	45.4
North Dakota	29.9	35.4	28.9	28.8	23.1	31.1
Ohio	32.8	32.7	35.9	28.4	29.3	33.0
Oklahoma	28.1	26.7	33.3	29.3	24.9	31.0
Oregon	40.4	35.1	37.3	42.4	36.0	43.0
Pennsylvania	32.5	32.5	35.3	39.6	33.3	25.7
Rhode Island	31.1	39.1	36.5	27.0	29.5	28.4
South Carolina	31.7	30.0	28.8	29.9	24.9	31.8
South Dakota	32.3	31.2	36.6	33.0	26.5	31.7
Tennessee	27.2	26.8	28.5	25.3	23.5	27.3
Texas	26.9	18.2	25.7	26.3	29.1	27.9
Utah	25.7	25.9	25.6	17.1	30.8	23.6
Vermont	36.6	42.3	37.9	31.0	32.3	36.8
Virginia	31.6	27.5	25.5	26.2	24.9	37.0
Washington	41.3	35.1	45.0	44.4	39.1	36.6
West Virginia	24.9	20.8	25.1	26.7	22.0	25.7
Wisconsin	31.6	39.1	36.1	34.1	25.3	29.8
Wyoming	23.7	20.2	23.2	22.9	17.5	28.0

Source: Compiled by New Strategist based on the Centers for Disease Control and Prevention Behavioral Risk Factor Surveillance System Survey, Internet site http://www.cdc.gov/brfss/index.htm

1.37 Colorectal Cancer Screening: Use of Home Blood Stool Test Kit by Sex, 1999

"Have you ever used a home blood stool test kit to determine
whether your stool contained blood?"

(percent of people aged 18 or older responding "yes," by state and sex, 1999)

	total	men	women
U.S. total	31.1%	26.6%	35.2%
Alabama	26.7	22.0	30.6
Alaska	21.5	18.0	25.2
Arizona	45.7	44.3	47.0
Arkansas	30.0	24.5	34.7
California	26.0	23.1	28.5
Colorado	33.6	27.9	38.8
Connecticut	34.6	29.2	39.2
Delaware	33.5	30.4	36.1
District of Columbia	42.5	42.0	42.9
Florida	34.7	31.1	37.8
Georgia	30.2	25.0	34.4
Hawaii	32.0	30.6	33.4
Idaho	30.1	23.6	36.0
Illinois	27.6	20.7	34.1
Indiana	27.1	24.0	29.7
Iowa	39.5	31.6	46.0
Kansas	28.7	28.7	71.3
Kentucky	30.8	30.8	69.2
Louisiana	29.4	25.4	32.9
Maine	36.0	25.0	45.3
Maryland	40.0	35.9	43.6
Massachusetts	33.1	29.7	36.1
Michigan	39.0	37.0	40.6
Minnesota	32.8	28.3	36.8
Mississippi	21.5	16.8	25.4
Missouri	30.2	26.5	33.3
Montana	30.8	25.9	35.4
Nebraska	31.2	26.2	35.6
Nevada	25.5	22.7	28.1
New Hampshire	34.7	33.0	36.3
New Jersey	33.6	29.3	37.3
New Mexico	29.1	26.7	31.2
New York	31.0	28.6	33.0
North Carolina	44.3	40.6	47.6
North Dakota	29.9	24.7	34.7
Ohio	32.8	27.6	37.3
Oklahoma	28.1	26.3	29.5
Oregon	40.4	32.5	47.5
Pennsylvania	32.5	28.0	36.1
Rhode Island	31.1	26.4	35.1
South Carolina	31.7	25.9	36.7
South Dakota	32.3	28.0	36.2
Tennessee	27.2	22.7	31.0
Texas	26.9	24.1	29.4
Utah	25.7	24.5	26.8
Vermont	36.6	30.5	42.2
Virginia	31.6	30.5	32.5
Washington	41.3	36.0	46.0
West Virginia	24.9	22.0	27.3
Wisconsin	31.6	27.5	35.3
Wyoming	23.7	22.0	25.2

Source: Compiled by New Strategist based on the Centers for Disease Control and Prevention Behavioral Risk Factor Surveillance System Survey, Internet site http://www.cdc.gov/brfss/index.htm

1.38 Dental Visit in Past Year by Age, 1999

"Have you visited the dentist or dental clinic within the past year?"

(percent of people aged 18 or older responding "yes," by state and age, 1999)

	total	18 to 24	25 to 34	35 to 44	45 to 54	55 to 64	65 or older
U.S. total	**68.1%**	**72.6%**	**66.2%**	**70.4%**	**73.1%**	**67.5%**	**62.3%**
West Virginia	56.4	58.7	64.9	68.0	63.0	59.8	48.5
Nevada	56.8	71.9	66.8	69.0	76.0	72.2	64.2
Arkansas	58.9	56.0	62.8	67.6	71.4	71.1	66.6
Mississippi	58.9	59.8	59.7	62.4	61.6	52.4	56.2
Oklahoma	59.1	66.3	61.3	65.2	75.5	66.3	69.0
Texas	59.7	68.1	62.3	70.4	70.5	71.7	63.8
Louisiana	60.6	78.7	74.0	78.5	81.7	85.5	73.1
Missouri	60.6	72.6	71.1	69.7	79.9	66.2	67.7
Alabama	60.7	78.2	76.3	74.4	72.6	73.6	64.7
New Mexico	62.5	68.6	59.9	68.7	69.1	67.7	68.9
Kentucky	63.0	72.6	67.3	66.2	73.1	60.9	55.0
Wyoming	63.5	75.5	65.0	75.9	78.0	80.0	75.3
Montana	63.6	67.3	60.6	69.2	70.3	66.4	56.7
Idaho	65.0	75.1	69.9	73.0	76.6	70.5	62.6
Arizona	66.0	70.4	65.1	69.5	79.5	62.8	53.8
North Dakota	66.2	75.8	65.2	76.7	74.1	69.0	63.5
South Dakota	66.2	74.2	68.9	70.5	72.1	64.2	60.3
Georgia	66.3	73.2	66.2	69.8	65.6	55.7	46.9
California	67.0	63.6	64.4	63.0	65.4	54.0	50.4
Indiana	67.0	78.4	63.1	74.6	73.4	63.8	54.9
Oregon	67.0	76.7	71.1	74.8	75.6	69.8	64.5
Florida	67.1	79.7	74.5	79.3	81.2	77.8	66.3
Washington	67.1	81.3	71.4	80.2	83.9	74.2	71.8
North Carolina	67.2	72.8	72.0	75.4	77.4	69.0	68.0
Colorado	67.8	67.3	58.2	61.8	59.1	57.8	49.3
Maine	67.9	60.1	59.3	68.1	66.0	58.8	49.9
Kansas	68.3	67.9	57.8	62.8	69.3	65.6	60.5
Ohio	68.9	76.5	69.7	75.1	78.7	73.3	63.8
Tennessee	69.3	53.1	50.0	57.7	58.9	64.1	57.9
South Carolina	69.6	73.8	70.0	76.2	78.9	69.6	64.1
New York	70.1	72.5	66.3	74.1	77.2	72.6	70.4
Alaska	70.2	60.0	58.2	63.6	66.3	67.9	60.3
Iowa	70.5	68.2	66.9	70.5	74.6	73.2	67.6
Illinois	71.0	70.5	64.5	73.7	66.1	67.2	59.9
Delaware	71.3	73.6	72.7	70.0	73.2	56.8	50.3
Pennsylvania	71.3	75.5	73.1	68.2	74.6	67.2	57.1
Virginia	71.9	61.2	62.0	64.7	62.5	53.9	48.8
Maryland	72.3	59.6	58.4	71.2	74.0	68.9	66.2
New Jersey	72.3	75.1	72.6	76.2	78.4	68.4	58.9
New Hampshire	72.4	75.0	73.4	81.1	81.9	74.8	64.5
Nebraska	72.5	78.1	72.4	69.7	71.3	60.7	63.4
Vermont	72.5	67.9	62.3	71.9	72.1	67.6	57.7
Minnesota	72.7	73.9	72.9	73.1	72.2	59.3	61.8
Utah	73.0	55.9	55.9	60.0	64.2	60.8	62.0
District of Columbia	73.1	72.8	73.4	76.1	77.8	69.2	65.0
Wisconsin	74.5	76.7	72.1	76.8	76.1	65.6	64.4
Hawaii	74.7	65.7	71.1	77.8	75.2	71.2	61.4
Rhode Island	75.0	65.9	64.9	67.4	71.7	70.3	62.7
Massachusetts	76.2	72.7	58.5	65.3	59.9	43.0	42.5
Michigan	77.2	73.1	71.5	78.6	77.3	77.2	69.2
Connecticut	78.2	66.2	54.4	64.6	69.2	65.4	62.1

Source: Compiled by New Strategist based on the Centers for Disease Control and Prevention Behavioral Risk Factor Surveillance System Survey, Internet site http://www.cdc.gov/brfss/index.htm

1.39 Dental Visit in Past Year by Education, 1999

"Have you visited the dentist or dental clinic within the past year?"

(percent of people aged 18 or older responding "yes," by state and educational attainment, 1999)

	total	less than high school	high school graduate	some college	college graduate
U.S. total	**68.1%**	**44.3%**	**64.3%**	**71.9%**	**80.4%**
Alabama	60.7	35.0	61.7	67.7	75.1
Alaska	70.2	54.1	65.6	70.6	81.1
Arizona	66.0	40.9	61.7	69.8	80.4
Arkansas	58.9	36.8	55.7	62.2	76.9
California	67.0	48.4	64.0	71.4	78.5
Colorado	67.8	44.8	60.4	71.6	78.0
Connecticut	78.2	60.7	73.0	78.8	87.3
Delaware	71.3	38.9	62.4	77.2	86.1
District of Columbia	73.1	54.1	70.3	72.7	80.4
Florida	67.1	48.2	62.6	69.5	78.5
Georgia	66.3	40.1	61.7	71.7	80.6
Hawaii	74.7	49.5	71.0	76.9	81.7
Idaho	65.0	43.1	60.2	67.1	78.2
Illinois	71.0	51.8	64.7	73.4	83.5
Indiana	67.0	43.8	64.9	66.0	82.4
Iowa	70.5	45.6	69.2	71.8	80.9
Kansas	68.3	42.2	62.3	74.3	78.8
Kentucky	63.0	36.9	61.8	73.1	81.7
Louisiana	60.6	42.2	62.3	74.3	78.8
Maine	67.9	36.9	61.8	73.1	81.7
Maryland	72.3	37.3	54.1	70.9	77.5
Massachusetts	76.2	37.7	61.7	73.2	83.7
Michigan	77.2	42.2	67.1	76.4	82.8
Minnesota	72.7	54.7	72.2	78.9	82.5
Mississippi	58.9	54.0	73.3	79.8	87.5
Missouri	60.6	57.9	68.3	74.3	79.7
Montana	63.6	34.0	59.7	63.1	75.0
Nebraska	72.5	37.1	58.0	62.2	77.2
Nevada	56.8	54.7	59.7	62.3	73.3
New Hampshire	72.4	56.7	70.0	74.5	79.4
New Jersey	72.3	30.9	52.5	59.4	73.3
New Mexico	62.5	44.6	66.0	76.5	81.0
New York	70.1	49.8	69.7	76.9	79.8
North Carolina	67.2	40.7	57.3	67.8	75.8
North Dakota	66.2	54.5	65.5	71.3	81.5
Ohio	68.9	44.4	64.6	70.7	81.8
Oklahoma	59.1	33.3	54.6	61.2	80.1
Oregon	67.0	38.0	62.3	68.8	80.4
Pennsylvania	71.3	43.2	68.8	75.5	83.3
Rhode Island	75.0	52.1	70.4	78.1	86.7
South Carolina	69.6	44.4	67.7	75.0	82.7
South Dakota	66.2	45.7	60.8	71.0	75.1
Tennessee	69.3	43.0	67.6	74.9	83.5
Texas	59.7	37.3	58.4	61.2	75.5
Utah	73.0	60.5	67.2	73.6	81.3
Vermont	72.5	41.9	67.3	75.8	86.2
Virginia	71.9	44.2	66.8	76.2	81.4
Washington	67.1	48.4	59.7	66.8	79.4
West Virginia	56.4	29.4	54.5	67.4	79.4
Wisconsin	74.5	57.9	72.0	75.0	82.8
Wyoming	63.5	38.2	59.0	66.3	73.2

Source: Compiled by New Strategist based on the Centers for Disease Control and Prevention Behavioral Risk Factor Surveillance System Survey. Internet site http://www.cdc.gov/brfss/index.htm

1.40 Dental Visit in Past Year by Household Income, 1999

"Have you visited the dentist or dental clinic within the past year?"

(percent of people aged 18 or older responding "yes," by state and household income, 1999)

	total	less than $15,000	$15,000 to $24,999	$25,000 to $34,999	$35,000 to $49,999	$50,000 or more
U.S. total	**68.1%**	**49.1%**	**55.9%**	**66.3%**	**72.0%**	**82.3%**
Alabama	60.7	33.9	55.9	58.5	71.7	78.4
Alaska	70.2	42.0	60.4	68.5	72.3	81.9
Arizona	66.0	43.6	49.9	64.5	81.6	84.0
Arkansas	58.9	37.6	49.9	59.4	64.6	74.5
California	67.0	49.6	56.5	67.0	71.9	79.6
Colorado	67.8	47.0	51.8	66.8	71.1	79.1
Connecticut	78.2	57.0	69.5	67.9	79.8	85.6
Delaware	71.3	52.5	50.6	62.8	71.4	85.4
District of Columbia	73.1	65.7	65.5	70.5	73.6	88.3
Florida	67.1	48.2	55.9	66.1	69.5	81.3
Georgia	66.3	36.2	56.1	59.0	68.1	82.7
Hawaii	74.7	56.8	65.7	74.4	70.8	84.6
Idaho	65.0	48.0	54.1	66.0	68.7	81.4
Illinois	71.0	52.2	55.7	72.5	72.7	81.6
Indiana	67.0	44.3	51.3	60.2	79.7	80.4
Iowa	70.5	50.3	60.7	67.4	73.8	82.9
Kansas	68.3	50.0	59.6	61.7	75.0	82.1
Kentucky	63.0	37.1	52.5	66.1	71.3	81.8
Louisiana	60.6	35.4	52.1	60.1	71.9	79.1
Maine	67.9	47.3	55.5	65.4	76.4	82.9
Maryland	72.3	49.1	54.6	68.2	75.2	83.2
Massachusetts	76.2	57.8	64.3	70.0	80.0	83.8
Michigan	77.2	53.3	65.6	76.6	79.4	88.3
Minnesota	72.7	51.0	60.7	68.5	73.9	81.4
Mississippi	58.9	41.6	47.9	58.3	69.6	78.3
Missouri	60.6	38.8	49.6	59.4	66.6	78.3
Montana	63.6	51.3	55.8	57.9	66.4	79.5
Nebraska	72.5	60.4	66.0	69.3	74.6	82.6
Nevada	56.8	42.6	42.9	50.2	48.2	73.8
New Hampshire	72.4	61.5	54.2	65.9	70.1	88.2
New Jersey	72.3	53.7	68.6	67.1	73.0	80.9
New Mexico	62.5	43.0	50.6	63.8	69.7	80.8
New York	70.1	53.5	55.9	71.5	71.4	82.5
North Carolina	67.2	49.1	48.9	66.3	76.4	85.1
North Dakota	66.2	45.0	58.8	66.3	69.6	80.6
Ohio	68.9	47.0	58.4	68.6	70.2	83.5
Oklahoma	59.1	40.9	49.3	59.6	71.3	82.7
Oregon	67.0	43.0	52.1	67.8	71.5	82.6
Pennsylvania	71.3	49.5	56.5	69.9	75.4	87.2
Rhode Island	75.0	58.5	63.4	72.1	75.9	89.2
South Carolina	69.6	53.6	60.1	67.6	77.5	82.8
South Dakota	66.2	52.3	56.0	63.2	71.6	79.7
Tennessee	69.3	47.0	58.2	70.9	74.2	84.8
Texas	59.7	34.5	48.5	62.0	65.1	76.3
Utah	73.0	58.0	63.4	69.2	78.1	80.8
Vermont	72.5	56.8	57.3	63.8	78.6	90.6
Virginia	71.9	52.7	50.0	69.0	75.4	82.8
Washington	67.1	44.3	54.4	58.5	69.3	80.4
West Virginia	56.4	30.0	44.8	57.2	72.2	83.3
Wisconsin	74.5	52.2	64.8	74.5	79.2	82.7
Wyoming	63.5	42.7	54.1	65.0	65.9	77.7

Source: Compiled by New Strategist based on the Centers for Disease Control and Prevention Behavioral Risk Factor Surveillance System Survey. Internet site http://www.cdc.gov/brfss/index.htm

1.41 Dental Visit in Past Year by Sex, 1999

"Have you visited the dentist or dental clinic within the past year?"

(percent of people aged 18 or older responding "yes," by state and sex, 1999)

	total	men	women
U.S. total	**68.1%**	**65.5%**	**70.5%**
Alabama	60.7	59.2	62.1
Alaska	70.2	67.8	72.8
Arizona	66.0	64.1	67.8
Arkansas	58.9	57.9	59.7
California	67.0	64.2	69.9
Colorado	67.8	63.8	71.7
Connecticut	78.2	74.4	81.6
Delaware	71.3	68.1	74.2
District of Columbia	73.1	70.6	75.2
Florida	67.1	64.7	69.3
Georgia	66.3	65.6	67.0
Hawaii	74.7	74.0	75.4
Idaho	65.0	62.3	67.5
Illinois	71.0	69.2	72.7
Indiana	67.0	66.0	68.0
Iowa	70.5	67.3	73.4
Kansas	68.3	64.7	71.7
Kentucky	63.0	62.0	63.8
Louisiana	60.6	58.7	62.2
Maine	67.9	65.4	70.2
Maryland	72.3	68.4	75.8
Massachusetts	76.2	73.2	78.9
Michigan	77.2	73.9	80.3
Minnesota	72.7	70.1	75.2
Mississippi	58.9	56.4	61.0
Missouri	60.6	55.6	65.2
Montana	63.6	60.4	66.7
Nebraska	72.5	69.0	75.8
Nevada	56.8	52.1	61.5
New Hampshire	72.4	69.6	75.0
New Jersey	72.3	71.1	73.4
New Mexico	62.5	60.1	64.7
New York	70.1	68.1	71.9
North Carolina	67.2	65.2	69.0
North Dakota	66.2	61.5	70.8
Ohio	68.9	69.8	68.1
Oklahoma	59.1	58.9	59.2
Oregon	67.0	65.2	68.6
Pennsylvania	71.3	71.1	71.4
Rhode Island	75.0	74.3	75.7
South Carolina	69.6	66.7	72.3
South Dakota	66.2	62.9	69.3
Tennessee	69.3	68.4	70.1
Texas	59.7	57.4	61.9
Utah	73.0	70.4	75.6
Vermont	72.5	70.8	74.1
Virginia	71.9	69.6	74.1
Washington	67.1	65.1	69.0
West Virginia	56.4	55.3	57.4
Wisconsin	74.5	73.1	75.8
Wyoming	63.5	61.7	65.2

Source: Compiled by New Strategist based on the Centers for Disease Control and Prevention Behavioral Risk Factor Surveillance System Survey, Internet site http://www.cdc.gov/brfss/index.htm

1.42 Dental: Teeth Cleaned in Past Year by Age, 1999

"Have you had your teeth cleaned by the dentist or dental hygienist within the past year?"

(percent of people aged 18 or older responding "yes," by state and age, 1999)

	total	18 to 24	25 to 34	35 to 44	45 to 54	55 to 64	65 or older
U.S. total	**71.5%**	**71.0%**	**65.6%**	**69.1%**	**73.5%**	**72.6%**	**73.1%**
Nevada	55.9	59.8	59.2	63.2	62.3	63.8	61.5
Texas	60.3	62.8	61.9	63.4	74.4	66.8	68.9
Arkansas	60.4	61.9	65.7	68.3	68.4	67.8	75.2
Mississippi	60.6	59.1	54.1	60.6	59.4	61.4	69.1
New Mexico	61.2	62.9	60.3	63.1	73.5	69.3	77.2
Alabama	61.5	67.2	60.1	66.4	69.7	72.0	72.3
Montana	61.7	79.1	74.0	78.8	84.0	86.2	84.6
West Virginia	62.5	73.4	69.1	71.9	81.0	71.5	78.8
Missouri	62.6	81.3	77.4	77.3	72.6	72.8	74.5
Wyoming	62.9	71.1	59.3	68.9	69.8	73.3	77.6
Oklahoma	63.8	70.8	63.5	63.9	73.0	70.0	68.0
Idaho	64.3	72.1	66.5	73.0	74.4	82.2	79.6
Louisiana	64.8	64.2	57.0	65.5	67.7	69.4	64.7
Alaska	65.7	73.5	68.8	72.1	76.8	75.6	67.2
California	66.8	67.9	64.8	67.0	80.2	69.3	69.6
South Dakota	67.0	74.2	61.5	74.6	76.0	73.6	74.5
Oregon	67.2	74.7	68.4	68.8	72.3	72.4	71.3
Colorado	67.3	73.9	63.2	68.9	67.2	72.4	67.6
Georgia	67.6	66.3	61.9	63.3	68.9	58.3	70.4
Arizona	68.0	72.0	63.9	74.6	74.4	75.9	76.3
Kentucky	68.3	75.9	69.8	72.8	74.7	73.8	76.1
North Carolina	68.8	78.9	75.8	80.0	82.5	84.4	79.4
North Dakota	69.3	83.9	70.9	80.0	83.6	74.6	83.1
Florida	69.8	71.0	72.4	75.4	76.0	76.2	78.8
Indiana	69.9	67.7	55.7	59.6	62.8	59.6	59.7
Kansas	70.9	60.0	55.7	65.2	65.4	61.3	67.5
Illinois	72.1	59.5	55.5	59.7	64.5	65.5	68.3
New Jersey	72.1	75.6	70.1	72.5	78.1	79.7	77.8
Tennessee	72.1	41.8	45.8	53.9	65.2	69.1	61.4
Utah	72.1	74.3	69.7	75.3	79.5	74.9	79.6
Iowa	72.3	72.7	65.6	70.8	75.8	74.5	74.9
Maine	72.5	54.7	55.6	60.1	62.1	68.4	71.7
New York	72.7	69.1	67.4	72.9	75.6	76.5	76.2
South Carolina	72.9	67.1	64.4	71.4	66.5	76.5	69.1
Ohio	73.0	71.5	70.1	67.5	71.4	62.6	70.6
Maryland	73.5	75.2	75.0	68.7	74.7	77.4	70.0
Virginia	73.8	64.5	62.2	60.7	66.0	66.9	64.4
Washington	74.0	56.4	57.2	67.4	74.4	75.4	72.7
Delaware	74.2	73.2	71.1	77.4	78.2	78.2	77.6
Hawaii	74.3	74.6	73.3	82.3	82.7	83.3	76.9
Wisconsin	74.8	79.5	70.3	68.4	72.0	71.8	79.3
Minnesota	74.9	64.7	62.4	70.0	69.3	68.4	67.6
Nebraska	75.1	75.5	70.0	69.3	75.9	67.9	74.6
New Hampshire	75.2	57.9	53.9	58.7	63.6	65.0	67.3
Pennsylvania	76.0	71.7	68.0	73.4	74.2	72.8	73.6
District of Columbia	76.1	76.1	70.9	77.1	80.2	77.1	80.0
Vermont	76.8	65.0	71.5	77.7	73.5	75.2	76.2
Rhode Island	78.9	69.9	67.4	74.0	76.7	78.9	78.6
Michigan	79.2	68.9	57.4	62.8	64.2	59.7	61.9
Massachusetts	79.9	71.4	70.7	78.0	76.6	76.2	74.7
Connecticut	80.7	61.6	52.3	60.8	67.0	73.5	69.3

Source: Compiled by New Strategist based on the Centers for Disease Control and Prevention Behavioral Risk Factor Surveillance System Survey, Internet site http://www.cdc.gov/brfss/index.htm

1.43 Dental: Teeth Cleaned in Past Year by Education, 1999

"Have you had your teeth cleaned by the dentist or dental hygienist within the past year?"

(percent of people aged 18 or older responding "yes," by state and educational attainment, 1999)

	total	less than high school	high school graduate	some college	college graduate
U.S. total	71.5	51.3	67.0	72.4	80.1
Alabama	61.5	36.7	59.9	68.1	73.5
Alaska	65.7	52.9	57.4	66.6	79.2
Arizona	68.0	49.7	63.2	69.1	83.2
Arkansas	60.4	37.5	56.8	62.7	75.2
California	66.8	51.3	62.7	69.5	77.4
Colorado	67.3	42.2	60.3	68.4	78.7
Connecticut	80.7	68.2	76.7	80.8	86.8
Delaware	74.2	44.5	68.1	77.8	84.5
District of Columbia	76.1	60.2	69.4	78.1	82.8
Florida	69.8	51.3	66.3	70.5	79.5
Georgia	67.6	39.9	63.3	72.7	78.4
Hawaii	74.3	58.5	69.0	76.3	80.1
Idaho	64.3	42.6	59.7	65.1	77.2
Illinois	72.1	54.5	66.5	72.0	82.9
Indiana	69.9	49.0	68.8	66.1	82.0
Iowa	72.3	54.8	72.1	71.3	78.7
Kansas	70.9	49.5	65.5	74.4	79.6
Kentucky	68.3	45.7	64.6	74.8	82.2
Louisiana	64.8	42.8	55.6	76.2	79.0
Maine	72.5	41.4	68.3	74.5	84.4
Maryland	73.5	52.0	67.7	74.4	82.6
Massachusetts	79.9	63.5	75.8	83.4	83.5
Michigan	79.2	55.6	77.4	81.2	86.1
Minnesota	74.9	64.0	72.1	74.8	80.1
Mississippi	60.6	36.5	61.3	61.3	74.5
Missouri	62.6	40.8	59.7	61.7	77.1
Montana	61.7	54.7	56.6	61.0	70.3
Nebraska	75.1	62.9	72.5	75.0	81.8
Nevada	55.9	27.8	51.7	56.4	74.6
New Hampshire	75.2	59.8	68.9	78.4	80.4
New Jersey	72.1	51.7	69.9	73.6	79.8
New Mexico	61.2	40.0	55.2	65.0	73.7
New York	72.7	60.3	69.7	71.1	81.9
North Carolina	68.8	46.8	64.8	72.2	81.0
North Dakota	69.3	53.2	63.5	73.2	76.5
Ohio	73.0	56.6	68.9	73.9	87.2
Oklahoma	63.8	39.9	59.9	62.6	81.4
Oregon	67.2	46.7	60.3	68.2	79.0
Pennsylvania	76.0	55.3	72.4	78.9	85.2
Rhode Island	78.9	63.8	74.8	79.3	87.1
South Carolina	72.9	53.4	68.9	75.5	84.1
South Dakota	67.0	50.3	62.3	70.4	72.9
Tennessee	72.1	46.2	71.6	74.5	84.4
Texas	60.3	37.2	57.1	62.1	75.1
Utah	72.1	65.0	67.5	72.1	77.9
Vermont	76.8	61.0	70.6	77.6	86.6
Virginia	73.8	49.6	68.4	76.3	82.2
Washington	74.0	54.1	68.7	71.6	84.4
West Virginia	62.5	38.1	57.9	70.9	78.6
Wisconsin	74.8	63.7	72.0	74.7	81.5
Wyoming	62.9	35.9	58.9	65.1	71.5

Source: Compiled by New Strategist based on the Centers for Disease Control and Prevention Behavioral Risk Factor Surveillance System Survey, Internet site http://www.cdc.gov/brfss/index.htm

1.44 Dental: Teeth Cleaned in Past Year by Household Income, 1999

"Have you had your teeth cleaned by the dentist or dental hygienist within the past year?"

(percent of people aged 18 or older responding "yes," by state and household income, 1999)

	total	less than $15,000	$15,000 to $24,999	$25,000 to $34,999	$35,000 to $49,999	$50,000 or more
U.S. total	**71.5%**	**51.8%**	**58.6%**	**67.0%**	**72.6%**	**82.2%**
Alabama	61.5	31.4	51.5	60.3	72.6	78.7
Alaska	65.7	37.6	59.1	61.7	62.1	77.9
Arizona	68.0	42.1	51.8	68.3	77.8	86.3
Arkansas	60.4	36.9	46.7	59.7	65.9	76.9
California	66.8	50.1	55.8	66.7	70.6	77.8
Colorado	67.3	49.2	50.0	61.1	70.6	78.6
Connecticut	80.7	61.0	72.1	73.1	79.6	86.0
Delaware	74.2	49.9	55.2	65.5	77.6	85.1
District of Columbia	76.1	56.5	67.4	72.9	76.1	90.3
Florida	69.8	52.7	57.4	66.9	72.0	82.2
Georgia	67.6	33.8	62.5	59.6	66.3	81.4
Hawaii	74.3	56.8	68.2	69.0	71.5	84.5
Idaho	64.3	46.9	51.5	63.9	67.3	80.4
Illinois	72.1	48.0	54.9	77.5	71.0	81.9
Indiana	69.9	45.0	56.1	64.0	78.9	80.6
Iowa	72.3	58.2	62.2	67.2	72.7	83.2
Kansas	70.9	54.2	60.4	63.3	75.5	82.6
Kentucky	68.3	44.8	58.1	66.0	72.8	82.3
Louisiana	64.8	42.3	57.6	62.3	69.0	80.9
Maine	72.5	54.7	61.2	68.5	76.7	86.5
Maryland	73.5	48.9	59.6	67.6	72.8	82.9
Massachusetts	79.9	64.4	73.9	69.5	80.9	86.0
Michigan	79.2	57.6	68.0	79.4	79.3	88.2
Minnesota	74.9	59.1	65.1	69.1	74.5	82.1
Mississippi	60.6	38.5	49.8	60.3	68.1	78.0
Missouri	62.6	44.0	51.9	58.9	66.5	75.6
Montana	61.7	45.0	53.7	52.9	65.3	76.2
Nebraska	75.1	68.1	69.5	69.1	74.4	84.2
Nevada	55.9	33.5	40.4	53.3	46.1	71.7
New Hampshire	75.2	66.1	62.4	65.8	70.8	87.3
New Jersey	72.1	55.7	67.2	67.5	69.5	80.2
New Mexico	61.2	41.7	47.7	59.7	67.1	80.5
New York	72.7	57.5	59.3	75.3	70.8	83.2
North Carolina	68.8	52.0	50.1	65.3	75.5	86.3
North Dakota	69.3	52.7	62.8	69.0	67.1	79.5
Ohio	73.0	51.7	66.3	73.7	71.1	82.9
Oklahoma	63.8	43.3	54.5	60.4	74.2	84.4
Oregon	67.2	40.6	53.1	68.8	70.7	81.1
Pennsylvania	76.0	58.0	63.0	71.7	77.1	87.9
Rhode Island	78.9	61.3	69.2	77.9	77.5	89.1
South Carolina	72.9	55.1	64.7	68.1	78.0	84.3
South Dakota	67.0	53.3	57.8	61.8	70.6	78.9
Tennessee	72.1	48.1	58.0	69.4	75.2	84.3
Texas	60.3	31.6	47.6	61.1	65.6	75.2
Utah	72.1	63.6	59.9	66.0	77.6	78.1
Vermont	76.8	67.9	62.7	71.0	76.3	90.6
Virginia	73.8	54.5	53.6	69.1	75.5	83.7
Washington	74.0	54.1	60.7	68.8	71.4	84.6
West Virginia	62.5	34.1	50.5	60.5	75.1	83.0
Wisconsin	74.8	52.0	63.9	72.7	81.3	82.2
Wyoming	62.9	44.8	53.7	62.8	65.8	74.8

Source: Compiled by New Strategist based on the Centers for Disease Control and Prevention Behavioral Risk Factor Surveillance System Survey, Internet site http://www.cdc.gov/brfss/index.htm

1.45 Dental: Teeth Cleaned in Past Year by Sex, 1999

"Have you had your teeth cleaned by the dentist or dental hygienist within the past year?"

(percent of people aged 18 or older responding "yes," by state and sex, 1999)

	total	men	women
U.S. total	**71.5%**	**68.2%**	**74.1%**
Alabama	61.5	59.5	63.3
Alaska	65.7	63.1	68.4
Arizona	68.0	65.5	70.3
Arkansas	60.4	58.0	62.6
California	66.8	63.6	70.1
Colorado	67.3	63.8	70.7
Connecticut	80.7	76.6	84.5
Delaware	74.2	70.0	78.0
District of Columbia	76.1	74.6	77.4
Florida	69.8	68.2	71.2
Georgia	67.6	65.6	69.5
Hawaii	74.3	73.3	75.3
Idaho	64.3	61.2	67.5
Illinois	72.1	69.8	74.4
Indiana	69.9	68.6	71.1
Iowa	72.3	67.5	76.8
Kansas	70.9	66.9	74.8
Kentucky	68.3	66.1	70.3
Louisiana	64.8	61.6	67.9
Maine	72.5	69.7	75.2
Maryland	73.5	70.0	76.8
Massachusetts	79.9	77.0	82.5
Michigan	79.2	74.9	83.2
Minnesota	74.9	72.2	77.5
Mississippi	60.6	59.0	62.0
Missouri	62.6	55.5	69.3
Montana	61.7	56.3	66.9
Nebraska	75.1	71.4	78.7
Nevada	55.9	52.6	59.1
New Hampshire	75.2	71.9	78.3
New Jersey	72.1	69.9	74.3
New Mexico	61.2	58.3	63.9
New York	72.7	69.7	75.5
North Carolina	68.8	66.8	70.6
North Dakota	˙69.3	63.3	75.4
Ohio	73.0	72.0	74.0
Oklahoma	63.8	63.3	64.2
Oregon	67.2	64.4	70.0
Pennsylvania	76.0	74.6	77.3
Rhode Island	78.9	77.4	80.2
South Carolina	72.9	70.1	75.6
South Dakota	67.0	62.8	71.2
Tennessee	72.1	71.0	73.1
Texas	60.3	58.0	62.4
Utah	72.1	68.2	75.9
Vermont	76.8	73.0	80.5
Virginia	73.8	71.0	76.6
Washington	74.0	70.8	77.0
West Virginia	62.5	62.4	62.5
Wisconsin	74.8	71.7	77.9
Wyoming	62.9	60.3	34.5

Source: Compiled by New Strategist based on the Centers for Disease Control and Prevention Behavioral Risk Factor Surveillance System Survey, Internet site http://www.cdc.gov/brfss/index.htm

1.46 Dental: Tooth Loss by Age, 1999

"Have you lost six or more teeth to decay or gum disease?"

(percent of people aged 18 or older responding "yes," by state and age, 1999)

	total	18 to 24	25 to 34	35 to 44	45 to 54	55 to 64	65 or older
U.S. total	**19.9%**	**0.5%**	**3.0%**	**9.0%**	**18.9%**	**38.9%**	**53.8%**
Utah	13.1	0.3	4.7	15.7	31.8	48.8	62.5
Hawaii	13.8	0.8	4.1	8.4	15.5	30.9	60.0
Alaska	14.2	4.4	2.5	5.1	11.8	31.2	52.7
Colorado	14.4	2.0	5.4	13.7	29.8	50.6	56.1
California	14.7	0.8	1.4	7.7	17.4	28.8	42.8
Washington	15.1	–	1.2	7.9	16.3	23.4	45.8
Texas	15.2	–	1.3	4.5	13.9	34.1	43.9
Connecticut	15.8	2.0	0.9	9.9	21.7	39.5	52.3
New Mexico	16.4	–	4.6	14.5	18.7	43.6	54.0
Wyoming	16.7	–	3.4	8.9	21.1	44.7	50.9
Kansas	17.2	–	2.7	13.1	27.1	48.0	57.2
Minnesota	17.3	1.5	0.6	3.4	11.2	25.3	41.9
Arizona	17.4	0.7	2.5	7.8	14.2	31.5	52.2
Oregon	17.4	–	1.8	9.1	19.1	47.0	55.0
Wisconsin	17.4	–	4.0	11.7	24.5	40.2	61.5
Idaho	17.7	–	1.6	6.7	14.5	36.5	51.5
Nebraska	17.7	–	3.2	7.5	12.7	34.7	47.6
New Jersey	18.2	1.0	3.8	16.5	35.2	55.4	71.2
Virginia	18.4	1.4	3.0	15.4	20.5	47.0	59.0
Massachusetts	18.6	3.2	5.1	12.3	21.6	45.3	61.4
Montana	18.9	1.0	4.1	7.4	18.6	37.4	56.3
Maryland	19.0	0.3	2.1	7.1	16.1	37.4	52.3
New York	19.1	1.8	2.5	10.0	20.2	36.8	49.6
Michigan	19.2	3.3	4.7	7.3	16.4	28.7	47.0
Iowa	19.3	0.4	5.2	18.1	32.0	54.7	64.3
Nevada	19.8	0.5	3.7	11.6	25.2	43.2	61.7
Rhode Island	20.1	1.3	1.5	6.5	18.2	34.6	49.9
Delaware	20.2	0.5	1.4	5.8	16.8	29.8	50.1
New Hampshire	20.4	0.7	3.0	10.3	21.0	44.4	46.6
Vermont	20.5	0.5	2.9	11.4	21.4	39.5	56.0
South Dakota	21.3	0.7	3.4	7.1	16.0	32.0	51.0
District of Columbia	21.7	–	3.0	5.3	15.4	28.5	53.6
Georgia	22.0	–	3.3	10.0	19.8	31.3	49.3
North Dakota	22.0	2.5	4.0	11.7	25.5	41.9	54.0
North Carolina	22.3	–	1.0	7.1	16.1	44.1	65.0
Illinois	22.4	–	0.6	13.1	28.5	50.8	58.6
Louisiana	22.6	0.9	4.5	12.6	22.8	45.8	65.0
Indiana	23.2	0.3	2.9	7.4	16.1	32.2	46.7
South Carolina	23.2	–	3.1	9.7	21.4	46.9	58.7
Tennessee	23.3	0.3	3.3	7.2	15.1	40.5	54.8
Florida	23.4	1.4	4.3	13.6	29.0	47.0	54.1
Pennsylvania	24.3	0.7	3.4	6.8	17.5	38.8	57.7
Maine	24.6	2.0	3.3	12.2	28.8	44.1	53.1
Missouri	24.6	0.5	1.9	8.2	13.6	33.7	45.7
Ohio	24.6	0.6	1.7	5.8	11.0	30.6	44.7
Oklahoma	25.3	0.4	3.2	10.9	22.1	39.1	54.0
Arkansas	26.7	0.4	2.9	10.7	19.8	34.1	56.9
Alabama	26.9	0.4	1.9	5.5	12.5	33.5	45.1
Mississippi	27.4	2.7	6.1	19.4	39.6	61.2	74.0
Kentucky	30.1	–	2.1	5.0	15.3	33.2	51.3
West Virginia	35.6	0.4	2.1	7.3	17.2	34.1	45.8

Note: (–) means less than 0.05 percent.
Source: Compiled by New Strategist based on the Centers for Disease Control and Prevention Behavioral Risk Factor
Surveillance System Survey, Internet site http://www.cdc.gov/brfss/index.htm

1.47 Dental: Tooth Loss by Education, 1999

"Have you lost six or more teeth to decay or gum disease?"

(percent of people aged 18 or older responding "yes," by state and educational attainment, 1999)

	total	less than high school	high school graduate	some college	college graduate
U.S. total	**19.9%**	**47.9%**	**24.3%**	**15.0%**	**8.6%**
Alabama	26.9	56.2	25.6	17.1	12.6
Alaska	14.2	46.6	14.5	10.4	8.3
Arizona	17.4	22.8	20.6	16.4	10.4
Arkansas	26.7	54.3	28.4	21.1	9.8
California	14.7	21.7	15.6	13.9	9.5
Colorado	14.4	25.9	21.8	12.8	6.4
Connecticut	15.8	32.0	22.3	12.9	7.4
Delaware	20.2	45.6	26.7	17.5	8.0
District of Columbia	21.7	49.2	30.0	15.3	11.2
Florida	23.4	43.7	27.6	19.4	13.2
Georgia	22.0	53.0	23.8	16.9	8.4
Hawaii	13.8	49.2	15.2	10.9	7.2
Idaho	17.7	36.3	22.3	14.5	7.6
Illinois	22.4	50.4	28.3	18.3	8.0
Indiana	23.2	55.0	27.4	16.2	7.9
Iowa	19.3	54.0	25.1	11.2	5.9
Kansas	17.2	40.7	23.0	13.2	5.8
Kentucky	30.1	61.3	29.5	19.0	9.9
Louisiana	22.6	50.0	23.4	14.7	8.8
Maine	24.6	56.3	29.5	17.8	11.0
Maryland	19.0	46.7	23.8	14.7	9.5
Massachusetts	18.6	39.3	25.9	18.3	7.8
Michigan	19.2	46.1	22.8	16.7	7.8
Minnesota	17.3	48.7	24.6	12.5	7.1
Mississippi	27.4	53.8	27.4	19.8	13.1
Missouri	24.6	50.5	30.8	16.2	8.3
Montana	18.9	41.5	24.6	15.7	6.7
Nebraska	17.7	47.2	23.3	11.8	5.8
Nevada	19.8	27.6	21.4	19.6	13.5
New Hampshire	20.4	66.2	28.1	13.7	10.0
New Jersey	18.2	27.1	26.4	15.6	8.9
New Mexico	16.4	30.9	18.0	13.8	8.2
New York	19.1	31.3	26.5	14.6	9.1
North Carolina	22.3	55.2	24.0	13.7	6.5
North Dakota	22.0	58.7	24.7	14.3	9.7
Ohio	24.6	54.6	27.4	18.6	7.5
Oklahoma	25.3	55.1	27.3	20.0	10.7
Oregon	17.4	27.8	21.1	16.4	9.6
Pennsylvania	24.3	52.0	28.7	17.7	11.2
Rhode Island	20.1	44.7	26.6	13.4	8.7
South Carolina	23.2	53.4	23.5	16.0	10.5
South Dakota	21.3	52.9	28.0	14.4	8.8
Tennessee	23.3	50.0	23.9	16.6	11.1
Texas	15.2	21.8	19.4	14.5	6.8
Utah	13.1	35.5	18.7	11.0	4.8
Vermont	20.5	54.6	24.7	15.6	8.6
Virginia	18.4	53.5	23.7	13.0	7.4
Washington	15.1	35.8	20.9	12.5	7.0
West Virginia	35.6	69.0	35.7	21.8	12.3
Wisconsin	17.4	45.4	21.4	13.8	6.7
Wyoming	16.7	42.2	21.1	12.7	8.8

Source: Compiled by New Strategist based on the Centers for Disease Control and Prevention Behavioral Risk Factor Surveillance System Survey, Internet site http://www.cdc.gov/brfss/index.htm

1.48 Dental: Tooth Loss by Household Income, 1999

"Have you lost six or more teeth to decay or gum disease?"

(percent of people aged 18 or older responding "yes," by state and household income, 1999)

	total	less than $15,000	$15,000 to $24,999	$25,000 to $34,999	$35,000 to $49,999	$50,000 or more
U.S. total	19.9%	38.9%	28.5%	20.6%	14.0%	8.3%
Alabama	26.9	45.1	31.6	21.8	19.1	13.1
Alaska	14.2	27.2	16.2	15.1	13.5	8.9
Arizona	17.4	23.8	19.3	14.2	13.9	24.9
Arkansas	26.7	54.8	33.0	23.0	18.6	11.8
California	14.7	22.3	20.5	12.4	13.0	8.2
Colorado	14.4	29.5	20.7	16.5	13.2	6.4
Connecticut	15.8	32.0	23.7	21.4	12.7	7.6
Delaware	20.2	31.0	39.6	22.5	18.8	9.4
District of Columbia	21.7	34.0	24.1	17.9	14.2	12.1
Florida	23.4	49.4	29.1	22.3	18.2	10.3
Georgia	22.0	42.9	28.8	20.6	17.2	12.4
Hawaii	13.8	27.7	16.3	11.1	15.5	6.8
Idaho	17.7	30.9	25.5	15.4	12.2	6.6
Illinois	22.4	41.2	32.3	24.0	21.3	9.6
Indiana	23.2	62.0	38.1	20.6	9.4	10.2
Iowa	19.3	47.2	27.7	22.6	12.0	6.2
Kansas	17.2	33.5	25.3	17.7	11.6	7.1
Kentucky	30.1	58.4	39.4	23.2	22.2	10.9
Louisiana	22.6	41.3	29.9	24.3	13.8	8.5
Maine	24.6	46.9	34.7	19.4	15.5	10.6
Maryland	19.0	41.0	34.3	25.8	12.9	9.2
Massachusetts	18.6	38.2	30.5	22.5	18.6	8.0
Michigan	19.2	44.9	27.2	24.7	14.0	8.3
Minnesota	17.3	41.8	32.9	20.9	13.9	8.0
Mississippi	27.4	48.3	35.2	23.9	19.8	11.7
Missouri	24.6	46.9	32.4	20.4	14.5	9.4
Montana	18.9	32.9	23.1	14.5	11.7	7.1
Nebraska	17.7	33.4	28.1	15.5	11.5	7.2
Nevada	19.8	42.1	24.6	21.1	15.5	10.8
New Hampshire	20.4	39.7	41.8	19.1	21.5	7.0
New Jersey	18.2	31.1	33.2	26.5	20.5	8.0
New Mexico	16.4	26.7	17.4	17.0	12.9	6.1
New York	19.1	31.6	27.6	21.6	14.6	10.5
North Carolina	22.3	46.9	31.3	18.9	15.4	6.7
North Dakota	22.0	46.0	27.3	18.2	14.1	9.5
Ohio	24.6	41.9	35.3	28.4	17.7	12.0
Oklahoma	25.3	35.2	35.6	23.9	16.0	8.9
Oregon	17.4	33.9	23.3	16.0	14.5	8.1
Pennsylvania	24.3	47.4	37.3	22.1	13.5	10.4
Rhode Island	20.1	38.4	33.2	24.9	14.3	7.6
South Carolina	23.2	43.6	26.6	22.9	16.2	12.0
South Dakota	21.3	32.2	32.4	20.2	13.4	8.3
Tennessee	23.3	48.3	28.2	19.2	12.4	9.4
Texas	15.2	23.8	19.3	14.9	12.1	8.0
Utah	13.1	24.2	22.0	15.2	10.2	5.6
Vermont	20.5	39.5	32.4	22.8	12.1	8.3
Virginia	18.4	38.1	30.6	23.4	15.3	7.9
Washington	15.1	26.6	25.7	16.5	13.4	6.5
West Virginia	35.6	61.6	45.6	26.8	18.3	12.5
Wisconsin	17.4	45.7	27.3	13.1	11.2	7.0
Wyoming	16.7	34.4	20.9	16.7	12.0	7.4

Source: Compiled by New Strategist based on the Centers for Disease Control and Prevention Behavioral Risk Factor Surveillance System Survey, Internet site http://www.cdc.gov/brfss/index.htm

1.49 Dental: Tooth Loss by Sex, 1999

"Have you lost six or more teeth to decay or gum disease?"

(percent of people aged 18 or older responding "yes," by state and sex, 1999)

	total	men	women
U.S. total	**19.9%**	**17.8%**	**21.4%**
Alabama	26.9	25.0	28.7
Alaska	14.2	13.1	15.4
Arizona	17.4	15.5	19.3
Arkansas	26.7	22.6	30.4
California	14.7	13.3	16.1
Colorado	14.4	12.8	16.0
Connecticut	15.8	14.8	16.8
Delaware	20.2	18.6	21.6
District of Columbia	21.7	20.7	22.5
Florida	23.4	21.8	24.9
Georgia	22.0	19.8	24.0
Hawaii	13.8	12.7	14.8
Idaho	17.7	16.3	19.0
Illinois	22.4	19.9	24.9
Indiana	23.2	20.8	25.5
Iowa	19.3	17.1	21.3
Kansas	17.2	16.3	18.1
Kentucky	30.1	29.1	31.0
Louisiana	22.6	18.5	26.2
Maine	24.6	22.7	26.3
Maryland	19.0	17.4	20.6
Massachusetts	18.6	17.2	19.8
Michigan	19.2	17.8	20.4
Minnesota	17.3	16.5	18.1
Mississippi	27.4	24.1	30.3
Missouri	24.6	22.5	26.5
Montana	18.9	16.9	20.8
Nebraska	17.7	15.9	19.3
Nevada	19.8	17.8	21.8
New Hampshire	20.4	19.4	21.3
New Jersey	18.2	16.7	19.6
New Mexico	16.4	15.2	17.6
New York	19.1	16.9	21.0
North Carolina	22.3	20.0	24.4
North Dakota	22.0	19.3	24.6
Ohio	24.6	21.9	27.1
Oklahoma	25.3	22.5	28.0
Oregon	17.4	14.6	20.1
Pennsylvania	24.3	21.6	26.6
Rhode Island	20.1	18.5	21.6
South Carolina	23.2	20.9	25.4
South Dakota	21.3	18.2	24.2
Tennessee	23.3	20.8	25.6
Texas	15.2	13.5	16.8
Utah	13.1	13.0	13.2
Vermont	20.5	18.8	22.2
Virginia	18.4	17.3	19.4
Washington	15.1	13.3	16.8
West Virginia	35.6	31.4	39.3
Wisconsin	17.4	15.3	19.4
Wyoming	16.7	14.5	18.9

Source: Compiled by New Strategist based on the Centers for Disease Control and Prevention Behavioral Risk Factor Surveillance System Survey, Internet site http://www.cdc.gov/brfss/index.htm

1.50 Diabetes by Age, 2001

"Have you ever been told by a doctor that you have diabetes?"

(percent of people aged 18 or older responding "yes," by state and age, 2001)

	total	18 to 24	25 to 34	35 to 44	45 to 54	55 to 64	65 or older
U.S. total	**6.5%**	**0.6%**	**1.5%**	**3.2%**	**7.4%**	**12.3%**	**14.9%**
Alabama	9.6	0.6	3.9	4.4	8.9	19.5	21.8
Alaska	4.0	0.1	1.4	1.0	5.8	8.6	14.6
Arizona	6.1	0.8	1.7	3.3	7.8	10.0	13.6
Arkansas	7.8	1.4	2.3	3.9	10.1	12.8	14.9
California	6.5	0.6	1.2	3.5	9.0	14.7	13.3
Colorado	4.6	0.9	1.3	1.5	3.7	10.3	13.5
Connecticut	6.3	0.6	0.9	3.5	6.5	11.3	14.3
Delaware	7.1	2.9	1.6	4.0	8.3	12.1	14.5
District of Columbia	8.3	1.4	1.8	3.7	8.7	15.3	22.1
Florida	8.2	2.0	2.1	3.4	8.8	13.0	15.4
Georgia	6.9	0.5	2.0	2.9	8.2	16.0	16.2
Hawaii	6.2	2.8	1.6	2.1	5.6	10.7	15.3
Idaho	5.4	1.4	1.6	2.8	5.0	10.1	12.7
Illinois	6.6	0.7	0.9	2.4	9.2	11.0	16.4
Indiana	6.5	0.6	2.5	3.6	7.8	11.8	13.5
Iowa	5.7	0.3	1.0	3.8	4.2	9.3	13.9
Kansas	5.8	1.6	1.3	2.4	5.9	9.9	14.2
Kentucky	6.7	0.3	1.7	4.9	7.8	12.9	12.8
Louisiana	7.6	0.5	1.7	4.9	8.3	16.1	17.3
Maine	6.7	–	1.5	3.1	9.8	8.1	16.1
Maryland	6.9	0.4	1.7	3.6	8.1	13.8	15.6
Massachusetts	5.6	0.5	1.2	2.3	4.8	10.4	14.9
Michigan	7.2	2.0	1.3	3.7	9.2	12.3	16.1
Minnesota	4.4	1.3	1.4	1.2	3.0	8.6	12.1
Mississippi	9.3	1.5	5.5	4.2	8.7	19.6	19.1
Missouri	6.6	1.1	1.9	2.5	7.1	15.2	12.6
Montana	5.6	0.3	2.0	2.5	6.5	7.9	13.0
Nebraska	5.2	0.7	0.4	1.4	5.1	13.2	11.8
Nevada	5.7	0.6	1.4	2.3	5.5	12.7	13.4
New Hampshire	5.4	–	1.2	2.6	5.3	9.9	15.0
New Jersey	7.1	1.6	1.7	3.8	7.3	13.7	15.1
New Mexico	6.2	0.3	1.0	3.0	9.3	11.7	13.7
New York	6.6	0.8	1.2	3.4	7.5	13.6	13.8
North Carolina	6.7	0.3	1.1	2.6	7.4	15.8	15.0
North Dakota	5.1	0.2	1.1	2.4	5.5	11.3	11.0
Ohio	7.2	0.3	2.3	3.2	8.1	15.4	14.9
Oklahoma	7.7	0.6	1.9	3.9	7.8	12.8	18.6
Oregon	5.7	0.3	1.1	3.3	5.5	8.0	14.7
Pennsylvania	6.7	0.4	1.4	2.3	6.3	12.9	15.4
Rhode Island	6.4	1.7	1.7	2.6	6.4	10.4	15.8
South Carolina	8.1	1.7	1.6	4.4	12.1	15.0	15.9
South Dakota	6.1	0.8	1.6	2.2	5.8	11.6	14.6
Tennessee	7.7	0.5	2.9	3.2	9.2	14.8	16.5
Texas	7.1	0.8	1.8	4.3	9.0	13.5	16.4
Utah	4.3	0.4	0.8	1.8	5.6	7.3	11.6
Vermont	5.1	–	0.6	1.7	3.3	11.2	15.9
Virginia	6.0	0.4	0.8	3.5	6.3	12.3	15.4
Washington	5.7	0.2	1.5	2.6	5.9	11.6	14.1
West Virginia	8.8	–	1.3	4.7	11.4	15.9	17.0
Wisconsin	5.6	–	1.2	2.3	6.2	9.0	14.5
Wyoming	4.5	1.1	1.2	2.2	2.9	9.6	11.7

Note: (–) means data are not available.
Source: Compiled by New Strategist based on the Centers for Disease Control and Prevention Behavioral Risk Factor Surveillance System Survey, Internet site http://www.cdc.gov/brfss/index.htm

1.51 Diabetes by Education, 2001

"Have you ever been told by a doctor that you have diabetes?"

(percent of people aged 18 or older responding "yes," by state and educational attainment, 2001)

	total	less than high school	high school graduate	some college	college graduate
U.S. total	**6.5%**	**12.5%**	**7.0%**	**5.9%**	**4.2%**
Alabama	9.6	18.3	9.3	7.6	6.3
Alaska	4.0	6.2	3.6	5.0	2.8
Arizona	6.1	10.4	6.0	6.3	4.0
Arkansas	7.8	15.9	6.7	5.9	6.0
California	6.5	8.2	7.0	7.6	4.1
Colorado	4.6	12.2	5.0	4.0	2.6
Connecticut	6.3	12.8	7.5	6.1	3.9
Delaware	7.1	14.9	7.9	6.0	5.2
District of Columbia	8.3	19.2	9.5	10.5	4.0
Florida	8.2	14.1	6.8	8.8	6.2
Georgia	6.9	13.0	8.2	5.1	4.0
Hawaii	6.2	13.7	6.5	6.7	3.8
Idaho	5.4	8.0	5.7	5.6	4.1
Illinois	6.6	9.7	7.4	6.8	4.7
Indiana	6.5	11.6	6.8	6.2	4.4
Iowa	5.7	12.6	6.5	5.3	2.2
Kansas	5.8	13.1	7.2	4.5	3.8
Kentucky	6.7	11.0	6.2	5.8	4.3
Louisiana	7.6	12.5	7.5	5.7	6.0
Maine	6.7	13.4	8.4	6.1	2.9
Maryland	6.9	13.4	8.4	5.9	4.8
Massachusetts	5.6	10.3	7.3	5.0	3.8
Michigan	7.2	13.3	8.6	6.1	4.3
Minnesota	4.4	8.7	5.8	4.1	2.3
Mississippi	9.3	16.6	7.3	7.7	7.9
Missouri	6.6	9.5	7.7	7.0	3.1
Montana	5.6	6.3	5.6	6.0	4.7
Nebraska	5.2	9.8	5.3	5.0	3.4
Nevada	5.7	12.3	5.2	4.9	5.3
New Hampshire	5.4	8.5	6.1	5.7	3.9
New Jersey	7.1	13.9	7.6	7.7	4.6
New Mexico	6.2	8.9	7.3	5.4	4.1
New York	6.6	13.0	6.3	5.9	4.8
North Carolina	6.7	12.1	6.6	7.0	3.5
North Dakota	5.1	7.4	7.0	4.5	3.1
Ohio	7.2	12.8	8.3	5.6	4.5
Oklahoma	7.7	12.5	8.5	5.8	5.8
Oregon	5.7	5.2	6.4	4.2	6.8
Pennsylvania	6.7	13.5	6.9	6.3	3.9
Rhode Island	6.4	10.3	7.0	6.3	4.3
South Carolina	8.1	14.4	7.9	8.0	4.7
South Dakota	6.1	12.3	7.0	4.8	4.2
Tennessee	7.7	13.5	8.8	5.4	5.2
Texas	7.1	11.4	7.1	6.9	4.0
Utah	4.3	7.1	5.4	3.4	3.4
Vermont	5.1	13.6	6.0	3.8	3.1
Virginia	6.0	15.6	6.1	3.9	4.5
Washington	5.7	7.7	6.2	6.0	4.5
West Virginia	8.8	17.9	7.0	7.4	5.2
Wisconsin	5.6	9.4	6.5	5.5	3.3
Wyoming	4.5	8.8	4.9	4.1	3.0

Source: Compiled by New Strategist based on the Centers for Disease Control and Prevention Behavioral Risk Factor Surveillance System Survey, Internet site http://www.cdc.gov/brfss/index.htm

1.52 Diabetes by Household Income, 2001

"Have you ever been told by a doctor that you have diabetes?"

(percent of people aged 18 or older responding "yes," by state and household income, 2001)

	total	less than $15,000	$15,000 to $24,999	$25,000 to $34,999	$35,000 to $49,999	$50,000 or more
U.S. total	**6.5%**	**11.8%**	**8.4%**	**5.9%**	**5.2%**	**4.1%**
Alabama	9.6	17.6	11.0	9.3	5.6	5.3
Alaska	4.0	7.4	5.3	5.1	1.8	3.7
Arizona	6.1	10.0	8.4	5.1	6.1	5.0
Arkansas	7.8	12.2	8.4	6.7	7.1	5.0
California	6.5	9.8	8.4	5.3	6.4	4.8
Colorado	4.6	10.8	7.9	5.5	3.1	2.6
Connecticut	6.3	11.7	9.6	8.7	5.9	3.8
Delaware	7.1	10.2	14.7	5.3	5.6	4.9
District of Columbia	8.3	13.3	11.6	12.1	6.4	4.7
Florida	8.2	16.3	9.3	7.0	5.6	5.5
Georgia	6.9	14.5	8.0	5.2	6.9	4.6
Hawaii	6.2	9.4	7.9	5.3	7.3	4.2
Idaho	5.4	9.2	7.1	5.9	3.2	4.0
Illinois	6.6	11.7	7.4	8.2	8.3	3.7
Indiana	6.5	14.6	11.5	5.9	4.9	3.1
Iowa	5.7	11.6	9.4	6.3	3.9	2.0
Kansas	5.8	9.0	10.0	5.9	4.5	3.4
Kentucky	6.7	12.5	8.0	5.5	5.4	3.9
Louisiana	7.6	13.0	8.5	5.6	5.4	5.5
Maine	6.7	13.4	9.9	10.5	3.2	3.0
Maryland	6.9	10.4	10.6	11.4	5.7	4.5
Massachusetts	5.6	10.9	7.9	7.2	5.2	3.6
Michigan	7.2	11.6	9.4	7.4	6.3	5.0
Minnesota	4.4	9.6	8.7	4.2	4.1	2.5
Mississippi	9.3	15.9	9.6	6.0	7.4	8.0
Missouri	6.6	12.5	9.8	6.4	5.5	3.3
Montana	5.6	9.1	4.9	2.9	5.3	4.8
Nebraska	5.2	9.2	6.9	5.7	4.2	3.1
Nevada	5.7	8.5	7.6	4.7	7.1	3.8
New Hampshire	5.4	13.2	9.0	7.1	5.1	3.1
New Jersey	7.1	16.1	8.5	8.4	5.9	4.6
New Mexico	6.2	10.1	7.3	4.6	4.9	4.9
New York	6.6	14.0	8.9	5.7	4.4	4.3
North Carolina	6.7	13.2	8.7	6.1	4.2	3.8
North Dakota	5.1	5.1	8.2	5.4	3.4	3.0
Ohio	7.2	11.9	10.8	8.2	7.7	3.9
Oklahoma	7.7	14.9	8.4	6.1	3.7	6.0
Oregon	5.7	7.4	5.7	7.0	6.3	4.2
Pennsylvania	6.7	16.3	7.7	3.2	5.6	4.6
Rhode Island	6.4	13.9	7.8	7.5	3.4	4.6
South Carolina	8.1	15.7	10.2	5.1	5.9	5.3
South Dakota	6.1	11.1	8.5	6.6	4.9	3.2
Tennessee	7.7	12.2	9.3	5.4	4.2	5.5
Texas	7.1	13.0	8.1	7.8	6.7	3.3
Utah	4.3	6.3	5.6	5.7	4.3	2.5
Vermont	5.1	10.3	8.6	4.1	3.9	2.1
Virginia	6.0	16.6	10.3	4.6	3.4	3.8
Washington	5.7	9.8	7.5	6.5	4.2	4.7
West Virginia	8.8	12.7	10.8	9.6	7.6	5.1
Wisconsin	5.6	7.3	9.4	4.4	4.0	3.9
Wyoming	4.5	9.2	6.6	3.8	2.6	2.2

Source: Compiled by New Strategist based on the Centers for Disease Control and Prevention Behavioral Risk Factor Surveillance System Survey, Internet site http://www.cdc.gov/brfss/index.htm

1.53 Diabetes by Sex, 2001

"Have you ever been told by a doctor that you have diabetes?"

(percent of people aged 18 or older responding "yes," by state and sex, 2001)

	total	men	women
U.S. total	**6.5%**	**6.6%**	**6.5%**
Alabama	9.6	10.5	8.8
Alaska	4.0	4.0	4.0
Arizona	6.1	7.3	4.9
Arkansas	7.8	8.4	7.2
California	6.5	5.8	7.1
Colorado	4.6	5.6	3.7
Connecticut	6.3	6.5	6.0
Delaware	7.1	7.5	6.7
District of Columbia	8.3	9.6	7.2
Florida	8.2	9.1	7.3
Georgia	6.9	6.5	7.2
Hawaii	6.2	6.8	5.6
Idaho	5.4	5.2	5.7
Illinois	6.6	6.7	6.6
Indiana	6.5	6.3	6.8
Iowa	5.7	5.8	5.6
Kansas	5.8	5.5	6.1
Kentucky	6.7	6.9	6.4
Louisiana	7.6	6.9	8.2
Maine	6.7	7.0	6.5
Maryland	6.9	7.1	6.6
Massachusetts	5.6	6.0	5.2
Michigan	7.2	6.8	7.6
Minnesota	4.4	4.4	4.3
Mississippi	9.3	8.8	9.7
Missouri	6.6	7.0	6.2
Montana	5.6	4.9	6.2
Nebraska	5.2	4.9	5.5
Nevada	5.7	5.2	6.2
New Hampshire	5.4	5.8	5.0
New Jersey	7.1	7.3	7.0
New Mexico	6.2	5.9	6.5
New York	6.6	6.4	6.8
North Carolina	6.7	6.8	6.7
North Dakota	5.1	4.7	5.6
Ohio	7.2	7.5	6.9
Oklahoma	7.7	8.3	7.2
Oregon	5.7	5.5	5.8
Pennsylvania	6.7	6.6	6.7
Rhode Island	6.4	7.4	5.6
South Carolina	8.1	8.4	7.7
South Dakota	6.1	6.6	5.6
Tennessee	7.7	7.6	7.9
Texas	7.1	7.0	7.2
Utah	4.3	4.3	4.2
Vermont	5.1	4.6	5.5
Virginia	6.0	6.2	5.8
Washington	5.7	6.2	5.2
West Virginia	8.8	8.9	8.8
Wisconsin	5.6	5.9	5.3
Wyoming	4.5	4.1	4.8

Source: Compiled by New Strategist based on the Centers for Disease Control and Prevention Behavioral Risk Factor Surveillance System Survey. Internet site http://www.cdc.gov/brfss/index.htm

1.54 Diabetes: Taking Insulin, 1999

If diagnosed as diabetic, "Are you now taking insulin?"

(percent of people aged 18 or older with diabetes responding "yes," by state, 1999)

	taking insulin
U.S. total	**32.1%**
Alabama	31.0
Alaska	29.9
Arizona	41.9
Arkansas	31.5
California	26.9
Colorado	36.0
Connecticut	35.2
District of Columbia	32.7
Florida	32.0
Georgia	35.1
Hawaii	18.8
Iowa	27.1
Kentucky	31.9
Louisiana	45.4
Maine	30.1
Massachusetts	32.1
Michigan	28.9
Minnesota	34.2
Montana	38.1
Nebraska	33.7
Nevada	40.5
New Hampshire	32.2
New Jersey	23.2
New Mexico	32.6
North Carolina	32.2
North Dakota	35.3
Ohio	36.2
Oklahoma	31.7
Pennsylvania	34.5
Rhode Island	24.9
Tennessee	38.0
Texas	26.5
Utah	30.7
Vermont	31.7
Virginia	25.6
West Virginia	26.4
Wisconsin	30.6
Wyoming	32.9

Source: Compiled by New Strategist based on the Centers for Disease Control and Prevention Behavioral Risk Factor Surveillance System Survey, Internet site http://www.cdc.gov/brfss/index.htm

1.55 Doctor Visits: Routine Checkup in Past Year by Age, 2000

"About how long has it been since you last visited a doctor for a routine checkup?"

(percent of people aged 18 or older who had visited a doctor for a routine checkup in the past year, by state and age, 2000)

	total	18 to 24	25 to 34	35 to 44	45 to 54	55 to 64	65 or older
U.S. total	**72.2%**	**68.3%**	**64.3%**	**65.6%**	**72.0%**	**80.2%**	**86.6%**
Alabama	69.9	71.3	65.7	57.3	67.7	80.4	83.0
Alaska	70.3	68.2	64.4	66.2	71.7	77.4	87.7
Arizona	74.6	59.6	61.3	74.0	76.4	86.0	89.8
Arkansas	67.7	62.0	54.5	59.8	68.1	76.3	84.0
California	62.9	57.5	53.5	55.5	63.9	72.4	83.1
Colorado	68.0	55.0	58.6	62.1	71.9	79.5	86.4
Connecticut	76.0	70.4	67.1	67.2	77.3	83.4	90.9
Delaware	77.7	76.6	73.9	71.7	70.2	86.2	91.1
District of Columbia	81.9	74.3	78.5	80.2	78.9	87.4	93.5
Florida	77.2	68.5	70.8	66.1	75.7	83.6	91.9
Georgia	72.1	66.6	67.2	67.2	71.8	77.2	87.2
Hawaii	77.6	75.9	72.1	70.9	77.8	81.7	89.6
Idaho	61.4	57.2	54.0	50.6	61.4	68.8	79.8
Illinois	73.3	68.2	62.9	67.7	72.8	82.4	89.3
Indiana	69.2	58.9	61.5	62.0	75.0	78.7	81.1
Iowa	71.2	66.4	60.2	63.7	68.7	79.9	86.9
Kansas	72.3	71.4	67.4	60.7	72.1	78.2	86.6
Kentucky	74.0	72.4	65.2	65.9	74.5	80.8	87.4
Louisiana	77.5	76.0	70.9	70.5	78.7	83.2	90.0
Maine	75.2	74.0	70.2	65.5	76.7	82.9	84.9
Maryland	78.4	79.2	71.7	72.9	78.2	82.0	91.4
Massachusetts	79.9	78.0	72.8	72.0	81.1	85.5	92.6
Michigan	75.4	74.5	68.3	67.5	75.0	82.6	88.6
Minnesota	68.4	59.9	63.3	63.6	67.6	74.9	82.4
Mississippi	69.8	65.1	63.0	67.0	70.2	75.6	79.5
Missouri	73.1	68.0	62.5	66.3	74.4	82.4	85.6
Montana	65.3	58.3	55.8	55.6	66.2	73.4	82.4
Nebraska	68.1	57.7	62.5	61.6	71.7	72.1	80.7
Nevada	67.2	58.4	59.9	57.0	65.9	85.0	82.9
New Hampshire	74.4	71.9	69.0	63.1	75.5	83.9	90.0
New Jersey	78.5	75.1	72.9	71.1	78.2	86.7	88.9
New Mexico	67.8	62.2	57.8	60.8	66.5	80.1	86.4
New York	80.3	79.7	71.6	69.8	84.6	87.1	92.2
North Carolina	74.4	68.2	67.2	69.5	74.9	82.5	86.7
North Dakota	70.9	71.3	65.1	64.1	65.9	74.7	84.3
Ohio	73.8	69.5	62.1	67.9	73.6	85.0	86.5
Oklahoma	67.0	61.8	64.3	58.6	69.5	68.8	79.0
Oregon	65.6	59.6	56.6	56.6	64.1	77.8	81.3
Pennsylvania	73.7	70.3	58.9	67.9	72.6	81.2	89.4
Rhode Island	81.2	79.3	72.2	73.8	79.7	89.4	94.5
South Carolina	76.7	73.1	73.2	70.3	76.0	80.5	89.4
South Dakota	72.0	74.7	60.9	62.4	72.6	78.3	85.5
Tennessee	76.8	75.2	69.8	72.5	76.1	82.8	86.1
Texas	66.6	55.8	57.6	60.3	70.4	75.8	85.1
Utah	61.9	53.9	55.5	58.0	64.0	71.8	75.6
Vermont	71.8	70.2	65.8	64.2	69.1	77.3	87.7
Virginia	70.6	64.9	65.2	65.8	68.8	73.7	88.7
Washington	66.4	60.2	62.3	60.0	66.3	69.2	82.1
West Virginia	72.6	70.7	61.5	62.4	71.8	78.4	88.8
Wisconsin	64.6	65.9	55.1	52.0	64.3	71.7	82.4
Wyoming	60.5	59.5	59.5	47.0	58.5	68.0	77.3

Source: Compiled by New Strategist based on the Centers for Disease Control and Prevention Behavioral Risk Factor Surveillance System Survey. Internet site http://www.cdc.gov/brfss/index.htm

1.56 Doctor Visits: Routine Checkup in Past Year by Education, 2000

"About how long has it been since you last visited a doctor for a routine checkup?"

(percent of people aged 18 or older who had visited a doctor for a routine checkup in the past year, by state and educational attainment, 2000)

	total	less than high school	high school graduate	some college	college graduate
U.S. total	**72.2%**	**73.5%**	**71.6%**	**72.7%**	**71.0%**
Alabama	69.9	64.9	71.5	70.3	71.0
Alaska	70.3	70.5	71.2	70.9	68.5
Arizona	74.6	74.0	70.2	75.0	80.1
Arkansas	67.7	69.9	64.5	68.7	70.4
California	62.9	62.1	64.9	63.0	61.7
Colorado	68.0	65.9	65.5	69.8	68.7
Connecticut	76.0	80.3	76.3	77.9	73.4
Delaware	77.7	82.2	78.8	79.5	74.1
District of Columbia	81.9	88.2	83.8	87.3	77.2
Florida	77.2	74.7	77.1	76.2	79.0
Georgia	72.1	73.0	72.0	73.1	70.8
Hawaii	77.6	80.3	75.3	78.0	78.9
Idaho	61.4	60.9	61.7	61.2	61.4
Illinois	73.3	75.9	74.1	72.7	72.1
Indiana	69.2	69.3	69.8	67.1	70.9
Iowa	71.2	72.6	70.7	71.9	70.4
Kansas	72.3	64.9	71.7	73.8	73.7
Kentucky	74.0	75.1	72.2	74.7	75.4
Louisiana	77.5	77.0	77.8	75.9	79.4
Maine	75.2	68.9	77.1	73.5	76.8
Maryland	78.4	80.0	80.4	78.9	76.1
Massachusetts	79.9	80.4	83.6	81.6	76.3
Michigan	75.4	75.9	75.2	75.4	74.9
Minnesota	68.4	65.0	70.1	67.8	68.2
Mississippi	69.8	69.2	69.8	70.6	69.9
Missouri	73.1	74.1	73.9	73.1	71.0
Montana	65.3	64.2	63.2	64.2	68.7
Nebraska	68.1	70.7	69.9	64.6	68.2
Nevada	67.2	59.0	65.4	68.9	70.8
New Hampshire	74.4	72.4	76.6	76.7	70.8
New Jersey	78.5	77.3	78.5	78.7	78.7
New Mexico	67.8	63.2	65.3	68.0	73.2
New York	80.3	80.8	81.6	80.3	78.7
North Carolina	74.4	71.6	72.6	76.3	76.5
North Dakota	70.9	77.5	71.1	69.2	70.2
Ohio	73.8	77.2	72.4	73.4	75.0
Oklahoma	67.0	70.5	65.2	63.0	73.6
Oregon	65.6	56.0	66.6	67.5	66.9
Pennsylvania	73.7	77.5	76.7	72.0	69.3
Rhode Island	81.2	82.9	83.4	80.9	78.4
South Carolina	76.7	75.5	76.6	77.7	76.5
South Dakota	72.0	78.5	70.6	72.5	70.7
Tennessee	76.8	79.4	77.7	72.7	79.2
Texas	66.6	61.3	65.9	66.9	70.8
Utah	61.9	61.7	62.0	62.7	60.9
Vermont	71.8	74.9	73.9	70.6	69.8
Virginia	70.6	75.0	66.7	72.9	70.9
Washington	66.4	68.0	62.8	67.5	67.8
West Virginia	72.6	76.2	70.0	75.6	71.1
Wisconsin	64.6	65.6	65.4	65.1	62.3
Wyoming	60.5	63.4	60.4	59.4	60.8

Source: Compiled by New Strategist based on the Centers for Disease Control and Prevention Behavioral Risk Factor Surveillance System Survey, Internet site http://www.cdc.gov/brfss/index.htm

1.57 Doctor Visits: Routine Checkup in Past Year by Household Income, 2000

"About how long has it been since you last visited a doctor for a routine checkup?"

(percent of people aged 18 or older who had visited a doctor for a routine checkup in the past year, by state and household income, 2000)

	total	less than $15,000	$15,000 to $24,999	$25,000 to $34,999	$35,000 to $49,999	$50,000 or more
U.S. total	**72.2%**	**74.6%**	**71.2%**	**71.0%**	**70.6%**	**71.2%**
Alabama	69.9	68.0	68.5	69.5	66.1	71.2
Alaska	70.3	61.6	73.2	68.9	69.9	70.1
Arizona	74.6	60.2	68.7	77.0	70.6	82.6
Arkansas	67.7	72.6	64.3	66.5	63.7	68.2
California	62.9	64.9	60.7	61.4	62.6	61.5
Colorado	68.0	65.1	70.0	65.4	63.7	68.0
Connecticut	76.0	86.3	76.1	71.9	77.2	74.2
Delaware	77.7	77.9	78.6	79.5	80.7	74.8
District of Columbia	81.9	84.6	86.0	77.2	85.2	76.8
Florida	77.2	75.5	73.1	78.5	75.0	79.5
Georgia	72.1	75.7	67.3	71.1	71.3	71.3
Hawaii	77.6	77.3	78.6	76.9	77.0	78.0
Idaho	61.4	58.9	56.4	62.8	59.6	64.1
Illinois	73.3	75.3	76.7	71.6	70.9	71.2
Indiana	69.2	63.7	68.7	69.2	66.9	70.0
Iowa	71.2	76.1	72.2	69.6	70.4	69.0
Kansas	72.3	71.0	71.6	71.3	72.8	72.8
Kentucky	74.0	76.9	70.2	71.8	72.2	75.3
Louisiana	77.5	81.2	76.2	73.9	75.7	77.6
Maine	75.2	76.7	67.6	74.5	76.3	78.3
Maryland	78.4	85.5	79.6	79.3	76.3	76.9
Massachusetts	79.9	84.0	81.2	81.4	79.4	77.5
Michigan	75.4	85.3	76.2	77.6	71.0	72.5
Minnesota	68.4	69.2	72.0	71.5	64.3	67.5
Mississippi	69.8	74.7	70.1	72.2	66.3	64.7
Missouri	73.1	75.2	71.1	72.7	66.8	74.2
Montana	65.3	63.6	61.3	63.6	65.4	68.5
Nebraska	68.1	72.7	65.3	68.6	63.8	70.2
Nevada	67.2	70.6	69.5	64.4	66.6	63.5
New Hampshire	74.4	84.1	72.6	66.4	75.5	76.6
New Jersey	78.5	82.0	73.7	78.5	80.5	80.1
New Mexico	67.8	68.5	62.1	67.0	68.0	72.8
New York	80.3	80.0	79.0	80.2	81.4	79.5
North Carolina	74.4	73.6	74.3	69.1	73.0	75.3
North Dakota	70.9	77.0	69.8	67.2	71.1	69.7
Ohio	73.8	68.6	74.9	71.0	71.3	73.9
Oklahoma	67.0	64.2	66.3	68.6	65.5	70.2
Oregon	65.6	62.1	63.6	63.6	66.1	67.8
Pennsylvania	73.7	78.9	75.6	72.9	70.4	70.6
Rhode Island	81.2	82.9	82.0	80.1	80.4	79.2
South Carolina	76.7	73.5	74.0	78.7	73.6	77.9
South Dakota	72.0	74.5	73.7	70.2	68.5	70.8
Tennessee	76.8	77.5	73.8	74.0	75.1	78.1
Texas	66.6	59.2	60.8	65.9	67.9	72.2
Utah	61.9	61.8	59.1	61.3	60.6	61.8
Vermont	71.8	76.9	69.5	69.9	68.0	71.1
Virginia	70.6	77.3	71.4	68.1	70.7	69.3
Washington	66.4	65.3	65.5	64.9	62.5	68.2
West Virginia	72.6	73.7	69.2	71.3	74.3	71.2
Wisconsin	64.6	67.4	62.0	65.5	61.5	64.3
Wyoming	60.5	63.9	60.5	57.8	57.4	59.9

Source: Compiled by New Strategist based on the Centers for Disease Control and Prevention Behavioral Risk Factor Surveillance System Survey, Internet site http://www.cdc.gov/brfss/index.htm

1.58 Doctor Visits: Routine Checkup in Past Year by Sex, 2000

"About how long has it been since you last visited a doctor for a routine checkup?"

(percent of people aged 18 or older who had visited a doctor for a routine checkup in the past year, by state and sex, 2000)

	total	men	women
U.S. total	**72.2%**	**63.4%**	**80.0%**
Alabama	69.9	63.4	75.8
Alaska	70.3	61.7	79.6
Arizona	74.6	68.6	80.5
Arkansas	67.7	59.5	75.1
California	62.9	54.9	70.7
Colorado	68.0	58.1	77.5
Connecticut	76.0	69.5	81.9
Delaware	77.7	72.2	82.8
District of Columbia	81.9	73.4	89.1
Florida	77.2	71.9	82.0
Georgia	72.1	64.7	78.9
Hawaii	77.6	71.1	84.1
Idaho	61.4	52.1	70.3
Illinois	73.3	63.5	82.4
Indiana	69.2	61.9	76.0
Iowa	71.2	61.6	80.0
Kansas	72.3	63.3	80.8
Kentucky	74.0	66.1	81.0
Louisiana	77.5	69.8	84.4
Maine	75.2	66.6	83.1
Maryland	78.4	71.5	84.7
Massachusetts	79.9	72.9	86.3
Michigan	75.4	67.6	82.4
Minnesota	68.4	60.1	76.2
Mississippi	69.8	61.9	76.7
Missouri	73.1	65.8	79.6
Montana	65.3	54.9	75.2
Nebraska	68.1	57.0	78.4
Nevada	67.2	59.1	75.3
New Hampshire	74.4	68.4	80.0
New Jersey	78.5	73.9	82.6
New Mexico	67.8	59.0	76.1
New York	80.3	74.7	85.2
North Carolina	74.4	67.2	81.0
North Dakota	70.9	61.5	80.1
Ohio	73.8	65.4	81.3
Oklahoma	67.0	57.2	76.0
Oregon	65.6	56.3	74.4
Pennsylvania	73.7	66.1	80.5
Rhode Island	81.2	74.7	86.9
South Carolina	76.7	68.5	84.2
South Dakota	72.0	62.1	81.3
Tennessee	76.8	70.0	82.8
Texas	66.6	57.9	74.8
Utah	61.9	53.5	69.9
Vermont	71.8	63.1	80.0
Virginia	70.6	63.0	77.6
Washington	66.4	58.2	74.3
West Virginia	72.6	65.8	78.6
Wisconsin	64.6	55.1	73.4
Wyoming	60.5	47.8	72.9

Source: Compiled by New Strategist based on the Centers for Disease Control and Prevention Behavioral Risk Factor Surveillance System Survey, Internet site http://www.cdc.gov/brfss/index.htm

1.59 Doctor Visits: Could Not See Doctor Because of Cost by Age, 2000

"Was there a time during the last 12 months when you needed
to see a doctor but could not because of the cost?"

(percent of people aged 18 or older responding "yes," by state and age, 2000)

	total	18 to 24	25 to 34	35 to 44	45 to 54	55 to 64	65 or older
U.S. total	**9.9%**	**13.6%**	**13.1%**	**11.5%**	**9.2%**	**8.1%**	**4.4%**
Alabama	12.3	22.5	15.0	11.5	9.1	9.1	3.7
Alaska	12.3	13.8	17.8	17.5	14.9	9.4	4.6
Arizona	11.8	17.4	18.8	13.4	12.6	9.6	2.6
Arkansas	13.0	13.0	17.2	8.9	8.6	8.5	3.0
California	12.8	13.6	10.5	6.6	8.2	4.1	4.7
Colorado	10.0	11.0	8.4	8.5	9.1	6.2	4.4
Connecticut	7.7	11.2	12.9	14.7	10.2	9.5	3.8
Delaware	8.0	18.2	17.5	17.3	13.2	9.2	3.9
District of Columbia	10.7	11.2	12.9	14.7	10.2	9.5	3.8
Florida	12.5	18.2	17.5	17.3	13.2	9.2	3.9
Georgia	11.9	13.1	13.3	14.6	11.8	10.3	6.6
Hawaii	6.4	9.8	7.6	7.0	7.0	3.8	2.5
Idaho	14.0	18.4	18.3	15.0	14.5	13.4	4.7
Illinois	7.2	5.5	10.2	8.0	6.6	7.2	5.0
Indiana	10.0	17.8	13.0	10.6	10.7	5.5	2.6
Iowa	5.8	10.5	5.3	7.6	5.6	5.1	2.2
Kansas	8.0	9.6	12.3	9.0	6.8	7.6	3.2
Kentucky	13.8	15.1	16.2	16.1	15.6	12.4	6.7
Louisiana	12.7	15.5	15.9	14.0	10.4	13.4	6.7
Maine	11.2	15.2	16.3	12.8	7.3	11.7	5.5
Maryland	8.9	13.1	9.8	8.2	9.1	7.0	7.2
Massachusetts	6.3	9.6	8.5	6.2	4.6	5.9	3.7
Michigan	9.0	16.3	9.5	11.5	6.2	6.0	4.7
Minnesota	7.7	12.0	9.4	8.7	6.7	5.9	3.6
Mississippi	16.3	19.8	19.0	18.3	14.2	17.3	8.9
Missouri	9.5	10.8	10.6	12.0	10.9	8.2	4.4
Montana	10.8	10.4	20.5	11.6	10.7	8.7	3.0
Nebraska	5.8	12.1	8.4	5.6	5.1	3.5	2.0
Nevada	14.3	23.3	15.3	12.2	13.6	13.2	12.0
New Hampshire	9.4	15.3	12.6	9.5	7.1	7.0	5.6
New Jersey	7.0	7.0	10.3	6.9	6.6	5.9	4.9
New Mexico	12.6	11.6	18.4	17.3	11.5	7.7	4.8
New York	8.8	11.3	14.0	9.5	6.3	8.8	3.6
North Carolina	12.0	9.8	13.4	16.8	12.5	10.9	6.6
North Dakota	7.1	10.5	9.5	6.6	8.7	4.9	2.9
Ohio	10.4	17.0	14.6	10.8	10.7	7.8	3.2
Oklahoma	9.9	13.9	13.1	12.6	9.7	8.1	2.5
Oregon	12.7	18.5	18.8	15.4	10.5	10.0	4.2
Pennsylvania	8.0	15.0	11.1	9.6	8.1	3.9	2.0
Rhode Island	7.2	12.4	7.8	9.0	7.6	2.9	3.3
South Carolina	12.3	15.5	14.0	13.1	14.1	10.3	5.9
South Dakota	7.2	8.3	7.7	10.0	7.6	5.4	3.6
Tennessee	9.4	10.3	14.7	9.1	9.3	9.7	4.0
Texas	15.1	19.7	18.6	16.7	15.5	13.1	5.5
Utah	10.8	14.9	13.2	13.7	8.2	6.9	3.1
Vermont	8.6	14.1	9.5	8.2	7.6	8.4	4.4
Virginia	9.5	15.3	10.4	11.9	8.2	4.5	5.8
Washington	8.8	16.4	12.9	8.4	6.9	6.0	3.2
West Virginia	16.4	22.4	21.1	22.1	16.3	14.5	5.5
Wisconsin	7.4	9.9	9.0	9.2	6.6	6.6	2.8
Wyoming	12.1	13.6	16.5	13.5	10.9	11.9	5.1

Source: Compiled by New Strategist based on the Centers for Disease Control and Prevention Behavioral Risk Factor Surveillance System Survey, Internet site http://www.cdc.gov/brfss/index.htm

1.60 Doctor Visits: Could Not See Doctor Because of Cost by Education, 2000

"Was there a time during the last 12 months when you needed
to see a doctor but could not because of the cost?"

(percent of people aged 18 or older responding "yes," by state and educational attainment, 2000)

	total	less than high school	high school graduate	some college	college graduate
U.S. total	**9.9%**	**16.5%**	**12.1%**	**9.8%**	**5.4%**
Alabama	12.3	20.7	14.1	10.9	5.0
Alaska	12.3	13.7	13.8	14.1	8.9
Arizona	11.8	19.2	15.9	10.3	5.5
Arkansas	13.0	16.2	14.5	13.6	7.8
California	12.8	24.4	12.1	12.1	6.4
Colorado	10.0	18.9	12.2	9.8	6.5
Connecticut	7.7	13.4	10.7	7.3	4.1
Delaware	8.0	15.3	9.5	7.5	5.2
District of Columbia	10.7	16.4	13.5	12.6	7.4
Florida	12.5	21.2	13.1	13.4	7.2
Georgia	11.9	20.1	13.6	10.4	6.9
Hawaii	6.4	8.9	7.3	6.0	4.9
Idaho	14.0	21.6	16.1	15.3	6.5
Illinois	7.2	14.1	6.0	9.9	3.7
Indiana	10.0	16.2	11.2	10.2	5.6
Iowa	5.8	11.2	6.9	4.7	4.0
Kansas	8.0	16.7	8.8	8.0	4.3
Kentucky	13.8	21.4	14.6	12.5	5.7
Louisiana	12.7	21.4	13.7	11.1	5.7
Maine	11.2	20.7	12.5	11.6	4.7
Maryland	8.9	18.1	10.7	9.8	4.9
Massachusetts	6.3	9.3	6.5	7.2	4.8
Michigan	9.0	15.0	9.7	9.1	5.2
Minnesota	7.7	11.3	9.0	8.2	4.9
Mississippi	16.3	28.4	18.1	13.7	7.1
Missouri	9.5	16.8	9.6	9.9	5.4
Montana	10.8	14.7	12.6	11.8	7.1
Nebraska	5.8	11.8	5.9	5.0	4.7
Nevada	14.3	30.4	18.2	9.2	9.1
New Hampshire	9.4	17.1	12.5	9.5	4.6
New Jersey	7.0	9.7	7.9	7.4	4.6
New Mexico	12.6	23.1	15.4	10.1	5.4
New York	8.8	12.8	9.6	9.0	6.2
North Carolina	12.0	19.6	13.4	11.3	6.0
North Dakota	7.1	6.7	7.3	8.5	5.0
Ohio	10.4	16.4	13.5	10.5	3.6
Oklahoma	9.9	18.1	11.4	7.6	4.9
Oregon	12.7	25.8	13.5	12.0	7.2
Pennsylvania	8.0	9.0	9.0	9.1	5.4
Rhode Island	7.2	7.6	9.0	7.9	4.4
South Carolina	12.3	19.5	15.0	10.7	6.6
South Dakota	7.2	9.0	8.1	7.3	5.1
Tennessee	9.4	13.8	10.7	9.1	3.4
Texas	15.1	25.7	16.5	14.1	7.4
Utah	10.8	20.3	12.4	11.3	6.4
Vermont	8.6	15.2	9.5	9.4	5.3
Virginia	9.5	17.6	14.5	7.1	4.2
Washington	8.8	16.4	11.5	8.3	5.6
West Virginia	16.4	23.8	18.2	14.2	8.5
Wisconsin	7.4	13.1	6.1	9.5	4.6
Wyoming	12.1	18.5	12.2	14.3	7.0

Source: Compiled by New Strategist based on the Centers for Disease Control and Prevention Behavioral Risk Factor Surveillance System Survey, Internet site http://www.cdc.gov/brfss/index.htm

1.61 Doctor Visits: Could Not See Doctor Because of Cost by Household Income, 2000

"Was there a time during the last 12 months when you needed
to see a doctor but could not because of the cost?"

(percent of people aged 18 or older responding "yes," by state and household income, 2000)

	total	less than $15,000	$15,000 to $24,999	$25,000 to $34,999	$35,000 to $49,999	$50,000 or more
U.S. total	**9.9%**	**22.3%**	**18.4%**	**11.9%**	**7.4%**	**3.3%**
Alabama	12.3	26.6	20.5	14.6	6.4	2.4
Alaska	12.3	32.9	20.5	15.2	12.4	5.2
Arizona	11.8	28.6	24.3	10.2	8.8	2.2
Arkansas	13.0	27.6	21.7	11.0	8.1	4.6
California	12.8	26.5	20.7	12.7	9.1	5.0
Colorado	10.0	21.0	20.8	11.9	10.7	2.5
Connecticut	7.7	11.6	15.9	12.8	10.0	3.5
Delaware	8.0	20.7	12.9	10.3	8.6	3.3
District of Columbia	10.7	22.5	18.2	10.8	8.6	5.4
Florida	12.5	26.3	21.6	12.0	9.8	4.3
Georgia	11.9	26.1	23.0	12.5	8.7	4.1
Hawaii	6.4	15.9	9.5	5.3	4.1	2.7
Idaho	14.0	28.3	22.5	15.0	9.5	4.6
Illinois	7.2	15.1	15.2	8.7	5.6	2.1
Indiana	10.0	30.0	18.6	14.0	6.4	2.4
Iowa	5.8	11.9	9.9	6.8	4.8	1.4
Kansas	8.0	20.6	14.1	8.9	5.5	1.8
Kentucky	13.8	30.5	23.4	11.8	7.4	4.0
Louisiana	12.7	26.9	19.8	13.1	6.3	3.2
Maine	11.2	26.8	16.9	12.3	6.0	3.0
Maryland	8.9	21.8	20.0	12.6	9.9	4.1
Massachusetts	6.3	10.9	11.6	9.5	6.4	3.4
Michigan	9.0	19.5	15.5	10.8	7.0	3.5
Minnesota	7.7	16.1	12.8	12.5	7.4	4.0
Mississippi	16.3	34.0	22.6	14.7	7.8	3.6
Missouri	9.5	16.9	14.2	11.2	10.1	3.3
Montana	10.8	22.1	19.5	13.6	5.5	3.8
Nebraska	5.8	12.1	11.7	7.7	2.7	1.9
Nevada	14.3	30.6	19.3	22.1	14.9	6.8
New Hampshire	9.4	27.1	22.4	12.8	7.0	2.5
New Jersey	7.0	20.3	10.1	11.0	8.4	3.3
New Mexico	12.6	27.9	20.7	13.1	6.0	1.9
New York	8.8	18.3	14.7	12.1	5.9	4.5
North Carolina	12.0	24.3	20.8	11.7	9.6	4.1
North Dakota	7.1	15.1	10.9	6.9	3.9	2.8
Ohio	10.4	29.3	20.1	16.2	6.3	3.0
Oklahoma	9.9	23.9	18.3	7.5	5.1	3.5
Oregon	12.7	27.1	23.7	13.7	9.2	2.7
Pennsylvania	8.0	14.2	16.8	9.0	6.9	2.7
Rhode Island	7.2	13.1	12.6	10.2	7.1	1.4
South Carolina	12.3	28.7	20.7	13.5	8.2	3.4
South Dakota	7.2	14.3	13.2	8.1	4.0	1.6
Tennessee	9.4	21.9	14.3	13.8	7.1	2.8
Texas	15.1	37.3	24.2	14.7	9.9	3.7
Utah	10.8	32.3	17.3	11.9	11.6	3.2
Vermont	8.6	18.4	16.8	11.1	6.0	2.6
Virginia	9.5	19.5	25.6	10.7	8.4	2.6
Washington	8.8	18.3	16.4	11.3	9.1	3.3
West Virginia	16.4	33.3	24.4	14.2	9.0	4.5
Wisconsin	7.4	17.3	14.0	11.5	3.7	2.1
Wyoming	12.1	23.3	20.9	13.8	9.0	3.6

Source: Compiled by New Strategist based on the Centers for Disease Control and Prevention Behavioral Risk Factor Surveillance System Survey, Internet site http://www.cdc.gov/brfss/index.htm

1.62 Doctor Visits: Could Not See Doctor Because of Cost by Sex, 2000

"Was there a time during the last 12 months when you needed
to see a doctor but could not because of the cost?"

(percent of people aged 18 or older responding "yes," by state and sex, 2000)

	total	men	women
U.S. total	**9.9%**	**8.1%**	**11.9%**
Alabama	12.3	12.1	12.4
Alaska	12.3	10.1	14.7
Arizona	11.8	9.4	14.1
Arkansas	13.0	9.6	16.1
California	12.8	10.8	14.8
Colorado	10.0	8.0	11.9
Connecticut	7.7	7.6	7.8
Delaware	8.0	6.4	9.4
District of Columbia	10.7	9.2	12.0
Florida	12.5	10.5	14.3
Georgia	11.9	8.8	14.8
Hawaii	6.4	6.1	6.6
Idaho	14.0	10.7	17.1
Illinois	7.2	5.7	8.6
Indiana	10.0	8.3	11.5
Iowa	5.8	4.7	6.9
Kansas	8.0	5.9	10.0
Kentucky	13.8	11.3	16.0
Louisiana	12.7	9.2	15.8
Maine	11.2	9.2	13.0
Maryland	8.9	7.0	10.6
Massachusetts	6.3	6.5	6.2
Michigan	9.0	6.4	11.3
Minnesota	7.7	6.3	8.9
Mississippi	16.3	9.9	21.9
Missouri	9.5	7.3	11.4
Montana	10.8	8.4	13.1
Nebraska	5.8	3.8	7.7
Nevada	14.3	12.7	16.0
New Hampshire	9.4	8.6	10.2
New Jersey	7.0	6.1	7.8
New Mexico	12.6	9.8	15.2
New York	8.8	8.4	9.2
North Carolina	12.0	8.2	15.5
North Dakota	7.1	5.5	8.6
Ohio	10.4	7.6	12.9
Oklahoma	9.9	7.5	12.0
Oregon	12.7	11.8	13.6
Pennsylvania	8.0	6.9	8.9
Rhode Island	7.2	6.6	7.7
South Carolina	12.3	7.7	16.5
South Dakota	7.2	5.0	9.3
Tennessee	9.4	8.2	10.5
Texas	15.1	11.6	18.4
Utah	10.8	8.6	12.8
Vermont	8.6	8.0	9.1
Virginia	9.5	6.5	12.3
Washington	8.8	6.7	10.7
West Virginia	16.4	14.9	17.8
Wisconsin	7.4	5.8	8.8
Wyoming	12.1	9.2	14.9

Source: Compiled by New Strategist based on the Centers for Disease Control and Prevention Behavioral Risk Factor Surveillance System Survey, Internet site http://www.cdc.gov/brfss/index.htm

1.63 Flu Shot in the Last 12 Months by Age, 2001

"During the past 12 months, have you had a flu shot?"

(percent of people aged 18 or older responding "yes," by state and age, 2001)

	total	18 to 24	25 to 34	35 to 44	45 to 54	55 to 64	65 or older
U.S. total	**31.8%**	**20.0%**	**16.5%**	**19.5%**	**27.7%**	**40.1%**	**66.1%**
Alabama	32.1	25.0	20.1	17.6	26.0	40.2	65.9
Alaska	32.1	25.7	25.7	25.9	29.3	44.6	62.8
Arizona	27.8	18.7	14.7	14.8	25.4	31.9	61.8
Arkansas	33.0	18.7	19.8	20.8	30.6	39.1	63.2
California	28.8	17.9	16.1	17.1	23.4	42.2	68.9
Colorado	33.3	21.3	16.8	20.9	32.1	44.2	77.4
Connecticut	32.6	23.1	16.0	18.8	29.2	39.1	69.1
Delaware	31.8	19.1	16.7	22.2	26.8	37.7	67.6
District of Columbia	28.7	17.2	17.5	21.7	29.2	33.3	55.5
Florida	26.9	16.2	14.6	11.2	17.9	30.9	54.9
Georgia	26.8	15.9	16.1	18.6	21.9	35.4	62.2
Hawaii	38.2	27.7	27.4	26.4	27.9	42.5	79.0
Idaho	29.4	16.9	16.4	14.9	25.4	39.9	65.1
Illinois	29.6	26.6	18.8	17.7	26.6	29.6	62.2
Indiana	30.6	18.2	15.4	17.5	28.5	40.1	65.7
Iowa	36.1	18.2	16.8	21.6	32.8	47.3	72.8
Kansas	33.0	22.9	16.4	19.8	27.2	43.8	68.5
Kentucky	29.2	21.5	15.6	15.6	26.6	37.2	60.9
Louisiana	25.9	22.5	18.0	15.0	19.3	29.7	56.1
Maine	35.0	23.7	18.4	21.3	30.8	44.8	71.5
Maryland	30.6	18.1	16.5	21.1	27.0	40.3	67.3
Massachusetts	32.0	19.7	15.9	19.0	27.5	38.7	70.6
Michigan	26.8	20.5	13.1	14.0	21.7	35.7	60.4
Minnesota	34.5	21.4	19.0	20.1	34.0	47.4	70.1
Mississippi	29.5	18.1	18.0	19.4	23.2	37.5	61.8
Missouri	34.3	17.9	16.3	22.1	30.8	47.8	67.5
Montana	35.3	23.5	15.3	23.8	29.8	44.0	73.1
Nebraska	35.5	25.1	17.9	21.4	31.7	47.6	70.1
Nevada	27.5	17.7	14.6	13.8	24.5	36.9	63.3
New Hampshire	29.8	20.0	15.5	15.8	25.8	39.8	69.8
New Jersey	29.6	20.4	18.1	16.6	23.1	34.6	64.5
New Mexico	31.8	20.5	15.8	20.7	30.3	40.3	70.0
New York	28.7	15.0	16.9	17.5	23.1	36.7	62.5
North Carolina	31.0	18.6	16.5	20.6	26.9	41.5	66.1
North Dakota	34.8	20.0	19.7	20.6	31.4	46.1	70.0
Ohio	29.5	14.6	14.5	16.3	26.3	43.0	63.4
Oklahoma	36.4	18.7	18.3	23.6	34.5	49.3	72.7
Oregon	33.4	20.1	14.7	23.2	29.1	39.8	71.1
Pennsylvania	29.7	20.9	10.2	16.4	23.4	37.7	63.8
Rhode Island	17.2	22.4	17.1	19.7	31.9	46.5	72.6
South Carolina	35.4	23.3	20.8	21.8	29.1	38.5	66.2
South Dakota	32.5	29.6	22.9	27.9	37.7	51.1	74.1
Tennessee	40.9	20.3	20.9	20.3	28.3	45.6	65.6
Texas	33.1	19.8	19.4	22.1	26.9	37.0	61.8
Utah	29.9	18.7	14.4	17.8	29.3	38.5	68.7
Vermont	28.6	18.9	14.0	18.3	26.1	42.6	71.5
Virginia	30.9	22.2	18.3	20.5	31.3	44.9	65.3
Washington	32.3	21.2	18.1	22.1	29.4	44.3	72.5
West Virginia	33.7	14.4	15.9	17.8	31.2	43.1	61.7
Wisconsin	31.9	13.7	17.1	20.5	27.9	45.7	70.4
Wyoming	32.7	22.1	15.3	19.4	28.3	44.1	69.6

Source: Compiled by New Strategist based on the Centers for Disease Control and Prevention Behavioral Risk Factor Surveillance System Survey. Internet site http://www.cdc.gov/brfss/index.htm

1.64 Flu Shot in the Last 12 Months by Education, 2001

"During the past 12 months, have you had a flu shot?"

(percent of people aged 18 or older responding "yes," by state and educational attainment, 2001)

	total	less than high school	high school graduate	some college	college graduate
U.S. total	**31.8%**	**32.9%**	**30.0%**	**29.7%**	**32.6%**
Alabama	32.1	37.5	31.4	28.9	33.4
Alaska	32.1	32.2	24.2	32.0	40.5
Arizona	27.8	24.4	29.4	24.9	31.2
Arkansas	33.0	36.6	30.0	31.7	36.7
California	28.8	25.7	27.1	28.8	32.1
Colorado	33.3	24.0	34.9	33.9	34.6
Connecticut	32.6	33.4	33.3	30.4	33.4
Delaware	31.8	30.3	30.0	29.2	35.6
District of Columbia	28.7	24.3	30.1	27.5	29.5
Florida	26.9	26.1	25.9	25.7	29.7
Georgia	26.8	27.5	25.2	24.7	29.3
Hawaii	38.2	50.3	38.2	38.4	35.5
Idaho	29.4	33.5	28.1	29.5	29.4
Illinois	29.6	30.3	28.8	30.4	29.3
Indiana	30.6	31.9	30.1	30.7	30.7
Iowa	36.1	39.2	38.0	33.3	34.7
Kansas	33.0	37.2	35.6	31.3	30.8
Kentucky	29.2	31.2	26.9	29.3	31.5
Louisiana	25.9	28.6	23.6	26.7	26.5
Maine	35.0	44.1	32.8	34.6	35.4
Maryland	30.6	36.0	27.1	29.8	32.5
Massachusetts	32.0	35.6	35.5	32.4	31.4
Michigan	26.8	32.2	24.4	27.0	27.2
Minnesota	34.5	42.7	35.4	33.6	32.8
Mississippi	29.5	27.2	28.6	29.6	32.1
Missouri	34.3	38.9	35.2	29.5	35.6
Montana	35.3	35.8	34.1	35.1	36.9
Nebraska	35.5	44.0	37.4	31.6	34.0
Nevada	27.5	26.2	24.2	27.0	32.3
New Hampshire	29.8	32.3	28.1	28.6	31.9
New Jersey	29.6	32.9	30.8	29.0	28.0
New Mexico	31.8	27.3	30.0	33.0	35.6
New York	28.7	32.6	28.0	28.4	28.2
North Carolina	31.0	34.3	30.4	29.5	31.3
North Dakota	34.8	48.5	36.0	27.7	36.9
Ohio	29.5	33.4	30.0	25.7	30.7
Oklahoma	36.4	32.2	37.6	32.2	42.5
Oregon	33.4	29.6	34.9	31.4	35.5
Pennsylvania	29.7	35.8	29.6	28.2	29.0
Rhode Island	17.2	41.5	37.3	31.2	34.4
South Carolina	35.4	34.4	29.8	33.7	33.4
South Dakota	32.5	49.7	39.3	39.9	40.8
Tennessee	40.9	37.5	31.1	30.9	37.0
Texas	33.1	26.1	29.0	29.8	33.6
Utah	29.9	32.9	28.7	25.5	31.1
Vermont	28.6	41.2	29.5	28.3	32.0
Virginia	30.9	37.4	28.9	32.8	33.3
Washington	32.3	30.3	33.5	30.9	37.5
West Virginia	33.7	35.4	28.9	32.1	35.7
Wisconsin	31.9	38.8	32.0	28.1	36.4
Wyoming	32.7	32.7	31.5	31.1	33.1

Source: Compiled by New Strategist based on the Centers for Disease Control and Prevention Behavioral Risk Factor Surveillance System Survey, Internet site http://www.cdc.gov/brfss/index.htm

1.65 Flu Shot in the Last 12 Months by Household Income, 2001

"During the past 12 months, have you had a flu shot?"

(percent of people aged 18 or older responding "yes," by state and household income, 2001)

	total	less than $15,000	$15,000 to $24,999	$25,000 to $34,999	$35,000 to $49,999	$50,000 or more
U.S. total	**31.8%**	**31.8%**	**32.6%**	**30.5%**	**28.6%**	**29.0%**
Alabama	32.1	31.4	32.8	27.9	31.9	28.9
Alaska	32.1	29.6	29.9	32.0	27.5	33.4
Arizona	27.8	25.8	34.5	33.0	29.3	31.3
Arkansas	33.0	30.0	30.5	28.3	24.5	27.2
California	28.8	29.2	31.9	31.7	37.1	30.8
Colorado	33.3	29.2	31.9	31.7	37.1	30.8
Connecticut	32.6	43.7	38.5	23.7	30.8	30.5
Delaware	31.8	31.1	33.3	23.7	30.8	30.5
District of Columbia	28.7	28.6	27.5	27.4	24.9	23.1
Florida	26.9	25.9	27.5	27.4	24.9	23.1
Georgia	26.8	27.0	27.9	24.3	25.9	25.9
Hawaii	38.2	37.3	41.6	36.5	39.5	33.3
Idaho	29.4	31.9	29.3	30.6	26.6	26.1
Illinois	29.6	30.0	35.7	34.0	24.1	24.9
Indiana	30.6	37.3	35.3	26.5	28.4	26.1
Iowa	36.1	39.1	43.5	33.8	33.7	30.6
Kansas	33.0	34.2	38.2	30.1	30.9	29.2
Kentucky	29.2	28.8	27.3	25.2	24.9	28.0
Louisiana	25.9	31.4	26.9	27.8	23.2	22.6
Maine	35.0	41.7	40.6	35.9	31.4	28.8
Maryland	30.6	25.3	31.2	31.1	31.9	29.1
Massachusetts	32.0	35.5	40.6	33.5	28.9	27.4
Michigan	26.8	32.6	30.1	27.4	25.5	22.2
Minnesota	34.5	45.3	41.5	36.9	32.7	30.2
Mississippi	29.5	30.4	32.7	26.6	27.6	28.8
Missouri	34.3	41.2	33.3	35.5	29.7	31.0
Montana	35.3	37.4	32.5	30.3	29.5	37.4
Nebraska	35.5	41.1	39.8	34.3	29.5	32.1
Nevada	27.5	35.3	29.8	27.1	24.4	24.6
New Hampshire	29.8	41.3	32.2	34.1	24.9	26.8
New Jersey	29.6	29.6	34.5	32.3	26.5	26.2
New Mexico	31.8	30.2	31.0	29.6	30.4	32.2
New York	28.7	31.4	31.3	30.4	24.9	25.6
North Carolina	31.0	36.9	30.6	34.2	25.4	29.4
North Dakota	34.8	31.4	31.3	30.4	24.9	25.6
Ohio	29.5	36.9	30.6	34.2	25.4	29.4
Oklahoma	36.4	35.0	37.1	34.2	31.3	32.5
Oregon	33.4	37.6	33.2	33.2	34.1	36.8
Pennsylvania	29.7	31.7	33.4	34.6	30.7	32.6
Rhode Island	17.2	31.1	36.7	31.2	28.4	23.1
South Carolina	35.4	37.0	43.1	38.1	29.9	30.5
South Dakota	32.5	33.7	30.7	28.1	31.3	33.9
Tennessee	40.9	44.5	42.8	39.1	36.5	38.9
Texas	33.1	33.1	31.2	28.8	27.2	33.7
Utah	29.9	30.4	31.6	30.7	27.5	26.2
Vermont	28.6	39.7	32.9	28.7	28.0	29.0
Virginia	30.9	38.3	34.4	26.9	26.7	32.9
Washington	32.3	29.7	34.3	32.5	30.7	32.6
West Virginia	33.7	29.5	32.5	28.9	30.6	32.4
Wisconsin	31.9	34.9	39.0	31.2	31.4	28.6
Wyoming	32.7	33.9	31.9	30.4	25.1	33.5

Source: Compiled by New Strategist based on the Centers for Disease Control and Prevention Behavioral Risk Factor Surveillance System Survey, Internet site http://www.cdc.gov/brfss/index.htm

1.66 Flu Shot in the Last 12 Months by Sex, 2001

"During the past 12 months, have you had a flu shot?"

(percent of people aged 18 or older responding "yes," by state and sex, 2001)

	total	men	women
U.S. total	**31.8%**	**30.6%**	**32.1%**
Alabama	32.1	32.4	31.9
Alaska	32.1	35.5	28.4
Arizona	27.8	27.1	28.5
Arkansas	33.0	32.2	33.8
California	28.8	27.8	29.8
Colorado	33.3	31.9	34.7
Connecticut	32.6	31.1	34.0
Delaware	31.8	32.1	31.5
District of Columbia	28.7	29.0	28.4
Florida	26.9	25.9	27.9
Georgia	26.8	27.3	26.3
Hawaii	38.2	36.7	39.7
Idaho	29.4	28.0	30.8
Illinois	29.6	29.7	29.5
Indiana	30.6	29.2	31.8
Iowa	36.1	32.5	39.4
Kansas	33.0	31.8	34.2
Kentucky	29.2	30.1	28.4
Louisiana	25.9	24.2	27.4
Maine	35.0	34.4	35.5
Maryland	30.6	30.6	30.5
Massachusetts	32.0	30.6	33.2
Michigan	26.8	25.8	27.7
Minnesota	34.5	30.1	38.8
Mississippi	29.5	28.8	30.1
Missouri	34.3	33.2	35.2
Montana	35.3	33.4	37.1
Nebraska	35.5	33.9	37.0
Nevada	27.5	27.7	27.3
New Hampshire	29.8	27.2	32.3
New Jersey	29.6	28.7	30.4
New Mexico	31.8	31.4	32.2
New York	28.7	28.5	28.9
North Carolina	31.0	29.5	32.4
North Dakota	34.8	30.7	38.8
Ohio	29.5	29.8	29.2
Oklahoma	36.4	35.2	37.5
Oregon	33.4	31.2	35.5
Pennsylvania	29.7	27.0	32.1
Rhode Island	17.2	32.0	38.5
South Carolina	35.4	33.6	31.5
South Dakota	32.5	37.6	44.1
Tennessee	40.9	32.5	33.7
Texas	33.1	30.6	29.4
Utah	29.9	26.5	30.6
Vermont	28.6	29.7	32.1
Virginia	30.9	30.7	33.8
Washington	32.3	32.9	34.4
West Virginia	33.7	31.6	32.2
Wisconsin	31.9	30.9	34.4
Wyoming	32.7	31.4	32.4

Source: Compiled by New Strategist based on the Centers for Disease Control and Prevention Behavioral Risk Factor Surveillance System Survey, Internet site http://www.cdc.gov/brfss/index.htm

1.67 Health Insurance by Age, 2001

"Do you have any kind of health care coverage?"

(percent of people aged 18 or older responding "yes," by state and age, 2001)

	total	18 to 24	25 to 34	35 to 44	45 to 54	55 to 64	65 or older
U.S. total	**86.7%**	**74.6%**	**81.9%**	**85.7%**	**88.5%**	**89.8%**	**98.2%**
Alabama	85.0	73.7	81.9	83.6	85.8	84.6	98.0
Alaska	81.2	74.3	78.6	79.3	86.4	76.9	96.5
Arizona	83.1	66.6	74.2	80.7	85.6	90.7	98.6
Arkansas	83.9	73.7	75.4	82.8	83.9	83.5	98.9
California	85.0	74.8	78.7	82.0	88.3	90.5	97.9
Colorado	84.7	69.0	77.3	85.0	87.8	88.1	98.7
Connecticut	90.5	76.2	86.1	91.8	91.6	93.8	98.3
Delaware	91.4	80.0	87.5	92.4	94.6	93.2	97.9
District of Columbia	87.7	81.2	84.7	87.0	87.1	88.3	97.2
Florida	83.2	63.6	77.1	81.4	80.6	84.9	97.4
Georgia	86.2	77.3	81.9	83.9	88.6	88.4	98.8
Hawaii	92.7	83.3	90.7	93.2	91.4	95.8	99.6
Idaho	85.2	69.7	79.1	82.3	89.5	87.9	99.4
Illinois	90.1	81.6	86.9	89.8	90.2	91.7	98.4
Indiana	86.3	70.5	80.6	87.7	88.5	89.5	98.0
Iowa	91.9	79.0	89.8	92.3	92.7	94.1	99.7
Kansas	89.9	79.5	86.2	90.3	91.1	91.0	98.3
Kentucky	84.9	73.6	78.3	83.1	87.4	86.7	97.8
Louisiana	77.9	65.1	70.6	77.0	77.9	83.7	94.7
Maine	87.1	73.8	82.6	86.6	88.4	89.8	97.2
Maryland	89.7	78.1	85.1	90.4	91.3	93.7	97.7
Massachusetts	92.1	82.4	88.7	91.8	94.6	93.8	98.5
Michigan	90.4	82.4	85.1	90.0	92.2	91.6	99.6
Minnesota	94.5	87.2	92.2	94.6	95.6	97.0	99.0
Mississippi	81.3	68.8	78.1	79.6	80.4	82.8	97.1
Missouri	89.4	77.4	85.9	85.4	92.7	93.2	98.6
Montana	83.1	77.8	73.8	79.3	83.8	82.7	98.6
Nebraska	86.0	68.8	81.4	86.0	87.2	93.2	96.7
Nevada	82.5	66.1	78.3	81.9	78.9	91.1	96.5
New Hampshire	88.5	76.1	84.2	88.1	91.1	91.4	98.3
New Jersey	88.7	74.5	84.1	88.0	90.6	91.6	97.9
New Mexico	77.5	61.8	65.4	75.6	81.5	83.2	98.3
New York	83.7	67.2	74.1	83.8	86.4	88.2	97.5
North Carolina	85.8	73.2	81.8	85.4	86.2	88.7	97.4
North Dakota	88.3	71.4	86.9	88.8	90.4	89.7	98.7
Ohio	88.9	82.8	84.7	85.9	91.2	90.3	97.8
Oklahoma	79.2	62.5	69.9	77.3	80.1	83.9	97.2
Oregon	86.1	73.7	79.4	84.4	87.9	89.2	98.3
Pennsylvania	90.8	82.3	87.0	88.5	91.6	92.8	98.8
Rhode Island	91.4	77.7	90.3	92.6	92.7	91.6	98.7
South Carolina	83.6	69.9	79.7	83.7	84.3	84.9	97.1
South Dakota	89.8	77.8	86.8	90.5	91.1	89.8	98.2
Tennessee	89.3	80.6	86.6	88.0	90.9	90.4	97.3
Texas	77.1	59.7	69.1	76.3	79.6	81.8	97.7
Utah	87.2	80.7	80.2	85.5	90.9	91.5	98.4
Vermont	88.5	74.5	84.7	89.7	90.3	92.2	98.6
Virginia	89.1	78.1	84.5	89.7	91.4	90.5	98.9
Washington	90.3	76.8	85.2	90.0	93.5	94.0	99.2
West Virginia	80.7	64.0	69.8	75.2	86.4	82.6	98.5
Wisconsin	90.2	78.5	88.0	90.3	92.9	88.9	98.7
Wyoming	83.3	66.6	79.6	83.5	85.1	82.8	98.0

Source: Compiled by New Strategist based on the Centers for Disease Control and Prevention Behavioral Risk Factor Surveillance System Survey, Internet site http://www.cdc.gov/brfss/index.htm

1.68 Health Insurance by Education, 2001

"Do you have any kind of health care coverage?"

(percent of people aged 18 or older responding "yes," by state and educational attainment, 2001)

	total	less than high school	high school graduate	some college	college graduate
U.S. total	**86.7%**	**76.4%**	**84.0%**	**87.4%**	**94.0%**
Alabama	85.0	76.3	82.5	85.6	95.1
Alaska	81.2	65.5	76.3	80.3	92.2
Arizona	83.1	60.6	78.6	85.4	94.6
Arkansas	83.9	76.0	78.8	85.1	95.6
California	85.0	65.9	84.5	87.0	94.0
Colorado	84.7	58.5	79.4	88.2	93.8
Connecticut	90.5	78.2	86.1	90.8	96.1
Delaware	91.4	81.7	89.1	91.5	95.9
District of Columbia	87.7	79.0	84.2	83.1	93.8
Florida	83.2	65.7	80.9	85.6	91.2
Georgia	86.2	75.3	83.8	86.4	93.4
Hawaii	92.7	87.2	91.3	92.9	95.3
Idaho	85.2	73.8	80.5	85.0	94.8
Illinois	90.1	78.0	87.9	91.2	95.1
Indiana	86.3	71.3	85.4	86.5	93.7
Iowa	91.9	86.0	90.2	91.8	96.7
Kansas	89.9	77.3	88.2	89.7	94.8
Kentucky	84.9	75.1	83.9	87.0	94.0
Louisiana	77.9	65.5	73.6	81.5	90.3
Maine	87.1	79.5	82.1	87.4	95.8
Maryland	89.7	73.2	86.1	90.7	95.8
Massachusetts	92.1	82.4	88.8	92.6	96.0
Michigan	90.4	82.8	86.8	92.2	95.9
Minnesota	94.5	90.0	92.7	94.8	96.9
Mississippi	81.3	69.7	77.4	84.2	93.0
Missouri	89.4	83.5	86.4	90.2	95.3
Montana	83.1	72.9	80.4	82.5	91.0
Nebraska	86.0	77.3	81.8	86.9	95.0
Nevada	82.5	63.1	81.1	84.4	88.0
New Hampshire	88.5	79.5	83.3	89.9	84.0
New Jersey	88.7	76.9	85.3	88.8	94.6
New Mexico	77.5	57.0	73.2	82.2	91.5
New York	83.7	60.8	84.2	85.8	90.8
North Carolina	85.8	72.4	84.6	87.5	93.3
North Dakota	88.3	85.7	85.2	87.4	93.6
Ohio	88.9	80.6	86.9	90.4	94.0
Oklahoma	79.2	64.7	76.5	81.3	89.6
Oregon	86.1	67.7	83.6	88.4	93.9
Pennsylvania	90.8	84.3	89.1	92.9	94.5
Rhode Island	91.4	84.4	87.7	94.1	95.9
South Carolina	83.6	71.2	81.8	82.8	93.5
South Dakota	89.8	87.9	85.4	89.5	96.0
Tennessee	89.3	85.1	88.0	88.7	95.4
Texas	77.1	50.8	75.7	82.5	92.2
Utah	87.2	78.2	81.7	88.1	93.9
Vermont	88.5	86.1	83.1	89.6	93.9
Virginia	89.1	71.6	86.4	90.6	95.9
Washington	90.3	76.6	85.4	91.6	96.2
West Virginia	80.7	77.3	77.4	81.9	91.9
Wisconsin	90.2	83.3	87.4	90.3	96.1
Wyoming	83.3	67.6	80.4	83.5	91.2

Source: Compiled by New Strategist based on the Centers for Disease Control and Prevention Behavioral Risk Factor Surveillance System Survey, Internet site http://www.cdc.gov/brfss/index.htm

1.69 Health Insurance by Household Income, 2001

"Do you have any kind of health care coverage?"

(percent of people aged 18 or older responding "yes," by state and household income, 2001)

	total	less than $15,000	$15,000 to $24,999	$25,000 to $34,999	$35,000 to $49,999	$50,000 or more
U.S. total	**86.7%**	**73.2%**	**75.5%**	**84.1%**	**91.6%**	**95.9%**
Alabama	85.0	73.2	74.8	82.2	87.9	98.3
Alaska	81.2	60.7	66.9	75.1	82.8	93.0
Arizona	83.1	62.2	64.4	79.6	90.2	94.4
Arkansas	83.9	77.3	72.2	80.4	90.1	94.0
California	85.0	67.4	72.1	86.0	87.5	95.3
Colorado	84.7	58.3	65.1	82.1	87.7	96.4
Connecticut	90.5	80.0	79.8	83.3	93.3	96.7
Delaware	91.4	82.7	84.2	82.1	90.6	97.5
District of Columbia	87.7	76.7	71.8	90.1	92.0	95.1
Florida	83.2	69.1	71.3	82.2	87.6	94.0
Georgia	86.2	71.4	69.6	80.9	93.0	96.9
Hawaii	92.7	79.9	90.8	94.6	95.1	97.6
Idaho	85.2	71.0	71.1	82.1	92.0	97.1
Illinois	90.1	75.7	78.9	86.7	94.1	97.0
Indiana	86.3	75.1	76.6	86.1	89.3	93.3
Iowa	91.9	79.9	84.1	91.5	94.2	98.8
Kansas	89.9	78.8	80.6	86.9	92.0	97.4
Kentucky	84.9	69.3	69.9	88.1	92.4	96.0
Louisiana	77.9	64.6	64.1	77.6	85.2	93.2
Maine	87.1	77.8	76.3	85.7	93.6	94.0
Maryland	89.7	72.1	79.4	82.0	92.6	97.7
Massachusetts	92.1	84.8	84.1	89.3	92.2	97.0
Michigan	90.4	82.0	76.5	88.5	94.8	95.9
Minnesota	94.5	88.4	88.5	88.5	95.9	97.8
Mississippi	81.3	68.8	76.5	81.7	91.6	94.7
Missouri	89.4	80.8	77.3	85.8	92.7	97.1
Montana	83.1	71.5	70.7	81.3	89.8	95.2
Nebraska	86.0	80.2	79.6	81.5	90.2	95.4
Nevada	82.5	63.2	62.6	83.9	87.5	91.4
New Hampshire	88.5	79.0	72.7	83.1	89.0	94.7
New Jersey	88.7	69.7	76.7	85.6	91.8	94.9
New Mexico	77.5	57.2	63.7	76.0	86.6	94.3
New York	83.7	68.6	71.2	83.4	86.4	94.7
North Carolina	85.8	73.3	74.5	83.3	90.5	96.3
North Dakota	88.3	69.9	80.5	89.1	92.1	96.5
Ohio	88.9	77.3	82.2	86.0	90.9	96.0
Oklahoma	79.2	62.8	67.1	76.8	86.4	92.6
Oregon	86.1	73.8	72.3	84.3	91.6	95.9
Pennsylvania	90.8	83.4	85.1	88.8	92.3	96.4
Rhode Island	91.4	83.5	86.2	87.1	93.5	97.8
South Carolina	83.6	66.2	70.2	82.2	88.7	95.1
South Dakota	89.8	77.3	82.6	88.7	93.9	96.9
Tennessee	89.3	79.0	81.4	88.5	94.3	94.6
Texas	77.1	52.1	62.1	73.9	86.2	95.1
Utah	87.2	68.0	75.5	83.6	91.8	94.8
Vermont	88.5	84.2	80.5	84.8	89.2	95.3
Virginia	89.1	72.6	75.5	89.2	92.1	97.1
Washington	90.3	78.2	76.0	88.9	92.5	96.5
West Virginia	80.7	68.2	70.7	79.6	89.6	96.0
Wisconsin	90.2	84.3	80.8	86.4	94.9	96.1
Wyoming	83.3	72.2	71.6	78.4	88.5	92.2

Source: Compiled by New Strategist based on the Centers for Disease Control and Prevention Behavioral Risk Factor Surveillance System Survey, Internet site http://www.cdc.gov/brfss/index.htm

1.70 Health Insurance by Sex, 2001

"Do you have any kind of health care coverage?"

(percent of people aged 18 or older responding "yes," by state and sex, 2001)

	total	men	women
U.S. total	**86.7%**	**85.0%**	**88.1%**
Alabama	85.0	85.3	84.7
Alaska	81.2	81.1	81.4
Arizona	83.1	82.9	83.3
Arkansas	83.9	84.3	83.6
California	85.0	84.1	85.9
Colorado	84.7	83.9	85.5
Connecticut	90.5	89.0	91.9
Delaware	91.4	89.1	93.5
District of Columbia	87.7	83.9	91.0
Florida	83.2	81.9	84.4
Georgia	86.2	84.8	87.5
Hawaii	92.7	91.1	94.3
Idaho	85.2	84.8	85.6
Illinois	90.1	89.4	90.7
Indiana	86.3	84.8	87.7
Iowa	91.9	92.1	91.8
Kansas	89.9	89.4	90.5
Kentucky	84.9	84.8	85.0
Louisiana	77.9	77.2	78.6
Maine	87.1	84.4	89.5
Maryland	89.7	88.7	90.7
Massachusetts	92.1	90.6	93.4
Michigan	90.4	89.8	90.9
Minnesota	94.5	93.0	95.9
Mississippi	81.3	80.5	82.0
Missouri	89.4	88.5	90.2
Montana	83.1	83.4	82.9
Nebraska	86.0	85.5	86.5
Nevada	82.5	79.6	85.4
New Hampshire	88.5	86.2	90.6
New Jersey	88.7	87.6	89.7
New Mexico	77.5	75.5	79.4
New York	83.7	80.7	86.4
North Carolina	85.8	84.3	87.0
North Dakota	88.3	86.4	90.1
Ohio	88.9	88.2	89.5
Oklahoma	79.2	77.5	80.8
Oregon	86.1	84.4	87.6
Pennsylvania	90.8	88.2	93.1
Rhode Island	91.4	88.9	93.8
South Carolina	83.6	83.0	84.1
South Dakota	89.8	88.3	91.2
Tennessee	89.3	86.4	91.9
Texas	77.1	77.2	77.0
Utah	87.2	85.6	88.6
Vermont	88.5	85.6	91.2
Virginia	89.1	88.0	90.2
Washington	90.3	89.5	91.1
West Virginia	80.7	79.1	82.2
Wisconsin	90.2	88.7	91.7
Wyoming	83.3	83.5	83.1

Source: Compiled by New Strategist based on the Centers for Disease Control and Prevention Behavioral Risk Factor Surveillance System Survey, Internet site http://www.cdc.gov/brfss/index.htm

1.71 Health Insurance Coverage Gaps in Past 12 Months by Age, 2001

Among those with health insurance, "During the past 12 months, was there any time that you did not have any health insurance or coverage?"

(percent of people aged 18 or older with health insurance responding "yes," by state and age, 2001)

	total	18 to 24	25 to 34	35 to 44	45 to 54	55 to 64	65 or older
U.S. total	**6.5%**	**14.4%**	**10.7%**	**6.3%**	**4.7%**	**3.6%**	**2.5%**
Alabama	5.7	11.4	8.0	6.5	4.8	3.7	1.9
Alaska	7.2	11.6	11.9	7.1	4.0	5.0	1.7
Arizona	8.8	22.8	12.7	8.2	9.6	3.6	2.6
Arkansas	7.1	17.2	11.4	9.0	4.6	4.6	1.5
California	8.2	22.8	12.1	7.9	4.7	4.3	2.9
Colorado	7.7	20.5	14.5	6.2	5.3	1.0	3.3
Connecticut	5.7	11.6	10.5	5.3	4.8	2.4	2.1
Delaware	5.8	8.9	8.6	6.5	4.7	3.0	3.5
District of Columbia	7.8	18.1	8.5	10.4	6.9	3.7	1.3
Florida	7.8	14.2	11.7	10.0	7.4	4.7	4.4
Georgia	7.2	13.0	10.5	6.8	7.3	2.9	2.9
Hawaii	4.9	8.2	7.3	4.7	3.3	3.6	3.4
Idaho	6.9	18.4	13.1	6.7	5.5	2.4	0.6
Illinois	6.0	16.0	9.0	6.1	4.0	3.7	0.7
Indiana	6.3	14.1	10.9	6.2	5.4	3.1	1.4
Iowa	4.5	13.8	7.5	4.6	2.5	1.5	0.9
Kansas	5.9	13.5	9.4	6.3	3.8	2.9	2.3
Kentucky	6.0	15.6	7.6	6.0	4.3	2.8	3.3
Louisiana	7.7	12.6	11.6	8.3	6.4	4.9	3.6
Maine	7.6	14.4	12.2	9.0	7.0	4.2	1.9
Maryland	5.5	12.1	9.6	4.6	4.0	3.9	2.0
Massachusetts	5.9	13.5	10.3	5.8	3.6	0.8	0.6
Michigan	5.4	13.5	10.3	5.8	3.6	0.8	0.6
Minnesota	5.5	18.7	7.6	4.4	3.8	2.3	0.4
Mississippi	8.6	20.6	10.1	8.6	5.5	3.8	5.4
Missouri	5.9	13.4	9.1	4.6	2.8	3.7	4.8
Montana	11.0	21.0	13.8	10.8	8.1	7.9	8.8
Nebraska	6.3	8.5	12.2	7.2	3.7	2.2	4.3
Nevada	8.0	16.6	12.8	10.1	7.0	3.9	1.3
New Hampshire	6.6	17.0	11.7	4.7	4.1	3.3	2.4
New Jersey	6.4	14.9	10.9	6.2	5.5	2.4	2.8
New Mexico	8.0	17.8	13.7	9.7	3.8	3.9	3.2
New York	8.1	19.0	11.7	8.9	6.2	4.8	3.8
North Carolina	7.1	15.5	10.5	5.1	6.4	3.9	4.3
North Dakota	4.2	12.8	6.4	4.3	2.3	1.4	1.0
Ohio	5.1	9.8	7.4	6.9	3.5	2.1	1.9
Oklahoma	7.1	11.1	11.3	6.3	7.8	5.0	4.0
Oregon	8.7	20.4	16.3	11.9	3.9	4.0	2.0
Pennsylvania	5.0	15.2	10.1	3.0	3.8	1.2	1.3
Rhode Island	4.9	12.3	7.3	5.3	4.7	1.6	0.8
South Carolina	6.0	11.5	10.2	6.0	3.7	2.8	3.5
South Dakota	5.4	14.8	6.9	4.8	2.8	3.6	3.1
Tennessee	6.0	8.1	6.9	6.6	5.7	3	5.9
Texas	7.5	18.8	11.1	7.7	4.3	3.7	2.9
Utah	6.6	11.5	11.4	6.3	4.8	3.4	1.5
Vermont	6.8	15.2	12.3	6.0	4.7	4.0	2.1
Virginia	5.4	14.4	8.9	4.5	2.9	4.6	1.0
Washington	6.0	11.5	11.5	6.5	4.7	2.8	1.3
West Virginia	9.0	23.8	13.0	8.6	6.4	4.7	5.8
Wisconsin	4.5	9.2	9.5	3.4	3.7	1.4	1.3
Wyoming	7.6	21.4	12.5	6.7	4.5	3.8	2.9

Source: Compiled by New Strategist based on the Centers for Disease Control and Prevention Behavioral Risk Factor Surveillance System Survey. Internet site http://www.cdc.gov/brfss/index.htm

1.72 Health Insurance Coverage Gaps in Past 12 Months by Education, 2001

Among those with health insurance, "During the past 12 months, was there
any time that you did not have any health insurance or coverage?"

(percent of people aged 18 or older responding "yes," by state and educational attainment, 2001)

	total	less than high school	high school graduate	some college	college graduate
U.S. total	6.5%	9.5%	7.1%	6.6%	4.7%
Alabama	5.7	8.1	7.0	5.9	2.2
Alaska	7.2	12.0	6.1	7.1	7.5
Arizona	8.8	14.0	8.8	9.2	6.3
Arkansas	7.1	7.5	8.5	7.5	4.9
California	8.2	13.1	9.3	9.0	5.3
Colorado	7.7	16.6	7.0	8.7	5.5
Connecticut	5.7	15.4	6.4	5.3	3.6
Delaware	5.8	9.7	6.1	5.3	5.1
District of Columbia	7.8	6.7	9.5	8.9	6.9
Florida	7.8	15.1	7.6	7.6	6.1
Georgia	7.2	7.2	8.7	8.5	4.9
Hawaii	4.9	7.2	4.9	5.6	3.8
Idaho	6.9	6.6	8.4	7.5	5.0
Illinois	6.0	4.0	6.4	8.1	4.5
Indiana	6.3	9.9	5.7	8.1	4.4
Iowa	4.5	6.7	4.2	5.8	3.0
Kansas	5.9	13.4	5.5	6.1	4.7
Kentucky	6.0	6.6	5.9	6.9	4.9
Louisiana	7.7	8.5	10.0	6.5	5.2
Maine	7.6	4.6	9.9	6.2	7.0
Maryland	5.5	11.9	5.9	6.5	3.6
Massachusetts	5.9	11.2	6.8	5.8	4.5
Michigan	5.4	4.8	5.5	6.9	3.9
Minnesota	5.5	5.4	7.4	6.3	3.2
Mississippi	8.6	11.6	8.9	9.2	5.7
Missouri	5.9	9.4	6.1	4.9	5.2
Montana	11.0	10.5	10.2	13.8	9.2
Nebraska	6.3	10.4	7.7	5.4	3.9
Nevada	8.0	5.9	12.0	6.8	6.1
New Hampshire	6.6	9.5	7.7	8.0	4.2
New Jersey	6.4	11.8	7.5	5.3	5.1
New Mexico	8.0	11.8	8.1	7.9	6.3
New York	8.1	16.4	7.9	7.9	6.1
North Carolina	7.1	10.6	6.4	9.1	4.7
North Dakota	4.2	4.9	4.4	4.9	3.0
Ohio	5.1	9.0	5.4	5.2	3.1
Oklahoma	7.1	10.2	8.0	7.1	4.3
Oregon	8.7	20.7	7.6	10.2	4.8
Pennsylvania	5.0	5.5	5.5	5.4	3.9
Rhode Island	4.9	5.8	5.8	6.2	2.7
South Carolina	6.0	9.7	6.9	6.5	3.2
South Dakota	5.4	9.4	5.3	5.8	3.8
Tennessee	6.0	9.6	6.7	5.0	4.1
Texas	7.5	10.8	8.0	8.7	4.7
Utah	6.6	11.9	6.5	6.1	6.3
Vermont	6.8	8.6	7.6	6.4	6.1
Virginia	5.4	4.8	7.3	6.2	3.7
Washington	6.0	11.9	6.9	6.1	4.3
West Virginia	9.0	12.9	8.3	10.0	5.6
Wisconsin	4.5	4.9	4.8	5.4	3.1
Wyoming	7.6	6.4	9.0	8.6	5.3

*Source: Compiled by New Strategist based on the Centers for Disease Control and Prevention Behavioral Risk Factor
Surveillance System Survey, Internet site http://www.cdc.gov/brfss/index.htm*

1.73 Health Insurance Coverage Gaps in Past 12 Months by Household Income, 2001

Among those with health insurance, "During the past 12 months, was there any time that you did not have any health insurance or coverage?"

(percent of people aged 18 or older responding "yes," by state and household income, 2001)

	total	less than $15,000	$15,000 to $24,999	$25,000 to $34,999	$35,000 to $49,999	$50,000 or more
U.S. total	**6.5%**	**10.7%**	**10.7%**	**9.0%**	**5.7%**	**3.4%**
Alabama	5.7	8.7	8.7	9.2	4.1	2.4
Alaska	7.2	18.2	9.5	12.8	5.7	4.8
Arizona	8.8	12.4	11.8	14.8	5.2	6.6
Arkansas	7.1	9.6	13.0	8.6	5.5	3.1
California	8.2	15.2	14.2	12.9	8.9	4.1
Colorado	7.7	12.3	16.4	10.7	7.3	4.3
Connecticut	5.7	11.3	11.3	9.1	4.8	3.2
Delaware	5.8	10.5	5.8	9.1	7.4	3.2
District of Columbia	7.8	15.7	10.6	7.4	5.8	6.2
Florida	7.8	10.8	10.6	12.4	6.6	4.4
Georgia	7.2	15.0	14.0	7.5	7.2	4.3
Hawaii	4.9	11.9	5.9	6.5	3.6	2.6
Idaho	6.9	10.6	13.0	8.5	6.1	3.3
Illinois	6.0	10.2	10.7	9.4	6.6	3.2
Indiana	6.3	10.8	11.5	9.4	4.8	3.4
Iowa	4.5	6.8	7.1	5.8	5.0	2.4
Kansas	5.9	10.0	10.0	9.0	5.3	3.2
Kentucky	6.0	7.3	10.3	9.3	6.3	2.5
Louisiana	7.7	9.5	12.1	11.4	5.0	5.0
Maine	7.6	10.9	9.6	11.6	7.7	5.1
Maryland	5.5	11.3	10.4	7.3	6.4	3.4
Massachusetts	5.9	9.1	9.7	8.4	6.8	4.0
Michigan	5.4	6.9	9.9	9.1	5.7	2.5
Minnesota	5.5	7.9	9.0	8.0	7.6	2.8
Mississippi	8.6	15.1	12.5	8.9	8.5	3.3
Missouri	5.9	11.0	10.1	8.6	5.1	2.3
Montana	11.0	14.7	17.4	11.2	13.5	6.1
Nebraska	6.3	9.2	11.2	7.5	6.2	2.8
Nevada	8.0	13.5	13.7	8.1	7.7	6.0
New Hampshire	6.6	11.5	12.3	7.1	6.4	4.4
New Jersey	6.4	15.5	11.0	10.1	6.1	3.7
New Mexico	8.0	8.6	15.2	9.4	7.6	3.6
New York	8.1	12.7	10.3	12.4	6.7	4.3
North Carolina	7.1	12.1	9.9	11.5	5.6	2.7
North Dakota	4.2	4.8	7.8	4.4	3.7	1.9
Ohio	5.1	10.0	8.4	7.5	4.2	2.4
Oklahoma	7.1	11.5	11.0	8.8	5.2	4.6
Oregon	8.7	19.2	17.0	9.6	5.2	3.9
Pennsylvania	5.0	7.5	8.4	8.1	4.4	2.6
Rhode Island	4.9	5.5	7.3	4.6	6.8	2.8
South Carolina	6.0	11.2	11.2	5.9	4.8	3.5
South Dakota	5.4	9.9	10.8	5.8	4.6	1.9
Tennessee	6.0	5.7	10.0	6.8	5.0	2.6
Texas	7.5	13.9	10.5	9.6	9.0	4.6
Utah	6.6	10.4	10.9	10.4	7.5	4.1
Vermont	6.8	11.3	13.7	9.0	7.0	2.4
Virginia	5.4	10.3	7.9	9.6	5.1	2.6
Washington	6.0	10.7	10.8	8.5	5.7	4.1
West Virginia	9.0	15.7	12.3	9.2	4.9	4.4
Wisconsin	4.5	9.1	5.3	9.1	3.9	1.8
Wyoming	7.6	10.6	17.3	9.0	7.0	3.5

Source: Compiled by New Strategist based on the Centers for Disease Control and Prevention Behavioral Risk Factor Surveillance System Survey, Internet site http://www.cdc.gov/brfss/index.htm

1.74 Health Insurance Coverage Gaps in Past 12 Months by Sex, 2001

Among those with health insurance, "During the past 12 months, was there any time that you did not have any health insurance or coverage?"

(percent of people aged 18 or older responding "yes," by state and sex, 2001)

	total	men	women
U.S. total	**6.5%**	**6.5%**	**6.5%**
Alabama	5.7	4.6	6.7
Alaska	7.2	5.9	8.6
Arizona	8.8	10.0	7.7
Arkansas	7.1	7.3	7.0
California	8.2	8.0	8.4
Colorado	7.7	7.7	7.6
Connecticut	5.7	5.7	5.6
Delaware	5.8	6.3	5.4
District of Columbia	7.8	9.5	6.5
Florida	7.8	8.1	7.5
Georgia	7.2	6.8	7.5
Hawaii	4.9	5.0	4.7
Idaho	6.9	6.5	7.4
Illinois	6.0	6.4	5.7
Indiana	6.3	6.9	5.8
Iowa	4.5	4.4	4.6
Kansas	5.9	6.6	5.3
Kentucky	6.0	5.5	6.5
Louisiana	7.7	7.4	8.0
Maine	7.6	8.1	7.2
Maryland	5.5	5.1	6.0
Massachusetts	5.9	6.2	5.8
Michigan	5.4	5.6	5.3
Minnesota	5.5	5.6	5.4
Mississippi	8.6	7.6	9.4
Missouri	5.9	4.8	6.9
Montana	11.0	10.3	11.7
Nebraska	6.3	6.8	5.8
Nevada	8.0	8.1	7.9
New Hampshire	6.6	6.2	7.0
New Jersey	6.4	6.4	6.4
New Mexico	8.0	7.2	8.7
New York	8.1	8.1	8.0
North Carolina	7.1	6.7	7.4
North Dakota	4.2	3.7	4.7
Ohio	5.1	5.1	5.1
Oklahoma	7.1	6.5	7.5
Oregon	8.7	9.0	8.5
Pennsylvania	5.0	5.6	4.6
Rhode Island	4.9	4.9	4.8
South Carolina	6.0	5.7	6.3
South Dakota	5.4	5.2	5.6
Tennessee	6.0	5.8	6.3
Texas	7.5	6.9	7.9
Utah	6.6	6.8	6.4
Vermont	6.8	7.8	6.0
Virginia	5.4	6.0	4.9
Washington	6.0	7.1	5.1
West Virginia	9.0	9.4	8.7
Wisconsin	4.5	5.1	3.9
Wyoming	7.6	7.5	7.7

Source: Compiled by New Strategist based on the Centers for Disease Control and Prevention Behavioral Risk Factor Surveillance System Survey, Internet site http://www.cdc.gov/brfss/index.htm

1.75 Health Status by Age, 2001

"How is your general health?"

(percent of people aged 18 or older responding "excellent/very good," by state and age, 2001)

	total	18 to 24	25 to 34	35 to 44	45 to 54	55 to 64	65 or older
U.S. total	**56.3%**	**64.1%**	**65.8%**	**62.5%**	**56.2%**	**48.6%**	**37.8%**
Alabama	50.2	71.1	68.1	56.6	44.7	39.4	22.1
Alaska	60.5	64.7	66.6	63.4	58.9	50.9	47.1
Arizona	55.9	62.9	63.3	54.7	55.6	60.5	43.2
Arkansas	47.5	56.5	61.8	54.7	46.4	38.7	30.0
California	56.0	62.1	63.6	59.5	53.1	47.7	45.5
Colorado	58.9	57.2	65.3	64.7	61.7	55.1	43.5
Connecticut	61.8	66.0	70.1	68.9	62.1	61.0	42.6
Delaware	57.5	61.0	69.5	62.8	58.7	46.1	43.5
District of Columbia	60.5	68.8	76.0	64.9	62.4	44.8	39.7
Florida	53.3	62.2	67.9	58.7	51.9	49.8	38.4
Georgia	55.3	67.2	69.2	60.1	52.4	42.1	32.4
Hawaii	54.8	59.4	62.0	61.4	57.4	49.1	37.7
Idaho	58.2	65.6	67.6	67.6	56.4	53.8	36.9
Illinois	55.1	62.0	65.2	62.7	53.6	45.8	38.1
Indiana	54.0	65.3	60.7	60.0	55.0	48.1	35.1
Iowa	57.2	66.1	70.6	64.1	62.0	52.4	33.4
Kansas	60.1	68.5	70.5	65.7	62.7	51.0	40.7
Kentucky	49.5	67.8	63.6	54.2	46.2	36.1	29.3
Louisiana	57.9	70.5	73.0	65.7	54.2	40.5	36.1
Maine	58.6	64.5	62.6	64.9	61.4	54.8	43.0
Maryland	60.3	64.9	70.7	66.6	61.0	54.6	38.1
Massachusetts	62.3	67.2	72.2	70.2	64.6	54.4	42.3
Michigan	53.9	59.3	61.7	59.4	54.7	49.5	36.8
Minnesota	62.8	65.6	73.2	69.0	67.4	56.1	41.6
Mississippi	46.5	63.4	59.5	49.1	41.1	35.2	26.7
Missouri	55.2	64.0	68.9	61.8	52.9	44.3	38.3
Montana	58.4	67.2	70.4	66.0	57.4	50.6	40.1
Nebraska	60.9	73.0	72.9	67.7	61.7	53.8	38.0
Nevada	55.3	60.0	58.8	62.3	52.2	51.1	45.4
New Hampshire	66.1	71.1	75.8	73.2	66.8	60.6	44.7
New Jersey	56.7	65.2	63.6	63.2	58.1	50.0	39.9
New Mexico	52.5	60.8	58.2	56.8	55.2	47.9	33.6
New York	53.8	62.1	62.8	59.4	54.8	46.3	37.0
North Carolina	55.3	65.8	70.7	60.9	54.6	41.3	35.2
North Dakota	55.3	66.9	69.3	64.7	57.9	46.6	27.7
Ohio	55.9	69.3	63.3	62.0	57.0	46.7	37.9
Oklahoma	52.5	66.9	67.0	62.9	49.2	38.8	29.4
Oregon	54.5	55.3	60.5	59.8	59.5	49.6	39.7
Pennsylvania	55.5	67.5	66.4	64.4	57.6	50.5	32.8
Rhode Island	57.3	62.3	68.2	64.3	59.3	52.0	38.3
South Carolina	54.6	64.8	63.0	58.3	56.7	43.7	37.9
South Dakota	58.4	65.4	72.1	66.4	62.7	51.4	33.8
Tennessee	50.6	65.6	67.4	55.7	44.4	36.3	34.7
Texas	47.5	49.7	54.6	52.9	48.0	42.7	31.3
Utah	60.3	73.3	69.7	64.8	57.3	50.8	34.9
Vermont	64.6	74.2	73.5	71.2	65.7	57.1	42.4
Virginia	60.8	65.5	73.5	66.6	61.8	55.1	37.2
Washington	60.2	68.3	66.8	67.2	61.2	57.7	38.3
West Virginia	45.2	56.8	57.7	53.8	42.8	33.0	30.8
Wisconsin	56.8	52.3	64.1	66.3	59.1	56.3	40.6
Wyoming	58.3	62.9	66.4	61.4	62.8	52.6	40.2

Source: Compiled by New Strategist based on the Centers for Disease Control and Prevention Behavioral Risk Factor Surveillance System Survey, Internet site http://www.cdc.gov/brfss/index.htm

1.76 Health Status by Education, 2001

"How is your general health?"

(percent of people aged 18 or older responding "excellent/very good," by state and educational attainment, 2001)

	total	less than high school	high school graduate	some college	college graduate
U.S. total	**56.3%**	**30.1%**	**49.3%**	**58.5%**	**70.8%**
Alabama	50.2	25.6	44.7	55.6	70.4
Alaska	60.5	34.2	57.1	59.2	73.1
Arizona	55.9	29.0	50.7	57.9	70.5
Arkansas	47.5	25.9	43.1	53.5	62.5
California	56.0	23.2	53.8	60.6	71.9
Colorado	58.9	25.0	50.2	61.3	73.6
Connecticut	61.8	31.4	52.3	61.0	75.8
Delaware	57.5	36.6	50.4	57.2	69.9
District of Columbia	60.5	29.3	47.7	55.8	77.7
Florida	53.3	30.2	46.7	58.1	66.5
Georgia	55.3	31.0	46.7	58.2	72.4
Hawaii	54.8	28.9	47.8	54.6	68.3
Idaho	58.2	33.2	51.3	61.7	71.0
Illinois	55.1	26.6	46.9	56.4	71.4
Indiana	54.0	29.7	50.0	56.1	68.6
Iowa	57.2	29.4	50.6	59.4	74.7
Kansas	60.1	34.4	52.1	61.5	72.9
Kentucky	49.5	26.6	45.2	59.4	69.1
Louisiana	57.9	37.4	53.4	65.3	72.9
Maine	58.6	33.2	50.0	61.6	74.8
Maryland	60.3	30.9	50.6	60.7	74.3
Massachusetts	62.3	32.7	49.9	63.1	76.1
Michigan	53.9	30.4	45.8	56.1	71.5
Minnesota	62.8	37.4	54.1	63.0	76.4
Mississippi	46.5	25.9	39.3	58.0	60.8
Missouri	55.2	33.6	47.0	61.2	69.9
Montana	58.4	38.6	52.8	57.8	73.7
Nebraska	60.9	40.0	57.7	65.0	69.6
Nevada	55.3	31.1	52.4	56.1	64.0
New Hampshire	66.1	38.2	59.3	66.9	78.1
New Jersey	56.7	30.8	49.6	56.4	69.6
New Mexico	52.5	29.6	48.9	54.6	69.8
New York	53.8	21.4	47.2	59.8	67.7
North Carolina	55.3	27.4	51.8	59.1	72.5
North Dakota	55.3	22.0	44.5	59.6	72.4
Ohio	55.9	32.2	50.0	61.5	69.9
Oklahoma	52.5	29.0	48.8	55.8	68.6
Oregon	54.5	30.3	47.5	57.6	68.4
Pennsylvania	55.5	33.0	46.6	63.8	71.1
Rhode Island	57.3	33.7	46.5	60.9	75.0
South Carolina	54.6	27.0	50.5	58.6	71.1
South Dakota	58.4	29.2	50.9	61.7	74.3
Tennessee	50.6	23.8	47.4	58.8	63.9
Texas	47.5	21.3	43.1	53.6	65.1
Utah	60.3	40.8	51.2	61.3	72.7
Vermont	64.6	31.6	58.0	67.2	77.1
Virginia	60.8	34.1	52.8	62.3	74.9
Washington	60.2	37.1	50.4	60.0	74.0
West Virginia	45.2	18.4	43.9	52.5	68.6
Wisconsin	56.8	35.9	46.9	59.9	73.7
Wyoming	58.3	35.6	50.4	59.5	73.4

Source: Compiled by New Strategist based on the Centers for Disease Control and Prevention Behavioral Risk Factor Surveillance System Survey, Internet site http://www.cdc.gov/brfss/index.htm

1.77 Health Status by Household Income, 2001

"How is your general health?"

(percent of people aged 18 or older responding "excellent/very good," by state and household income. 2001)

	total	less than $15,000	$15,000 to $24,999	$25,000 to $34,999	$35,000 to $49,999	$50,000 or more
U.S. total	**56.3%**	**33.2%**	**41.7%**	**51.6%**	**61.2%**	**71.0%**
Alabama	50.2	28.1	38.9	52.0	58.0	69.6
Alaska	60.5	30.6	46.2	56.3	67.1	70.8
Arizona	55.9	25.8	42.0	50.1	59.8	72.6
Arkansas	47.5	27.8	37.3	45.8	54.2	68.1
California	56.0	36.5	38.5	47.6	58.2	72.2
Colorado	58.9	22.9	44.7	53.3	61.6	73.7
Connecticut	61.8	29.8	41.5	56.4	63.6	75.0
Delaware	57.5	45.2	34.9	57.2	60.6	67.9
District of Columbia	60.5	39.4	47.7	54.8	59.6	77.7
Florida	53.3	32.8	39.9	52.3	57.3	72.9
Georgia	55.3	35.1	41.1	47.4	64.9	70.2
Hawaii	54.8	36.5	50.1	55.1	54.3	66.4
Idaho	58.2	38.2	45.2	55.7	64.8	73.5
Illinois	55.1	27.5	41.6	48.6	54.8	69.6
Indiana	54.0	38.3	35.5	49.7	58.8	68.6
Iowa	57.2	35.1	42.0	52.8	64.4	73.5
Kansas	60.1	46.9	42.8	55.2	65.2	71.1
Kentucky	49.5	29.4	39.8	47.9	57.9	69.4
Louisiana	57.9	38.2	52.0	59.1	65.8	72.2
Maine	58.6	29.1	42.5	57.8	66.6	74.9
Maryland	60.3	37.0	46.0	51.5	61.0	71.5
Massachusetts	62.3	32.7	45.2	51.0	62.9	75.7
Michigan	53.9	37.1	39.2	47.6	54.3	66.9
Minnesota	62.8	31.7	46.1	54.6	63.4	74.7
Mississippi	46.5	27.4	36.3	48.3	55.3	64.2
Missouri	55.2	33.0	40.5	50.7	62.4	69.6
Montana	58.4	44.5	52.5	62.1	66.1	71.6
Nebraska	60.9	41.8	50.9	61.0	66.2	75.4
Nevada	55.3	32.3	40.3	48.9	62.4	63.7
New Hampshire	66.1	31.6	53.3	56.7	65.6	77.3
New Jersey	56.7	26.0	40.5	48.4	54.9	70.7
New Mexico	52.5	32.9	39.4	52.1	60.4	71.9
New York	53.8	31.7	37.1	42.9	57.1	72.5
North Carolina	55.3	30.5	45.2	52.1	61.7	73.1
North Dakota	55.3	42.5	41.6	52.2	58.4	73.3
Ohio	55.9	33.9	39.5	50.0	59.6	71.1
Oklahoma	52.5	33.0	43.4	54.3	60.7	70.5
Oregon	54.5	31.2	44.4	52.2	57.4	70.2
Pennsylvania	55.5	38.0	36.9	53.9	58.5	73.1
Rhode Island	57.3	33.9	43.5	54.5	57.1	74.5
South Carolina	54.6	31.2	43.4	54.4	59.6	72.5
South Dakota	58.4	39.8	43.1	58.9	65.1	74.9
Tennessee	50.6	32.4	39.0	51.8	62.4	67.0
Texas	47.5	22.9	32.5	47.3	53.3	66.8
Utah	60.3	39.6	50.2	50.6	62.4	71.6
Vermont	64.6	41.2	51.7	63.8	67.6	79.3
Virginia	60.8	34.6	49.2	55.3	66.7	71.8
Washington	60.2	32.4	47.6	53.1	62.5	72.3
West Virginia	45.2	27.4	32.7	44.2	56.1	65.8
Wisconsin	56.8	42.4	36.3	51.2	58.2	72.7
Wyoming	58.3	39.8	45.3	56.8	64.2	70.5

Source: Compiled by New Strategist based on the Centers for Disease Control and Prevention Behavioral Risk Factor Surveillance System Survey, Internet site http://www.cdc.gov/brfss/index.htm

1.78 Health Status by Sex, 2001

"How is your general health?"

(percent of people aged 18 or older responding "excellent/very good," by state and sex, 2001)

	total	men	women
U.S. total	**56.3%**	**57.3%**	**55.6%**
Alabama	50.2	53.6	47.1
Alaska	60.5	63.6	57.3
Arizona	55.9	60.3	51.7
Arkansas	47.5	48.6	46.7
California	56.0	57.0	54.9
Colorado	58.9	57.7	60.1
Connecticut	61.8	62.5	61.1
Delaware	57.5	59.0	56.1
District of Columbia	60.5	62.2	59.0
Florida	53.3	54.5	52.1
Georgia	55.3	56.5	54.0
Hawaii	54.8	56.6	52.9
Idaho	58.2	59.0	57.3
Illinois	55.1	55.4	54.8
Indiana	54.0	54.7	53.5
Iowa	57.2	59.3	55.3
Kansas	60.1	61.8	58.4
Kentucky	49.5	50.4	48.8
Louisiana	57.9	60.8	55.3
Maine	58.6	58.3	58.7
Maryland	60.3	62.4	58.4
Massachusetts	62.3	63.2	61.5
Michigan	53.9	55.6	52.2
Minnesota	62.8	62.7	63.0
Mississippi	46.5	49.5	43.7
Missouri	55.2	57.0	53.5
Montana	58.4	62.8	54.2
Nebraska	60.9	62.0	59.8
Nevada	55.3	55.9	54.6
New Hampshire	66.1	66.7	65.6
New Jersey	56.7	58.9	54.6
New Mexico	52.5	54.1	50.8
New York	53.8	53.6	53.9
North Carolina	55.3	58.2	52.5
North Dakota	55.3	55.4	55.2
Ohio	55.9	55.7	55.9
Oklahoma	52.5	54.5	50.5
Oregon	54.5	55.3	53.7
Pennsylvania	55.5	56.5	54.7
Rhode Island	57.3	58.5	56.3
South Carolina	54.6	56.1	53.1
South Dakota	58.4	58.6	58.2
Tennessee	50.6	53.5	48.1
Texas	47.5	47.6	47.4
Utah	60.3	60.8	59.8
Vermont	64.6	64.4	64.7
Virginia	60.8	63.4	58.3
Washington	60.2	60.2	60.3
West Virginia	45.2	44.5	45.9
Wisconsin	56.8	56.2	57.4
Wyoming	58.3	58.4	58.2

Source: Compiled by New Strategist based on the Centers for Disease Control and Prevention Behavioral Risk Factor Surveillance System Survey, Internet site http://www.cdc.gov/brfss/index.htm

1.79 Health Status: Poor Physical Health by Age, 2001

"For how many days during the last 30 days was your physical health not good?"

(percent of people aged 18 or older responding "one or more," by state and age, 2001)

	total	18 to 24	25 to 34	35 to 44	45 to 54	55 to 64	65 or older
U.S. total	**33.8%**	**37.0%**	**31.8%**	**33.5%**	**33.7%**	**32.6%**	**34.5%**
Alabama	37.4	39.4	33.3	35.5	36.6	38.7	42.7
Alaska	38.0	43.5	37.9	39.8	35.3	39.6	29.2
Arizona	36.2	38.5	31.5	45.1	32.6	27.9	38.8
Arkansas	36.6	32.6	32.6	34.8	37.7	41.7	41.0
California	35.3	35.6	32.4	36.1	35.7	32.4	39.8
Colorado	35.1	39.6	31.8	33.3	34.0	35.8	38.4
Connecticut	33.3	40.3	31.5	32.9	32.1	31.6	33.9
Delaware	33.7	42.7	29.6	31.7	32.3	32.7	35.0
District of Columbia	32.9	34.3	31.5	31.3	33.8	33.8	35.3
Florida	31.1	31.6	28.7	26.7	33.9	35.7	31.8
Georgia	32.6	32.8	31.4	32.4	31.6	33.0	35.8
Hawaii	24.5	32.1	23.7	24.0	24.9	22.7	21.8
Idaho	35.3	37.6	38.5	34.3	34.9	34.3	31.9
Illinois	33.6	36.0	33.8	31.7	32.5	31.4	35.8
Indiana	35.7	37.3	37.0	33.8	34.9	32.3	39.7
Iowa	33.9	44.8	34.1	35.2	32.2	29.8	30.2
Kansas	31.6	35.6	30.8	29.7	31.5	30.9	31.7
Kentucky	29.2	25.6	30.4	28.2	31.5	30.7	28.5
Louisiana	28.6	27.3	23.6	27.5	28.6	33.8	34.8
Maine	33.8	38.7	33.6	35.5	31.6	29.7	34.0
Maryland	33.7	35.4	33.0	33.7	32.4	35.7	33.6
Massachusetts	35.5	44.4	33.0	35.3	32.9	34.3	35.9
Michigan	37.0	42.9	36.4	34.6	35.1	35.9	38.0
Minnesota	37.3	48.1	37.2	36.7	31.9	35.9	36.5
Mississippi	32.4	24.1	29.7	32.2	36.8	34.8	37.8
Missouri	35.6	36.7	35.3	34.3	38.5	36.1	33.3
Montana	30.9	40.9	26.8	28.8	31.3	31.6	29.5
Nebraska	27.8	30.3	28.1	30.1	28.7	24.9	25.2
Nevada	39.8	44.7	39.7	44.9	40.0	34.6	33.3
New Hampshire	33.4	41.5	33.1	31.4	35.4	28.0	33.1
New Jersey	31.8	40.7	28.0	30.5	32.2	29.9	32.8
New Mexico	33.9	35.7	32.3	33.5	35.0	30.4	36.3
New York	35.3	40.4	33.5	33.2	35.6	33.0	37.3
North Carolina	32.6	28.1	31.9	30.5	33.1	33.0	39.4
North Dakota	32.6	40.2	31.7	29.3	30.0	34.1	32.4
Ohio	34.7	38.0	34.9	34.4	30.5	37.3	35.0
Oklahoma	33.8	35.4	32.0	27.9	35.6	36.1	37.6
Oregon	37.6	42.4	36.5	37.7	37.8	35.6	36.8
Pennsylvania	35.2	38.7	32.5	33.2	36.3	35.8	36.0
Rhode Island	38.0	45.5	36.5	36.9	37.6	37.8	36.7
South Carolina	33.9	33.2	31.1	32.6	35.8	36.2	35.8
South Dakota	30.9	36.7	31.1	30.5	27.8	28.3	32.0
Tennessee	29.1	32.7	25.6	30.3	30.0	30.5	27.2
Texas	32.1	30.7	29.3	30.7	32.5	35.0	37.6
Utah	60.5	46.2	40.1	37.5	40.1	39.2	34.7
Vermont	65.6	37.5	35.5	33.8	33.4	31.1	35.5
Virginia	63.9	44.2	33.6	34.8	36.2	28.2	41.0
Washington	62.6	40.6	38.3	40.7	34.1	30.4	38.7
West Virginia	58.9	37.3	38.7	38.2	42.0	46.4	44.2
Wisconsin	61.5	44.2	35.4	36.0	40.6	35.4	40.4
Wyoming	67.5	42.1	29.7	34.6	28.7	29.9	33.2

Source: Compiled by New Strategist based on the Centers for Disease Control and Prevention Behavioral Risk Factor Surveillance System Survey. Internet site http://www.cdc.gov/brfss/index.htm

1.80 Health Status: Poor Physical Health by Education, 2001

"For how many days during the last 30 days was your physical health not good?"

(percent of people aged 18 or older responding "one or more," by state and educational attainment, 2001)

	total	less than high school	high school graduate	some college	college graduate
U.S. total	**33.8%**	**38.7%**	**33.4%**	**35.5%**	**30.8%**
Alabama	37.4	52.6	36.2	35.8	31.0
Alaska	38.0	43.6	37.4	41.9	32.5
Arizona	36.2	40.5	36.5	39.7	30.0
Arkansas	36.6	50.1	35.5	36.2	30.6
California	35.3	36.8	36.0	38.0	31.9
Colorado	35.1	41.0	31.9	35.9	35.0
Connecticut	33.3	38.6	33.4	36.6	30.2
Delaware	33.7	38.4	33.1	37.6	29.8
District of Columbia	32.9	46.0	31.5	35.2	29.4
Florida	31.1	32.7	31.1	32.7	29.0
Georgia	32.6	38.7	33.7	33.2	28.7
Hawaii	24.5	29.7	22.7	28.8	20.8
Idaho	35.3	41.7	33.9	36.8	32.7
Illinois	33.6	33.5	34.0	35.4	31.1
Indiana	35.7	44.3	35.6	35.3	33.0
Iowa	33.9	40.5	32.6	34.7	33.2
Kansas	31.6	31.6	31.9	33.1	29.7
Kentucky	29.2	38.6	29.8	26.6	22.5
Louisiana	28.6	38.6	26.7	29.8	23.8
Maine	33.8	39.2	36.7	33.8	28.3
Maryland	33.7	39.2	36.7	33.8	28.3
Massachusetts	35.5	45.0	35.9	39.0	31.3
Michigan	37.0	42.2	36.8	38.5	33.1
Minnesota	37.3	46.1	40.7	37.1	32.4
Mississippi	32.4	42.4	30.4	30.3	30.5
Missouri	35.6	43.0	35.2	35.7	32.7
Montana	30.9	31.8	30.3	31.8	30.3
Nebraska	27.8	29.3	26.8	27.8	29.3
Nevada	39.8	45.6	43.8	36.8	37.5
New Hampshire	33.4	34.8	35.3	32.1	32.8
New Jersey	31.8	38.1	31.5	35.3	28.3
New Mexico	33.9	29.7	36.8	35.2	32.7
New York	35.3	46.2	33.6	38.0	30.2
North Carolina	32.6	42.8	30.4	31.4	30.7
North Dakota	32.6	37.1	32.2	34.4	29.9
Ohio	34.7	40.6	35.3	34.7	31.0
Oklahoma	33.8	36.6	32.1	38.1	29.6
Oregon	37.6	37.3	34.5	43.0	35.2
Pennsylvania	35.2	41.7	33.2	37.6	33.6
Rhode Island	38.0	43.8	39.6	38.2	33.8
South Carolina	33.9	45.8	33.2	34.5	27.7
South Dakota	30.9	33.1	28.5	33.4	30.5
Tennessee	29.1	34.4	27.6	34.6	21.6
Texas	32.1	32.5	31.2	33.5	31.6
Utah	60.5	44.4	39.3	44.5	33.2
Vermont	65.6	46.3	34.0	36.8	30.6
Virginia	63.9	39.5	38.1	37.7	32.1
Washington	62.6	42.5	40.7	37.8	33.4
West Virginia	58.9	51.8	39.1	42.1	33.1
Wisconsin	61.5	48.3	40.4	36.7	34.6
Wyoming	67.5	42.0	31.6	34.1	29.2

Source: Compiled by New Strategist based on the Centers for Disease Control and Prevention Behavioral Risk Factor Surveillance System Survey, Internet site http://www.cdc.gov/brfss/index.htm

1.81 Health Status: Poor Physical Health by Household Income, 2001

"For how many days during the past 30 days was your physical health not good?"

(percent of people aged 18 or older responding "one or more," by state and household income, 2001)

	total	less than $15,000	$15,000 to $24,999	$25,000 to $34,999	$35,000 to $49,999	$50,000 or more
U.S. total	**33.8%**	**47.9%**	**38.4%**	**34.1%**	**32.0%**	**29.1%**
Alabama	37.4	53.2	42.1	30.9	36.8	30.2
Alaska	38.0	57.2	45.0	40.2	34.7	33.7
Arizona	36.2	50.7	42.4	37.3	38.0	29.9
Arkansas	36.6	53.0	40.3	36.0	32.3	25.6
California	35.3	45.5	37.5	38.3	34.0	30.7
Colorado	35.1	56.8	37.5	35.0	37.5	28.8
Connecticut	33.3	42.7	37.0	37.0	34.3	29.8
Delaware	33.7	34.6	47.8	30.9	35.1	29.8
District of Columbia	32.9	43.3	39.4	31.8	26.4	30.6
Florida	31.1	43.9	36.1	30.8	30.9	26.2
Georgia	32.6	44.4	37.8	33.1	31.3	28.6
Hawaii	24.5	29.0	27.3	24.5	27.9	21.9
Idaho	35.3	46.6	40.9	38.1	31.5	28.7
Illinois	33.6	49.1	38.1	27.1	33.1	32.3
Indiana	35.7	50.2	46.1	35.7	31.1	30.2
Iowa	33.9	50.0	39.8	30.9	28.4	30.1
Kansas	31.6	51.4	38.5	32.1	31.1	26.0
Kentucky	29.2	43.0	36.3	31.8	26.9	22.8
Louisiana	28.6	40.6	33.9	27.5	26.8	22.9
Maine	33.8	63.3	43.9	32.9	26.2	25.7
Maryland	33.7	46.4	33.4	34.1	31.2	31.6
Massachusetts	35.5	50.7	41.6	38.1	34.9	30.8
Michigan	37.0	46.2	43.7	39.6	36.4	31.6
Minnesota	37.3	53.0	45.4	39.7	36.6	32.5
Mississippi	32.4	45.9	37.3	30.6	24.9	26.8
Missouri	35.6	52.1	42.6	35.6	34.1	29.1
Montana	30.9	52.5	29.0	34.7	31.5	21.1
Nebraska	27.8	36.0	32.4	25.7	27.1	27.0
Nevada	39.8	60.1	50.8	38.1	41.4	33.1
New Hampshire	33.4	53.7	39.5	38.3	34.3	28.4
New Jersey	31.8	47.7	32.6	29.2	33.2	29.0
New Mexico	33.9	42.8	35.6	32.2	31.8	30.5
New York	35.3	47.3	40.8	37.1	34.1	28.6
North Carolina	32.6	48.6	34.4	32.0	32.3	26.9
North Dakota	32.6	44.0	39.7	31.6	30.3	23.7
Ohio	34.7	52.0	41.7	35.9	33.0	28.8
Oklahoma	33.8	45.8	39.9	33.9	32.8	26.7
Oregon	37.6	49.9	41.2	37.0	35.9	31.1
Pennsylvania	35.2	46.6	40.3	35.7	34.6	28.5
Rhode Island	38.0	50.4	45.1	40.3	36.4	31.2
South Carolina	33.9	54.5	39.3	32.2	31.3	27.5
South Dakota	30.9	40.5	37.0	29.4	28.1	27.1
Tennessee	29.1	49.6	36.9	27.1	27.2	24.2
Texas	32.1	38.8	35.0	32.3	30.6	29.5
Utah	60.5	52.7	43.1	40.7	41.8	35.9
Vermont	65.6	50.4	41.4	35.1	30.7	28.4
Virginia	63.9	56.5	41.8	38.0	32.6	31.9
Washington	62.6	52.8	43.2	38.0	35.9	33.1
West Virginia	58.9	54.8	46.1	43.3	31.8	33.3
Wisconsin	61.5	48.7	47.7	41.6	38.3	31.8
Wyoming	67.5	47.2	36.7	35.6	31.7	24.8

Source: Compiled by New Strategist based on the Centers for Disease Control and Prevention Behavioral Risk Factor Surveillance System Survey, Internet site http://www.cdc.gov/brfss/index.htm

1.82 Health Status: Poor Physical Health by Sex, 2001

"For how many days during the past 30 days was your physical health not good?"

(percent of people aged 18 or older responding "one or more," by state and sex, 2001)

	total	men	women
U.S. total	**33.8%**	**30.0%**	**37.7%**
Alabama	37.4	32.0	42.3
Alaska	38.0	32.7	43.6
Arizona	36.2	31.6	40.4
Arkansas	36.6	33.3	39.7
California	35.3	29.5	41.2
Colorado	35.1	31.4	31.4
Connecticut	33.3	30.3	36.1
Delaware	33.7	29.2	37.6
District of Columbia	32.9	30.6	34.8
Florida	31.1	27.8	34.1
Georgia	32.6	27.9	37.0
Hawaii	24.5	22.2	26.7
Idaho	35.3	31.4	38.9
Illinois	33.6	29.3	37.5
Indiana	35.7	30.1	41.1
Iowa	33.9	31.4	36.6
Kansas	31.6	27.8	35.1
Kentucky	29.2	27.3	31.1
Louisiana	28.6	24.9	32.0
Maine	33.8	31.9	35.6
Maryland	33.7	30.3	37.0
Massachusetts	35.5	32.1	38.6
Michigan	37.0	33.6	40.1
Minnesota	37.3	33.7	40.5
Mississippi	32.4	28.4	36.2
Missouri	35.6	30.9	40.0
Montana	30.9	23.4	38.0
Nebraska	27.8	24.8	30.6
Nevada	39.8	34.4	45.2
New Hampshire	33.4	30.7	36.2
New Jersey	31.8	28.6	34.8
New Mexico	33.9	31.8	36.1
New York	35.3	33.4	36.8
North Carolina	32.6	28.1	36.9
North Dakota	32.6	28.7	36.3
Ohio	34.7	32.9	36.2
Oklahoma	33.8	29.8	37.6
Oregon	37.6	32.0	43.0
Pennsylvania	35.2	32.0	38.0
Rhode Island	38.0	33.6	42.0
South Carolina	33.9	28.6	38.7
South Dakota	30.9	26.3	35.3
Tennessee	29.1	27.4	30.9
Texas	32.1	28.1	36.1
Utah	60.5	34.4	44.5
Vermont	65.6	31.9	36.8
Virginia	63.9	31.9	39.9
Washington	62.6	31.8	42.8
West Virginia	58.9	38.1	43.8
Wisconsin	61.5	33.7	42.9
Wyoming	67.5	26.9	38.1

Source: Compiled by New Strategist based on the Centers for Disease Control and Prevention Behavioral Risk Factor Surveillance System Survey, Internet site http://www.cdc.gov/brfss/index.htm

1.83 Health Status: Poor Mental Health by Age, 2001

"For how many days during the past 30 days was your mental health not good?"

(percent of people aged 18 or older responding "one or more," by state and age, 2001)

	total	18 to 24	25 to 34	35 to 44	45 to 54	55 to 64	65 or older
U.S. total	**33.9%**	**46.7%**	**40.7%**	**37.8%**	**33.7%**	**24.2%**	**16.4%**
Alabama	38.9	50.4	42.7	38.9	44.1	36.3	22.9
Alaska	36.6	46.7	40.7	38.3	34.9	30.3	19.1
Arizona	36.0	45.6	42.9	43.2	35.4	26.4	20.4
Arkansas	35.0	54.4	41.1	40.4	35.0	28.4	16.6
California	37.8	54.8	44.0	41.2	37.2	26.7	20.0
Colorado	35.9	46.6	43.4	42.3	38.6	27.6	11.1
Connecticut	33.1	49.5	39.4	36.5	35.5	24.1	16.5
Delaware	32.8	53.5	39.6	36.0	33.0	22.8	13.6
District of Columbia	33.7	50.0	42.2	36.3	30.1	25.4	17.8
Florida	29.9	44.2	40.3	33.5	30.7	24.9	16.3
Georgia	34.6	50.9	40.4	40.7	31.3	24.1	14.3
Hawaii	15.8	28.6	16.2	17.4	18.2	8.4	8.7
Idaho	36.4	52.8	43.8	44.2	35.3	23.6	18.4
Illinois	33.9	47.4	40.8	37.5	36.1	25.0	16.4
Indiana	36.9	52.5	45.6	43.0	37.3	26.4	16.4
Iowa	31.7	50.9	42.1	36.2	31.7	20.5	13.3
Kansas	30.5	45.3	36.8	32.3	32.1	25.0	14.4
Kentucky	28.2	28.5	29.3	30.8	33.3	27.6	18.3
Louisiana	25.1	31.7	28.1	28.9	27.7	21.0	12.8
Maine	32.9	47.5	40.7	36.8	35.6	22.5	15.6
Maryland	33.0	51.5	39.1	33.2	33.6	24.1	18.7
Massachusetts	34.7	51.0	41.8	39.0	33.9	27.1	17.7
Michigan	38.5	55.4	48.6	40.2	38.4	30.8	18.2
Minnesota	39.8	63.3	48.6	45.2	39.2	28.0	15.3
Mississippi	30.1	37.9	34.1	34.6	32.7	22.8	16.5
Missouri	33.5	51.3	40.4	40.2	36.5	19.6	15.4
Montana	22.8	34.5	22.9	27.5	22.2	20.8	11.6
Nebraska	24.4	31.2	27.1	28.7	28.5	19.5	12.9
Nevada	39.7	63.5	48.0	43.8	39.7	26.1	19.5
New Hampshire	33.7	49.5	43.9	37.0	31.7	24.9	14.2
New Jersey	32.9	48.2	35.7	38.5	36.0	26.3	16.7
New Mexico	34.6	47.1	38.5	39.2	35.5	28.0	18.4
New York	35.5	49.2	43.1	39.9	37.4	27.0	17.8
North Carolina	26.2	31.7	31.4	28.7	27.6	19.0	17.3
North Dakota	32.8	44.2	43.2	37.6	32.4	24.1	14.9
Ohio	34.6	56.5	42.5	37.4	31.2	30.0	14.5
Oklahoma	29.0	35.2	32.7	31.0	35.5	25.5	15.4
Oregon	38.4	55.5	47.7	44.0	37.8	32.2	17.1
Pennsylvania	36.8	54.2	45.0	40.5	41.0	27.9	17.9
Rhode Island	37.0	52.9	47.1	42.1	35.0	30.7	19.3
South Carolina	31.8	43.9	33.7	37.5	30.3	24.1	20.2
South Dakota	28.7	40.7	38.0	34.0	27.4	21.1	13.3
Tennessee	29.1	37.9	34.9	34.3	32.0	22.9	12.5
Texas	33.2	48.2	37.6	36.5	32.3	23.6	17.7
Utah	43.1	58.1	46.0	48.3	44.8	34.7	18.1
Vermont	35.6	52.5	45.0	38.8	34.0	24.7	17.5
Virginia	36.8	54.4	44.5	40.1	33.6	27.6	19.2
Washington	38.8	58.0	48.6	42.7	39.3	21.4	21.6
West Virginia	35.1	42.8	45.4	40.0	39.7	29.0	17.3
Wisconsin	40.3	59.2	45.0	45.9	42.0	26.4	23.5
Wyoming	35.2	50.0	44.7	41.2	31.7	27.9	16.1

Source: Compiled by New Strategist based on the Centers for Disease Control and Prevention Behavioral Risk Factor Surveillance System Survey, Internet site http://www.cdc.gov/brfss/index.htm

1.84 Health Status: Poor Mental Health by Education, 2001

"For how many days during the last 30 days was your mental health not good?"

(percent of people aged 18 or older responding "one or more," by state and educational attainment, 2001)

	total	less than high school	high school graduate	some college	college graduate
U.S. total	**33.9%**	**33.0%**	**32.6%**	**36.7%**	**31.8%**
Alabama	38.9	42.2	37.3	42.8	34.0
Alaska	36.6	34.8	34.1	40.8	34.6
Arizona	36.0	40.2	34.1	38.4	33.4
Arkansas	35.0	34.8	34.0	40.0	31.0
California	37.8	36.5	36.4	43.4	35.2
Colorado	35.9	34.6	32.4	39.7	35.8
Connecticut	33.1	30.5	33.0	36.3	31.6
Delaware	32.8	32.8	30.1	34.8	34.0
District of Columbia	33.7	37.5	33.0	37.0	32.0
Florida	29.9	27.6	30.0	32.1	29.0
Georgia	34.6	37.1	33.9	36.4	32.4
Hawaii	15.8	16.2	14.7	18.1	14.7
Idaho	36.4	36.8	38.1	37.4	33.1
Illinois	33.9	29.9	31.9	37.6	33.7
Indiana	36.9	38.5	35.8	39.8	35.1
Iowa	31.7	31.7	27.6	36.2	32.6
Kansas	30.5	27.4	29.3	34.0	29.2
Kentucky	28.2	33.1	27.9	29.5	22.4
Louisiana	25.1	25.4	24.8	28.3	22.7
Maine	32.9	25.7	34.7	36.0	29.9
Maryland	33.0	31.2	32.8	38.3	30.4
Massachusetts	34.7	39.3	33.2	37.6	33.0
Michigan	38.5	35.1	36.2	44.9	35.5
Minnesota	39.8	38.8	35.3	42.4	41.4
Mississippi	30.1	36.2	26.6	30.5	30.2
Missouri	33.5	37.4	32.1	33.8	33.7
Montana	22.8	22.5	21.2	26.6	20.9
Nebraska	24.4	21.9	22.7	25.3	27.9
Nevada	39.7	41.6	42.1	41.4	34.6
New Hampshire	33.7	34.9	33.5	36.0	32.0
New Jersey	32.9	33.9	31.3	36.5	31.9
New Mexico	34.6	27.4	36.2	40.5	32.1
New York	35.5	33.6	32.9	39.1	35.8
North Carolina	26.2	25.6	25.2	27.2	26.5
North Dakota	32.8	26.5	29.4	35.8	34.7
Ohio	34.6	32.3	36.2	37.0	30.3
Oklahoma	29.0	24.1	28.9	34.4	26.6
Oregon	38.4	35.8	38.5	40.9	36.5
Pennsylvania	36.8	31.7	35.8	42.2	35.9
Rhode Island	37.0	40.1	36.9	40.8	32.8
South Carolina	31.8	38.2	27.1	37.0	28.6
South Dakota	28.7	22.9	29.5	30.9	27.0
Tennessee	29.1	28.7	29.1	32.8	25.1
Texas	33.2	31.7	33.4	36.4	31.4
Utah	43.1	41.5	45.4	48.6	34.2
Vermont	35.6	38.1	34.4	36.1	35.7
Virginia	36.8	33.8	36.5	39.9	35.9
Washington	38.8	47.3	40.0	39.2	35.5
West Virginia	35.1	36.1	35.4	37.3	30.1
Wisconsin	40.3	41.4	38.6	44.1	38.4
Wyoming	35.2	41.7	32.0	38.8	33.1

Source: Compiled by New Strategist based on the Centers for Disease Control and Prevention Behavioral Risk Factor Surveillance System Survey, Internet site http://www.cdc.gov/brfss/index.htm

1.85 Health Status: Poor Mental Health by Household Income, 2001

"For how many days during the past 30 days was your mental health not good?"

(percent of people aged 18 or older responding "one or more," by state and household income, 2001)

	total	less than $15,000	$15,000 to $24,999	$25,000 to $34,999	$35,000 to $49,999	$50,000 or more
U.S. total	**33.9%**	**41.9%**	**36.3%**	**33.9%**	**33.0%**	**31.5%**
Alabama	38.9	51.8	49.6	30.9	35.8	35.3
Alaska	36.6	48.7	44.2	33.5	37.2	33.8
Arizona	36.0	48.7	35.9	39.5	30.8	36.0
Arkansas	35.0	38.2	40.6	33.7	35.4	32.0
California	37.8	45.0	38.0	36.4	38.2	36.7
Colorado	35.9	44.3	37.8	36.6	33.3	36.6
Connecticut	33.1	38.1	37.2	34.5	32.7	33.0
Delaware	32.8	36.9	38.0	38.0	31.6	34.1
District of Columbia	33.7	37.9	36.6	36.9	35.1	30.0
Florida	29.9	41.6	31.7	30.9	35.2	26.8
Georgia	34.6	45.9	33.5	36.6	35.3	32.9
Hawaii	15.8	20.3	17.4	18.7	20.1	14.0
Idaho	36.4	48.4	41.0	40.2	34.3	30.4
Illinois	33.9	43.3	35.8	33.2	33.6	34.4
Indiana	36.9	46.8	43.8	36.9	35.5	35.3
Iowa	31.7	40.7	31.7	31.6	32.3	31.9
Kansas	30.5	48.1	36.7	31.7	30.1	29.2
Kentucky	28.2	41.0	33.4	30.4	25.7	24.6
Louisiana	25.1	31.8	28.6	23.0	24.4	24.4
Maine	32.9	37.7	36.3	34.3	28.9	33.4
Maryland	33.0	44.9	35.6	34.3	34.9	31.0
Massachusetts	34.7	45.8	37.3	33.4	36.4	33.3
Michigan	38.5	43.2	43.8	41.1	37.0	36.6
Minnesota	39.8	44.5	39.1	37.8	38.6	41.3
Mississippi	30.1	42.9	34.1	32.1	26.0	24.4
Missouri	33.5	42.6	33.9	35.4	34.2	32.6
Montana	22.8	47.2	24.9	19.1	16.5	21.8
Nebraska	24.4	37.5	26.6	21.1	25.9	24.8
Nevada	39.7	51.2	47.4	42.2	42.8	36.2
New Hampshire	33.7	39.8	38.6	36.0	34.8	32.9
New Jersey	32.9	41.8	32.8	29.5	36.6	33.2
New Mexico	34.6	39.8	37.0	37.1	34.2	30.5
New York	35.5	45.5	35.7	34.9	36.6	34.8
North Carolina	26.2	29.5	29.2	30.5	22.2	24.3
North Dakota	32.8	40.4	35.0	32.6	32.4	30.7
Ohio	34.6	38.8	37.9	42.4	33.7	31.3
Oklahoma	29.0	34.7	31.1	31.2	30.5	28.9
Oregon	38.4	43.8	40.4	38.2	40.2	35.0
Pennsylvania	36.8	45.7	38.6	38.4	36.9	35.4
Rhode Island	37.0	44.3	43.4	38.6	41.0	31.9
South Carolina	31.8	48.0	40.6	33.2	27.3	26.4
South Dakota	28.7	33.4	31.8	31.1	27.2	26.9
Tennessee	29.1	50.5	31.4	32.2	29.6	29.5
Texas	33.2	37.6	36.5	37.7	33.0	30.2
Utah	43.1	54.0	52.2	42.7	44.1	40.1
Vermont	35.6	48.5	41.9	34.4	34.6	31.5
Virginia	36.8	51.1	39.3	39.8	34.8	35.5
Washington	38.8	53.8	45.7	41.6	39.8	34.4
West Virginia	35.1	44.3	38.8	32.1	32.1	31.1
Wisconsin	40.3	53.4	48.2	39.5	40.7	37.0
Wyoming	35.2	45.9	40.4	33.5	37.2	31.2

Source: Compiled by New Strategist based on the Centers for Disease Control and Prevention Behavioral Risk Factor Surveillance System Survey, Internet site http://www.cdc.gov/brfss/index.htm

1.86 Health Status: Poor Mental Health by Sex, 2001

"For how many days during the past 30 days was your mental health not good?"

(percent of people aged 18 or older responding "one or more," by state and sex, 2001)

	total	men	women
U.S. total	**33.9%**	**28.3%**	**38.1%**
Alabama	38.9	33.8	43.3
Alaska	36.6	28.9	44.7
Arizona	36.0	31.3	40.4
Arkansas	35.0	32.3	37.2
California	37.8	31.5	44.0
Colorado	35.9	30.1	41.6
Connecticut	33.1	28.2	37.5
Delaware	32.8	26.6	38.7
District of Columbia	33.7	28.5	38.3
Florida	29.9	26.1	33.6
Georgia	34.6	29.9	38.8
Hawaii	15.8	12.9	18.6
Idaho	36.4	29.0	43.4
Illinois	33.9	28.3	38.9
Indiana	36.9	31.4	42.0
Iowa	31.7	26.8	36.1
Kansas	30.5	24.7	35.9
Kentucky	28.2	23.0	32.9
Louisiana	25.1	19.3	30.6
Maine	32.9	27.8	37.6
Maryland	33.0	27.5	38.0
Massachusetts	34.7	30.2	38.9
Michigan	38.5	31.9	44.6
Minnesota	39.8	35.5	44.0
Mississippi	30.1	22.3	37.1
Missouri	33.5	28.3	38.5
Montana	22.8	14.7	30.7
Nebraska	24.4	19.9	28.7
Nevada	39.7	32.8	46.8
New Hampshire	33.7	28.9	38.3
New Jersey	32.9	28.1	37.5
New Mexico	34.6	29.8	39.2
New York	35.5	31.7	38.9
North Carolina	26.2	19.4	32.5
North Dakota	32.8	27.8	37.5
Ohio	34.6	29.0	39.7
Oklahoma	29.0	22.8	34.9
Oregon	38.4	33.0	43.4
Pennsylvania	36.8	31.6	41.5
Rhode Island	37.0	31.8	41.7
South Carolina	31.8	25.6	37.3
South Dakota	28.7	24.6	32.6
Tennessee	29.1	25.6	32.5
Texas	33.2	27.0	39.0
Utah	43.1	36.6	49.2
Vermont	35.6	30.8	39.8
Virginia	36.8	28.8	44.3
Washington	38.8	33.1	44.2
West Virginia	35.1	29.3	40.4
Wisconsin	40.3	33.4	46.8
Wyoming	35.2	28.7	41.8

Source: Compiled by New Strategist based on the Centers for Disease Control and Prevention Behavioral Risk Factor Surveillance System Survey, Internet site http://www.cdc.gov/brfss/index.htm

1.87 Health Status: Poor Health Disrupted Usual Activity by Age, 2001

"For how many days of the last 30 did poor physical or mental
health keep you from doing your usual activities?"

(percent of people aged 18 or older responding "one or more," by state and age, 2001)

	total	18 to 24	25 to 34	35 to 44	45 to 54	55 to 64	65 or older
U.S. total	19.3%	21.4%	19.4%	19.5%	19.7%	18.5%	15.8%
Alabama	22.4	21.7	21.6	22.3	24.4	24.0	20.6
Alaska	23.5	23.6	22.6	25.7	23.3	24.8	18.5
Arizona	21.1	23.8	20.3	28.4	21.0	13.2	17.8
Arkansas	21.4	23.2	20.0	21.6	22.3	22.9	19.3
California	22.0	22.2	24.4	23.9	19.8	19.8	20.8
Colorado	20.9	22.6	23.4	21.5	20.4	19.0	17.6
Connecticut	17.2	23.8	17.8	17.2	18.1	14.0	13.2
Delaware	17.9	19.4	15.0	19.5	18.9	19.4	14.8
District of Columbia	19.3	25.5	20.1	19.0	20.1	18.7	15.0
Florida	17.9	20.4	17.7	17.6	21.0	20.0	13.8
Georgia	19.6	24.8	18.2	19.4	21.5	16.8	16.5
Hawaii	14.4	16.4	15.0	14.4	15.9	11.9	13.3
Idaho	21.1	27.3	23.0	22.3	19.8	20.0	16.1
Illinois	17.8	17.0	20.1	18.6	17.5	14.8	17.8
Indiana	18.6	21.6	21.7	18.8	20.5	15.0	13.7
Iowa	17.7	28.0	20.2	16.8	19.0	11.9	12.5
Kansas	16.7	22.8	16.6	14.5	17.1	17.3	13.6
Kentucky	19.0	12.7	17.6	19.8	20.7	22.9	19.1
Louisiana	17.5	16.0	15.1	18.4	19.7	20.5	15.9
Maine	18.4	24.5	19.4	17.5	20.3	12.9	16.6
Maryland	19.4	24.1	21.3	18.1	19.9	19.8	14.9
Massachusetts	20.1	24.2	20.6	20.2	19.2	20.5	18.1
Michigan	21.1	26.0	23.0	20.5	22.7	17.3	16.7
Minnesota	21.4	29.2	23.2	21.4	21.2	18.4	15.6
Mississippi	19.7	19.0	18.5	18.1	20.8	22.8	21.1
Missouri	22.1	23.0	25.4	21.5	22.5	23.7	17.8
Montana	18.4	18.8	17.1	16.0	19.6	21.9	19.0
Nebraska	15.4	16.9	18.3	15.5	15.6	14.7	12.7
Nevada	21.6	24.6	22.1	24.7	21.3	22.3	15.1
New Hampshire	17.8	21.9	17.0	15.9	22.0	15.7	15.0
New Jersey	18.6	26.4	20.2	17.8	18.2	17.2	14.5
New Mexico	20.5	19.4	20.0	22.5	24.2	18.1	17.0
New York	19.7	22.6	20.1	18.9	22.1	17.1	17.2
North Carolina	18.0	13.1	18.6	18.4	16.5	16.1	24.3
North Dakota	16.7	18.1	19.2	16.8	13.9	18.1	14.9
Ohio	19.4	24.2	20.1	19.6	17.8	22.3	14.1
Oklahoma	19.3	18.2	18.3	17.4	22.2	20.9	18.8
Oregon	23.3	25.8	24.6	25.0	22.8	22.9	18.6
Pennsylvania	20.3	24.8	19.9	22.6	21.7	17.4	16.8
Rhode Island	21.3	25.4	23.0	23.1	19.6	21.0	17.8
South Carolina	19.4	19.5	15.7	21.2	20.8	20.9	18.6
South Dakota	15.9	17.5	16.8	16.8	14.9	14.9	15.0
Tennessee	16.8	15.7	15.5	19.8	20.9	15.0	11.9
Texas	19.2	23.6	20.4	18.8	17.1	20.5	16.1
Utah	21.5	26.9	23.0	21.5	21.6	22.3	13.5
Vermont	19.3	21.5	21.6	20.2	18.3	19.0	16.0
Virginia	20.0	25.8	18.5	18.5	21.1	16.8	20.2
Washington	22.1	26.6	22.6	24.3	21.7	19.1	17.8
West Virginia	24.2	22.5	23.0	23.4	26.9	28.4	21.6
Wisconsin	19.6	23.7	19.9	19.0	19.7	19.0	17.2
Wyoming	17.5	20.6	18.6	20.1	15.1	16.7	14.7

*Source: Compiled by New Strategist based on the Centers for Disease Control and Prevention Behavioral Risk Factor
Surveillance System Survey, Internet site http://www.cdc.gov/brfss/index.htm*

1.88 Health Status: Poor Health Disrupted Usual Activity by Education, 2001

"For how many days of the last 30 did poor physical or mental
health keep you from doing your usual activities?"

(percent of people aged 18 or older responding "one or more," by state and educational attainment, 2001)

	total	less than high school	high school graduate	some college	college graduate
U.S. total	**19.3%**	**22.5%**	**18.3%**	**19.9%**	**17.3%**
Alabama	22.4	36.2	21.4	20.2	16.9
Alaska	23.5	27.6	22.6	26.5	19.7
Arizona	21.1	27.2	21.0	22.0	17.7
Arkansas	21.4	30.1	20.1	20.5	18.3
California	22.0	23.4	19.6	25.3	20.1
Colorado	20.9	19.3	20.2	23.6	19.7
Connecticut	17.2	18.5	17.4	18.8	15.5
Delaware	17.9	24.7	16.3	19.1	16.8
District of Columbia	19.3	25.0	20.9	15.8	18.6
Florida	17.9	19.6	16.8	18.2	18.1
Georgia	19.6	23.7	19.1	20.7	17.4
Hawaii	14.4	14.7	12.6	17.4	13.2
Idaho	21.1	29.4	18.3	22.9	19.9
Illinois	17.8	17.5	18.6	18.2	17.0
Indiana	18.6	24.2	16.5	20.6	17.1
Iowa	17.7	19.6	16.5	19.7	16.9
Kansas	16.7	17.9	16.2	18.2	15.3
Kentucky	19.0	29.5	18.7	16.7	12.0
Louisiana	17.5	22.4	16.4	18.8	14.0
Maine	18.4	21.4	19.7	18.2	16.2
Maryland	19.4	19.6	18.7	22.4	18.3
Massachusetts	20.1	26.1	20.5	21.2	18.1
Michigan	21.1	24.6	19.5	22.6	20.0
Minnesota	21.4	28.5	22.3	20.5	19.7
Mississippi	19.7	27.8	17.7	18.6	17.8
Missouri	22.1	26.8	20.4	22.4	21.4
Montana	18.4	21.3	18.2	20.9	15.3
Nebraska	15.4	19.7	15.2	13.6	16.8
Nevada	21.6	22.9	22.3	23.2	19.2
New Hampshire	17.8	17.0	18.4	18.1	17.3
New Jersey	18.6	23.6	18.1	21.0	16.0
New Mexico	20.5	18.6	20.3	21.6	20.8
New York	19.7	25.4	17.7	20.4	18.5
North Carolina	18.0	25.5	17.4	15.9	16.4
North Dakota	16.7	20.0	16.4	16.8	15.8
Ohio	19.4	23.5	19.5	19.0	17.6
Oklahoma	19.3	23.1	17.7	23.7	14.3
Oregon	23.3	23.8	22.2	24.5	22.5
Pennsylvania	20.3	24.8	19.0	22.8	18.8
Rhode Island	21.3	22.5	21.9	21.8	20.0
South Carolina	19.4	28.2	18.8	19.2	15.3
South Dakota	15.9	18.9	15.2	15.9	15.7
Tennessee	16.8	19.9	16.3	18.7	13.1
Texas	19.2	20.8	18.0	20.9	17.7
Utah	21.5	23.2	22.8	22.7	18.5
Vermont	19.3	25.1	16.8	21.8	18.7
Virginia	20.0	23.1	21.0	20.4	17.7
Washington	22.1	25.5	23.6	22.7	19.1
West Virginia	24.2	32.9	22.4	25.0	17.5
Wisconsin	19.6	26.5	18.3	19.9	18.7
Wyoming	17.5	21.8	16.4	18.7	16.2

Source: Compiled by New Strategist based on the Centers for Disease Control and Prevention Behavioral Risk Factor Surveillance System Survey, Internet site http://www.cdc.gov/brfss/index.htm

1.89 Health Status: Poor Health Disrupted Usual Activity by Household Income, 2001

"For how many days of the last 30 did poor physical or mental
health keep you from doing your usual activities?"

(percent of people aged 18 or older responding "one or more," by state and household income, 2001)

	total	less than $15,000	$15,000 to $24,999	$25,000 to $34,999	$35,000 to $49,999	$50,000 or more
U.S. total	**19.3%**	**31.7%**	**22.7%**	**18.6%**	**17.5%**	**15.3%**
Alabama	22.4	38.2	29.3	19.4	16.4	15.2
Alaska	23.5	44.2	27.7	25.1	22.8	20.5
Arizona	21.1	33.3	28.1	24.0	16.4	15.1
Arkansas	21.4	33.1	28.4	19.2	16.2	13.3
California	22.0	29.7	24.9	22.6	16.0	20.2
Colorado	20.9	35.6	23.2	27.1	18.7	16.5
Connecticut	17.2	28.3	23.0	17.6	16.3	15.1
Delaware	17.9	23.2	25.1	16.7	18.2	15.6
District of Columbia	19.3	26.7	25.4	19.5	18.7	15.8
Florida	17.9	29.4	20.0	16.9	17.8	14.8
Georgia	19.6	29.9	22.0	22.1	16.9	17.4
Hawaii	14.4	20.7	12.9	16.0	16.4	13.7
Idaho	21.1	34.3	25.0	20.7	18.1	17.0
Illinois	17.8	31.2	21.4	16.7	16.8	15.7
Indiana	18.6	28.6	25.8	18.6	16.6	15.1
Iowa	17.7	28.8	20.2	14.3	16.5	16.4
Kansas	16.7	33.0	20.6	15.4	15.6	12.9
Kentucky	19.0	36.6	27.3	19.1	15.0	10.8
Louisiana	17.5	28.1	21.0	15.2	16.1	13.1
Maine	18.4	40.6	25.3	15.6	11.2	14.0
Maryland	19.4	30.5	24.1	20.0	17.2	17.5
Massachusetts	20.1	36.0	23.7	20.5	20.5	16.9
Michigan	21.1	32.0	24.7	21.7	22.0	16.6
Minnesota	21.4	35.1	24.7	27.8	19.6	18.9
Mississippi	19.7	33.2	21.5	15.6	15.5	15.8
Missouri	22.1	35.2	27.0	22.9	17.0	19.7
Montana	18.4	35.2	19.4	19.7	15.9	11.3
Nebraska	15.4	27.4	17.2	13.1	15.0	14.9
Nevada	21.6	45.1	22.5	24.9	21.1	18.7
New Hampshire	17.8	35.5	19.8	19.3	18.2	15.1
New Jersey	18.6	31.3	20.3	17.7	17.8	16.0
New Mexico	20.5	28.9	20.4	18.0	19.5	19.6
New York	19.7	32.6	22.0	19.5	22.2	14.8
North Carolina	18.0	33.1	19.6	15.2	15.7	14.0
North Dakota	16.7	21.7	19.5	17.5	17.9	11.3
Ohio	19.4	32.9	20.5	21.0	20.0	15.1
Oklahoma	19.3	30.2	23.6	21.2	17.6	12.8
Oregon	23.3	33.5	25.3	20.4	25.2	18.2
Pennsylvania	20.3	33.0	25.4	18.1	19.8	16.9
Rhode Island	21.3	34.8	28.8	19.5	20.1	16.9
South Carolina	19.4	38.0	26.6	16.9	16.4	13.0
South Dakota	15.9	22.0	19.5	14.0	15.2	14.2
Tennessee	16.8	38.1	22.9	14.7	14.3	14.2
Texas	19.2	27.7	23.1	16.2	17.6	16.4
Utah	21.5	36.1	26.1	22.6	20.6	19.9
Vermont	19.3	31.8	24.0	18.5	16.6	17.1
Virginia	20.0	36.1	24.1	24.7	16.5	16.9
Washington	22.1	37.3	29.7	22.1	20.2	18.1
West Virginia	24.2	38.8	27.8	24.3	20.2	16.2
Wisconsin	19.6	29.3	25.1	22.4	17.6	15.2
Wyoming	17.5	30.3	19.8	18.5	16.1	12.9

Source: Compiled by New Strategist based on the Centers for Disease Control and Prevention Behavioral Risk Factor Surveillance System Survey, Internet site http://www.cdc.gov/brfss/index.htm

1.90 Health Status: Poor Health Disrupted Usual Activity by Sex, 2001

"For how many days of the last 30 did poor physical or mental health keep you from doing your usual activities?"

(percent of people aged 18 or older responding "one or more," by state and sex, 2001)

	total	men	women
U.S. total	**19.3%**	**16.8%**	**21.6%**
Alabama	22.4	19.5	25.0
Alaska	23.5	20.6	26.6
Arizona	21.1	18.5	23.5
Arkansas	21.4	21.1	21.4
California	22.0	18.1	25.9
Colorado	20.9	19.2	22.5
Connecticut	17.2	16.1	17.9
Delaware	17.9	14.6	20.9
District of Columbia	19.3	15.8	22.5
Florida	17.9	16.4	19.1
Georgia	19.6	18.0	21.1
Hawaii	14.4	13.0	15.9
Idaho	21.1	18.6	23.7
Illinois	17.8	16.1	19.5
Indiana	18.6	15.0	21.9
Iowa	17.7	16.0	19.4
Kansas	16.7	14.7	18.5
Kentucky	19.0	17.5	20.3
Louisiana	17.5	14.1	20.5
Maine	18.4	16.5	20.3
Maryland	19.4	16.8	21.9
Massachusetts	20.1	18.3	21.8
Michigan	21.1	18.6	23.6
Minnesota	21.4	19.0	23.6
Mississippi	19.7	17.1	22.0
Missouri	22.1	19.7	24.1
Montana	18.4	12.5	24.4
Nebraska	15.4	13.4	17.5
Nevada	21.6	16.7	26.7
New Hampshire	17.8	15.6	19.8
New Jersey	18.6	15.6	21.2
New Mexico	20.5	18.6	22.4
New York	19.7	19.4	19.8
North Carolina	18.0	14.2	21.7
North Dakota	16.7	12.9	20.4
Ohio	19.4	18.1	20.5
Oklahoma	19.3	18.0	20.5
Oregon	23.3	19.7	26.4
Pennsylvania	20.3	18.0	22.6
Rhode Island	21.3	19.2	23.3
South Carolina	19.4	17.3	21.1
South Dakota	15.9	14.2	17.6
Tennessee	16.8	14.3	19.1
Texas	19.2	16.0	22.3
Utah	21.5	17.0	25.9
Vermont	19.3	17.5	21.1
Virginia	20.0	16.6	23.0
Washington	22.1	18.6	25.3
West Virginia	24.2	22.2	25.9
Wisconsin	19.6	17.7	21.4
Wyoming	17.5	14.1	20.9

Source: Compiled by New Strategist based on the Centers for Disease Control and Prevention Behavioral Risk Factor Surveillance System Survey, Internet site http://www.cdc.gov/brfss/index.htm

1.91 Heart Attack by Sex, 2000

"Has a doctor ever told you that you had a heart attack or myocardial infarction?"

(percent of people aged 18 or older responding "yes," by state and sex, 2000)

	total	men	women
Delaware	4.2%	4.9%	3.4%
District of Columbia	3.0	2.8	3.2
Georgia	3.7	4.6	2.9
Indiana	5.2	6.4	4.0
Iowa	4.1	5.7	2.6
Kentucky	5.4	7.0	3.9
Mississippi	5.3	6.2	4.6
Montana	3.4	4.3	2.6
Ohio	5.4	7.4	3.6
Oklahoma	4.0	4.1	3.9
Pennsylvania	4.6	5.4	3.7
South Carolina	4.5	5.6	3.5
Virginia	4.2	5.3	3.1
West Virginia	7.6	9.5	6.0

Source: Compiled by New Strategist based on the Centers for Disease Control and Prevention Behavioral Risk Factor Surveillance System Survey, Internet site http://www.cdc.gov/brfss/index.htm

1.92 High Blood Pressure by Age, 2001

"Have you ever been told by a doctor, nurse, or other health professional that you have high blood pressure?"

(percent of people aged 18 or older responding "yes," by state and age, 2001)

	total	18 to 24	25 to 34	35 to 44	45 to 54	55 to 64	65 or older
U.S. total	**25.6%**	**6.0%**	**9.7%**	**15.8%**	**27.9%**	**41.9%**	**53.0%**
Alabama	31.6	7.5	14.9	22.1	37.1	51.0	57.9
Alaska	21.8	4.3	10.1	15.2	26.4	41.0	59.2
Arizona	23.6	5.8	11.4	19.4	25.5	35.1	44.6
Arkansas	29.7	4.5	13.6	19.4	34.7	43.5	55.3
California	23.3	6.4	9.4	15.9	26.6	41.2	48.8
Colorado	21.6	8.0	7.4	12.4	17.9	37.9	56.0
Connecticut	24.0	5.1	9.4	13.3	24.8	36.6	53.0
Delaware	27.2	7.3	13.2	15.7	28.6	49.6	52.8
District of Columbia	29.0	6.7	9.7	16.5	30.7	51.4	67.7
Florida	26.9	5.7	8.5	13.2	25.8	43.3	50.5
Georgia	26.9	7.7	10.3	19.5	31.7	49.1	54.1
Hawaii	24.1	4.2	7.2	15.1	24.6	38.5	55.3
Idaho	24.6	4.1	10.8	16.2	27.8	41.9	48.2
Illinois	24.8	4.7	7.6	13.7	29.8	44.2	55.8
Indiana	25.8	4.7	10.4	19.4	30.7	38.4	50.5
Iowa	25.5	3.0	9.0	15.8	25.6	38.7	55.1
Kansas	23.9	5.0	9.4	14.2	26.9	39.1	49.3
Kentucky	30.1	7.8	12.9	22.4	33.3	46.1	58.2
Louisiana	27.6	7.3	12.1	18.6	32.7	46.3	55.5
Maine	25.2	3.8	9.1	14.9	27.3	39.3	55.0
Maryland	26.3	7.8	9.2	15.8	29.3	44.2	57.8
Massachusetts	23.6	4.8	8.7	14.3	24.1	39.0	51.3
Michigan	27.3	6.1	13.1	19.0	29.2	42.7	54.8
Minnesota	22.3	4.5	6.9	13.6	23.6	37.5	50.8
Mississippi	31.3	5.0	15.1	22.6	39.2	51.5	59.9
Missouri	26.5	8.1	10.1	16.4	28.7	44.8	50.5
Montana	26.8	8.4	10.1	17.7	29.3	39.5	52.6
Nebraska	22.6	5.5	6.8	11.0	23.7	38.7	50.0
Nevada	25.6	8.2	10.7	16.5	29.4	39.4	50.6
New Hampshire	22.8	6.2	10.8	13.0	24.3	38.7	49.7
New Jersey	26.1	4.7	8.9	14.4	28.1	45.6	53.5
New Mexico	20.0	5.8	6.3	15.0	22.5	34.5	40.6
New York	26.0	6.9	10.7	15.0	24.9	42.0	57.6
North Carolina	27.2	7.5	8.4	19.2	30.7	45.2	54.9
North Dakota	24.1	4.4	9.3	14.0	25.2	39.5	52.1
Ohio	26.6	7.8	12.3	13.9	26.1	46.6	55.5
Oklahoma	28.5	6.3	13.6	17.3	31.1	48.5	54.1
Oregon	24.9	6.4	9.3	14.5	25.3	42.0	51.7
Pennsylvania	28.1	8.9	8.1	17.8	29.0	42.4	55.6
Rhode Island	25.4	7.3	9.7	17.2	24.3	40.4	52.4
South Carolina	28.8	7.7	12.1	20.0	31.8	47.5	58.9
South Dakota	24.1	5.1	8.2	13.8	24.1	41.4	50.8
Tennessee	29.3	5.9	14.3	18.7	33.8	46.9	56.0
Texas	25.6	6.8	8.8	17.8	29.8	45.2	55.0
Utah	22.3	5.4	8.7	15.1	27.6	37.9	52.8
Vermont	21.4	5.0	8.5	12.2	21.9	36.3	49.6
Virginia	25.8	9.7	10.4	16.6	30.2	40.7	54.2
Washington	24.4	6.7	10.0	14.8	26.8	40.4	51.5
West Virginia	32.5	7.3	15.1	19.5	40.3	45.7	57.9
Wisconsin	24.1	5.7	9.0	12.9	24.8	41.6	52.1
Wyoming	22.4	4.9	8.4	14.3	22.2	37.6	51.2

Source: Compiled by New Strategist based on the Centers for Disease Control and Prevention Behavioral Risk Factor Surveillance System Survey, Internet site http://www.cdc.gov/brfss/index.htm

1.93 High Blood Pressure by Education, 2001

"Have you ever been told by a doctor, nurse, or other health professional that you have high blood pressure?"

(percent of people aged 18 or older responding "yes," by state and educational attainment, 2001)

	total	less than high school	high school graduate	some college	college graduate
U.S. total	**25.6%**	**36.3%**	**27.9%**	**23.6%**	**20.1%**
Alabama	31.6	48.2	32.2	27.5	23.5
Alaska	21.8	32.3	20.4	21.9	20.1
Arizona	23.6	28.7	22.9	23.7	22.2
Arkansas	29.7	40.3	28.4	25.0	29.7
California	23.3	25.4	22.5	26.8	19.7
Colorado	21.6	26.0	20.5	21.9	20.8
Connecticut	24.0	35.9	27.4	24.4	18.8
Delaware	27.2	39.2	29.0	26.4	22.9
District of Columbia	29.0	56.4	34.0	27.3	19.6
Florida	26.9	29.9	27.5	27.6	24.6
Georgia	26.9	40.8	28.9	25.5	19.3
Hawaii	24.1	47.2	24.4	23.3	19.9
Idaho	24.6	33.0	27.3	22.1	21.4
Illinois	24.8	37.9	30.2	21.3	18.9
Indiana	25.8	30.1	27.2	27.2	20.6
Iowa	25.5	39.0	28.6	22.8	19.2
Kansas	23.9	32.9	28.1	22.3	21.4
Kentucky	30.1	45.4	31.6	22.3	21.4
Louisiana	27.6	42.0	27.0	23.9	21.1
Maine	25.2	37.9	26.1	23.8	21.3
Maryland	26.3	45.0	28.3	23.4	19.0
Massachusetts	23.6	30.4	28.3	23.4	19.0
Michigan	27.3	36.3	31.5	24.3	21.6
Minnesota	22.3	35.6	26.5	20.7	17.1
Mississippi	31.3	43.0	31.3	26.9	26.5
Missouri	26.5	36.3	30.8	23.3	19.6
Montana	26.8	29.9	29.2	26.3	23.1
Nebraska	22.6	34.2	25.0	19.0	18.8
Nevada	25.6	30.0	24.4	23.3	28.4
New Hampshire	22.8	30.0	25.6	23.6	18.1
New Jersey	26.1	33.6	29.4	25.0	21.8
New Mexico	20.0	21.9	21.4	20.0	17.5
New York	26.0	36.3	27.5	23.9	21.8
North Carolina	27.2	38.6	30.4	25.0	18.5
North Dakota	24.1	40.6	28.0	20.7	18.8
Ohio	26.6	36.9	29.1	23.6	21.2
Oklahoma	28.5	36.3	29.8	27.4	23.2
Oregon	24.9	24.6	29.0	23.5	22.3
Pennsylvania	28.1	37.1	32.8	25.3	19.6
Rhode Island	25.4	34.5	29.3	23.0	19.9
South Carolina	28.8	45.0	28.1	28.4	20.9
South Dakota	24.1	38.2	25.4	22.4	19.4
Tennessee	29.3	45.9	28.9	29.4	18.7
Texas	25.6	28.9	25.5	25.6	23.3
Utah	22.3	24.9	23.5	20.5	22.7
Vermont	21.4	34.9	22.7	20.0	17.9
Virginia	25.8	40.7	29.0	24.2	19.8
Washington	24.4	25.4	27.9	25.6	20.1
West Virginia	32.5	49.9	30.5	28.6	23.3
Wisconsin	24.1	35.3	26.9	22.5	18.5
Wyoming	22.4	28.1	25.8	20.2	19.1

Source: Compiled by New Strategist based on the Centers for Disease Control and Prevention Behavioral Risk Factor Surveillance System Survey, Internet site http://www.cdc.gov/brfss/index.htm

1.94 High Blood Pressure by Household Income, 2001

"Have you ever been told by a doctor, nurse, or other health professional that you have high blood pressure?"

(percent of people aged 18 or older responding "yes," by state and household income, 2001)

	total	less than $15,000	$15,000 to $24,999	$25,000 to $34,999	$35,000 to $49,999	$50,000 or more
U.S. total	25.6%	34.0%	29.5%	25.8%	23.5%	20.4%
Alabama	31.6	39.9	35.1	29.4	26.4	24.8
Alaska	21.8	31.6	25.7	19.8	21.6	20.3
Arizona	23.6	31.9	26.6	23.9	25.2	18.7
Arkansas	29.7	38.5	32.0	25.3	27.0	23.0
California	23.3	29.7	25.9	25.5	23.9	18.8
Colorado	21.6	26.5	25.3	23.3	23.9	16.7
Connecticut	24.0	35.1	31.4	27.2	22.8	19.2
Delaware	27.2	29.1	36.9	19.5	26.0	22.7
District of Columbia	29.0	38.8	35.6	29.5	26.0	20.9
Florida	26.9	28.4	30.0	26.2	23.2	22.8
Georgia	26.9	42.9	30.0	28.1	22.8	20.0
Hawaii	24.1	28.2	21.6	19.3	25.5	23.1
Idaho	24.6	34.3	25.7	26.0	21.9	20.4
Illinois	24.8	40.4	27.8	25.0	23.4	19.1
Indiana	25.8	41.0	30.9	27.6	22.7	20.4
Iowa	25.5	32.6	33.0	25.7	23.5	18.9
Kansas	23.9	32.1	29.8	24.6	22.7	19.9
Kentucky	30.1	40.0	31.9	35.5	24.7	21.0
Louisiana	27.6	43.4	28.7	26.4	22.0	21.8
Maine	25.2	38.4	29.1	28.6	20.0	20.3
Maryland	26.3	36.5	34.1	29.3	24.2	21.1
Massachusetts	23.6	33.0	33.1	28.7	21.9	17.9
Michigan	27.3	32.6	32.7	29.0	24.2	22.5
Minnesota	22.3	35.6	28.8	24.5	21.9	16.8
Mississippi	31.3	44.1	35.3	26.7	24.9	25.3
Missouri	26.5	43.6	34.1	26.3	20.4	19.0
Montana	26.8	30.5	27.8	29.2	23.8	20.4
Nebraska	22.6	31.9	25.7	22.3	20.4	15.3
Nevada	25.6	32.9	24.6	22.0	22.4	24.1
New Hampshire	22.8	39.0	29.2	25.4	22.7	18.1
New Jersey	26.1	34.6	31.2	28.7	25.1	21.3
New Mexico	20.0	21.0	22.3	20.8	14.8	18.6
New York	26.0	37.8	27.9	31.7	25.5	21.5
North Carolina	27.2	40.0	33.9	25.5	21.3	20.5
North Dakota	24.1	32.3	26.9	23.7	20.2	18.1
Ohio	26.6	37.3	31.8	25.6	25.9	21.3
Oklahoma	28.5	39.7	31.2	22.6	26.5	22.3
Oregon	24.9	28.8	25.6	23.9	27.5	21.2
Pennsylvania	28.1	33.8	35.4	29.0	24.8	22.4
Rhode Island	25.4	33.3	32.2	27.4	25.5	19.1
South Carolina	28.8	44.2	33.3	26.0	24.4	21.8
South Dakota	24.1	30.8	27.4	23.9	20.2	18.2
Tennessee	29.3	41.0	34.0	28.3	19.1	21.9
Texas	25.6	29.2	26.2	26.4	23.5	22.1
Utah	22.3	25.1	24.5	26.7	22.7	19.0
Vermont	21.4	27.5	25.3	22.2	17.9	17.9
Virginia	25.8	40.8	30.4	23.4	25.3	21.3
Washington	24.4	32.8	28.3	27.4	22.8	20.7
West Virginia	32.5	42.0	34.5	33.8	28.9	24.9
Wisconsin	24.1	27.1	29.1	26.5	24.5	17.8
Wyoming	22.4	30.3	25.9	22.5	16.9	20.0

Source: Compiled by New Strategist based on the Centers for Disease Control and Prevention Behavioral Risk Factor Surveillance System Survey, Internet site http://www.cdc.gov/brfss/index.htm

1.95 High Blood Pressure by Sex, 2001

"Have you ever been told by a doctor, nurse, or other health
professional that you have high blood pressure?"

(percent of people aged 18 or older responding "yes." by state and sex, 2001)

	total	men	women
U.S. total	**25.6%**	**24.9%**	**26.2%**
Alabama	31.6	29.8	33.3
Alaska	21.8	20.6	23.0
Arizona	23.6	25.7	21.7
Arkansas	29.7	29.4	30.0
California	23.3	22.2	24.3
Colorado	21.6	21.8	21.4
Connecticut	24.0	23.9	24.2
Delaware	27.2	27.2	27.3
District of Columbia	29.0	26.4	31.1
Florida	26.9	26.6	27.2
Georgia	26.9	25.7	28.1
Hawaii	24.1	24.0	24.1
Idaho	24.6	24.8	24.4
Illinois	24.8	22.8	26.5
Indiana	25.8	24.5	26.9
Iowa	25.5	24.9	26.1
Kansas	23.9	23.1	24.6
Kentucky	30.1	31.0	29.3
Louisiana	27.6	25.2	29.7
Maine	25.2	25.3	25.1
Maryland	26.3	26.3	26.3
Massachusetts	23.6	23.5	23.6
Michigan	27.3	27.0	27.5
Minnesota	22.3	22.6	22.0
Mississippi	31.3	28.8	33.6
Missouri	26.5	26.3	26.7
Montana	26.8	26.4	27.2
Nebraska	22.6	21.5	23.7
Nevada	25.6	25.4	25.8
New Hampshire	22.8	23.9	21.8
New Jersey	26.1	24.7	27.3
New Mexico	20.0	19.9	20.2
New York	26.0	26.5	25.5
North Carolina	27.2	25.4	28.9
North Dakota	24.1	23.5	24.7
Ohio	26.6	25.8	27.3
Oklahoma	28.5	29.1	28.0
Oregon	24.9	24.3	25.5
Pennsylvania	28.1	27.2	28.8
Rhode Island	25.4	25.7	25.2
South Carolina	28.8	28.6	29.1
South Dakota	24.1	23.9	24.3
Tennessee	29.3	28.4	30.1
Texas	25.6	23.8	27.3
Utah	22.3	22.5	22.2
Vermont	21.4	21.0	21.8
Virginia	25.8	24.8	26.7
Washington	24.4	25.5	23.5
West Virginia	32.5	32.5	32.4
Wisconsin	24.1	23.6	24.7
Wyoming	22.4	23.2	21.7

*Source: Compiled by New Strategist based on the Centers for Disease Control and Prevention Behavioral Risk Factor
Surveillance System Survey, Internet site http://www.cdc.gov/brfss/index.htm*

1.96 HIV: Ever Tested by Age, 2000

"Have you ever been tested for HIV?"

(percent of people aged 18 or older responding "yes," by state and age, 2000)

	total	18 to 24	25 to 34	35 to 44	45 to 54	55 to 64
U.S. total	**45.7%**	**42.4%**	**61.6%**	**50.3%**	**37.7%**	**27.3%**
Alabama	50.6	61.8	69.9	50.3	40.4	34.5
Alaska	53.6	45.7	74.5	55.7	44.7	36.2
Arizona	38.1	40.8	49.1	40.1	33.9	22.5
Arkansas	49.2	57.2	65.0	54.9	41.4	28.6
California	49.2	38.7	60.1	54.5	45.8	35.8
Colorado	50.3	57.1	61.4	60.1	34.7	29.8
Connecticut	47.2	48.6	64.1	55.9	38.1	23.6
Delaware	50.4	39.7	65.3	58.4	43.4	38.8
District of Columbia	71.0	53.1	78.8	77.8	73.7	60.5
Florida	54.9	45.7	72.0	62.4	51.0	38.6
Georgia	54.8	51.7	77.0	57.5	44.8	35.2
Hawaii	36.8	40.5	50.3	39.5	31.8	19.1
Idaho	43.2	38.8	61.3	45.9	34.2	31.2
Illinois	41.8	36.5	57.4	50.3	32.3	24.1
Indiana	44.2	45.6	61.7	47.0	36.5	28.8
Iowa	31.8	34.1	45.5	33.7	30.0	11.7
Kansas	39.3	38.8	56.8	42.0	30.1	25.9
Kentucky	39.0	40.4	57.5	42.7	31.8	19.7
Louisiana	46.5	46.5	64.0	49.3	38.6	29.5
Maine	38.8	46.5	51.7	42.5	32.4	21.7
Maryland	57.7	56.3	75.2	65.2	47.7	37.0
Massachusetts	46.7	40.1	64.2	54.3	38.6	29.4
Michigan	49.5	39.0	67.0	59.8	41.0	31.2
Minnesota	26.7	24.5	40.4	25.3	18.8	21.8
Mississippi	54.2	63.7	73.1	54.8	42.5	34.2
Missouri	43.7	46.6	60.4	45.4	40.9	25.1
Montana	38.8	37.2	61.5	42.2	29.1	23.7
Nebraska	35.1	33.5	53.0	37.3	25.3	21.9
Nevada	61.6	56.1	71.0	67.7	58.7	47.3
New Hampshire	41.1	42.4	59.8	45.7	32.1	21.6
New Jersey	46.8	40.0	62.9	54.9	40.7	27.4
New Mexico	46.6	41.2	62.8	52.9	37.5	27.2
New York	47.8	42.5	61.7	54.3	43.5	29.7
North Carolina	43.2	52.0	58.1	48.8	33.8	21.5
North Dakota	33.8	29.7	56.0	33.8	23.0	22.3
Ohio	43.2	49.6	63.8	45.8	32.0	23.9
Oklahoma	35.3	37.1	54.8	38.6	26.1	18.8
Oregon	46.0	40.9	61.2	50.2	40.6	32.8
Pennsylvania	43.0	34.6	59.6	51.6	36.0	29.2
Rhode Island	47.2	42.8	63.6	58.2	38.7	23.7
South Carolina	51.7	54.0	71.3	54.0	40.5	36.4
South Dakota	33.1	31.7	50.9	37.5	22.9	19.0
Tennessee	47.7	50.7	60.7	53.5	39.9	29.4
Texas	50.5	45.4	62.5	58.0	45.2	31.3
Utah	38.0	26.5	52.7	42.9	37.9	22.6
Vermont	38.7	33.0	55.3	49.3	31.9	20.2
Virginia	55.3	49.9	67.7	64.1	48.2	40.6
Washington	49.2	43.2	66.2	59.2	41.5	28.5
West Virginia	35.5	37.8	49.6	43.3	25.6	21.5
Wisconsin	41.8	42.5	57.5	47.0	33.5	22.5
Wyoming	45.5	44.9	67.7	51.5	34.0	25.8

Source: Compiled by New Strategist based on the Centers for Disease Control and Prevention Behavioral Risk Factor Surveillance System Survey. Internet site http://www.cdc.gov/brfss/index.htm

1.97 HIV: Ever Tested by Education, 2000

"Have you ever been tested for HIV?"

(percent of people aged 18 or older responding "yes," by state and educational attainment, 2000)

	total	less than high school	high school graduate	some college	college graduate
U.S. total	**45.7%**	**44.4%**	**41.8%**	**46.6%**	**46.4%**
Alabama	50.6	47.5	52.9	53.9	46.4
Alaska	53.6	50.2	51.5	58.0	52.3
Arizona	38.1	41.6	34.9	36.5	42.9
Arkansas	49.2	44.4	47.1	54.9	49.7
California	49.2	43.7	46.1	52.1	53.8
Colorado	50.3	49.0	45.9	54.6	50.7
Connecticut	47.2	52.1	48.7	46.3	45.0
Delaware	50.4	44.6	49.8	52.2	51.5
District of Columbia	71.0	72.0	72.0	79.6	66.7
Florida	54.9	53.4	52.9	58.9	53.7
Georgia	54.8	50.7	53.6	56.2	58.5
Hawaii	36.8	27.9	33.8	39.8	39.4
Idaho	43.2	39.5	43.0	44.2	43.7
Illinois	41.8	32.6	39.6	44.1	45.1
Indiana	44.2	47.9	41.6	45.9	44.9
Iowa	31.8	36.4	27.3	36.6	30.7
Kansas	39.3	45.7	36.4	43.1	36.4
Kentucky	39.0	37.3	36.3	42.5	43.1
Louisiana	46.5	47.5	42.0	47.8	52.7
Maine	38.8	33.0	37.1	40.6	42.7
Maryland	57.7	50.9	55.5	61.7	58.6
Massachusetts	46.7	55.8	41.7	48.2	46.8
Michigan	49.5	47.3	47.9	54.7	45.9
Minnesota	26.7	29.2	26.6	23.9	29.6
Mississippi	54.2	56.1	51.3	58.1	52.6
Missouri	43.7	41.6	38.4	51.9	42.3
Montana	38.8	28.3	34.2	41.5	43.6
Nebraska	35.1	32.0	31.1	35.6	41.1
Nevada	61.6	68.2	58.7	59.7	65.7
New Hampshire	41.1	40.4	33.4	45.3	45.7
New Jersey	46.8	49.9	42.5	48.8	46.4
New Mexico	46.6	44.4	42.7	45.4	55.6
New York	47.8	54.0	43.2	49.6	48.8
North Carolina	43.2	43.8	40.1	47.4	42.8
North Dakota	33.8	30.3	29.8	36.7	35.9
Ohio	43.2	42.8	41.2	46.3	42.8
Oklahoma	35.3	33.4	31.4	37.0	42.6
Oregon	46.0	39.6	43.2	47.0	52.8
Pennsylvania	43.0	43.1	38.6	43.7	49.4
Rhode Island	47.2	48.4	44.9	46.2	49.9
South Carolina	51.7	55.1	48.9	52.5	53.8
South Dakota	33.1	32.8	31.0	31.6	38.6
Tennessee	47.7	47.5	45.4	48.4	52.0
Texas	50.5	45.5	48.4	52.9	55.7
Utah	38.0	42.3	41.7	33.1	39.3
Vermont	38.7	42.8	34.7	39.3	41.6
Virginia	55.3	50.5	51.5	59.2	58.1
Washington	49.2	57.6	51.8	46.2	48.5
West Virginia	35.5	36.3	32.2	39.3	38.3
Wisconsin	41.8	41.8	40.6	41.1	44.3
Wyoming	45.5	51.5	36.4	49.5	51.2

Source: Compiled by New Strategist based on the Centers for Disease Control and Prevention Behavioral Risk Factor Surveillance System Survey, Internet site http://www.cdc.gov/brfss/index.htm

1.98 HIV: Ever Tested by Household Income, 2000

"Have you ever been tested for HIV?"

(percent of people aged 18 or older responding "yes," by state and household income, 2000)

	total	less than $15,000	$15,000 to $24,999	$25,000 to $34,999	$35,000 to $49,999	$50,000 or more
U.S. total	**45.7%**	**50.1%**	**49.7%**	**46.5%**	**45.0%**	**45.0%**
Alabama	50.6	55.8	63.0	51.7	46.7	44.8
Alaska	53.6	59.0	54.0	56.1	61.5	49.2
Arizona	38.1	56.7	31.7	39.7	32.2	43.2
Arkansas	49.2	61.1	53.0	48.9	42.1	47.5
California	49.2	47.5	50.1	51.6	45.1	51.7
Colorado	50.3	55.5	42.2	50.6	54.7	51.5
Connecticut	47.2	53.4	59.3	53.5	45.8	44.9
Delaware	50.4	55.9	52.9	56.3	54.8	50.2
District of Columbia	71.0	70.1	72.6	74.6	69.6	70.2
Florida	54.9	62.4	59.4	54.7	54.1	51.0
Georgia	54.8	59.2	58.3	60.3	53.8	53.1
Hawaii	36.8	46.2	42.2	43.9	34.9	36.8
Idaho	43.2	50.0	44.1	47.9	38.6	43.7
Illinois	41.8	42.5	42.2	41.3	40.1	44.3
Indiana	44.2	57.6	54.2	40.7	40.1	44.4
Iowa	31.8	43.2	32.8	33.2	28.0	32.8
Kansas	39.3	43.6	44.3	40.7	40.9	40.5
Kentucky	39.0	50.6	43.9	35.9	33.9	37.6
Louisiana	46.5	45.6	50.0	45.3	51.6	47.1
Maine	38.8	44.6	41.8	36.2	40.7	38.5
Maryland	57.7	60.4	64.1	64.7	59.4	55.8
Massachusetts	46.7	48.3	54.7	46.2	47.3	46.7
Michigan	49.5	61.6	58.5	44.7	52.7	47.0
Minnesota	26.7	44.7	32.0	24.7	22.2	28.9
Mississippi	54.2	50.7	59.2	56.0	51.1	55.5
Missouri	43.7	49.5	38.3	47.1	40.3	47.2
Montana	38.8	42.1	39.2	40.6	44.9	35.6
Nebraska	35.1	43.0	42.5	32.3	40.2	33.3
Nevada	61.6	73.7	66.5	61.9	50.6	66.2
New Hampshire	41.1	47.4	48.8	39.9	36.9	44.7
New Jersey	46.8	48.2	50.3	42.1	45.9	45.2
New Mexico	46.6	50.9	45.2	54.1	40.7	45.8
New York	47.8	56.5	55.1	45.3	46.9	45.6
North Carolina	43.2	54.9	49.9	49.4	38.6	39.5
North Dakota	33.8	39.7	41.3	39.4	31.9	26.7
Ohio	43.2	50.3	52.8	44.1	49.5	36.5
Oklahoma	35.3	45.3	39.0	42.6	30.5	39.6
Oregon	46.0	49.2	49.5	46.1	42.1	47.9
Pennsylvania	43.0	50.5	44.5	45.9	47.3	40.7
Rhode Island	47.2	55.4	54.5	49.4	41.6	48.0
South Carolina	51.7	55.5	52.6	55.3	53.3	46.8
South Dakota	33.1	35.7	36.5	33.2	33.7	34.0
Tennessee	47.7	50.5	44.4	53.5	52.8	46.8
Texas	50.5	47.0	47.6	55.2	51.3	53.1
Utah	38.0	48.3	40.9	37.7	36.4	36.1
Vermont	38.7	40.5	44.5	36.9	36.0	39.5
Virginia	55.3	58.9	56.2	56.0	60.7	55.1
Washington	49.2	49.8	54.9	56.3	53.9	47.8
West Virginia	35.5	42.9	38.5	35.9	32.8	31.6
Wisconsin	41.8	38.6	52.5	46.9	38.6	38.2
Wyoming	45.5	65.6	40.2	47.0	47.6	42.2

Source: Compiled by New Strategist based on the Centers for Disease Control and Prevention Behavioral Risk Factor Surveillance System Survey, Internet site http://www.cdc.gov/brfss/index.htm

1.99 HIV: Ever Tested by Sex, 2000

"Have you ever been tested for HIV?"

(percent of people aged 18 or older responding "yes," by state and sex, 2000)

	total	men	women
U.S. total	**45.7%**	**44.3%**	**46.5%**
Alabama	50.6	49.5	51.6
Alaska	53.6	52.9	54.3
Arizona	38.1	34.0	41.7
Arkansas	49.2	48.9	49.6
California	49.2	46.1	51.9
Colorado	50.3	50.5	50.0
Connecticut	47.2	48.9	45.7
Delaware	50.4	48.9	51.6
District of Columbia	71.0	73.1	69.3
Florida	54.9	52.9	56.5
Georgia	54.8	54.8	54.9
Hawaii	36.8	37.2	36.4
Idaho	43.2	39.9	46.2
Illinois	41.8	40.9	42.5
Indiana	44.2	41.1	46.6
Iowa	31.8	29.8	33.6
Kansas	39.3	36.5	41.8
Kentucky	39.0	33.6	43.6
Louisiana	46.5	45.6	47.2
Maine	38.8	38.8	38.9
Maryland	57.7	55.5	59.6
Massachusetts	46.7	47.6	46.0
Michigan	49.5	45.1	53.3
Minnesota	26.7	22.3	30.9
Mississippi	54.2	52.6	55.5
Missouri	43.7	43.1	44.1
Montana	38.8	38.6	39.1
Nebraska	35.1	35.7	34.6
Nevada	61.6	61.7	61.6
New Hampshire	41.1	38.5	43.4
New Jersey	46.8	46.3	47.2
New Mexico	46.6	45.5	47.7
New York	47.8	44.9	50.4
North Carolina	43.2	40.4	45.5
North Dakota	33.8	34.0	33.7
Ohio	43.2	42.7	43.7
Oklahoma	35.3	32.1	38.2
Oregon	46.0	44.7	47.2
Pennsylvania	43.0	42.7	43.3
Rhode Island	47.2	46.1	48.1
South Carolina	51.7	48.1	54.4
South Dakota	33.1	32.7	33.5
Tennessee	47.7	46.9	48.3
Texas	50.5	46.1	54.1
Utah	38.0	38.4	37.6
Vermont	38.7	38.1	39.1
Virginia	55.3	53.8	56.6
Washington	49.2	48.4	50.0
West Virginia	35.5	36.3	34.9
Wisconsin	41.8	36.8	46.4
Wyoming	45.5	44.0	46.9

Source: Compiled by New Strategist based on the Centers for Disease Control and Prevention Behavioral Risk Factor Surveillance System Survey. Internet site http://www.cdc.gov/brfss/index.htm

1.100 HIV Test Past 12 Months, 2001

"Have you been tested for HIV in the past 12 months?"

(percent of people aged 18 or older responding "yes," by state, 2001)

	tested in past 12 months
U.S. total	**32.1%**
Alabama	35.4
Alaska	28.5
Arizona	39.8
Arkansas	33.6
California	31.8
Colorado	30.8
Connecticut	33.9
Delaware	37.4
District of Columbia	45.5
Florida	36.3
Georgia	37.2
Hawaii	36.8
Idaho	28.5
Illinois	35.5
Indiana	28.8
Iowa	32.1
Kansas	31.2
Kentucky	35.3
Louisiana	35.0
Maine	25.2
Maryland	34.2
Massachusetts	30.4
Michigan	29.4
Minnesota	26.6
Mississippi	38.8
Missouri	34.6
Montana	29.2
Nebraska	33.3
Nevada	31.5
New Hampshire	26.6
New Jersey	34.2
New Mexico	29.0
New York	39.8
North Carolina	40.3
North Dakota	29.6
Ohio	31.3
Oklahoma	28.5
Oregon	25.8
Pennsylvania	32.8
Rhode Island	34.2
South Carolina	38.2
South Dakota	31.7
Tennessee	32.1
Texas	36.0
Utah	28.4
Vermont	27.1
Virginia	33.9
Washington	25.9
West Virginia	31.3
Wisconsin	28.5
Wyoming	24.9

Source: Compiled by New Strategist based on the Centers for Disease Control and Prevention Behavioral Risk Factor Surveillance System Survey, Internet site http://www.cdc.gov/brfss/index.htm

1.101 HIV Risk by Age, 2000

"What are your chances of getting infected with HIV, the virus that causes AIDS?"

(percent of people aged 18 to 64 responding "medium/high," by state and age, 2000)

	total	18 to 24	25 to 34	35 to 44	45 to 54	55 to 64
U.S. total	**5.9%**	**9.7%**	**6.1%**	**5.6%**	**4.9%**	**3.3%**
Alabama	6.0	10.4	6.5	5.2	3.8	4.7
Alaska	5.6	14.2	6.3	4.7	3.7	0.8
Arizona	5.1	5.9	4.6	5.4	4.3	5.6
Arkansas	6.1	8.9	6.2	6.4	4.9	4.3
California	11.8	17.9	16.2	10.2	9.0	4.4
Colorado	5.5	6.1	5.0	4.8	6.5	5.5
Connecticut	6.2	11.2	7.5	4.8	4.3	4.5
Delaware	6.1	12.2	6.8	3.8	5.0	3.8
District of Columbia	11.8	15.0	11.5	12.9	11.9	6.0
Florida	7.6	11.2	8.2	8.0	6.0	5.3
Georgia	6.6	9.3	6.9	6.1	7.1	3.4
Hawaii	7.9	14.5	8.9	7.0	6.4	3.8
Idaho	4.3	6.2	4.3	4.2	4.4	2.5
Illinois	6.8	11.8	5.6	7.1	6.4	4.1
Indiana	5.1	9.0	5.3	4.3	4.7	2.7
Iowa	5.2	10.3	5.4	3.3	4.2	4.0
Kansas	5.1	8.7	5.0	4.7	4.5	2.5
Kentucky	5.7	7.8	6.0	5.9	4.9	3.5
Louisiana	6.2	9.8	6.3	7.0	3.9	4.1
Maine	5.0	6.4	7.6	4.0	4.6	1.8
Maryland	6.1	10.8	6.3	5.4	5.2	4.1
Massachusetts	6.6	13.8	5.9	5.5	4.6	4.8
Michigan	6.5	8.9	7.7	5.3	6.4	4.2
Minnesota	6.8	12.1	4.9	6.9	6.9	3.7
Mississippi	6.3	8.0	8.7	6.4	4.8	2.0
Missouri	6.1	12.0	6.8	5.8	5.6	0.4
Montana	4.2	5.9	5.4	4.3	3.0	2.3
Nebraska	4.9	5.5	6.4	5.1	3.7	3.4
Nevada	8.7	14.8	10.5	6.6	7.2	6.6
New Hampshire	5.2	14.0	3.1	3.5	5.6	2.1
New Jersey	5.7	9.0	6.3	5.4	4.7	3.8
New Mexico	7.0	8.7	8.2	8.2	4.8	4.4
New York	7.7	10.4	7.8	7.2	8.0	5.7
North Carolina	5.1	9.7	4.8	4.8	3.0	4.3
North Dakota	5.7	8.3	5.5	6.0	6.2	1.4
Ohio	6.4	9.7	6.0	7.6	5.8	2.4
Oklahoma	4.2	5.8	4.7	4.3	3.4	3.2
Oregon	6.1	14.6	5.2	5.9	3.6	3.7
Pennsylvania	5.9	11.1	5.5	4.8	6.7	2.2
Rhode Island	4.8	8.0	5.4	4.9	3.2	2.6
South Carolina	6.3	9.5	6.5	5.4	6.8	2.6
South Dakota	5.1	8.5	4.7	6.3	3.3	2.4
Tennessee	6.4	10.9	7.3	5.6	5.4	2.9
Texas	9.2	13.1	11.4	7.8	8.2	5.2
Utah	4.6	4.1	6.5	4.4	3.5	3.7
Vermont	6.0	14.5	4.4	6.0	3.9	1.6
Virginia	5.2	8.1	3.5	5.8	6.3	1.8
Washington	5.2	8.3	6.0	4.9	4.0	3.2
West Virginia	4.4	4.0	7.1	4.4	4.6	1.3
Wisconsin	2.5	10.2	7.7	8.0	4.6	4.1
Wyoming	1.6	8.1	7.3	6.2	4.9	3.0

Source: Compiled by New Strategist based on the Centers for Disease Control and Prevention Behavioral Risk Factor Surveillance System Survey. Internet site http://www.cdc.gov/brfss/index.htm

1.102 HIV Risk by Education, 2000

"What are your chances of getting infected with HIV, the virus that causes AIDS?"

(percent of people aged 18 or older responding "medium/high," by state and educational attainment, 2000)

	total	less than high school	high school graduate	some college	college graduate
U.S. total	**5.9%**	**7.6%**	**6.1%**	**6.4%**	**4.5%**
Alabama	6.0	3.8	6.7	7.3	4.7
Alaska	5.6	8.5	7.9	5.5	3.0
Arizona	5.1	2.4	6.9	5.4	3.7
Arkansas	6.1	7.0	6.5	7.1	3.8
California	11.8	30.3	11.6	7.5	5.1
Colorado	5.5	9.9	7.2	5.6	3.3
Connecticut	6.2	9.0	7.7	5.3	5.0
Delaware	6.1	10.3	5.4	7.8	4.5
District of Columbia	11.8	15.3	16.7	12.1	8.6
Florida	7.6	10.4	6.5	9.3	5.8
Georgia	6.6	7.3	6.4	5.5	7.7
Hawaii	7.9	10.2	11.3	6.3	5.7
Idaho	4.3	5.4	4.3	5.2	2.9
Illinois	6.8	8.8	9.2	7.4	3.7
Indiana	5.1	4.3	5.0	7.8	3.0
Iowa	5.2	3.6	4.6	5.9	5.4
Kansas	5.1	7.9	5.7	4.8	4.0
Kentucky	5.7	6.5	5.0	6.9	4.8
Louisiana	6.2	5.8	6.0	6.1	7.1
Maine	5.0	3.9	4.8	7.3	3.2
Maryland	6.1	7.1	5.6	8.6	4.6
Massachusetts	6.6	7.9	7.2	9.2	4.4
Michigan	6.5	12.2	7.7	4.9	4.8
Minnesota	6.8	6.1	8.7	7.2	4.7
Mississippi	6.3	2.7	5.9	7.8	6.3
Missouri	6.1	4.2	7.4	5.6	5.5
Montana	4.2	4.2	4.4	4.0	4.1
Nebraska	4.9	3.9	4.9	5.9	4.2
Nevada	8.7	14.1	8.6	7.4	8.6
New Hampshire	5.2	16.4	6.5	3.9	3.1
New Jersey	5.7	7.0	5.2	6.3	5.2
New Mexico	7.0	11.8	8.7	5.7	4.3
New York	7.7	6.8	9.9	8.0	5.9
North Carolina	5.1	5.5	4.3	6.8	4.4
North Dakota	5.7	7.0	4.3	7.0	4.9
Ohio	6.4	8.1	6.5	7.1	5.1
Oklahoma	4.2	4.4	3.7	4.5	5.0
Oregon	6.1	15.7	6.0	4.5	3.8
Pennsylvania	5.9	9.3	6.7	6.8	3.5
Rhode Island	4.8	4.0	4.4	5.8	4.7
South Carolina	6.3	10.1	5.8	6.3	5.2
South Dakota	5.1	7.4	4.5	5.2	5.1
Tennessee	6.4	9.7	5.8	6.9	4.4
Texas	9.2	19.2	7.8	8.9	4.6
Utah	4.6	11.6	6.2	3.3	3.4
Vermont	6.0	10.3	6.3	7.0	4.1
Virginia	5.2	12.4	2.8	6.2	4.7
Washington	5.2	12.0	6.0	5.0	3.7
West Virginia	4.4	4.1	2.8	6.1	6.0
Wisconsin	2.5	10.2	8.6	5.5	6.2
Wyoming	1.6	10.6	5.0	5.9	6.3

Source: Compiled by New Strategist based on the Centers for Disease Control and Prevention Behavioral Risk Factor Surveillance System Survey, Internet site http://www.cdc.gov/brfss/index.htm

1.103 HIV Risk by Household Income, 2000

"What are your chances of getting infected with HIV, the virus that causes AIDS?"

(percent of people aged 18 or older responding "medium/high," by state and household income, 2000)

	total	less than $15,000	$15,000 to $24,999	$25,000 to $34,999	$35,000 to $49,999	$50,000 or more
U.S. total	**5.9%**	**7.3%**	**6.9%**	**6.6%**	**5.6%**	**4.9%**
Alabama	6.0	8.2	4.2	4.3	8.3	6.3
Alaska	5.6	11.5	9.9	8.4	6.4	2.0
Arizona	5.1	2.6	5.2	2.3	10.1	5.5
Arkansas	6.1	8.0	6.8	6.2	6.7	4.5
California	11.8	21.7	19.0	12.7	7.4	6.5
Colorado	5.5	14.5	6.1	6.7	4.2	4.5
Connecticut	6.2	8.6	11.5	7.2	7.0	4.6
Delaware	6.1	3.8	10.2	5.5	5.4	4.8
District of Columbia	11.8	9.9	13.8	19.9	7.1	8.5
Florida	7.6	9.4	8.0	8.4	7.6	4.9
Georgia	6.6	7.2	10.6	8.4	4.6	5.3
Hawaii	7.9	8.8	9.7	8.4	7.6	5.7
Idaho	4.3	5.8	5.6	6.3	3.2	3.4
Illinois	6.8	11.4	10.1	7.4	5.8	5.6
Indiana	5.1	7.0	9.3	4.1	5.0	4.1
Iowa	5.2	3.7	7.7	4.2	5.3	4.6
Kansas	5.1	8.2	6.0	4.9	3.1	4.8
Kentucky	5.7	6.2	7.9	5.6	6.5	2.7
Louisiana	6.2	5.3	6.4	5.7	6.4	6.7
Maine	5.0	4.8	4.3	7.3	6.1	3.1
Maryland	6.1	8.0	9.3	9.4	7.8	3.8
Massachusetts	6.6	14.6	7.9	6.2	7.5	5.0
Michigan	6.5	10.9	8.0	5.9	6.0	4.7
Minnesota	6.8	9.3	9.6	8.5	6.7	5.5
Mississippi	6.3	9.6	6.4	6.9	4.6	5.4
Missouri	6.1	8.4	6.0	7.0	5.6	6.1
Montana	4.2	2.6	4.4	3.6	4.3	4.7
Nebraska	4.9	6.0	6.4	5.8	5.1	4.0
Nevada	8.7	8.4	16.8	12.1	9.3	5.7
New Hampshire	5.2	9.2	9.6	6.7	5.1	4.3
New Jersey	5.7	6.2	8.5	12.1	5.7	4.6
New Mexico	7.0	11.0	8.3	7.8	5.7	4.8
New York	7.7	7.0	9.3	10.4	5.3	6.5
North Carolina	5.1	7.0	6.5	5.8	4.9	5.0
North Dakota	5.7	6.1	6.2	7.2	5.2	4.9
Ohio	6.4	8.9	5.6	7.2	8.3	5.5
Oklahoma	4.2	3.1	6.7	4.7	2.6	4.7
Oregon	6.1	10.3	7.5	8.5	4.7	3.5
Pennsylvania	5.9	10.5	7.5	7.1	7.1	3.9
Rhode Island	4.8	5.4	5.3	8.6	4.8	3.6
South Carolina	6.3	9.4	7.2	6.7	6.5	5.0
South Dakota	5.1	6.4	5.1	7.3	4.8	4.3
Tennessee	6.4	7.3	8.4	3.7	7.7	5.5
Texas	9.2	14.9	13.1	12.8	8.0	3.9
Utah	4.6	5.7	2.7	8.5	3.3	4.5
Vermont	6.0	5.0	8.6	5.3	5.6	4.6
Virginia	5.2	5.0	9.2	7.7	2.2	3.9
Washington	5.2	10.7	7.9	6.3	4.5	4.4
West Virginia	4.4	7.0	4.0	3.8	3.9	4.5
Wisconsin	2.5	11.5	6.7	10.3	7.2	4.4
Wyoming	1.6	7.2	8.2	4.6	4.5	6.3

Source: Compiled by New Strategist based on the Centers for Disease Control and Prevention Behavioral Risk Factor Surveillance System Survey, Internet site http://www.cdc.gov/brfss/index.htm

1.104   HIV Risk by Sex, 2000

"What are your chances of getting infected with HIV, the virus that causes AIDS?"

(percent of people aged 18 or older responding "medium/high," by state and sex, 2000)

	total	men	women
U.S. total	**5.9%**	**6.5%**	**5.1%**
Alabama	6.0	6.6	5.3
Alaska	5.6	6.4	4.8
Arizona	5.1	4.9	5.2
Arkansas	6.1	6.3	5.9
California	11.8	13.9	9.5
Colorado	5.5	4.7	6.3
Connecticut	6.2	7.2	5.1
Delaware	6.1	6.4	5.9
District of Columbia	11.8	15.4	8.4
Florida	7.6	8.0	7.1
Georgia	6.6	7.7	5.6
Hawaii	7.9	9.0	6.7
Idaho	4.3	4.9	3.8
Illinois	6.8	7.9	5.9
Indiana	5.1	5.0	5.3
Iowa	5.2	5.6	4.9
Kansas	5.1	5.2	4.9
Kentucky	5.7	6.1	5.2
Louisiana	6.2	7.0	5.5
Maine	5.0	5.9	3.9
Maryland	6.1	6.9	5.3
Massachusetts	6.6	7.9	5.2
Michigan	6.5	6.2	6.8
Minnesota	6.8	7.9	5.6
Mississippi	6.3	7.7	4.9
Missouri	6.1	7.3	4.8
Montana	4.2	4.5	3.9
Nebraska	4.9	5.0	4.8
Nevada	8.7	10.1	7.1
New Hampshire	5.2	6.1	4.5
New Jersey	5.7	7.2	4.2
New Mexico	7.0	7.4	6.7
New York	7.7	9.2	6.3
North Carolina	5.1	5.7	4.7
North Dakota	5.7	5.0	6.3
Ohio	6.4	7.1	5.7
Oklahoma	4.2	4.4	4.1
Oregon	6.1	7.5	4.7
Pennsylvania	5.9	6.3	5.6
Rhode Island	4.8	5.4	4.3
South Carolina	6.3	7.2	5.3
South Dakota	5.1	5.6	4.7
Tennessee	6.4	7.3	5.5
Texas	9.2	10.0	8.5
Utah	4.6	5.8	3.3
Vermont	6.0	6.3	5.7
Virginia	5.2	5.8	4.5
Washington	5.2	6.2	4.2
West Virginia	4.4	3.9	4.9
Wisconsin	2.5	7.0	6.9
Wyoming	1.6	6.0	6.0

Source: Compiled by New Strategist based on the Centers for Disease Control and Prevention Behavioral Risk Factor Surveillance System Survey. Internet site http://www.cdc.gov/brfss/index.htm

1.105 Physical Activity by Age, 2001

"During the past month, did you participate in any physical activities?"

(percent of people aged 18 or older responding "yes," by state and age, 2001)

	total	18 to 24	25 to 34	35 to 44	45 to 54	55 to 64	65 or older
U.S. total	**74.2%**	**81.1%**	**79.0%**	**76.3%**	**74.5%**	**72.1%**	**65.5%**
Alabama	68.8	77.8	75.6	69.0	70.0	63.9	57.1
Alaska	78.9	86.5	82.7	77.9	80.3	75.9	63.6
Arizona	78.1	83.2	81.8	77.0	77.2	77.8	72.7
Arkansas	68.5	78.9	74.2	71.7	66.4	60.0	61.5
California	73.4	72.0	75.6	76.2	70.6	72.2	72.2
Colorado	80.8	83.7	80.1	81.9	86.1	79.6	72.4
Connecticut	76.0	78.6	78.2	79.4	76.4	77.7	66.7
Delaware	74.3	80.1	79.7	73.2	74.4	71.3	67.9
District of Columbia	75.8	79.0	79.7	75.3	80.1	73.4	66.5
Florida	72.3	76.1	77.3	75.6	69.0	70.5	67.7
Georgia	72.7	80.9	78.3	76.8	70.2	63.3	62.6
Hawaii	81.1	86.3	81.6	81.9	77.6	77.6	81.8
Idaho	79.0	86.9	83.0	80.9	78.9	71.8	71.5
Illinois	73.5	81.1	79.5	75.7	72.3	66.2	65.3
Indiana	73.8	79.6	76.0	78.4	71.9	72.6	64.0
Iowa	74.1	82.6	80.4	74.3	76.7	70.7	62.9
Kansas	73.3	83.8	77.6	75.5	74.3	70.1	60.4
Kentucky	66.6	79.3	70.4	67.2	63.5	62.2	58.4
Louisiana	64.4	73.3	72.4	67.4	60.5	59.5	51.2
Maine	76.8	93.5	80.9	78.7	74.2	73.7	63.4
Maryland	75.8	83.8	80.1	76.4	74.9	75.1	65.4
Massachusetts	77.2	82.7	80.5	77.9	78.9	75.6	68.3
Michigan	76.6	87.0	79.3	80.0	73.6	75.0	66.2
Minnesota	82.9	87.5	84.9	87.2	83.9	79.5	73.4
Mississippi	66.6	77.6	67.6	67.7	65.2	64.0	58.0
Missouri	72.5	80.1	78.0	75.3	71.3	66.2	65.2
Montana	78.1	86.6	82.7	81.0	77.1	73.7	69.5
Nebraska	68.6	77.8	69.5	69.8	69.8	70.1	60.6
Nevada	77.4	79.7	82.7	75.9	80.1	77.6	68.4
New Hampshire	80.5	84.0	83.3	82.1	80.6	80.1	72.4
New Jersey	73.4	80.7	75.8	75.9	75.3	72.0	63.3
New Mexico	74.2	81.1	75.2	73.1	75.3	73.3	67.7
New York	71.3	78.8	70.9	69.1	73.9	73.6	63.8
North Carolina	73.6	77.6	78.7	75.7	72.5	67.0	68.7
North Dakota	76.8	84.0	82.4	77.4	78.1	74.4	65.7
Ohio	73.8	76.7	78.2	74.1	74.7	69.3	69.0
Oklahoma	67.2	75.8	74.9	69.6	63.0	61.8	59.1
Oregon	79.2	86.1	82.4	80.0	79.1	77.4	72.4
Pennsylvania	75.3	81.4	79.1	79.9	76.3	74.8	63.9
Rhode Island	75.1	82.8	78.9	77.8	75.6	74.3	64.3
South Carolina	73.6	82.8	77.1	75.0	71.3	70.0	64.8
South Dakota	74.6	87.7	80.1	78.2	73.6	68.9	62.1
Tennessee	64.9	72.8	71.8	71.3	63.5	55.5	53.3
Texas	72.9	80.9	74.0	73.7	72.0	70.9	65.9
Utah	83.5	92.1	86.5	83.3	82.3	78.6	74.9
Vermont	79.7	88.9	83.5	83.4	80.7	75.4	64.3
Virginia	76.8	87.6	80.5	77.2	77.2	72.1	65.8
Washington	82.9	87.6	85.6	84.5	84.6	82.5	72.7
West Virginia	68.3	78.9	70.4	70.9	64.5	66.4	62.8
Wisconsin	79.3	85.0	82.2	81.0	77.5	77.7	73.3
Wyoming	78.8	87.0	84.1	79.1	81.5	71.3	68.3

Source: Compiled by New Strategist based on the Centers for Disease Control and Prevention Behavioral Risk Factor Surveillance System Survey. Internet site http://www.cdc.gov/brfss/index.htm

1.106 Physical Activity by Education, 2001

"During the past month, did you participate in any physical activities?"

(percent of people aged 18 or older responding "yes," by state and educational attainment, 2001)

	total	less than high school	high school graduate	some college	college graduate
U.S. total	**74.2%**	**54.3%**	**67.6%**	**78.4%**	**86.5%**
Alabama	68.8	48.8	63.9	74.7	84.4
Alaska	78.9	56.0	72.8	81.4	88.4
Arizona	78.1	54.9	74.3	80.5	88.9
Arkansas	68.5	52.8	61.7	77.2	80.1
California	73.4	50.1	67.6	78.9	85.7
Colorado	80.8	57.3	73.8	85.2	89.3
Connecticut	76.0	54.0	66.9	77.6	86.5
Delaware	74.3	52.8	65.2	78.5	85.1
District of Columbia	75.8	51.4	62.7	77.5	88.8
Florida	72.3	53.6	66.4	77.4	82.4
Georgia	72.7	53.0	66.0	75.2	86.7
Hawaii	81.1	72.8	75.2	84.6	85.9
Idaho	79.0	57.7	74.8	83.3	86.6
Illinois	73.5	51.4	64.4	78.4	85.3
Indiana	73.8	58.7	66.7	77.4	87.1
Iowa	74.1	57.5	66.9	77.7	86.5
Kansas	73.3	52.2	65.9	76.4	83.0
Kentucky	66.6	45.6	64.1	74.5	82.6
Louisiana	64.4	43.9	60.0	71.5	79.6
Maine	76.8	54.1	71.9	80.1	87.4
Maryland	75.8	54.5	68.9	77.1	85.1
Massachusetts	77.2	54.2	67.1	78.8	87.6
Michigan	76.6	60.5	70.9	78.5	88.7
Minnesota	82.9	66.0	75.7	84.8	91.2
Mississippi	66.6	51.6	62.2	71.3	80.6
Missouri	72.5	52.7	68.4	75.1	85.4
Montana	78.1	61.3	71.6	81.7	88.9
Nebraska	68.6	54.2	57.5	76.0	83.2
Nevada	77.4	65.8	70.8	77.5	88.1
New Hampshire	80.5	61.7	72.7	83.0	89.7
New Jersey	73.4	47.9	65.5	77.0	84.6
New Mexico	74.2	57.7	66.6	79.5	88.3
New York	71.3	52.2	65.3	74.3	82.2
North Carolina	73.6	58.3	65.6	79.9	87.0
North Dakota	76.8	58.5	71.3	76.6	88.6
Ohio	73.8	60.6	67.1	77.5	86.6
Oklahoma	67.2	50.7	63.2	69.9	80.3
Oregon	79.2	57.1	74.2	83.6	89.0
Pennsylvania	75.3	53.0	71.3	80.9	85.7
Rhode Island	75.1	54.6	68.7	78.6	87.2
South Carolina	73.6	55.8	67.0	78.6	86.4
South Dakota	74.6	52.2	69.0	77.0	86.6
Tennessee	64.9	37.8	59.2	73.2	82.0
Texas	72.9	54.6	68.9	77.6	85.8
Utah	83.5	66.9	77.8	86.5	89.5
Vermont	79.7	51.2	71.9	83.4	91.7
Virginia	76.8	53.6	69.7	80.5	87.2
Washington	82.9	68.7	75.7	83.7	91.4
West Virginia	68.3	50.1	65.7	79.5	79.8
Wisconsin	79.3	65.3	74.2	81.3	88.5
Wyoming	78.8	62.1	74.5	80.2	87.5

Source: Compiled by New Strategist based on the Centers for Disease Control and Prevention Behavioral Risk Factor Surveillance System Survey, Internet site http://www.cdc.gov/brfss/index.htm

1.107 Physical Activity by Household Income, 2001

"During the past month, did you participate in any physical activities?"

(percent of people aged 18 or older responding "yes," by state and household income, 2001)

	total	less than $15,000	$15,000 to $24,999	$25,000 to $34,999	$35,000 to $49,999	$50,000 or more
U.S. total	**74.2%**	**60.9%**	**65.2%**	**72.0%**	**77.8%**	**84.8%**
Alabama	68.8	48.6	61.6	70.9	74.2	82.7
Alaska	78.9	57.3	69.6	72.8	82.3	85.6
Arizona	78.1	58.9	68.7	76.6	82.9	87.5
Arkansas	68.5	55.8	58.7	72.1	73.3	81.6
California	73.4	57.4	65.0	65.9	77.0	84.4
Colorado	80.8	66.5	68.7	78.3	83.0	89.5
Connecticut	76.0	55.6	60.7	69.7	76.7	85.1
Delaware	74.3	61.7	59.0	74.7	76.3	82.9
District of Columbia	75.8	66.2	60.7	72.3	80.3	89.1
Florida	72.3	53.5	60.5	76.9	76.6	84.4
Georgia	72.7	53.7	52.0	68.3	74.6	84.5
Hawaii	81.1	71.0	82.0	77.5	80.0	86.8
Idaho	79.0	72.6	75.3	77.9	79.3	87.4
Illinois	73.5	57.2	64.9	69.3	74.3	83.1
Indiana	73.8	61.6	62.8	75.6	75.5	82.2
Iowa	74.1	65.3	64.9	67.0	78.0	84.1
Kansas	73.3	65.5	65.4	66.6	78.5	81.6
Kentucky	66.6	49.1	58.2	67.8	74.2	80.4
Louisiana	64.4	46.3	58.6	63.8	68.4	78.7
Maine	76.8	55.4	68.3	72.5	81.1	86.4
Maryland	75.8	58.5	62.0	69.6	76.3	84.4
Massachusetts	77.2	62.5	63.5	70.6	77.0	86.4
Michigan	76.6	68.9	66.4	76.4	78.2	84.1
Minnesota	82.9	70.1	73.3	78.1	82.7	89.3
Mississippi	66.6	53.0	61.6	65.3	75.2	81.2
Missouri	72.5	63.1	59.7	68.4	74.9	84.0
Montana	78.1	68.2	74.7	79.5	83.7	86.5
Nebraska	68.6	65.0	64.7	63.1	68.9	82.1
Nevada	77.4	65.3	69.8	72.4	78.8	83.5
New Hampshire	80.5	64.6	67.2	73.4	80.3	88.3
New Jersey	73.4	53.0	59.6	66.8	72.4	85.0
New Mexico	74.2	61.3	64.7	74.5	79.5	86.4
New York	71.3	56.6	63.5	64.5	75.4	81.7
North Carolina	73.6	57.3	64.4	71.4	80.1	86.8
North Dakota	76.8	69.6	69.1	78.5	77.1	85.3
Ohio	73.8	58.7	65.8	74.7	74.8	81.7
Oklahoma	67.2	54.3	62.2	67.8	71.5	81.3
Oregon	79.2	64.2	75.5	71.4	84.8	88.6
Pennsylvania	75.3	58.6	65.7	72.5	79.2	87.9
Rhode Island	75.1	61.6	62.5	72.0	78.5	87.5
South Carolina	73.6	53.3	67.9	72.7	81.0	84.6
South Dakota	74.6	61.4	67.2	74.0	77.6	84.7
Tennessee	64.9	53.3	57.9	65.2	71.7	82.9
Texas	72.9	60.3	65.4	69.7	75.6	85.6
Utah	83.5	75.1	80.4	79.1	84.0	88.3
Vermont	79.7	63.0	74.8	74.6	81.1	89.5
Virginia	76.8	61.4	63.5	71.8	77.1	86.6
Washington	82.9	75.2	76.5	78.5	82.2	88.7
West Virginia	68.3	49.1	65.5	67.4	76.6	80.6
Wisconsin	79.3	66.2	69.2	77.0	82.8	87.2
Wyoming	78.8	65.1	69.8	79.2	81.9	86.9

Source: Compiled by New Strategist based on the Centers for Disease Control and Prevention Behavioral Risk Factor Surveillance System Survey, Internet site http://www.cdc.gov/brfss/index.htm

1.108 Physical Activity by Sex, 2001

"During the past month, did you participate in any physical activities?"

(percent of people aged 18 or older responding "yes," by state and sex, 2001)

	total	men	women
U.S. total	**74.2%**	**76.9%**	**71.9%**
Alabama	68.8	72.4	65.6
Alaska	78.9	81.5	76.1
Arizona	78.1	82.4	74.0
Arkansas	68.5	70.6	66.6
California	73.4	76.1	70.8
Colorado	80.8	82.7	78.9
Connecticut	76.0	78.9	73.4
Delaware	74.3	78.3	70.8
District of Columbia	75.8	79.3	72.7
Florida	72.3	74.5	70.3
Georgia	72.7	76.5	69.3
Hawaii	81.1	84.2	77.8
Idaho	79.0	80.5	77.6
Illinois	73.5	76.8	70.6
Indiana	73.8	76.6	71.1
Iowa	74.1	76.1	72.1
Kansas	73.3	75.8	71.0
Kentucky	66.6	69.7	63.7
Louisiana	64.4	67.9	61.2
Maine	76.8	77.3	76.3
Maryland	75.8	78.9	72.9
Massachusetts	77.2	80.4	74.2
Michigan	76.6	79.7	73.8
Minnesota	82.9	84.2	81.6
Mississippi	66.6	72.4	61.5
Missouri	72.5	75.7	69.5
Montana	78.1	80.0	76.4
Nebraska	68.6	68.0	69.3
Nevada	77.4	80.9	73.8
New Hampshire	80.5	82.4	78.7
New Jersey	73.4	76.2	70.8
New Mexico	74.2	75.8	72.6
New York	71.3	73.8	69.0
North Carolina	73.6	77.0	70.5
North Dakota	76.8	76.3	77.2
Ohio	73.8	77.1	70.9
Oklahoma	67.2	69.2	65.4
Oregon	79.2	81.2	77.4
Pennsylvania	75.3	77.6	73.3
Rhode Island	75.1	78.9	71.7
South Carolina	73.6	76.8	70.6
South Dakota	74.6	75.5	73.7
Tennessee	64.9	69.2	61.1
Texas	72.9	75.4	70.6
Utah	83.5	84.6	82.5
Vermont	79.7	79.8	79.5
Virginia	76.8	80.0	73.8
Washington	82.9	85.1	80.8
West Virginia	68.3	71.8	65.2
Wisconsin	79.3	80.6	78.0
Wyoming	78.8	79.6	77.9

Source: Compiled by New Strategist based on the Centers for Disease Control and Prevention Behavioral Risk Factor Surveillance System Survey, Internet site http://www.cdc.gov/brfss/index.htm

1.109 Physical Activity: At Risk Due to Lack of Physical Activity by Age, 2001

At risk for health problems related to lack of regular and sustained physical activity.

(percent of people aged 18 or older who reported no leisure-time physical activity in the past month, by state and age, 2001)

	total	18 to 24	25 to 34	35 to 44	45 to 54	55 to 64	65 or older
U.S. total	**25.7%**	**18.9%**	**21.0%**	**23.7%**	**25.4%**	**27.8%**	**34.4%**
Alabama	31.2	22.2	24.4	31.0	30.0	36.1	42.9
Alaska	21.1	13.5	17.3	22.1	19.7	24.1	36.4
Arizona	21.9	16.8	18.2	23.0	22.8	22.2	27.3
Arkansas	31.5	21.1	25.8	28.3	33.6	40.0	38.5
California	26.6	28.0	24.4	23.8	29.4	27.8	27.8
Colorado	19.2	16.3	19.9	18.1	13.9	20.4	27.6
Connecticut	24.0	21.4	21.8	20.6	23.6	22.3	33.3
Delaware	25.7	19.9	20.3	26.8	25.6	28.7	32.1
District of Columbia	24.2	21.0	20.3	24.7	19.9	26.6	33.5
Florida	27.7	23.9	22.7	24.4	31.0	29.5	32.3
Georgia	27.3	19.1	21.7	23.2	29.8	36.7	37.4
Hawaii	18.9	13.7	18.4	18.1	22.4	22.4	18.2
Idaho	21.0	13.1	17.0	19.1	21.1	28.2	28.5
Illinois	26.5	18.9	20.5	24.3	27.7	33.8	34.7
Indiana	26.2	20.4	24.0	21.6	28.1	27.4	36.0
Iowa	25.9	17.4	19.6	25.7	23.3	29.3	37.1
Kansas	26.7	16.2	22.4	24.5	25.7	29.9	39.6
Kentucky	33.4	20.7	29.6	32.8	36.5	37.8	41.6
Louisiana	35.6	26.7	27.6	32.6	39.5	40.5	48.8
Maine	23.2	6.5	19.1	21.3	25.8	26.3	36.6
Maryland	24.2	16.2	19.9	23.6	25.1	24.9	34.6
Massachusetts	22.8	17.3	19.5	22.1	21.1	24.4	31.7
Michigan	23.4	13.0	20.7	20.0	26.4	25.0	33.8
Minnesota	17.1	12.5	15.1	12.8	16.1	20.5	26.6
Mississippi	33.4	22.4	32.4	32.3	34.8	36.0	42.0
Missouri	27.5	19.9	22.0	24.7	28.7	33.8	34.8
Montana	21.9	13.4	17.3	19.0	22.9	26.3	30.5
Nebraska	31.4	22.2	30.5	30.2	30.2	29.9	39.4
Nevada	22.6	20.3	17.3	24.1	19.9	22.4	31.6
New Hampshire	19.5	16.0	16.7	17.9	19.4	19.9	27.6
New Jersey	26.6	19.3	24.2	24.1	24.7	28.0	36.7
New Mexico	25.8	18.9	24.8	26.9	24.7	26.7	32.3
New York	28.7	21.2	29.1	30.9	26.1	26.4	36.2
North Carolina	26.4	22.4	21.3	24.3	27.5	33.0	31.3
North Dakota	23.2	16.0	17.6	22.6	21.9	25.6	34.3
Ohio	26.2	23.3	21.8	25.9	25.3	30.7	31.0
Oklahoma	32.8	24.2	25.1	30.4	37.0	38.2	40.9
Oregon	20.8	13.9	17.6	20.0	20.9	22.6	27.6
Pennsylvania	24.7	18.6	20.9	20.1	23.7	25.2	36.1
Rhode Island	24.9	17.2	21.1	22.2	24.4	25.7	35.7
South Carolina	26.4	17.2	22.9	25.0	28.7	30.0	35.2
South Dakota	25.4	12.3	19.9	21.8	26.4	31.1	37.9
Tennessee	35.1	27.2	28.2	28.7	36.5	44.5	46.7
Texas	27.1	19.1	26.0	26.3	28.0	29.1	34.1
Utah	16.5	7.9	13.5	16.7	17.7	21.4	25.1
Vermont	20.3	11.1	16.5	16.6	19.3	24.6	35.7
Virginia	23.2	12.4	19.5	22.8	22.8	27.9	34.2
Washington	17.1	12.4	14.4	15.5	15.4	17.5	27.3
West Virginia	31.7	21.1	29.6	29.1	35.5	33.6	37.2
Wisconsin	20.7	15.0	17.8	19.0	22.5	22.3	26.7
Wyoming	21.1	13.0	15.9	20.9	18.5	28.7	31.7

Source: Compiled by New Strategist based on the Centers for Disease Control and Prevention Behavioral Risk Factor Surveillance System Survey. Internet site http://www.cdc.gov/brfss/index.htm

1.110   Physical Activity: At Risk Due to Lack of Physical Activity by Education, 2001

At risk for health problems related to lack of regular and sustained physical activity.

(percent of people aged 18 or older who reported no leisure-time physical activity in the past month, by state and education, 2001)

	total	less than high school	high school graduate	some college	college graduate
U.S. total	**25.7%**	**45.6%**	**32.3%**	**21.5%**	**13.4%**
Alabama	31.2	51.2	36.1	25.3	15.6
Alaska	21.1	44.0	27.2	18.6	11.6
Arizona	21.9	45.1	25.7	19.5	11.1
Arkansas	31.5	47.2	38.3	22.8	19.9
California	26.6	49.9	32.4	21.1	14.3
Colorado	19.2	42.7	26.2	14.8	10.7
Connecticut	24.0	46.0	33.1	22.4	13.5
Delaware	25.7	47.2	34.8	21.5	14.9
District of Columbia	24.2	48.6	37.3	22.5	11.2
Florida	27.7	46.4	33.6	22.6	17.6
Georgia	27.3	47.0	34.0	24.8	13.3
Hawaii	18.9	27.2	24.8	15.4	14.1
Idaho	21.0	42.3	25.2	16.7	13.4
Illinois	26.5	48.6	35.6	21.6	14.7
Indiana	26.2	41.3	33.3	22.6	12.9
Iowa	25.9	42.5	33.1	22.3	13.5
Kansas	26.7	47.8	34.1	23.6	17.0
Kentucky	33.4	54.4	35.9	25.5	17.4
Louisiana	35.6	56.1	40.0	28.5	20.4
Maine	23.2	45.9	28.1	19.9	12.6
Maryland	24.2	45.5	31.1	22.9	14.9
Massachusetts	22.8	45.8	32.9	21.2	12.4
Michigan	23.4	39.5	29.1	21.5	11.3
Minnesota	17.1	34.0	24.3	15.2	8.8
Mississippi	33.4	48.4	37.8	28.7	19.4
Missouri	27.5	47.3	31.6	24.9	14.6
Montana	21.9	38.7	28.4	18.3	11.1
Nebraska	31.4	45.8	42.5	24.0	16.8
Nevada	22.6	34.2	29.2	22.5	11.9
New Hampshire	19.5	38.3	27.3	17.0	10.3
New Jersey	26.6	52.1	34.5	23.0	15.4
New Mexico	25.8	42.3	33.4	20.5	11.7
New York	28.7	47.8	34.7	25.7	17.8
North Carolina	26.4	41.7	34.4	20.1	13.0
North Dakota	23.2	41.5	28.7	23.4	11.4
Ohio	26.2	39.4	32.9	22.5	13.4
Oklahoma	32.8	49.3	36.8	30.1	19.7
Oregon	20.8	42.9	25.8	16.4	11.0
Pennsylvania	24.7	47.0	28.7	19.1	14.3
Rhode Island	24.9	45.4	31.3	21.4	12.8
South Carolina	26.4	44.2	33.0	21.4	13.6
South Dakota	25.4	47.8	31.0	23.0	13.4
Tennessee	35.1	62.2	40.8	26.8	18.0
Texas	27.1	45.4	31.1	22.4	14.2
Utah	16.5	33.1	22.2	13.5	10.5
Vermont	20.3	48.8	28.1	16.6	8.3
Virginia	23.2	46.4	30.3	19.5	12.8
Washington	17.1	31.3	24.3	16.3	8.6
West Virginia	31.7	49.9	34.3	20.5	20.2
Wisconsin	20.7	34.7	25.8	18.7	11.5
Wyoming	21.1	37.9	25.5	19.8	12.5

Source: Compiled by New Strategist based on the Centers for Disease Control and Prevention Behavioral Risk Factor Surveillance System Survey, Internet site http://www.cdc.gov/brfss/index.htm

1.111 Physical Activity: At Risk Due to Lack of Physical Activity by Household Income, 2001

At risk for health problems related to lack of regular and sustained physical activity.

(percent of people aged 18 or older who reported no leisure-time physical activity in the past month, by state and household income, 2001)

	total	less than $15,000	$15,000 to $24,999	$25,000 to $34,999	$35,000 to $49,999	$50,000 or more
U.S. total	**25.7%**	**39.0%**	**34.8%**	**27.9%**	**22.2%**	**15.1%**
Alabama	31.2	51.4	38.4	29.1	25.8	17.3
Alaska	21.1	42.7	30.4	27.2	17.7	14.4
Arizona	21.9	41.1	31.3	23.4	17.1	12.5
Arkansas	31.5	44.2	41.3	27.9	26.7	18.4
California	26.6	42.6	35.0	34.1	23.0	15.6
Colorado	19.2	33.5	31.3	21.7	17.0	10.5
Connecticut	24.0	44.4	39.3	30.3	23.3	14.9
Delaware	25.7	38.3	41.0	25.3	23.7	17.1
District of Columbia	24.2	33.8	39.3	27.7	19.7	10.9
Florida	27.7	46.5	39.5	23.1	23.4	15.6
Georgia	27.3	46.3	38.0	31.7	25.4	15.5
Hawaii	18.9	29.0	18.0	22.5	20.0	13.2
Idaho	21.0	27.4	24.7	22.1	20.7	12.6
Illinois	26.5	42.8	35.1	30.7	25.7	16.9
Indiana	26.2	38.4	37.2	24.4	24.5	17.8
Iowa	25.9	34.7	35.1	33.0	22.0	15.9
Kansas	26.7	34.5	34.6	33.4	21.5	18.4
Kentucky	33.4	50.9	41.8	32.2	25.8	19.6
Louisiana	35.6	53.7	41.4	36.2	31.6	21.3
Maine	23.2	44.6	31.7	27.5	18.9	13.6
Maryland	24.2	41.5	38.0	30.4	23.7	15.6
Massachusetts	22.8	37.5	36.5	29.4	23.0	13.6
Michigan	23.4	31.1	33.6	23.6	21.8	15.9
Minnesota	17.1	29.9	26.7	21.9	17.3	10.7
Mississippi	33.4	47.0	38.4	34.7	24.8	18.8
Missouri	27.5	36.9	40.3	31.6	25.1	16.0
Montana	21.9	31.8	25.3	20.5	16.3	13.5
Nebraska	31.4	35.0	35.3	36.9	31.1	17.9
Nevada	22.6	34.7	30.2	27.6	21.2	16.5
New Hampshire	19.5	35.4	32.8	26.6	19.7	11.7
New Jersey	26.6	47.0	40.4	33.2	27.6	15.0
New Mexico	25.8	38.7	35.3	25.5	20.5	13.6
New York	28.7	43.4	36.5	35.5	24.6	18.3
North Carolina	26.4	42.7	35.6	28.6	19.9	13.2
North Dakota	23.2	30.4	30.9	21.5	22.9	14.7
Ohio	26.2	41.3	34.2	25.3	25.2	18.3
Oklahoma	32.8	45.7	37.8	32.2	28.5	18.7
Oregon	20.8	35.8	24.5	28.6	15.2	11.4
Pennsylvania	24.7	41.4	34.3	27.5	20.8	12.1
Rhode Island	24.9	38.4	37.5	28.0	21.5	12.5
South Carolina	26.4	46.7	32.1	27.3	19.0	15.4
South Dakota	25.4	38.6	32.8	26.0	22.4	15.3
Tennessee	35.1	46.7	42.1	34.8	28.3	17.1
Texas	27.1	39.7	34.6	30.3	24.4	14.4
Utah	16.5	24.9	19.6	20.9	16.0	11.7
Vermont	20.3	37.0	25.2	25.4	18.9	10.5
Virginia	23.2	38.6	36.5	28.2	22.9	13.4
Washington	17.1	24.8	23.5	21.5	17.8	11.3
West Virginia	31.7	50.9	34.5	32.6	23.4	19.4
Wisconsin	20.7	33.8	30.8	23.0	17.2	12.8
Wyoming	21.1	34.9	30.2	20.8	18.1	13.1

Source: Compiled by New Strategist based on the Centers for Disease Control and Prevention Behavioral Risk Factor Surveillance System Survey, Internet site http://www.cdc.gov/brfss/index.htm

1.112 Physical Activity: At Risk Due to Lack of Physical Activity by Sex, 2001

At risk for health problems related to lack of regular and sustained physical activity.

(percent of people aged 18 or older who reported no leisure-time physical activity in the past month, by state and sex, 2001)

	total	men	women
U.S. total	**25.7%**	**23.1%**	**28.1%**
Alabama	31.2	27.6	34.4
Alaska	21.1	18.5	23.9
Arizona	21.9	17.6	26.0
Arkansas	31.5	29.4	33.4
California	26.6	23.9	29.2
Colorado	19.2	17.3	21.1
Connecticut	24.0	21.1	26.6
Delaware	25.7	21.7	29.2
District of Columbia	24.2	20.7	27.3
Florida	27.7	25.5	29.7
Georgia	27.3	23.5	30.7
Hawaii	18.9	15.8	22.2
Idaho	21.0	19.5	22.4
Illinois	26.5	23.2	29.4
Indiana	26.2	23.4	28.9
Iowa	25.9	23.9	27.9
Kansas	26.7	24.2	29.0
Kentucky	33.4	30.3	36.3
Louisiana	35.6	32.1	38.8
Maine	23.2	22.7	23.7
Maryland	24.2	21.1	27.1
Massachusetts	22.8	19.6	25.8
Michigan	23.4	20.3	26.2
Minnesota	17.1	15.8	18.4
Mississippi	33.4	27.6	38.5
Missouri	27.5	24.3	30.5
Montana	21.9	20.0	23.6
Nebraska	31.4	32.0	30.7
Nevada	22.6	19.1	26.2
New Hampshire	19.5	17.6	21.3
New Jersey	26.6	23.8	29.2
New Mexico	25.8	24.2	27.4
New York	28.7	26.2	31.0
North Carolina	26.4	23.0	29.5
North Dakota	23.2	23.7	22.8
Ohio	26.2	22.9	29.1
Oklahoma	32.8	30.8	34.6
Oregon	20.8	18.8	22.6
Pennsylvania	24.7	22.4	26.7
Rhode Island	24.9	21.1	28.3
South Carolina	26.4	23.2	29.4
South Dakota	25.4	24.5	26.3
Tennessee	35.1	30.8	38.9
Texas	27.1	24.6	29.4
Utah	16.5	15.4	17.5
Vermont	20.3	20.2	20.5
Virginia	23.2	20.0	26.2
Washington	17.1	14.9	19.2
West Virginia	31.7	28.2	34.8
Wisconsin	20.7	19.4	22.0
Wyoming	21.1	20.4	22.1

Source: Compiled by New Strategist based on the Centers for Disease Control and Prevention Behavioral Risk Factor Surveillance System Survey, Internet site http://www.cdc.gov/brfss/index.htm

1.113 Pneumonia Vaccination: Ever Had by Age, 2001

"Have you ever had a pneumonia vaccination?"

(percent of people aged 18 or older responding "yes," by state and age, 2001)

	total	18 to 24	25 to 34	35 to 44	45 to 54	55 to 64	65 or older
U.S. total	**21.8%**	**17.7%**	**9.5%**	**8.7%**	**12.2%**	**24.0%**	**61.2%**
Alabama	24.4	21.8	14.0	9.8	14.5	26.0	60.3
Alaska	19.2	14.0	13.2	9.2	11.2	31.4	65.3
Arizona	25.7	19.8	13.2	11.0	16.0	27.9	65.6
Arkansas	24.4	20.8	12.1	8.0	14.5	24.9	59.0
California	21.4	20.3	11.4	10.6	13.2	22.1	59.6
Colorado	24.7	26.9	12.7	10.2	15.6	27.7	68.6
Connecticut	21.1	18.1	8.2	6.8	11.7	17.4	63.3
Delaware	22.4	18.0	7.1	7.9	10.3	22.6	68.9
District of Columbia	19.0	19.8	13.8	10.2	12.1	11.9	49.0
Florida	24.9	17.8	10.3	8.4	12.8	22.3	58.1
Georgia	20.9	18.3	11.2	9.9	13.9	24.5	57.9
Hawaii	20.8	16.9	9.6	8.7	10.7	17.4	63.7
Idaho	22.9	22.8	9.2	8.0	14.3	25.9	60.3
Illinois	21.0	22.6	9.4	10.8	11.8	18.8	56.7
Indiana	22.9	17.0	12.7	8.9	12.3	25.0	60.2
Iowa	24.2	16.9	7.8	8.0	11.5	25.5	65.9
Kansas	22.1	12.8	9.2	7.0	13.6	23.9	62.9
Kentucky	18.6	11.1	5.6	6.6	10.4	23.5	55.1
Louisiana	18.8	16.0	9.1	7.4	12.8	23.8	49.5
Maine	22.7	14.1	9.4	7.3	12.8	25.1	65.0
Maryland	22.3	24.9	13.1	9.8	11.1	22.6	62.3
Massachusetts	21.6	14.4	10.1	8.5	11.1	17.6	63.5
Michigan	20.7	19.2	9.2	7.5	13.3	21.2	56.6
Minnesota	20.0	15.9	7.2	5.1	9.5	23.1	62.9
Mississippi	21.2	13.4	9.9	10.9	11.0	27.4	55.7
Missouri	19.7	11.0	3.5	6.5	12.6	23.4	56.0
Montana	24.5	15.9	9.3	7.6	15.5	28.3	67.9
Nebraska	20.2	8.2	3.7	6.6	11.7	24.9	61.2
Nevada	27.8	20.3	13.8	12.7	21.1	35.4	66.3
New Hampshire	20.3	22.6	8.3	6.9	8.4	20.1	62.7
New Jersey	20.0	16.9	8.4	6.8	10.4	17.2	58.9
New Mexico	23.1	19.5	10.6	13.3	13.6	24.1	62.7
New York	21.0	18.8	9.8	8.2	12.7	20.2	55.9
North Carolina	21.1	11.9	7.0	8.9	10.7	25.7	65.8
North Dakota	24.2	17.3	9.0	10.7	12.1	25.0	64.2
Ohio	21.4	17.2	8.4	8.1	11.2	25.2	59.3
Oklahoma	24.8	11.9	6.0	9.6	19.6	32.5	66.1
Oregon	27.3	28.3	12.5	11.1	14.9	26.2	70.9
Pennsylvania	23.8	17.7	12.4	9.1	11.9	22.6	59.5
Rhode Island	24.7	21.4	9.4	7.3	11.7	26.8	67.0
South Carolina	21.0	13.1	9.5	9.9	14.6	22.5	57.9
South Dakota	21.2	15.2	5.6	7.9	11.1	22.7	59.2
Tennessee	19.8	10.2	7.7	8.8	12.0	25.4	55.4
Texas	21.3	17.6	11.9	10.9	12.6	23.2	58.0
Utah	23.5	19.5	12.0	10.6	16.2	27.5	67.3
Vermont	22.1	19.4	9.0	8.1	9.4	24.0	67.3
Virginia	22.1	29.5	11.8	6.5	11.3	24.7	60.1
Washington	24.4	22.4	11.8	11.3	13.8	23.2	66.8
West Virginia	24.7	15.6	7.9	9.2	16.5	29.6	61.3
Wisconsin	24.1	16.5	16.6	7.9	11.5	22.4	65.6
Wyoming	24.7	18.2	12.3	10.2	14.8	29.6	68.4

Source: Compiled by New Strategist based on the Centers for Disease Control and Prevention Behavioral Risk Factor Surveillance System Survey, Internet site http://www.cdc.gov/brfss/index.htm

1.114 Pneumonia Vaccination: Ever Had by Education, 2001

"Have you ever had a pneumonia vaccination?"

(percent of people aged 18 or older responding "yes." by state and educational attainment, 2001)

	total	less than high school	high school graduate	some college	college graduate
U.S. total	**21.8%**	**30.1%**	**23.6%**	**21.6%**	**17.3%**
Alabama	24.4	33.8	24.9	21.4	20.6
Alaska	19.2	33.9	17.3	21.8	14.4
Arizona	25.7	20.9	30.1	25.9	23.4
Arkansas	24.4	33.4	23.7	23.9	20.1
California	21.4	17.8	24.8	24.1	18.7
Colorado	24.7	25.5	27.7	26.5	20.7
Connecticut	21.1	31.0	24.3	21.5	16.4
Delaware	22.4	29.6	25.1	20.7	19.4
District of Columbia	19.0	20.7	22.3	20.7	16.0
Florida	24.9	26.5	26.2	23.6	23.8
Georgia	20.9	26.3	22.7	18.4	18.6
Hawaii	20.8	32.4	22.6	20.9	16.6
Idaho	22.9	31.9	24.3	22.9	18.3
Illinois	21.0	24.0	23.4	18.9	19.8
Indiana	22.9	30.6	24.2	24.1	16.5
Iowa	24.2	34.0	29.1	21.4	16.1
Kansas	22.1	28.9	29.0	19.7	15.8
Kentucky	18.6	27.2	18.9	16.3	12.4
Louisiana	18.8	26.6	18.3	18.1	14.2
Maine	22.7	36.4	25.6	19.2	17.3
Maryland	22.3	30.6	26.2	22.8	17.3
Massachusetts	21.6	31.7	26.0	22.3	16.4
Michigan	20.7	28.3	19.9	22.3	16.4
Minnesota	20.0	40.1	24.0	17.3	14.5
Mississippi	21.2	24.9	22.0	20.6	17.4
Missouri	19.7	30.1	21.6	18.7	13.2
Montana	24.5	31.3	25.8	25.1	19.5
Nebraska	20.2	30.6	22.4	17.5	15.6
Nevada	27.8	29.2	23.6	26.2	33.8
New Hampshire	20.3	29.1	22.2	20.9	16.4
New Jersey	20.0	25.3	22.5	18.8	17.2
New Mexico	23.1	23.6	23.0	23.7	22.3
New York	21.0	23.3	24.4	21.2	17.0
North Carolina	21.1	32.5	20.8	20.2	15.7
North Dakota	24.2	50.9	26.4	20.0	18.2
Ohio	21.4	32.8	22.2	19.1	17.5
Oklahoma	24.8	31.5	27.2	22.6	19.8
Oregon	27.3	24.1	30.6	28.7	23.9
Pennsylvania	23.8	36.8	23.6	23.5	18.6
Rhode Island	24.7	35.4	26.2	22.4	20.8
South Carolina	21.0	29.8	19.2	21.9	17.1
South Dakota	21.2	37.3	22.5	21.6	13.3
Tennessee	19.8	30.0	19.1	17.1	17.6
Texas	21.3	20.7	21.0	24.7	18.9
Utah	23.5	33.3	26.1	21.6	21.1
Vermont	22.1	39.6	23.9	21.3	16.9
Virginia	22.1	30.1	22.3	24.8	17.3
Washington	24.4	26.7	26.2	24.7	22.1
West Virginia	24.7	38.0	22.5	21.9	20.2
Wisconsin	24.1	37.9	25.6	23.1	18.7
Wyoming	24.7	39.2	24.8	23.7	21.6

Source: Compiled by New Strategist based on the Centers for Disease Control and Prevention Behavioral Risk Factor Surveillance System Survey, Internet site http://www.cdc.gov/brfss/index.htm

1.115 Pneumonia Vaccination: Ever Had by Household Income, 2001

"Have you ever had a pneumonia vaccination?"

(percent of people aged 18 or older responding "yes," by state and household income, 2001)

	total	less than $15,000	$15,000 to $24,999	$25,000 to $34,999	$35,000 to $49,999	$50,000 or more
U.S. total	**21.8%**	**32.1%**	**28.2%**	**24.0%**	**18.7%**	**14.3%**
Alabama	24.4	31.8	28.2	25.8	18.7	13.5
Alaska	19.2	23.1	27.1	19.1	18.8	14.9
Arizona	25.7	25.1	28.9	27.3	29.5	18.1
Arkansas	24.4	32.2	28.4	23.2	18.7	15.4
California	21.4	21.6	30.2	23.6	19.8	16.7
Colorado	24.7	30.3	26.1	25.3	30.3	20.3
Connecticut	21.1	33.6	31.7	26.6	20.1	13.5
Delaware	22.4	32.0	35.4	18.7	22.7	13.8
District of Columbia	19.0	21.8	19.9	17.3	20.7	15.3
Florida	24.9	26.8	27.4	27.5	21.7	17.2
Georgia	20.9	23.8	24.7	25.4	20.5	14.1
Hawaii	20.8	20.3	27.1	19.8	15.9	15.9
Idaho	22.9	38.1	27.5	24.6	16.6	14.3
Illinois	21.0	26.1	27.0	28.6	15.3	14.8
Indiana	22.9	37.0	30.3	25.7	18.0	12.6
Iowa	24.2	33.6	37.3	27.1	19.5	12.9
Kansas	22.1	33.4	29.2	24.6	18.0	15.1
Kentucky	18.6	28.0	19.2	16.3	13.0	10.1
Louisiana	18.8	27.8	19.2	20.4	13.8	12.2
Maine	22.7	36.3	33.0	26.8	15.8	12.9
Maryland	22.3	36.4	29.5	27.0	21.5	15.2
Massachusetts	21.6	32.9	35.2	24.6	19.6	14.4
Michigan	20.7	29.5	28.2	23.0	18.1	14.3
Minnesota	20.0	35.5	34.2	23.5	16.9	11.8
Mississippi	21.2	26.8	25.4	21.0	17.2	13.2
Missouri	19.7	33.7	27.1	23.4	11.7	11.6
Montana	24.5	36.3	25.7	23.7	18.7	15.4
Nebraska	20.2	22.9	26.9	21.7	12.4	13.0
Nevada	27.8	45.3	28.0	27.8	23.8	23.3
New Hampshire	20.3	40.9	31.4	25.4	18.0	12.0
New Jersey	20.0	31.3	26.7	22.5	14.9	14.3
New Mexico	23.1	27.4	23.7	24.5	20.3	17.6
New York	21.0	25.7	27.7	26.8	18.5	14.8
North Carolina	21.1	32.5	28.4	21.4	11.6	11.5
North Dakota	24.2	35.3	32.6	22.9	19.8	14.2
Ohio	21.4	35.1	31.4	24.4	17.7	11.5
Oklahoma	24.8	34.5	28.2	21.8	19.4	14.3
Oregon	27.3	34.8	31.7	28.8	25.2	18.2
Pennsylvania	23.8	35.2	32.7	24.6	20.8	12.3
Rhode Island	24.7	32.8	32.9	26.2	19.8	16.0
South Carolina	21.0	32.6	21.5	17.0	21.5	15.0
South Dakota	21.2	34.7	30.5	21.5	15.3	10.5
Tennessee	19.8	28.0	22.3	18.7	15.2	9.8
Texas	21.3	26.8	21.7	20.8	19.9	17.5
Utah	23.5	30.9	32.8	27.4	22.8	15.7
Vermont	22.1	35.0	32.6	19.5	17.2	14.8
Virginia	22.1	31.7	26.6	26.8	17.5	15.8
Washington	24.4	37.5	33.3	28.1	25.2	16.0
West Virginia	24.7	29.8	29.1	21.3	21.1	16.1
Wisconsin	24.1	37.3	40.6	25.3	19.1	14.3
Wyoming	24.7	34.4	29.6	25.9	20.4	18.7

Source: Compiled by New Strategist based on the Centers for Disease Control and Prevention Behavioral Risk Factor Surveillance System Survey, Internet site http://www.cdc.gov/brfss/index.htm

1.116 Pneumonia Vaccination: Ever Had by Sex, 2001

"Have you ever had a pneumonia vaccination?"

(percent of people aged 18 or older responding "yes," by state and sex, 2001)

	total	men	women
U.S. total	**21.8%**	**22.2%**	**21.6%**
Alabama	24.4	24.9	24.0
Alaska	19.2	21.2	17.3
Arizona	25.7	25.1	26.2
Arkansas	24.4	27.4	21.8
California	21.4	22.1	20.7
Colorado	24.7	26.3	23.2
Connecticut	21.1	21.1	21.1
Delaware	22.4	21.4	23.2
District of Columbia	19.0	20.8	17.5
Florida	24.9	24.4	25.3
Georgia	20.9	22.2	19.8
Hawaii	20.8	21.5	20.2
Idaho	22.9	23.0	22.9
Illinois	21.0	21.6	20.5
Indiana	22.9	22.6	23.1
Iowa	24.2	24.1	24.3
Kansas	22.1	20.7	23.4
Kentucky	18.6	19.4	17.9
Louisiana	18.8	18.8	18.7
Maine	22.7	22.5	22.8
Maryland	22.3	24.1	20.8
Massachusetts	21.6	20.9	22.3
Michigan	20.7	21.3	20.1
Minnesota	20.0	20.1	20.0
Mississippi	21.2	21.2	21.2
Missouri	19.7	19.5	19.9
Montana	24.5	24.7	24.4
Nebraska	20.2	19.6	20.8
Nevada	27.8	30.6	25.2
New Hampshire	20.3	21.3	19.5
New Jersey	20.0	19.9	20.1
New Mexico	23.1	24.1	22.2
New York	21.0	20.4	21.5
North Carolina	21.1	20.5	21.7
North Dakota	24.2	26.9	21.7
Ohio	21.4	21.0	21.8
Oklahoma	24.8	24.6	24.9
Oregon	27.3	28.8	26.1
Pennsylvania	23.8	25.2	22.6
Rhode Island	24.7	24.5	24.8
South Carolina	21.0	22.2	19.9
South Dakota	21.2	21.3	21.1
Tennessee	19.8	19.3	20.2
Texas	21.3	23.5	19.4
Utah	23.5	24.3	22.8
Vermont	22.1	24.1	20.4
Virginia	22.1	24.0	20.3
Washington	24.4	25.2	23.6
West Virginia	24.7	26.6	23.1
Wisconsin	24.1	25.5	22.9
Wyoming	24.7	27.2	22.4

Source: Compiled by New Strategist based on the Centers for Disease Control and Prevention Behavioral Risk Factor Surveillance System Survey, Internet site http://www.cdc.gov/brfss/index.htm

1.117 Seat Belt Use by Age, 1997

"How often do you use seatbelts when you drive or ride in the car?"

(percent of people aged 18 or older responding "always," by state and age, 1997)

	total	18 to 24	25 to 34	35 to 44	45 to 54	55 to 64	65 or older
U.S. total	**69.3%**	**58.9%**	**66.3%**	**69.5%**	**70.9%**	**70.3%**	**74.4%**
Alabama	66.2	53.8	63.2	66.2	70.7	67.7	73.2
Alaska	65.3	52.6	66.1	70.4	61.5	71.8	65.4
Arizona	80.5	70.5	75.6	76.0	85.9	83.5	91.5
Arkansas	65.5	47.8	68.6	66.5	62.7	69.1	72.1
California	87.2	83.9	87.4	86.5	87.1	88.8	90.0
Colorado	71.4	55.7	72.7	74.0	73.7	73.0	74.0
Connecticut	69.1	58.2	65.9	70.9	69.8	67.2	78.2
Delaware	69.9	56.5	68.0	70.2	74.4	68.3	78.2
District of Columbia	78.0	57.8	74.5	84.1	84.4	77.5	84.9
Florida	76.1	60.0	72.5	75.5	78.2	74.6	85.5
Georgia	75.4	56.4	74.3	76.1	78.9	81.0	84.6
Hawaii	87.1	79.0	86.0	87.2	88.9	93.5	88.3
Idaho	59.6	48.6	60.1	61.8	54.9	64.0	65.9
Illinois	68.1	55.4	61.5	68.3	76.5	64.4	78.5
Indiana	61.9	48.2	56.8	63.0	66.4	61.1	72.7
Iowa	67.2	61.2	61.2	67.3	70.2	66.5	73.6
Kansas	53.8	34.8	52.3	55.5	55.6	55.1	63.5
Kentucky	65.4	55.2	65.2	64.5	68.3	66.2	70.9
Louisiana	74.3	62.8	75.2	71.4	74.2	76.9	84.4
Maine	69.5	66.2	69.2	73.0	66.6	64.0	73.8
Maryland	76.1	67.9	74.0	76.3	78.3	82.3	77.7
Massachusetts	62.7	62.6	63.6	63.3	57.3	65.4	64.4
Michigan	72.3	61.6	67.8	73.5	73.8	75.7	80.0
Minnesota	59.8	51.4	55.3	61.8	59.9	61.7	66.7
Mississippi	56.5	49.8	52.8	59.2	56.2	58.3	62.3
Missouri	61.9	53.9	61.8	60.9	62.6	59.2	68.2
Montana	57.6	46.6	50.9	56.7	58.5	63.1	67.1
Nebraska	57.7	48.0	58.8	55.2	60.1	55.0	64.6
Nevada	73.7	67.0	65.5	72.8	80.5	78.3	78.1
New Hampshire	58.3	53.7	64.6	59.6	58.7	60.6	49.0
New Jersey	72.2	62.3	71.1	73.4	75.3	73.3	74.8
New Mexico	83.5	74.6	82.8	84.5	83.0	85.9	88.3
New York	73.8	60.9	71.7	75.9	74.5	75.7	80.2
North Carolina	84.8	82.2	80.4	85.7	82.7	86.8	90.9
North Dakota	40.2	40.9	39.0	38.1	39.5	37.9	45.0
Ohio	70.0	62.7	65.4	68.9	71.4	72.1	78.3
Oklahoma	63.1	51.5	65.6	64.3	59.6	65.2	68.4
Oregon	84.0	75.0	86.1	84.2	83.9	84.5	87.1
Pennsylvania	67.3	54.9	66.4	67.2	65.4	71.9	73.9
Rhode Island	56.8	37.8	57.3	58.2	59.1	59.6	63.1
South Carolina	80.5	69.0	77.2	80.1	82.8	85.4	88.3
South Dakota	42.0	38.3	44.0	41.4	38.4	39.4	47.7
Tennessee	66.4	59.6	59.8	68.2	70.9	67.4	71.6
Texas	81.3	75.2	79.6	84.1	78.3	79.9	88.3
Utah	65.0	60.0	63.4	65.7	62.9	68.4	71.3
Vermont	73.7	66.2	72.6	73.9	72.8	75.1	81.4
Virginia	71.7	61.7	66.8	75.8	74.4	71.6	77.4
Washington	75.8	61.5	73.1	77.2	76.8	80.1	83.4
West Virginia	70.6	59.9	71.2	66.7	70.9	75.3	77.1
Wisconsin	61.3	48.8	56.1	63.4	64.6	57.8	71.9
Wyoming	50.2	41.1	47.1	49.7	53.3	53.7	55.6

Source: Compiled by New Strategist based on the Centers for Disease Control and Prevention Behavioral Risk Factor Surveillance System Survey, Internet site http://www.cdc.gov/brfss/index.htm

1.118 Seat Belt Use by Education, 1997

"How often do you use seatbelts when you drive or ride in a car?"

(percent of people aged 18 or older responding "always," by state and educational attainment. 1997)

	total	less than high school	high school graduate	some college	college graduate
U.S. total	**69.3%**	**60.7%**	**64.9%**	**68.9%**	**78.2%**
Alabama	66.2	60.6	64.9	62.1	78.0
Alaska	65.3	56.7	60.3	66.5	73.1
Arizona	80.5	77.4	73.2	83.8	86.6
Arkansas	65.5	60.8	64.4	67.2	71.0
California	87.2	86.6	86.8	87.0	88.2
Colorado	71.4	58.1	64.9	72.0	79.9
Connecticut	69.1	60.5	65.0	66.3	77.4
Delaware	69.9	56.1	62.0	73.6	82.5
District of Columbia	78.0	74.5	78.1	69.3	84.8
Florida	76.1	66.6	72.5	77.8	83.8
Georgia	75.4	66.0	74.3	76.7	80.2
Hawaii	87.1	83.9	86.8	86.5	88.9
Idaho	59.6	51.5	53.9	60.2	70.5
Illinois	68.1	66.2	61.1	64.3	80.0
Indiana	61.9	54.9	58.6	62.3	71.5
Iowa	67.2	62.4	65.8	67.4	71.6
Kansas	53.8	51.9	47.4	52.7	66.4
Kentucky	65.4	58.9	61.6	67.8	78.3
Louisiana	74.3	77.6	68.2	74.5	82.2
Maine	69.5	60.9	63.6	70.8	81.1
Maryland	76.1	63.8	72.6	76.1	84.0
Massachusetts	62.7	47.0	54.7	61.6	74.3
Michigan	72.3	65.5	71.7	69.8	80.1
Minnesota	59.8	51.0	56.1	57.5	70.0
Mississippi	56.5	53.7	54.5	53.6	67.8
Missouri	61.9	52.9	58.1	63.0	71.8
Montana	57.6	49.4	52.5	60.3	63.9
Nebraska	57.7	50.6	52.9	60.6	64.0
Nevada	73.7	60.9	75.7	73.6	75.3
New Hampshire	58.3	34.2	49.9	58.4	73.8
New Jersey	72.2	64.1	70.2	73.7	75.8
New Mexico	83.5	79.9	83.3	84.0	85.1
New York	73.8	68.9	72.5	71.0	79.5
North Carolina	84.8	83.8	84.5	83.5	87.1
North Dakota	40.2	33.9	30.2	43.3	54.5
Ohio	70.0	59.8	65.9	72.1	81.0
Oklahoma	63.1	55.2	62.1	62.6	69.5
Oregon	84.0	80.1	83.0	83.5	87.4
Pennsylvania	67.3	60.3	64.7	68.1	74.4
Rhode Island	56.8	53.4	48.7	58.5	67.4
South Carolina	80.5	77.4	75.0	81.7	90.2
South Dakota	42.0	30.2	36.4	43.6	56.8
Tennessee	66.4	55.9	61.6	70.3	78.8
Texas	81.3	80.8	79.8	81.9	82.4
Utah	65.0	57.0	56.5	66.1	73.4
Vermont	73.7	68.5	66.5	75.3	83.6
Virginia	71.7	63.1	66.8	73.2	79.0
Washington	75.8	66.7	73.2	75.9	80.8
West Virginia	70.6	68.0	70.1	69.9	76.8
Wisconsin	61.3	57.6	53.5	61.5	73.3
Wyoming	50.2	44.1	45.0	47.0	64.1

Source: Compiled by New Strategist based on the Centers for Disease Control and Prevention Behavioral Risk Factor Surveillance System Survey. Internet site http://www.cdc.gov/brfss/index.htm

1.119 Seat Belt Use by Household Income, 1997

"How often do you use seatbelts when you drive or ride in a car?"

(percent of people aged 18 or older responding "always," by state and household income, 1997)

	total	less than $15,000	$15,000 to $24,999	$25,000 to $34,999	$35,000 to $49,999	$50,000 or more
U.S. total	**69.3%**	**64.7%**	**64.6%**	**65.1%**	**70.9%**	**73.6%**
Alabama	66.2	57.7	61.0	64.6	70.1	72.8
Alaska	65.3	50.7	67.0	65.4	71.1	64.6
Arizona	80.5	48.3	77.9	82.4	82.3	91.8
Arkansas	65.5	63.7	63.0	64.8	64.6	69.6
California	87.2	88.1	86.7	82.4	88.7	87.4
Colorado	71.4	65.7	63.2	68.1	74.5	77.2
Connecticut	69.1	63.7	68.7	62.5	65.1	72.2
Delaware	69.9	67.3	65.2	64.0	67.9	76.1
District of Columbia	78.0	71.0	78.5	76.5	85.4	75.0
Florida	76.1	73.0	78.0	71.2	76.3	81.1
Georgia	75.4	68.6	66.8	72.3	77.2	82.3
Hawaii	87.1	87.0	88.9	88.9	83.6	89.2
Idaho	59.6	54.1	57.8	55.4	61.8	65.8
Illinois	68.1	56.0	68.0	61.4	72.4	72.7
Indiana	61.9	59.1	59.4	51.7	63.2	68.8
Iowa	67.2	68.2	67.4	60.1	66.8	70.9
Kansas	53.8	48.4	43.1	47.4	55.2	66.3
Kentucky	65.4	63.2	62.0	64.5	66.5	71.6
Louisiana	74.3	75.7	70.2	74.5	71.0	75.4
Maine	69.5	68.1	62.5	67.7	72.8	73.9
Maryland	76.1	75.4	70.5	75.2	74.4	80.6
Massachusetts	62.7	48.5	54.2	62.2	62.5	66.7
Michigan	72.3	72.7	67.7	69.8	72.8	75.0
Minnesota	59.8	58.7	56.5	57.5	57.2	63.3
Mississippi	56.5	54.7	51.4	55.8	53.2	66.7
Missouri	61.9	61.2	58.3	54.8	56.6	70.5
Montana	57.6	56.4	53.4	57.5	57.5	62.0
Nebraska	57.7	52.7	52.2	55.1	59.4	64.1
Nevada	73.7	70.5	62.9	76.4	77.8	69.8
New Hampshire	58.3	47.9	54.0	49.7	53.4	69.3
New Jersey	72.2	66.3	67.8	68.4	71.0	76.9
New Mexico	83.5	85.3	82.6	83.0	85.2	80.0
New York	73.8	74.7	70.0	73.7	72.8	76.4
North Carolina	84.8	82.8	83.8	85.9	81.8	86.2
North Dakota	40.2	36.0	37.1	41.7	40.8	43.7
Ohio	70.0	60.9	64.8	70.2	72.1	75.8
Oklahoma	63.1	57.4	58.5	63.5	66.9	68.6
Oregon	84.0	80.4	83.3	81.8	87.0	84.3
Pennsylvania	67.3	63.7	63.5	61.9	66.4	73.3
Rhode Island	56.8	43.9	49.5	54.0	56.8	63.3
South Carolina	80.5	80.5	76.8	75.8	81.8	84.8
South Dakota	42.0	37.9	36.2	36.7	44.6	56.0
Tennessee	66.4	56.9	60.7	63.4	70.8	77.3
Texas	81.3	84.2	80.4	79.8	82.3	80.9
Utah	65.0	61.7	63.6	61.7	63.4	69.5
Vermont	73.7	71.4	69.2	70.6	77.0	78.4
Virginia	71.7	66.6	64.4	66.9	72.1	76.6
Washington	75.8	71.2	75.7	71.4	72.8	79.3
West Virginia	70.6	67.8	69.5	69.5	69.7	78.3
Wisconsin	61.3	67.2	55.7	54.1	60.9	68.2
Wyoming	50.2	43.6	42.4	47.5	51.6	59.3

Source: Compiled by New Strategist based on the Centers for Disease Control and Prevention Behavioral Risk Factor Surveillance System Survey, Internet site http://www.cdc.gov/brfss/index.htm

1.120 Seat Belt Use by Sex, 1997

"How often do you use seatbelts when you drive or ride in a car?"

(percent of people aged 18 or older responding "always," by state and sex, 1997)

	total	men	women
U.S. total	**69.3%**	**61.9%**	**74.8%**
Alabama	66.2	56.5	74.8
Alaska	65.3	60.2	71.0
Arizona	80.5	80.3	80.7
Arkansas	65.5	57.8	72.3
California	87.2	85.1	89.3
Colorado	71.4	68.1	74.5
Connecticut	69.1	62.9	74.8
Delaware	69.9	62.1	77.0
District of Columbia	78.0	72.6	82.6
Florida	76.1	68.1	83.5
Georgia	75.4	68.9	81.4
Hawaii	87.1	84.0	90.4
Idaho	59.6	51.1	67.8
Illinois	68.1	62.9	72.7
Indiana	61.9	52.9	70.0
Iowa	67.2	58.9	74.7
Kansas	53.8	46.7	60.5
Kentucky	65.4	54.9	75.0
Louisiana	74.3	66.2	81.5
Maine	69.5	61.7	76.7
Maryland	76.1	68.7	82.8
Massachusetts	62.7	56.8	68.0
Michigan	72.3	65.0	78.9
Minnesota	59.8	51.1	67.8
Mississippi	56.5	47.9	64.2
Missouri	61.9	54.7	68.3
Montana	57.6	48.7	66.1
Nebraska	57.7	49.4	65.4
Nevada	73.7	62.4	85.2
New Hampshire	58.3	48.1	67.8
New Jersey	72.2	65.5	78.3
New Mexico	83.5	79.2	87.5
New York	73.8	66.1	80.7
North Carolina	84.8	78.4	90.5
North Dakota	40.2	29.0	51.0
Ohio	70.0	65.7	73.9
Oklahoma	63.1	56.7	69.0
Oregon	84.0	79.0	88.7
Pennsylvania	67.3	59.4	74.3
Rhode Island	56.8	52.3	60.9
South Carolina	80.5	74.0	86.3
South Dakota	42.0	33.6	50.0
Tennessee	66.4	60.3	71.9
Texas	81.3	75.5	86.7
Utah	65.0	56.9	72.6
Vermont	73.7	66.2	80.8
Virginia	71.7	65.2	77.8
Washington	75.8	69.2	82.1
West Virginia	70.6	60.7	79.4
Wisconsin	61.3	51.0	70.9
Wyoming	50.2	44.0	56.3

Source: Compiled by New Strategist based on the Centers for Disease Control and Prevention Behavioral Risk Factor Surveillance System Survey, Internet site http://www.cdc.gov/brfss/index.htm

1.121 Seat Belt Use by Children, 1997

"How often does the child (under 16 years old) in your household
use an appropriate restraint when riding in a car?"

(percent of people aged 18 or older living in households with children under age 16 responding "always," by state, 1997)

	child always uses restraint
U.S. total	**85.4%**
Alabama	79.7
Alaska	82.8
Arizona	94.0
Arkansas	80.1
California	92.2
Colorado	85.0
Connecticut	90.1
Delaware	87.4
District of Columbia	88.5
Florida	87.8
Georgia	89.1
Hawaii	80.3
Idaho	71.4
Illinois	82.1
Indiana	79.6
Iowa	76.3
Kansas	76.5
Kentucky	85.8
Louisiana	83.7
Maine	96.3
Maryland	89.6
Massachusetts	87.6
Michigan	84.7
Minnesota	74.4
Mississippi	70.2
Missouri	77.6
Montana	74.6
Nebraska	73.5
Nevada	86.8
New Hampshire	90.7
New Jersey	87.0
New Mexico	89.6
New York	88.3
North Carolina	89.6
North Dakota	69.8
Ohio	87.4
Oklahoma	82.2
Oregon	91.5
Pennsylvania	88.0
Rhode Island	90.1
South Carolina	91.1
South Dakota	61.5
Tennessee	84.8
Texas	80.5
Utah	68.2
Vermont	93.5
Virginia	86.3
Washington	86.4
West Virginia	87.0
Wisconsin	78.0
Wyoming	68.6

Source: Compiled by New Strategist based on the Centers for Disease Control and Prevention Behavioral Risk Factor Surveillance System Survey, Internet site http://www.cdc.gov/brfss/index.htm

1.122 Smoke Detector by Age, 1999

"Do you have a smoke detector in your home?"

(percent of people aged 18 or older responding "yes," by state and age, 1999)

	total	18 to 24	25 to 34	35 to 44	45 to 54	55 to 64	65 or older
U.S. total	**96.0%**	**96.4%**	**97.0%**	**97.1%**	**96.1%**	**94.9%**	**93.5%**
Alabama	94.2	97.4	96.2	94.1	92.7	92.9	91.9
Alaska	97.6	97.9	98.2	96.6	98.8	97.4	95.3
Arizona	94.3	89.7	91.9	95.5	93.7	98.1	96.6
Arkansas	92.0	92.2	95.7	94.1	91.1	86.6	90.6
California	95.9	95.2	96.3	97.0	95.1	95.1	95.9
Colorado	93.3	92.5	96.0	95.4	94.0	90.2	88.1
Connecticut	97.5	95.6	99.1	99.4	99.4	93.8	94.9
Delaware	98.1	97.8	99.0	98.1	97.6	96.1	99.1
District of Columbia	99.0	100.0	98.0	99.0	98.5	99.3	100.0
Florida	93.4	91.0	93.8	95.3	92.7	92.5	93.1
Georgia	95.0	93.1	97.0	95.8	96.4	93.7	91.5
Hawaii	87.0	93.7	85.7	90.2	88.4	83.9	80.5
Idaho	94.3	95.8	96.4	95.7	95.0	91.5	90.5
Illinois	98.2	94.8	99.2	99.1	98.6	97.4	98.0
Indiana	97.4	99.6	98.8	98.6	96.1	95.0	95.6
Iowa	95.4	97.7	95.9	97.9	93.6	96.2	92.3
Kansas	95.2	95.0	96.3	97.1	95.1	93.9	92.8
Kentucky	95.4	95.9	98.1	96.2	94.8	94.2	92.7
Louisiana	88.6	93.6	90.4	88.6	92.4	89.3	78.6
Maine	97.4	99.5	98.4	99.2	96.5	94.8	95.8
Maryland	98.7	97.6	98.7	99.3	99.3	99.2	97.6
Massachusetts	97.4	96.4	98.9	98.0	98.1	95.8	96.1
Michigan	98.0	96.8	97.7	98.4	98.5	97.9	98.0
Minnesota	98.2	98.9	99.2	98.9	98.3	98.3	95.4
Mississippi	90.8	92.2	94.4	95.6	90.6	88.1	81.6
Missouri	96.2	96.3	98.2	97.9	96.2	95.2	93.2
Montana	94.8	95.6	95.4	95.6	95.5	93.3	93.1
Nebraska	92.7	93.3	96.1	94.5	92.7	90.3	88.5
Nevada	92.2	87.8	91.1	94.5	93.4	96.6	88.0
New Hampshire	98.5	98.8	98.8	99.1	97.5	97.8	98.6
New Jersey	97.4	98.0	98.6	98.7	96.4	95.8	96.1
New Mexico	89.9	88.8	93.5	92.8	90.1	87.1	83.1
New York	94.9	91.1	94.8	96.8	97.3	95.3	92.1
North Carolina	97.6	98.3	98.1	98.7	98.5	96.9	94.6
North Dakota	96.2	97.3	98.6	98.4	95.8	93.0	93.3
Ohio	96.8	96.7	99.4	97.3	95.8	96.2	95.2
Oklahoma	94.3	96.4	95.1	95.5	94.8	93.8	91.0
Oregon	98.7	99.4	98.1	99.4	98.6	97.7	98.8
Pennsylvania	96.4	97.1	96.5	97.6	97.6	96.2	93.9
Rhode Island	97.6	98.0	98.6	98.0	96.5	97.9	96.7
South Carolina	97.4	97.3	99.1	97.7	96.8	97.4	95.5
South Dakota	92.9	97.4	96.8	94.8	92.8	88.7	87.1
Tennessee	96.6	96.8	97.4	98.3	96.8	93.9	95.3
Texas	90.6	90.4	94.0	93.0	89.8	85.4	86.9
Utah	94.1	93.9	95.2	95.6	95.7	91.0	90.2
Vermont	96.5	95.0	97.1	98.8	97.4	95.6	93.5
Virginia	96.3	96.6	98.0	97.1	97.2	92.7	93.9
Washington	97.8	97.9	98.4	99.0	98.3	96.7	95.8
West Virginia	94.9	92.9	96.7	96.0	94.7	94.7	93.6
Wisconsin	98.2	98.0	97.7	99.5	98.5	97.0	97.9
Wyoming	94.0	96.8	95.8	95.4	96.2	93.5	85.9

Source: Compiled by New Strategist based on the Centers for Disease Control and Prevention Behavioral Risk Factor Surveillance System Survey, Internet site http://www.cdc.gov/brfss/index.htm

1.123 Smoke Detector by Education, 1999

"Do you have a smoke detector in your home?"

(percent of people aged 18 or older responding "yes," by state and educational attainment, 1999)

	total	less than high school	high school graduate	some college	college graduate
U.S. total	**96.0%**	**91.0%**	**95.5%**	**96.9%**	**97.9%**
Alabama	94.2	89.7	93.7	95.9	96.9
Alaska	97.6	90.8	97.3	98.6	98.5
Arizona	94.3	80.4	94.8	95.0	98.4
Arkansas	92.0	86.8	90.8	93.6	95.9
California	95.9	91.9	95.9	96.8	97.9
Colorado	93.3	83.5	91.3	94.2	97.0
Connecticut	97.5	95.3	96.9	98.0	98.4
Delaware	98.1	96.0	96.9	98.9	99.4
District of Columbia	99.0	99.5	98.7	100.0	98.6
Florida	93.4	85.2	93.1	94.7	96.2
Georgia	95.0	89.4	94.1	96.1	97.9
Hawaii	87.0	74.8	85.3	88.6	89.7
Idaho	94.3	90.6	93.0	95.3	96.3
Illinois	98.2	96.1	97.5	98.2	99.7
Indiana	97.4	90.7	97.5	99.1	98.6
Iowa	95.4	90.0	93.4	97.1	98.6
Kansas	95.2	88.7	95.1	96.1	96.5
Kentucky	95.4	90.8	95.3	97.4	98.0
Louisiana	88.6	75.5	88.3	93.1	94.6
Maine	97.4	96.0	97.6	96.9	98.3
Maryland	98.7	97.7	98.7	98.4	99.3
Massachusetts	97.4	95.1	97.6	97.3	98.0
Michigan	98.0	95.5	98.9	97.9	97.7
Minnesota	98.2	95.7	98.0	98.2	99.2
Mississippi	90.8	81.5	91.3	93.3	94.9
Missouri	96.2	91.0	96.4	96.9	98.4
Montana	94.8	87.9	95.8	94.4	96.0
Nebraska	92.7	81.3	91.0	95.9	95.6
Nevada	92.2	70.3	94.4	94.8	96.8
New Hampshire	98.5	95.2	98.7	98.2	99.3
New Jersey	97.4	93.0	97.2	98.5	98.5
New Mexico	89.9	81.5	89.5	91.1	93.8
New York	94.9	91.0	95.5	95.0	96.1
North Carolina	97.6	95.5	97.4	97.7	99.0
North Dakota	96.2	91.4	95.3	97.3	98.4
Ohio	96.8	97.5	96.5	96.6	97.3
Oklahoma	94.3	87.3	93.6	97.1	96.5
Oregon	98.7	97.7	98.0	98.8	99.6
Pennsylvania	96.4	95.4	95.7	96.5	97.9
Rhode Island	97.6	95.3	97.5	97.5	98.8
South Carolina	97.4	92.6	98.0	98.2	98.5
South Dakota	92.9	87.7	91.5	94.1	95.3
Tennessee	96.6	92.9	96.2	97.4	99.2
Texas	90.6	78.6	90.0	93.9	96.4
Utah	94.1	87.8	94.8	94.0	94.7
Vermont	96.5	95.1	95.6	97.4	97.1
Virginia	96.3	94.8	94.7	97.9	97.0
Washington	97.8	95.5	96.8	98.4	98.9
West Virginia	94.9	92.1	95.4	95.4	96.0
Wisconsin	98.2	96.6	97.8	98.3	99.2
Wyoming	94.0	87.1	93.6	95.3	94.7

Source: Compiled by New Strategist based on the Centers for Disease Control and Prevention Behavioral Risk Factor Surveillance System Survey, Internet site http://www.cdc.gov/brfss/index.htm

1.124 Smoke Detector by Household Income, 1999

"Do you have a smoke detector in your home?"

(percent of people aged 18 or older responding "yes," by state and household income, 1999)

	total	less than $15,000	$15,000 to $24,999	$25,000 to $34,999	$35,000 to $49,999	$50,000 or more
U.S. total	**96.0%**	**92.7%**	**94.8%**	**96.1%**	**97.1%**	**98.1%**
Alabama	94.2	90.5	92.6	93.3	97.2	98.0
Alaska	97.6	94.3	96.8	96.0	97.9	99.4
Arizona	94.3	90.0	87.0	97.9	96.9	99.5
Arkansas	92.0	87.0	88.5	93.6	94.0	96.8
California	95.9	93.2	95.9	95.6	97.1	97.8
Colorado	93.3	84.0	89.9	94.5	94.9	96.9
Connecticut	97.5	98.9	98.3	98.4	98.5	97.8
Delaware	98.1	93.2	97.2	97.8	98.6	99.3
District of Columbia	99.0	100.0	98.3	100.0	99.4	98.1
Florida	93.4	87.4	89.2	94.7	96.2	96.8
Georgia	95.0	88.4	94.4	96.2	97.2	96.9
Hawaii	87.0	74.1	87.4	87.3	84.9	92.8
Idaho	94.3	90.2	90.7	94.3	96.5	97.3
Illinois	98.2	99.6	95.4	97.4	97.5	99.0
Indiana	97.4	97.5	94.9	97.1	97.1	99.9
Iowa	95.4	88.7	95.0	95.7	94.9	97.9
Kansas	95.2	91.3	94.4	92.7	97.2	98.1
Kentucky	95.4	90.1	94.7	96.5	97.1	98.5
Louisiana	88.6	75.8	85.2	89.2	93.0	96.1
Maine	97.4	95.8	96.9	97.4	99.6	98.2
Maryland	98.7	96.4	98.1	98.6	98.8	99.3
Massachusetts	97.4	96.3	95.9	97.5	97.2	98.9
Michigan	98.0	95.9	96.3	98.0	98.1	99.2
Minnesota	98.2	95.4	96.2	98.1	99.0	99.1
Mississippi	90.8	85.2	88.5	91.9	94.5	95.9
Missouri	96.2	92.0	95.2	97.5	98.1	98.3
Montana	94.8	90.5	93.4	96.8	96.8	99.0
Nebraska	92.7	85.8	88.4	93.0	95.3	98.0
Nevada	92.2	94.9	85.5	86.0	91.0	98.1
New Hampshire	98.5	98.1	97.5	99.0	98.2	98.5
New Jersey	97.4	95.8	98.6	93.1	98.8	98.5
New Mexico	89.9	84.5	88.1	89.2	92.3	97.4
New York	94.9	89.8	94.0	94.5	96.2	96.9
North Carolina	97.6	95.5	96.2	98.0	99.2	99.0
North Dakota	96.2	95.4	93.1	95.8	98.8	98.2
Ohio	96.8	94.4	97.0	96.2	96.5	98.7
Oklahoma	94.3	89.2	91.4	94.5	97.7	96.9
Oregon	98.7	95.4	98.3	99.4	98.6	99.5
Pennsylvania	96.4	94.6	94.9	96.2	98.3	97.8
Rhode Island	97.6	94.7	97.4	97.9	98.0	98.4
South Carolina	97.4	93.6	97.4	97.2	98.5	99.2
South Dakota	92.9	89.1	91.6	91.9	94.6	97.3
Tennessee	96.6	92.7	96.3	97.6	96.8	98.8
Texas	90.6	78.1	87.2	90.8	94.9	97.2
Utah	94.1	86.1	93.4	92.0	96.9	96.5
Vermont	96.5	94.1	96.1	97.0	97.7	96.9
Virginia	96.3	92.7	90.6	94.2	96.1	99.2
Washington	97.8	96.8	96.4	98.1	98.0	99.0
West Virginia	94.9	90.9	93.9	95.4	95.6	98.5
Wisconsin	98.2	96.9	98.7	98.4	98.3	99.2
Wyoming	94.0	90.5	91.5	94.9	94.6	96.6

Source: Compiled by New Strategist based on the Centers for Disease Control and Prevention Behavioral Risk Factor Surveillance System Survey, Internet site http://www.cdc.gov/brfss/index.htm

1.125 Smoke Detector by Sex, 1999

"Do you have a smoke detector in your home?"

(percent of people aged 18 or older responding "yes," by state and sex, 1999)

	total	men	women
U.S. total	**96.0%**	**95.9%**	**95.8%**
Alabama	94.2	93.8	94.5
Alaska	97.6	97.2	98.0
Arizona	94.3	93.6	95.0
Arkansas	92.0	91.8	92.2
California	95.9	96.4	95.5
Colorado	93.3	92.8	93.8
Connecticut	97.5	97.3	97.6
Delaware	98.1	97.0	99.1
District of Columbia	99.0	98.3	99.7
Florida	93.4	92.8	93.9
Georgia	95.0	95.0	94.9
Hawaii	87.0	87.2	86.8
Idaho	94.3	94.4	94.2
Illinois	98.2	97.9	98.4
Indiana	97.4	97.1	97.6
Iowa	95.4	94.9	95.9
Kansas	95.2	95.7	94.7
Kentucky	95.4	95.8	95.0
Louisiana	88.6	88.2	89.0
Maine	97.4	97.1	97.8
Maryland	98.7	99.0	98.5
Massachusetts	97.4	97.2	97.7
Michigan	98.0	97.4	98.4
Minnesota	98.2	97.9	98.5
Mississippi	90.8	91.4	90.2
Missouri	96.2	96.3	96.2
Montana	94.8	93.8	95.8
Nebraska	92.7	92.0	93.3
Nevada	92.2	90.9	93.4
New Hampshire	98.5	98.6	98.4
New Jersey	97.4	97.1	97.6
New Mexico	89.9	90.8	88.9
New York	94.9	94.7	95.1
North Carolina	97.6	98.3	96.9
North Dakota	96.2	96.3	96.2
Ohio	96.8	98.2	95.6
Oklahoma	94.3	94.2	94.5
Oregon	98.7	98.8	98.5
Pennsylvania	96.4	96.3	96.6
Rhode Island	97.6	97.1	98.0
South Carolina	97.4	97.0	97.7
South Dakota	92.9	92.4	93.4
Tennessee	96.6	96.4	96.8
Texas	90.6	90.4	90.8
Utah	94.1	93.9	94.2
Vermont	96.5	95.6	97.3
Virginia	96.3	96.0	96.6
Washington	97.8	97.7	97.9
West Virginia	94.9	94.2	95.4
Wisconsin	98.2	98.1	98.4
Wyoming	94.0	94.0	94.0

Source: Compiled by New Strategist based on the Centers for Disease Control and Prevention Behavioral Risk Factor Surveillance System Survey. Internet site http://www.cdc.gov/brfss/index.htm

1.126 Smoke Detector Tested in Past Six Months, 2001

"When was the last time you or someone else deliberately
tested all of the smoke detectors in your home?"

(percent of people aged 18 or older responding "past month" or "past six months," by state, 2001)

	tested in past month or six months
U.S. total	**68.9%**
Alabama	68.7
Alaska	67.4
Arizona	69.4
Arkansas	70.3
California	62.5
Colorado	57.2
Connecticut	70.0
Delaware	70.0
District of Columbia	66.1
Florida	64.8
Georgia	66.1
Hawaii	48.1
Idaho	58.7
Illinois	70.7
Indiana	68.3
Iowa	64.2
Kansas	74.9
Kentucky	77.5
Louisiana	70.4
Maine	77.7
Maryland	68.2
Massachusetts	66.9
Michigan	71.5
Minnesota	58.7
Mississippi	66.9
Missouri	73.1
Montana	61.2
Nebraska	70.1
Nevada	59.8
New Hampshire	65.5
New Jersey	70.8
New Mexico	62.1
New York	71.7
North Carolina	74.6
North Dakota	65.1
Ohio	81.8
Oklahoma	79.8
Oregon	63.5
Pennsylvania	72.8
Rhode Island	72.6
South Carolina	77.0
South Dakota	59.1
Tennessee	81.1
Texas	63.5
Utah	61.7
Vermont	68.1
Virginia	67.6
Washington	62.3
West Virginia	76.6
Wisconsin	70.7
Wyoming	64.9

Source: Compiled by New Strategist based on the Centers for Disease Control and Prevention Behavioral Risk Factor Surveillance System Survey, Internet site http://www.cdc.gov/brfss/index.htm

1.127 Smoking by Age, 2001

"Do you smoke cigarettes now?"

(percent of people aged 18 or older responding "yes," by state and age, 2001)

	total	18 to 24	25 to 34	35 to 44	45 to 54	55 to 64	65 or older
U.S. total	**22.8%**	**30.7%**	**26.5%**	**27.6%**	**24.6%**	**20.1%**	**10.0%**
Alabama	23.8	25.1	30.2	31.7	25.7	19.6	9.0
Alaska	26.2	36.3	28.8	28.8	24.9	14.4	14.2
Arizona	21.5	28.2	23.4	26.6	21.2	22.6	8.7
Arkansas	25.5	34.6	28.8	30.9	27.9	24.1	11.1
California	17.2	34.6	28.8	30.9	27.9	24.1	11.1
Colorado	22.3	22.2	17.7	19.7	17.6	17.2	8.4
Connecticut	20.6	37.3	21.7	37.6	18.4	20.5	10.2
Delaware	25.0	28.8	21.5	23.1	23.6	16.8	12.4
District of Columbia	20.8	32.8	29.8	32.4	23.7	21.4	10.1
Florida	22.4	24.7	26.3	30.7	26.7	22.2	9.8
Georgia	23.7	30.3	20.7	28.8	28.0	19.7	12.0
Hawaii	20.5	30.7	23.7	21.8	20.6	19.4	9.7
Idaho	19.6	24.4	22.2	21.4	21.5	20.3	8.9
Illinois	23.7	31.6	29.6	23.9	27.8	20.1	9.2
Indiana	27.4	35.8	33.7	35.3	26.4	22.1	11.1
Iowa	22.1	30.8	26.1	27.3	26.6	16.1	8.6
Kansas	22.2	25.9	26.4	24.3	26.9	20.5	10.0
Kentucky	30.9	38.5	34.1	38.6	30.6	28.6	15.0
Louisiana	24.6	28.5	27.5	30.5	27.0	20.9	11.8
Maine	23.9	32.5	28.6	29.5	27.4	15.4	9.9
Maryland	21.1	22.1	24.1	24.7	23.8	20.7	9.3
Massachusetts	19.5	28.0	24.2	22.3	19.7	15.9	8.6
Michigan	25.6	33.7	30.7	33.6	26.2	19.4	8.6
Minnesota	22.2	38.4	23.7	26.5	20.4	17.5	8.6
Mississippi	25.3	33.4	27.9	27.7	30.4	20.9	11.7
Missouri	25.9	35.7	30.6	31.4	29.3	19.3	10.4
Montana	21.9	31.5	21.6	24.2	22.0	25.3	11.2
Nebraska	20.2	28.5	23.2	24.6	19.7	19.0	9.3
Nevada	26.9	29.5	28.0	32.2	28.6	27.2	14.7
New Hampshire	24.1	34.7	31.1	28.4	19.9	18.1	11.2
New Jersey	21.1	25.2	26.2	24.3	22.3	19.5	10.8
New Mexico	23.8	29.4	26.8	27.5	24.9	22.5	10.9
New York	23.2	33.0	28.7	26.3	25.5	17.2	10.8
North Carolina	25.7	30.8	27.9	31.2	29.6	21.0	13.0
North Dakota	22.1	32.9	22.2	29.9	20.5	20.1	8.4
Ohio	27.6	37.0	34.5	32.3	30.1	22.7	10.1
Oklahoma	28.7	34.8	30.1	33.5	34.6	26.5	14.3
Oregon	20.5	29.0	22.9	27.8	19.0	15.5	9.6
Pennsylvania	24.5	35.0	27.4	30.3	28.6	21.0	9.2
Rhode Island	23.9	28.7	31.7	29.4	22.9	19.3	12.2
South Carolina	26.0	33.2	27.6	32.3	30.8	21.3	9.6
South Dakota	22.3	33.1	26.1	26.0	22.8	19.1	9.9
Tennessee	24.4	30.0	26.0	31.5	25.6	24.0	9.5
Texas	22.4	26.5	23.9	27.2	22.9	20.5	11.3
Utah	13.2	12.3	15.7	18.1	14.8	12.2	2.6
Vermont	22.4	34.7	27.4	24.6	21.0	17.5	9.5
Virginia	22.5	27.4	24.9	26.7	24.4	18.4	10.8
Washington	22.5	30.5	26.7	26.0	24.0	15.7	11.0
West Virginia	28.2	41.1	35.0	35.4	28.1	23.7	11.2
Wisconsin	23.6	33.7	31.6	27.9	25.8	16.9	6.2
Wyoming	22.2	27.9	25.5	24.0	22.9	20.2	12.4

Source: Compiled by New Strategist based on the Centers for Disease Control and Prevention Behavioral Risk Factor Surveillance System Survey, Internet site http://www.cdc.gov/brfss/index.htm

1.128 Smoking by Education, 2001

"Do you smoke cigarettes now?"

(percent of people aged 18 or older responding "yes," by state and educational attainment, 2001)

	total	less than high school	high school graduate	some college	college graduate
U.S. total	**22.8%**	**32.0%**	**28.6%**	**24.5%**	**12.4%**
Alabama	23.8	31.4	28.0	22.4	13.0
Alaska	26.2	38.8	36.8	27.9	9.6
Arizona	21.5	24.2	27.2	23.8	12.5
Arkansas	25.5	31.2	29.7	28.2	12.7
California	17.2	22.5	21.6	18.7	9.6
Colorado	22.3	31.0	26.7	26.6	12.9
Connecticut	20.6	27.8	28.5	22.4	12.3
Delaware	25.0	39.9	31.2	26.4	14.4
District of Columbia	20.8	29.6	24.6	22.5	15.6
Florida	22.4	29.1	27.3	21.9	14.5
Georgia	23.7	36.4	28.2	24.1	13.1
Hawaii	20.5	26.1	27.2	20.6	11.8
Idaho	19.6	28.6	26.8	17.1	10.8
Illinois	23.7	28.2	29.5	25.7	14.7
Indiana	27.4	42.1	32.5	27.2	14.0
Iowa	22.1	30.5	25.8	23.6	12.0
Kansas	22.2	30.1	27.9	25.6	11.6
Kentucky	30.9	37.9	35.4	31.0	14.7
Louisiana	24.6	32.0	28.2	24.6	14.1
Maine	23.9	28.2	29.4	26.2	13.2
Maryland	21.1	32.1	29.9	24.2	10.3
Massachusetts	19.5	27.5	27.3	22.2	11.1
Michigan	25.6	40.4	30.6	25.1	13.5
Minnesota	22.2	29.5	30.0	23.8	11.8
Mississippi	25.3	31.2	30.4	23.8	14.8
Missouri	25.9	34.8	29.9	25.9	16.3
Montana	21.9	37.0	23.5	24.7	11.0
Nebraska	20.2	30.6	21.5	22.8	11.4
Nevada	26.9	37.9	30.7	28.9	17.3
New Hampshire	24.1	41.1	33.2	25.4	11.0
New Jersey	21.1	25.5	27.4	24.1	12.9
New Mexico	23.8	32.9	26.7	24.8	13.8
New York	23.2	29.7	27.9	25.3	14.8
North Carolina	25.7	37.4	31.1	24.5	13.6
North Dakota	22.1	28.2	27.0	25.7	10.8
Ohio	27.6	38.0	32.7	29.0	13.5
Oklahoma	28.7	44.4	31.7	27.8	15.7
Oregon	20.5	28.9	25.6	20.7	11.4
Pennsylvania	24.5	33.6	28.9	25.1	13.5
Rhode Island	23.9	33.1	29.8	24.8	13.5
South Carolina	26.0	33.7	33.7	24.9	13.4
South Dakota	22.3	29.6	28.5	22.2	12.4
Tennessee	24.4	33.2	29.7	22.7	11.2
Texas	22.4	27.5	27.0	24.5	12.2
Utah	13.2	32.5	18.1	11.1	6.5
Vermont	22.4	37.8	29.8	23.4	10.5
Virginia	22.5	39.3	29.1	22.7	11.8
Washington	22.5	39.0	30.9	22.9	11.2
West Virginia	28.2	33.6	30.7	28.0	15.9
Wisconsin	23.6	33.2	28.3	26.9	10.7
Wyoming	22.2	38.1	28.7	22.3	9.3

Source: Compiled by New Strategist based on the Centers for Disease Control and Prevention Behavioral Risk Factor Surveillance System Survey. Internet site http://www.cdc.gov/brfss/index.htm

1.129 Smoking by Household Income, 2001

"Do you smoke cigarettes now?"

(percent of people aged 18 or older responding "yes," by state and household income, 2001)

	total	less than $15,000	$15,000 to $24,999	$25,000 to $34,999	$35,000 to $49,999	$50,000 or more
U.S. total	**22.8%**	**29.9%**	**29.6%**	**28.1%**	**24.6%**	**17.7%**
Alabama	23.8	30.1	30.5	29.0	24.6	16.8
Alaska	26.2	38.0	36.3	30.2	24.8	19.5
Arizona	21.5	23.3	28.3	29.6	21.6	15.2
Arkansas	25.5	32.9	30.9	29.6	23.2	18.4
California	17.2	22.2	20.8	21.2	19.0	14.0
Colorado	22.3	31.3	31.5	25.5	25.4	17.2
Connecticut	20.6	30.1	25.1	28.5	27.0	16.1
Delaware	25.0	38.5	34.6	37.0	29.0	18.6
District of Columbia	20.8	25.8	24.5	26.4	27.0	15.5
Florida	22.4	26.8	28.7	21.9	24.6	19.9
Georgia	23.7	27.4	28.1	25.6	24.7	20.0
Hawaii	20.5	29.6	23.9	23.1	19.7	14.7
Idaho	19.6	31.0	26.9	19.4	16.1	13.4
Illinois	23.7	33.5	25.1	26.1	26.4	21.0
Indiana	27.4	32.5	36.5	31.9	28.1	22.2
Iowa	22.1	24.5	29.4	23.3	18.3	20.2
Kansas	22.2	25.8	29.2	26.2	23.5	17.8
Kentucky	30.9	37.6	40.6	35.5	32.1	22.5
Louisiana	24.6	31.5	29.9	25.2	26.6	18.2
Maine	23.9	29.1	30.5	28.4	24.5	16.6
Maryland	21.1	27.5	28.4	23.3	24.0	16.8
Massachusetts	19.5	26.2	24.7	28.4	23.1	15.4
Michigan	25.6	31.1	38.0	31.4	28.9	18.7
Minnesota	22.2	32.8	28.1	28.1	24.5	17.9
Mississippi	25.3	27.0	31.2	26.5	24.9	17.3
Missouri	25.9	29.5	35.5	29.2	27.1	19.5
Montana	21.9	33.1	27.2	24.5	16.0	15.5
Nebraska	20.2	26.4	26.5	17.9	21.0	18.0
Nevada	26.9	33.9	29.4	30.4	28.6	24.7
New Hampshire	24.1	34.7	36.2	30.3	25.4	17.7
New Jersey	21.1	24.9	25.3	25.1	26.5	19.0
New Mexico	23.8	28.5	30.9	28.9	21.1	15.8
New York	23.2	25.4	25.0	27.8	25.9	20.5
North Carolina	25.7	30.1	33.9	29.3	28.8	19.5
North Dakota	22.1	30.0	29.0	23.6	21.1	15.4
Ohio	27.6	36.3	32.7	31.7	28.3	23.9
Oklahoma	28.7	33.6	37.3	30.9	23.0	24.8
Oregon	20.5	27.4	26.6	24.5	20.9	12.8
Pennsylvania	24.5	32.7	29.8	28.1	27.5	18.1
Rhode Island	23.9	24.9	29.9	32.5	28.6	17.7
South Carolina	26.0	31.1	33.8	29.9	29.5	17.7
South Dakota	22.3	27.2	31.3	25.6	22.0	14.1
Tennessee	24.4	37.1	33.4	29.9	23.1	17.5
Texas	22.4	26.3	26.0	27.5	27.2	16.5
Utah	13.2	23.2	17.3	17.3	14.8	8.4
Vermont	22.4	29.9	30.2	30.3	22.6	12.5
Virginia	22.5	28.2	28.4	28.7	26.0	16.0
Washington	22.5	30.3	31.5	27.1	26.1	15.9
West Virginia	28.2	35.4	33.5	31.0	23.6	19.3
Wisconsin	23.6	23.8	26.3	28.8	24.7	20.4
Wyoming	22.2	38.5	30.4	21.8	22.0	15.6

Source: Compiled by New Strategist based on the Centers for Disease Control and Prevention Behavioral Risk Factor Surveillance System Survey, Internet site http://www.cdc.gov/brfss/index.htm

1.130 Smoking by Sex, 2001

"Do you smoke cigarettes now?"

(percent of people aged 18 or older responding "yes," by state and sex, 2001)

	total	men	women
U.S. total	**22.9%**	**25.5%**	**21.3%**
Alabama	23.8	25.8	22.1
Alaska	26.2	26.4	25.9
Arizona	21.5	23.1	20.1
Arkansas	25.5	27.2	24.0
California	17.2	20.6	14.0
Colorado	22.3	23.7	20.9
Connecticut	20.6	21.2	20.1
Delaware	25.0	28.2	22.1
District of Columbia	20.8	24.9	17.3
Florida	22.4	25.6	19.4
Georgia	23.7	25.7	21.8
Hawaii	20.5	24.7	16.3
Idaho	19.6	21.0	18.2
Illinois	23.7	26.7	20.9
Indiana	27.4	29.7	25.3
Iowa	22.1	24.2	20.3
Kansas	22.2	22.5	22.0
Kentucky	30.9	31.9	30.0
Louisiana	24.6	28.7	21.0
Maine	23.9	27.0	21.1
Maryland	21.1	24.6	17.9
Massachusetts	19.5	20.4	18.7
Michigan	25.6	26.7	24.5
Minnesota	22.2	24.8	19.6
Mississippi	25.3	29.3	21.7
Missouri	25.9	27.6	24.4
Montana	21.9	21.7	22.1
Nebraska	20.2	20.6	19.8
Nevada	26.9	27.8	26.0
New Hampshire	24.1	25.6	22.7
New Jersey	21.1	21.6	20.7
New Mexico	23.8	27.9	20.0
New York	23.2	26.1	20.7
North Carolina	25.7	28.6	23.1
North Dakota	22.1	24.6	19.7
Ohio	27.6	29.1	26.3
Oklahoma	28.7	31.1	26.4
Oregon	20.5	21.4	19.7
Pennsylvania	24.5	26.3	22.8
Rhode Island	23.9	25.8	22.1
South Carolina	26.0	27.9	24.3
South Dakota	22.3	23.2	21.4
Tennessee	24.4	26.1	22.8
Texas	22.4	25.1	19.8
Utah	13.2	14.6	12.0
Vermont	22.4	24.4	20.5
Virginia	22.5	23.5	21.6
Washington	22.5	24.5	20.5
West Virginia	28.2	28.9	27.6
Wisconsin	23.6	25.3	21.9
Wyoming	22.2	22.5	21.8

Source: Compiled by New Strategist based on the Centers for Disease Control and Prevention Behavioral Risk Factor Surveillance System Survey. Internet site http://www.cdc.gov/brfss/index.htm

1.131 Smoking: Tried to Quit, 2000

"During the past 12 months, have you quit smoking for one day or longer?"

(among people aged 18 or older who smoke every day, percent responding "yes." by state, 2000)

	tried to quit smoking
U.S. total	**49.4%**
Alabama	49.7
Alaska	51.4
Arizona	49.3
Arkansas	44.4
California	56.1
Colorado	52.8
Connecticut	52.0
Delaware	49.4
District of Columbia	59.8
Florida	49.6
Georgia	53.0
Hawaii	64.4
Idaho	48.1
Illinois	53.2
Indiana	49.4
Iowa	48.7
Kansas	46.0
Kentucky	48.2
Louisiana	52.7
Maine	52.3
Maryland	50.5
Massachusetts	55.8
Michigan	58.6
Minnesota	46.1
Mississippi	46.6
Missouri	46.8
Montana	52.4
Nebraska	44.9
Nevada	43.4
New Hampshire	53.2
New Jersey	51.1
New Mexico	51.8
New York	50.4
North Carolina	51.9
North Dakota	46.5
Ohio	45.6
Oklahoma	49.2
Oregon	51.8
Pennsylvania	44.5
Rhode Island	49.1
South Carolina	44.0
South Dakota	48.2
Tennessee	45.3
Texas	52.7
Utah	53.6
Vermont	49.1
Virginia	48.9
Washington	49.4
West Virginia	44.1
Wisconsin	48.3
Wyoming	48.4

Source: Compiled by New Strategist based on the Centers for Disease Control and Prevention Behavioral Risk Factor Surveillance System Survey. Internet site http://www.cdc.gov/brfss/index.htm

1.132 Stroke by Sex, 2000

"Has a doctor ever told you that you had a stroke?"

(percent of people aged 18 or older responding "yes," by state and sex, 2000)

	total	men	women
Delaware	2.3%	2.3%	2.2%
District of Columbia	2.7	2.2	3.1
Georgia	2.2	2.5	1.9
Indiana	2.5	2.4	2.6
Iowa	1.9	1.6	2.2
Kentucky	2.8	2.6	3.0
Mississippi	2.6	1.8	3.4
Montana	2.3	2.1	2.5
Ohio	2.5	2.2	2.7
Oklahoma	1.7	1.4	2.0
Pennsylvania	2.4	2.5	2.4
South Carolina	1.7	1.7	1.7
Virginia	2.1	1.8	2.3
West Virginia	3.1	2.9	3.2

Source: Compiled by New Strategist based on the Centers for Disease Control and Prevention Behavioral Risk Factor Surveillance System Survey, Internet site http://www.cdc.gov/brfss/index.htm

1.133 Weight: Overweight by Age, 2001

At risk for health problems related to being overweight
(defined as having a body mass index of 25.0 or higher).

(percent of people aged 18 or older with a body mass index of 25.0 or higher, by state and age, 2001)

	total	18 to 24	25 to 34	35 to 44	45 to 54	55 to 64	65 or older
U.S. total	**59.1%**	**37.6%**	**54.9%**	**60.6%**	**66.6%**	**68.6%**	**59.8%**
Alabama	61.6	38.3	57.0	64.2	73.8	71.3	62.1
Alaska	63.3	49.9	64.3	60.0	69.4	69.5	68.6
Arizona	56.0	36.8	54.2	60.1	63.4	62.2	55.7
Arkansas	59.5	42.0	58.1	62.5	68.1	65.7	58.2
California	59.4	38.4	55.7	63.9	65.7	68.7	59.5
Colorado	51.7	28.9	47.6	55.8	57.4	58.5	54.4
Connecticut	55.1	37.9	50.8	56.2	64.2	62.5	55.0
Delaware	59.1	38.1	56.1	62.5	65.3	72.8	58.5
District of Columbia	52.1	29.3	44.4	54.4	58.2	68.8	56.4
Florida	55.8	35.3	50.6	54.7	63.2	67.4	57.1
Georgia	59.4	40.5	58.4	61.4	66.4	71.4	56.7
Hawaii	51.4	40.6	54.7	55.1	54.8	57.6	42.0
Idaho	59.3	32.4	58.0	60.9	70.7	69.9	59.8
Illinois	58.6	36.4	54.6	59.4	65.0	70.5	63.3
Indiana	60.0	37.9	53.6	63.7	68.4	67.6	65.4
Iowa	59.8	35.2	55.9	60.4	69.1	72.9	63.5
Kansas	57.0	38.1	53.7	59.3	66.2	62.0	59.7
Kentucky	62.1	43.6	60.7	64.8	69.9	68.4	61.5
Louisiana	60.3	35.9	57.5	61.9	68.8	72.3	65.7
Maine	58.7	48.0	52.9	56.9	69.6	67.9	56.4
Maryland	57.0	37.2	52.9	58.6	63.4	64.8	59.8
Massachusetts	54.4	34.9	49.1	57.8	60.7	65.9	56.3
Michigan	60.2	33.4	54.2	61.5	69.4	71.0	67.6
Minnesota	60.5	42.6	55.6	60.9	66.8	73.4	62.2
Mississippi	63.8	48.0	62.4	69.4	70.1	69.4	63.0
Missouri	59.4	34.5	53.8	61.7	68.8	69.1	64.4
Montana	56.8	32.4	52.3	60.2	64.4	67.6	58.1
Nebraska	59.1	38.2	53.7	60.8	68.8	72.4	59.8
Nevada	56.5	41.3	49.3	52.5	68.6	69.5	55.3
New Hampshire	56.0	36.7	48.6	56.6	65.3	68.1	59.7
New Jersey	57.7	36.3	52.6	56.1	66.0	70.1	61.4
New Mexico	57.1	31.4	59.3	61.5	64.3	66.3	54.7
New York	56.0	33.8	47.3	60.4	63.6	64.6	61.5
North Carolina	58.8	41.4	54.7	62.4	67.3	68.2	56.2
North Dakota	61.5	47.7	55.5	63.3	67.6	69.7	65.5
Ohio	60.1	38.3	56.4	64.7	64.2	68.6	65.3
Oklahoma	61.6	40.6	59.6	64.1	67.6	73.0	62.8
Oregon	58.2	35.0	55.1	62.0	64.3	68.3	57.9
Pennsylvania	60.4	35.8	55.8	60.1	70.1	70.0	64.7
Rhode Island	56.0	37.7	48.5	58.5	61.8	66.7	62.0
South Carolina	59.8	37.5	61.8	61.2	67.6	66.9	61.7
South Dakota	59.4	40.1	53.2	62.0	67.5	71.9	61.9
Tennessee	58.9	36.3	57.0	64.1	67.8	65.7	56.9
Texas	61.3	39.6	60.0	65.6	68.0	71.8	59.9
Utah	54.8	35.8	47.5	55.3	67.8	72.0	56.3
Vermont	52.1	25.5	51.0	52.8	57.7	65.1	59.3
Virginia	57.6	38.5	55.1	58.3	65.8	66.3	59.5
Washington	56.0	37.1	48.8	58.4	63.1	65.0	60.6
West Virginia	63.0	44.7	57.5	67.0	70.5	68.7	65.5
Wisconsin	59.1	40.9	51.7	59.6	66.3	71.1	62.9
Wyoming	55.6	28.5	55.6	59.9	62.5	63.3	56.6

Note: Body mass index is calculated by dividing weight in kilograms by height in meters squared.
Source: Compiled by New Strategist based on the Centers for Disease Control and Prevention Behavioral Risk Factor
Surveillance System Survey, Internet site http://www.cdc.gov/brfss/index.htm

1.134 Weight: Overweight by Education, 2001

At risk for health problems related to being overweight
(defined as having a body mass index of 25.0 or higher).

(percent of people aged 18 or older with a body mass index of 25.0 or higher, by state and educational attainment, 2001)

	total	less than high school	high school graduate	some college	college graduate
U.S. total	**59.1%**	**62.5%**	**61.1%**	**58.1%**	**54.7%**
Alabama	61.6	63.8	63.8	59.7	59.3
Alaska	63.3	66.6	65.3	63.3	60.2
Arizona	56.0	58.6	54.9	58.3	53.6
Arkansas	59.5	61.0	59.8	58.2	59.5
California	59.4	73.9	62.8	57.2	51.4
Colorado	51.7	58.4	54.2	51.1	48.4
Connecticut	55.1	62.5	58.0	55.4	51.4
Delaware	59.1	61.4	61.1	57.9	57.8
District of Columbia	52.1	66.2	59.6	57.7	41.9
Florida	55.8	59.0	57.3	55.3	53.5
Georgia	59.4	63.3	66.5	60.0	50.3
Hawaii	51.4	47.0	56.1	50.7	47.8
Idaho	59.3	65.9	56.9	59.1	60.1
Illinois	58.6	65.5	61.4	57.4	55.1
Indiana	60.0	60.8	62.5	58.4	57.5
Iowa	59.8	59.9	62.5	60.6	54.7
Kansas	57.0	61.9	59.1	56.6	54.2
Kentucky	62.1	60.9	64.4	61.7	59.2
Louisiana	60.3	65.9	62.3	56.5	56.7
Maine	58.7	59.0	61.0	61.3	53.2
Maryland	57.0	62.5	62.8	57.8	51.0
Massachusetts	54.4	64.5	58.0	55.0	49.7
Michigan	60.2	62.3	60.6	60.5	58.7
Minnesota	60.5	58.6	65.4	59.7	57.4
Mississippi	63.8	67.5	64.1	64.1	60.0
Missouri	59.4	62.5	61.8	58.0	56.8
Montana	56.8	67.5	64.1	64.1	60.0
Nebraska	59.1	62.5	61.8	58.0	56.8
Nevada	56.5	62.8	53.1	55.5	59.2
New Hampshire	56.0	57.4	58.1	57.0	53.0
New Jersey	57.7	68.2	61.2	57.8	52.0
New Mexico	57.1	69.2	55.5	59.8	49.1
New York	56.0	66.5	59.8	54.8	49.6
North Carolina	58.8	57.5	62.1	61.2	53.5
North Dakota	61.5	66.6	63.8	59.8	59.2
Ohio	60.1	54.4	63.7	57.7	59.2
Oklahoma	61.6	61.5	63.4	61.2	59.6
Oregon	58.2	68.6	59.1	56.7	54.7
Pennsylvania	60.4	65.0	63.2	59.9	54.5
Rhode Island	56.0	57.7	58.7	58.3	50.8
South Carolina	59.8	65.6	63.7	59.6	51.8
South Dakota	59.4	60.2	60.0	58.8	59.2
Tennessee	58.9	63.9	61.0	55.2	57.0
Texas	61.3	70.2	61.2	59.5	57.4
Utah	54.8	55.0	54.1	53.8	56.6
Vermont	52.1	62.0	57.3	48.9	46.7
Virginia	57.6	67.3	61.9	54.5	53.3
Washington	56.0	52.9	59.0	59.0	51.2
West Virginia	63.0	63.6	65.7	61.2	58.1
Wisconsin	59.1	63.0	65.1	58.4	50.5
Wyoming	55.6	55.8	59.6	54.2	52.4

Note: Body mass index is calculated by dividing weight in kilograms by height in meters squared.
Source: Compiled by New Strategist based on the Centers for Disease Control and Prevention Behavioral Risk Factor Surveillance System Survey. Internet site http://www.cdc.gov/brfss/index.htm

1.135 Weight: Overweight by Household Income, 2001

At risk for health problems related to being overweight
(defined as having a body mass index of 25.0 or higher).

(percent of people aged 18 or older with a body mass index of 25.0 or higher, by state and household income, 2001)

	total	less than $15,000	$15,000 to $24,999	$25,000 to $34,999	$35,000 to $49,999	$50,000 or more
U.S. total	**59.1%**	**56.9%**	**59.7%**	**60.0%**	**60.9%**	**58.4%**
Alabama	61.6	59.7	64.7	59.0	61.0	63.5
Alaska	63.3	64.8	62.7	62.4	61.1	66.1
Arizona	56.0	65.2	57.1	57.1	60.1	57.3
Arkansas	59.5	58.2	59.1	60.6	62.4	60.5
California	59.4	60.1	62.5	63.8	63.0	56.8
Colorado	51.7	40.3	53.4	52.1	56.7	50.8
Connecticut	55.1	58.0	52.8	58.2	56.7	56.0
Delaware	59.1	60.0	55.5	62.7	62.7	60.7
District of Columbia	52.1	56.7	60.2	57.8	52.7	48.7
Florida	55.8	56.7	59.5	54.7	56.0	55.5
Georgia	59.4	63.3	61.0	55.5	65.3	56.5
Hawaii	51.4	51.7	54.3	53.5	52.2	52.0
Idaho	59.3	56.5	54.4	62.0	62.2	62.8
Illinois	58.6	62.6	61.1	59.9	58.7	57.2
Indiana	60.0	61.3	65.1	56.8	63.4	58.7
Iowa	59.8	49.4	59.9	59.7	62.6	62.0
Kansas	57.0	51.9	59.2	59.1	58.3	57.8
Kentucky	62.1	58.5	63.6	67.5	64.7	64.0
Louisiana	60.3	63.5	59.8	62.7	60.7	61.5
Maine	58.7	61.2	65.0	59.9	60.8	58.1
Maryland	57.0	53.2	52.8	61.2	58.9	56.8
Massachusetts	54.4	57.0	55.6	56.1	53.1	55.8
Michigan	60.2	58.5	57.2	64.0	61.8	61.4
Minnesota	60.5	53.1	58.6	64.7	63.6	61.4
Mississippi	63.8	65.0	62.3	63.8	66.1	66.1
Missouri	59.4	56.8	61.3	60.9	62.9	59.1
Montana	56.8	52.1	55.5	60.7	58.8	59.2
Nebraska	59.1	47.6	61.3	62.8	65.0	56.1
Nevada	56.5	50.2	53.3	53.1	59.3	60.9
New Hampshire	56.0	50.8	55.6	58.3	58.1	57.4
New Jersey	57.7	60.6	59.8	64.6	59.6	56.9
New Mexico	57.1	55.1	58.6	60.8	58.9	57.8
New York	56.0	58.3	58.2	62.2	55.8	54.4
North Carolina	58.8	57.4	62.1	59.9	59.0	61.1
North Dakota	61.5	55.2	63.2	62.7	62.4	62.0
Ohio	60.1	55.9	62.0	58.6	65.8	61.1
Oklahoma	61.6	62.9	61.3	63.0	63.7	63.7
Oregon	58.2	58.1	57.2	60.1	57.0	60.4
Pennsylvania	60.4	55.7	62.0	60.2	63.7	62.3
Rhode Island	56.0	53.5	58.8	55.7	57.4	56.2
South Carolina	59.8	57.4	62.8	64.2	57.6	58.7
South Dakota	59.4	54.8	59.7	58.8	63.0	61.8
Tennessee	58.9	56.1	60.3	63.9	59.6	60.4
Texas	61.3	65.4	63.7	60.5	62.1	59.8
Utah	54.8	48.3	53.5	55.4	58.5	55.8
Vermont	52.1	49.1	51.6	55.3	56.6	52.0
Virginia	57.6	54.4	61.5	55.2	62.1	57.2
Washington	56.0	49.6	55.5	55.7	58.6	58.5
West Virginia	63.0	63.5	63.6	65.4	67.3	60.5
Wisconsin	59.1	52.6	58.6	62.7	61.6	58.2
Wyoming	55.6	45.0	56.0	55.5	57.5	58.3

Note: Body mass index is calculated by dividing weight in kilograms by height in meters squared.
Source: Compiled by New Strategist based on the Centers for Disease Control and Prevention Behavioral Risk Factor Surveillance System Survey, Internet site http://www.cdc.gov/brfss/index.htm

1.136 Weight: Overweight by Sex, 2001

At risk for health problems related to being overweight
(defined as having a body mass index of 25.0 or higher).

(percent of people aged 18 or older with a body mass index of 25.0 or higher, by state and sex, 2001)

	total	men	women
U.S. total	**59.1%**	**67.0%**	**50.3%**
Alabama	61.6	69.1	54.7
Alaska	63.3	68.9	56.7
Arizona	56.0	63.9	47.9
Arkansas	59.5	67.1	52.3
California	59.4	67.6	51.0
Colorado	51.7	61.5	41.7
Connecticut	55.1	66.0	44.4
Delaware	59.1	68.5	50.0
District of Columbia	52.1	53.6	50.8
Florida	55.8	64.1	47.9
Georgia	59.4	65.3	53.6
Hawaii	51.4	61.6	40.7
Idaho	59.3	68.5	49.9
Illinois	58.6	64.6	53.0
Indiana	60.0	67.8	52.7
Iowa	59.8	68.1	51.6
Kansas	57.0	67.3	46.6
Kentucky	62.1	70.1	54.5
Louisiana	60.3	65.8	55.0
Maine	58.7	67.3	50.2
Maryland	57.0	64.5	49.8
Massachusetts	54.4	65.4	43.8
Michigan	60.2	67.4	53.2
Minnesota	60.5	69.4	51.6
Mississippi	63.8	70.3	57.7
Missouri	59.4	69.4	49.8
Montana	56.8	66.6	46.9
Nebraska	59.1	68.2	50.2
Nevada	56.5	68.5	43.9
New Hampshire	56.0	67.0	44.8
New Jersey	57.7	66.5	49.3
New Mexico	57.1	65.8	48.7
New York	56.0	63.2	49.2
North Carolina	58.8	67.5	50.4
North Dakota	61.5	73.4	49.2
Ohio	60.1	67.7	52.6
Oklahoma	61.6	70.3	53.1
Oregon	58.2	64.1	52.3
Pennsylvania	60.4	68.0	53.4
Rhode Island	56.0	66.4	46.1
South Carolina	59.8	66.2	53.6
South Dakota	59.4	69.4	49.4
Tennessee	58.9	66.1	52.0
Texas	61.3	69.2	53.4
Utah	54.8	61.5	47.9
Vermont	52.1	60.2	44.1
Virginia	57.6	66.1	49.3
Washington	56.0	64.4	47.5
West Virginia	63.0	70.4	55.9
Wisconsin	59.1	66.1	52.2
Wyoming	55.6	63.6	47.5

Note: Body mass index is calculated by dividing weight in kilograms by height in meters squared.
Source: Compiled by New Strategist based on the Centers for Disease Control and Prevention Behavioral Risk Factor Surveillance System Survey, Internet site http://www.cdc.gov/brfss/index.htm

1.137 Weight: Obesity, 2001

At risk for health problems related to being obese
(defined as having a body mass index of 30.0 or higher)

(percent of people aged 18 or older with a body mass index of 30.0 or higher, by state, 2001)

	obese (BMI of 30.0 or higher)
U.S. total	**21.0%**
Alabama	24.5
Alaska	22.1
Arizona	18.5
Arkansas	22.4
California	21.9
Colorado	14.9
Connecticut	17.9
Delaware	20.8
District of Columbia	20.0
Florida	18.8
Georgia	22.7
Hawaii	17.9
Idaho	20.5
Illinois	21.0
Indiana	24.5
Iowa	22.5
Kansas	21.6
Kentucky	24.6
Louisiana	24.0
Maine	19.5
Maryland	20.5
Massachusetts	16.6
Michigan	25.0
Minnesota	19.9
Mississippi	26.5
Missouri	23.2
Montana	18.8
Nebraska	20.7
Nevada	19.5
New Hampshire	19.4
New Jersey	19.6
New Mexico	19.7
New York	20.3
North Carolina	22.9
North Dakota	20.4
Ohio	22.4
Oklahoma	22.6
Oregon	21.1
Pennsylvania	22.1
Rhode Island	17.7
South Carolina	22.5
South Dakota	21.2
Tennessee	23.4
Texas	24.6
Utah	19.1
Vermont	17.6
Virginia	20.9
Washington	19.3
West Virginia	25.1
Wisconsin	22.4
Wyoming	19.7

Note: Body mass index is calculated by dividing weight in kilograms by height in meters squared.

1.138 Weight: Trying to Lose Weight by Age, 2000

"Are you now trying to lose weight?"

(percent of people aged 18 or older responding "yes," by state and age, 2000)

	total	18 to 24	25 to 34	35 to 44	45 to 54	55 to 64	65 or older
U.S. total	**38.0%**	**30.2%**	**38.0%**	**40.4%**	**44.7%**	**42.6%**	**30.6%**
Alabama	37.0	34.5	36.8	40.3	47.2	36.3	26.3
Alaska	36.8	30.8	30.3	39.7	43.7	41.6	32.5
Arizona	38.3	25.4	36.2	37.7	52.3	48.5	30.7
Arkansas	37.5	34.5	38.2	45.5	40.6	41.1	26.7
California	44.3	39.7	39.6	45.4	53.3	50.3	37.8
Colorado	36.4	30.5	36.5	38.7	40.0	42.6	28.7
Connecticut	39.9	24.4	38.6	42.6	44.2	48.5	37.3
Delaware	38.7	21.4	41.9	38.9	48.8	43.8	34.7
District of Columbia	37.0	26.7	33.8	42.7	49.2	39.2	26.4
Florida	36.9	25.4	38.7	40.7	40.6	42.2	31.2
Georgia	36.2	32.3	35.2	41.9	40.7	36.7	26.6
Hawaii	38.0	32.8	35.6	40.9	42.4	43.0	32.5
Idaho	37.6	28.3	37.0	41.4	43.1	43.6	30.6
Illinois	37.9	27.9	38.8	38.8	44.2	45.2	31.8
Indiana	39.0	37.1	37.0	43.7	43.8	40.6	30.3
Iowa	38.1	28.5	36.5	40.4	43.5	49.0	32.5
Kansas	36.5	31.9	34.8	34.8	48.2	42.3	28.8
Kentucky	35.7	35.2	36.4	40.5	42.7	35.0	23.0
Louisiana	35.4	27.5	35.2	39.3	43.9	39.2	26.8
Maine	41.4	35.7	41.9	40.5	47.9	44.4	37.3
Maryland	38.8	27.3	38.2	40.1	45.0	46.7	32.6
Massachusetts	40.4	30.8	38.0	41.3	50.3	46.6	34.8
Michigan	44.9	34.2	44.7	46.7	53.0	47.4	40.6
Minnesota	32.4	23.4	33.2	31.0	37.7	36.7	30.6
Mississippi	37.9	40.2	40.2	38.8	41.6	39.5	27.6
Missouri	34.0	31.0	38.0	34.7	37.0	36.9	26.4
Montana	35.5	25.5	33.5	36.9	44.9	38.8	30.3
Nebraska	35.7	27.7	38.6	36.7	46.2	39.6	27.2
Nevada	39.6	29.8	44.6	39.6	43.5	40.1	34.9
New Hampshire	39.2	27.5	36.4	41.5	46.2	51.1	32.3
New Jersey	41.7	34.8	40.5	42.3	48.9	50.4	33.9
New Mexico	37.1	32.6	36.9	38.2	41.6	46.0	27.8
New York	40.1	24.5	40.2	43.3	48.9	47.0	33.5
North Carolina	36.9	28.7	39.4	41.8	40.1	41.6	27.9
North Dakota	36.1	28.6	38.0	32.2	39.9	46.3	35.2
Ohio	38.3	32.3	40.8	40.4	45.4	41.1	28.0
Oklahoma	31.6	27.8	32.9	40.3	40.4	29.0	17.4
Oregon	38.3	32.9	36.3	40.0	45.8	43.8	30.4
Pennsylvania	39.1	33.2	38.0	42.6	45.7	45.6	30.8
Rhode Island	40.9	28.3	38.3	40.6	48.9	52.3	38.4
South Carolina	35.0	25.2	39.1	37.2	41.3	40.3	25.5
South Dakota	36.6	30.0	37.6	40.4	42.7	38.7	29.8
Tennessee	33.4	28.1	36.0	38.5	36.6	36.6	23.3
Texas	39.3	33.0	39.9	43.4	47.4	42.2	26.8
Utah	40.6	34.8	39.2	44.3	46.6	44.8	31.4
Vermont	38.2	24.7	36.9	41.5	44.6	47.5	32.9
Virginia	38.9	28.8	38.9	39.4	45.1	45.7	33.3
Washington	39.9	31.6	39.6	42.9	45.9	42.6	33.7
West Virginia	38.7	35.2	45.5	36.5	47.6	42.3	26.7
Wisconsin	39.9	36.5	36.2	36.9	47.3	48.7	36.6
Wyoming	37.3	24.3	36.8	39.5	47.7	42.7	27.8

Source: Compiled by New Strategist based on the Centers for Disease Control and Prevention Behavioral Risk Factor Surveillance System Survey, Internet site http://www.cdc.gov/brfss/index.htm

1.139 Weight: Trying to Lose Weight by Education, 2000

"Are you now trying to lose weight?"

(percent of people aged 18 or older responding "yes," by state and educational attainment, 2000)

	total	less than high school	high school graduate	some college	college graduate
U.S. total	**38.0%**	**31.9%**	**36.3%**	**40.2%**	**39.7%**
Alabama	37.0	28.0	38.4	37.3	41.7
Alaska	36.8	33.9	35.0	37.1	39.0
Arizona	38.3	41.7	34.0	40.2	39.9
Arkansas	37.5	35.0	35.4	39.1	40.6
California	44.3	36.8	45.4	46.3	46.2
Colorado	36.4	31.6	31.8	42.2	36.2
Connecticut	39.9	38.9	37.8	41.1	41.2
Delaware	38.7	26.8	31.9	43.9	44.2
District of Columbia	37.0	32.4	33.6	41.7	38.1
Florida	36.9	29.7	35.9	38.4	39.2
Georgia	36.2	30.7	33.8	40.5	38.2
Hawaii	38.0	29.7	37.4	39.9	38.9
Idaho	37.6	29.7	36.8	42.2	35.9
Illinois	37.9	31.3	36.1	42.0	37.7
Indiana	39.0	32.3	35.1	42.0	44.2
Iowa	38.1	34.2	36.5	40.9	38.1
Kansas	36.5	31.8	33.0	39.2	39.1
Kentucky	35.7	28.4	34.5	38.2	42.7
Louisiana	35.4	28.4	35.6	36.0	40.0
Maine	41.4	32.2	39.5	45.5	43.9
Maryland	38.8	29.1	40.1	39.1	39.8
Massachusetts	40.4	41.2	39.8	39.1	41.5
Michigan	44.9	40.2	46.5	43.9	45.7
Minnesota	32.4	26.6	32.8	31.1	34.8
Mississippi	37.9	30.6	35.5	41.7	42.6
Missouri	34.0	30.8	31.5	38.4	34.1
Montana	35.5	26.6	34.3	39.1	35.6
Nebraska	35.7	33.0	33.2	37.6	38.4
Nevada	39.6	42.1	37.5	41.0	39.4
New Hampshire	39.2	26.3	38.1	42.5	40.8
New Jersey	41.7	41.6	39.1	42.9	43.5
New Mexico	37.1	33.8	35.8	38.2	39.2
New York	40.1	37.8	38.4	42.0	41.1
North Carolina	36.9	25.7	37.7	40.3	39.7
North Dakota	36.1	33.1	37.2	36.6	35.2
Ohio	38.3	26.8	38.2	40.3	40.5
Oklahoma	31.6	24.1	30.7	31.9	37.5
Oregon	38.3	36.0	36.4	40.8	38.7
Pennsylvania	39.1	35.3	41.2	38.5	38.3
Rhode Island	40.9	43.2	39.3	40.5	41.7
South Carolina	35.0	27.8	34.8	36.8	37.8
South Dakota	36.6	27.2	34.7	40.2	38.2
Tennessee	33.4	27.8	32.0	37.0	35.8
Texas	39.3	39.2	37.2	39.1	41.3
Utah	40.6	28.2	39.8	42.9	40.9
Vermont	38.2	34.7	38.2	39.3	38.4
Virginia	38.9	36.9	35.9	39.2	41.9
Washington	39.9	32.8	37.1	43.0	40.6
West Virginia	38.7	31.2	36.2	43.6	45.3
Wisconsin	39.9	31.5	40.1	41.7	40.8
Wyoming	37.3	32.0	35.2	39.2	39.1

Source: Compiled by New Strategist based on the Centers for Disease Control and Prevention Behavioral Risk Factor Surveillance System Survey, Internet site http://www.cdc.gov/brfss/index.htm

1.140 Weight: Trying to Lose Weight by Household Income, 2000

"Are you now trying to lose weight?"

(percent of people aged 18 or older responding "yes," by state and household income, 2000)

	total	less than $15,000	$15,000 to $24,999	$25,000 to $34,999	$35,000 to $49,999	$50,000 or more
U.S. total	**38.0%**	**34.7%**	**36.0%**	**36.4%**	**38.8%**	**41.6%**
Alabama	37.0	33.2	32.4	37.7	37.8	42.6
Alaska	36.8	35.4	41.5	32.7	34.4	38.4
Arizona	38.3	32.8	35.0	42.0	36.8	47.2
Arkansas	37.5	37.3	32.2	38.3	38.8	41.5
California	44.3	40.8	35.7	46.6	48.5	48.4
Colorado	36.4	26.9	36.3	38.6	35.5	39.4
Connecticut	39.9	34.7	35.4	35.5	42.2	42.2
Delaware	38.7	30.6	33.5	41.8	37.0	42.1
District of Columbia	37.0	33.7	32.6	33.8	43.3	39.7
Florida	36.9	40.0	31.6	36.6	38.3	40.2
Georgia	36.2	31.0	34.1	28.9	40.7	40.6
Hawaii	38.0	34.7	37.0	39.2	39.0	40.1
Idaho	37.6	36.0	35.9	36.4	38.8	40.1
Illinois	37.9	28.3	27.0	34.1	50.4	39.6
Indiana	39.0	35.3	35.4	40.2	39.5	42.0
Iowa	38.1	33.0	37.0	37.3	39.8	40.3
Kansas	36.5	34.1	32.6	33.6	39.4	40.9
Kentucky	35.7	31.3	33.6	35.4	38.4	41.7
Louisiana	35.4	35.9	32.2	34.1	34.9	41.9
Maine	41.4	42.0	39.5	45.3	39.6	43.9
Maryland	38.8	29.6	41.0	33.7	37.5	42.8
Massachusetts	40.4	38.7	38.1	36.7	40.3	42.2
Michigan	44.9	37.0	41.2	43.0	45.3	47.9
Minnesota	32.4	28.9	32.2	32.8	27.2	35.2
Mississippi	37.9	31.3	35.0	40.3	42.7	41.9
Missouri	34.0	34.5	31.3	34.1	33.2	37.3
Montana	35.5	34.7	37.9	30.6	45.1	37.5
Nebraska	35.7	32.5	34.9	37.1	38.8	39.4
Nevada	39.6	36.4	39.1	34.0	39.2	42.6
New Hampshire	39.2	25.3	40.5	41.2	36.5	42.3
New Jersey	41.7	42.0	41.1	48.6	44.8	43.7
New Mexico	37.1	36.3	34.6	35.7	37.3	41.1
New York	40.1	35.3	38.7	38.4	39.7	43.7
North Carolina	36.9	26.7	37.0	32.6	40.8	41.0
North Dakota	36.1	35.4	36.6	32.7	36.3	39.5
Ohio	38.3	39.8	37.6	37.5	40.4	40.4
Oklahoma	31.6	28.1	31.1	28.8	34.9	40.9
Oregon	38.3	33.2	35.1	34.5	38.3	43.1
Pennsylvania	39.1	42.5	36.5	35.5	41.9	41.0
Rhode Island	40.9	40.6	38.4	42.6	40.4	41.0
South Carolina	35.0	30.4	37.0	33.3	38.2	36.0
South Dakota	36.6	33.2	33.8	36.1	38.4	42.5
Tennessee	33.4	30.4	35.9	33.0	33.3	40.2
Texas	39.3	43.5	36.1	39.6	36.4	43.2
Utah	40.6	40.9	33.1	40.9	42.5	42.8
Vermont	38.2	33.2	39.1	34.6	41.1	42.2
Virginia	38.9	42.5	36.9	35.6	37.7	41.0
Washington	39.9	36.4	40.5	39.7	36.4	43.6
West Virginia	38.7	38.8	35.0	36.5	42.5	45.0
Wisconsin	39.9	35.3	39.4	40.4	38.9	42.0
Wyoming	37.3	33.1	36.1	32.9	36.3	45.0

Source: Compiled by New Strategist based on the Centers for Disease Control and Prevention Behavioral Risk Factor Surveillance System Survey, Internet site http://www.cdc.gov/brfss/index.htm

1.141 Weight: Trying to Lose Weight by Sex, 2000

"Are you now trying to lose weight?"

(percent of people aged 18 or older responding "yes," by state and sex, 2000)

	total	men	women
U.S. total	38.0%	30.6%	44.9%
Alabama	37.0	30.6	42.8
Alaska	36.8	28.6	45.8
Arizona	38.3	33.1	43.2
Arkansas	37.5	29.2	44.9
California	44.3	38.0	50.6
Colorado	36.4	29.5	43.1
Connecticut	39.9	32.7	46.5
Delaware	38.7	30.6	46.2
District of Columbia	37.0	29.3	43.6
Florida	36.9	30.4	42.8
Georgia	36.2	28.0	43.9
Hawaii	38.0	32.6	43.5
Idaho	37.6	29.5	45.5
Illinois	37.9	30.1	45.3
Indiana	39.0	32.1	45.2
Iowa	38.1	29.7	45.7
Kansas	36.5	29.6	43.0
Kentucky	35.7	28.9	41.8
Louisiana	35.4	26.0	43.9
Maine	41.4	34.8	47.5
Maryland	38.8	33.1	44.0
Massachusetts	40.4	34.9	45.4
Michigan	44.9	38.4	50.8
Minnesota	32.4	24.8	39.5
Mississippi	37.9	31.8	43.2
Missouri	34.0	26.6	40.7
Montana	35.5	28.2	42.3
Nebraska	35.7	27.5	43.2
Nevada	39.6	32.3	46.9
New Hampshire	39.2	32.2	45.8
New Jersey	41.7	35.7	47.2
New Mexico	37.1	30.7	43.1
New York	40.1	33.6	46.0
North Carolina	36.9	27.7	45.3
North Dakota	36.1	27.3	44.6
Ohio	38.3	31.8	44.1
Oklahoma	31.6	25.2	37.5
Oregon	38.3	31.3	44.9
Pennsylvania	39.1	32.6	45.0
Rhode Island	40.9	33.2	47.7
South Carolina	35.0	27.8	41.6
South Dakota	36.6	26.7	46.0
Tennessee	33.4	27.4	38.8
Texas	39.3	32.9	45.3
Utah	40.6	30.6	50.1
Vermont	38.2	31.4	44.5
Virginia	38.9	30.8	46.4
Washington	39.9	33.3	46.3
West Virginia	38.7	32.3	44.4
Wisconsin	39.9	30.8	48.5
Wyoming	37.3	28.9	45.5

Source: Compiled by New Strategist based on the Centers for Disease Control and Prevention Behavioral Risk Factor Surveillance System Survey. Internet site http://www.cdc.gov/brfss/index.htm

1.142 Weight: Advised by Medical Professional to Lose Weight by Age, 2000

"In the past 12 months, has a doctor, nurse, or other health professional given you advice about your weight?"

(percent of people aged 18 or older responding "yes, to lose weight," by state and age, 2000)

	total	18 to 24	25 to 34	35 to 44	45 to 54	55 to 64	65 or older
U.S. total	**11.7%**	**4.0%**	**8.4%**	**11.3%**	**16.0%**	**17.7%**	**11.2%**
Alabama	13.6	10.6	10.1	12.7	16.7	17.9	14.9
Alaska	10.0	3.5	5.4	9.9	15.4	17.2	11.5
Arizona	12.4	2.5	10.5	12.3	19.2	14.0	14.6
Arkansas	11.1	6.5	8.3	11.4	15.7	14.9	9.7
California	12.0	5.9	7.3	11.2	18.3	20.1	11.3
Colorado	9.2	1.0	5.1	9.1	12.8	18.9	9.5
Connecticut	13.4	4.8	7.4	13.5	19.6	21.4	13.2
Delaware	11.9	4.8	7.4	13.5	19.6	21.4	13.2
District of Columbia	15.4	1.6	7.9	12.1	18.6	19.4	11.9
Florida	11.9	6.8	9.6	18.9	20.3	20.0	15.8
Georgia	13.9	3.5	7.3	12.8	15.6	17.5	12.4
Hawaii	12.4	6.2	7.7	15.5	21.1	19.7	13.7
Idaho	8.9	4.4	9.9	13.7	15.6	19.1	10.8
Illinois	12.0	4.3	6.8	9.5	12.9	10.4	8.8
Indiana	10.8	4.1	8.7	11.7	15.3	22.6	11.1
Iowa	8.9	3.6	7.7	11.2	15.6	16.1	10.6
Kansas	11.0	4.6	6.2	9.4	11.6	14.0	8.2
Kentucky	13.5	4.3	8.7	9.7	16.7	17.3	10.0
Louisiana	11.0	9.8	9.4	10.3	21.4	19.0	11.8
Maine	11.8	4.8	7.9	10.7	15.1	15.5	12.9
Maryland	14.3	3.3	9.8	9.7	18.4	17.3	11.8
Massachusetts	13.6	4.4	10.7	14.0	17.9	24.7	13.4
Michigan	12.6	6.1	9.1	12.8	18.0	22.6	13.9
Minnesota	7.6	4.0	8.5	11.2	20.4	17.1	13.6
Mississippi	14.2	2.3	4.1	8.8	10.0	12.6	7.8
Missouri	10.4	7.7	11.9	15.8	18.3	18.3	13.9
Montana	9.4	4.2	7.3	10.5	15.0	17.3	8.2
Nebraska	9.5	5.1	9.5	8.4	10.3	12.1	10.4
Nevada	12.2	4.0	7.0	9.8	15.1	15.0	7.9
New Hampshire	11.7	1.6	7.8	12.0	13.4	18.0	18.5
New Jersey	13.7	6.3	9.1	11.3	13.4	19.9	11.7
New Mexico	9.6	3.0	9.8	12.2	19.2	23.9	13.4
New York	13.8	4.0	7.1	9.7	12.5	14.4	9.9
North Carolina	12.6	4.3	8.6	12.8	16.3	19.2	14.7
North Dakota	8.4	3.2	8.9	7.0	9.5	15.0	8.6
Ohio	9.3	1.3	5.7	10.8	13.7	16.8	7.9
Oklahoma	8.1	3.9	8.5	8.5	11.6	10.0	5.7
Oregon	11.3	2.1	7.6	11.3	16.6	19.5	10.1
Pennsylvania	12.5	5.1	7.4	14.3	16.6	16.8	13.5
Rhode Island	14.2	4.3	8.9	14.5	19.3	24.3	15.0
South Carolina	12.4	4.8	11.0	12.4	18.0	18.7	9.5
South Dakota	9.2	3.3	6.9	9.5	13.9	10.6	9.7
Tennessee	11.5	3.9	9.9	13.6	17.5	14.2	8.5
Texas	12.4	3.5	8.4	13.5	20.3	19.8	10.0
Utah	10.5	3.0	5.6	11.7	18.0	16.9	9.6
Vermont	11.0	3.7	8.1	9.2	14.4	18.7	13.2
Virginia	10.2	2.7	6.5	12.6	13.0	16.0	9.7
Washington	9.2	1.5	9.0	10.0	11.8	10.4	10.3
West Virginia	13.1	2.1	9.8	8.7	23.2	20.6	12.9
Wisconsin	9.0	4.1	5.9	6.3	12.0	18.2	9.3
Wyoming	9.4	2.4	10.5	8.1	12.9	14.5	6.9

Source: Compiled by New Strategist based on the Centers for Disease Control and Prevention Behavioral Risk Factor Surveillance System Survey, Internet site http://www.cdc.gov/brfss/index.htm

1.143 Weight: Advised by Medical Professional to Lose Weight by Education, 2000

"In the past 12 months, has a doctor, nurse, or other health professional
given you advice about your weight?"

(percent of people aged 18 or older responding "yes, to lose weight," by state and educational attainment, 2000)

	total	less than high school	high school graduate	some college	college graduate
U.S. total	**11.7%**	**11.7%**	**11.6%**	**11.5%**	**10.9%**
Alabama	13.6	13.5	13.6	14.7	12.8
Alaska	10.0	11.1	9.0	11.2	9.5
Arizona	12.4	11.6	14.6	11.6	11.1
Arkansas	11.1	13.3	10.8	10.8	10.7
California	12.0	11.8	11.7	13.6	10.8
Colorado	9.2	13.0	8.5	9.5	8.6
Connecticut	13.4	16.9	14.0	12.7	12.6
Delaware	11.9	11.4	10.2	14.2	12.0
District of Columbia	15.4	21.2	18.2	14.9	12.6
Florida	11.9	13.9	11.6	11.7	11.5
Georgia	13.9	14.3	13.6	14.9	13.0
Hawaii	12.4	13.3	10.9	14.4	11.6
Idaho	8.9	8.6	7.8	9.7	9.7
Illinois	12.0	10.9	13.6	11.6	10.9
Indiana	10.8	11.3	10.2	10.5	11.9
Iowa	8.9	9.5	8.1	8.6	10.1
Kansas	11.0	11.1	11.0	11.1	10.6
Kentucky	13.5	13.5	13.0	14.0	13.7
Louisiana	11.0	11.8	11.4	10.4	10.2
Maine	11.8	11.3	12.2	12.4	10.9
Maryland	14.3	13.4	15.3	14.5	13.5
Massachusetts	13.6	17.2	14.0	13.3	12.6
Michigan	12.6	12.4	12.0	12.2	13.7
Minnesota	7.6	7.0	6.6	8.0	8.3
Mississippi	14.2	16.7	14.1	15.7	10.9
Missouri	10.4	9.7	9.2	13.8	8.3
Montana	9.4	8.7	8.4	10.8	9.2
Nebraska	9.5	10.1	8.8	9.4	10.7
Nevada	12.2	15.9	13.4	9.0	13.2
New Hampshire	11.7	9.0	12.6	12.9	10.6
New Jersey	13.7	18.0	14.0	13.3	11.9
New Mexico	9.6	11.2	8.4	10.4	9.0
New York	13.8	14.5	11.6	17.1	12.7
North Carolina	12.6	13.4	12.7	12.4	11.9
North Dakota	8.4	10.7	8.9	7.7	7.8
Ohio	9.3	7.8	9.1	10.0	9.6
Oklahoma	8.1	10.3	6.6	7.5	10.2
Oregon	11.3	8.6	10.6	14.0	10.5
Pennsylvania	12.5	13.3	12.5	11.1	13.1
Rhode Island	14.2	17.4	12.0	14.2	14.7
South Carolina	12.4	14.0	12.7	11.4	11.9
South Dakota	9.2	8.5	8.4	10.3	9.0
Tennessee	11.5	11.5	10.9	11.3	13.5
Texas	12.4	10.6	13.0	13.4	12.4
Utah	10.5	5.3	8.9	10.9	12.8
Vermont	11.0	13.4	11.9	9.8	10.2
Virginia	10.2	13.2	11.7	8.3	9.5
Washington	9.2	7.4	7.6	10.3	9.8
West Virginia	13.1	16.1	12.7	13.4	11.0
Wisconsin	9.0	9.3	9.6	9.9	6.7
Wyoming	9.4	5.7	8.5	11.4	8.9

Source: Compiled by New Strategist based on the Centers for Disease Control and Prevention Behavioral Risk Factor Surveillance System Survey, Internet site http://www.cdc.gov/brfss/index.htm

1.144 Weight: Advised by Medical Professional to Lose Weight by Household Income, 2000

"In the past 12 months, has a doctor, nurse, or other health professional given you advice about your weight?"

(percent of people aged 18 or older responding "yes, to lose weight," by state and household income, 2000)

	total	less than $15,000	$15,000 to $24,999	$25,000 to $34,999	$35,000 to $49,999	$50,000 or more
U.S. total	**11.7%**	**14.4%**	**11.8%**	**11.1%**	**11.6%**	**11.4%**
Alabama	13.6	12.1	13.5	18.1	12.1	12.7
Alaska	10.0	15.3	13.3	9.2	8.7	8.8
Arizona	12.4	21.2	9.9	13.5	14.5	11.3
Arkansas	11.1	14.6	10.4	11.3	11.9	10.2
California	12.0	10.9	10.1	14.8	12.1	12.9
Colorado	9.2	16.3	10.7	6.4	6.7	10.3
Connecticut	13.4	18.4	12.8	13.9	15.6	11.8
Delaware	11.9	15.7	12.3	15.1	12.6	11.3
District of Columbia	15.4	21.5	19.8	13.3	17.5	11.5
Florida	11.9	19.4	13.6	12.5	10.2	9.3
Georgia	13.9	18.9	13.8	9.6	17.4	12.5
Hawaii	12.4	12.2	13.1	13.3	14.2	12.7
Idaho	8.9	10.4	8.4	8.4	10.1	8.9
Illinois	12.0	10.3	14.3	11.3	14.3	11.0
Indiana	10.8	13.0	12.6	10.3	9.9	10.0
Iowa	8.9	9.8	9.0	10.6	9.5	7.6
Kansas	11.0	15.5	10.2	10.8	12.3	11.3
Kentucky	13.5	15.6	13.7	15.6	12.5	13.4
Louisiana	11.0	14.2	11.3	8.8	10.7	10.5
Maine	11.8	14.4	9.8	12.7	13.3	11.9
Maryland	14.3	18.6	13.8	14.6	13.2	14.6
Massachusetts	13.6	15.2	11.6	12.5	15.6	13.0
Michigan	12.6	14.4	13.3	12.2	11.5	13.2
Minnesota	7.6	9.1	6.5	8.3	6.4	8.2
Mississippi	14.2	14.3	14.2	13.6	14.6	14.8
Missouri	10.4	12.1	9.1	11.3	11.2	11.5
Montana	9.4	6.9	10.8	9.2	10.2	8.9
Nebraska	9.5	14.6	11.1	9.3	9.4	10.9
Nevada	12.2	18.8	13.6	9.0	9.2	12.6
New Hampshire	11.7	16.7	15.2	10.8	11.1	12.1
New Jersey	13.7	14.5	14.9	15.7	16.2	12.9
New Mexico	9.6	12.4	8.4	10.1	9.7	10.1
New York	13.8	18.6	12.1	17.2	13.4	13.4
North Carolina	12.6	15.8	14.2	12.6	13.5	10.0
North Dakota	8.4	6.4	9.0	10.1	7.8	8.9
Ohio	9.3	13.7	10.5	7.6	9.5	10.0
Oklahoma	8.1	6.4	7.9	7.4	7.5	12.2
Oregon	11.3	9.9	10.6	11.1	11.2	13.2
Pennsylvania	12.5	17.2	12.0	10.6	10.5	12.8
Rhode Island	14.2	16.8	15.8	16.4	10.5	13.5
South Carolina	12.4	12.1	15.1	10.8	12.5	12.0
South Dakota	9.2	11.4	9.4	8.2	9.8	9.9
Tennessee	11.5	12.4	13.5	9.7	12.1	12.4
Texas	12.4	14.6	9.8	12.7	14.7	13.0
Utah	10.5	9.4	8.3	11.2	11.7	11.0
Vermont	11.0	12.2	12.6	11.8	9.6	11.3
Virginia	10.2	14.4	12.3	9.5	10.2	9.4
Washington	9.2	11.5	8.7	8.0	8.0	10.7
West Virginia	13.1	20.2	11.5	11.3	16.1	9.7
Wisconsin	9.0	7.7	9.3	8.3	8.6	8.6
Wyoming	9.4	7.4	8.6	5.6	12.5	11.9

Source: Compiled by New Strategist based on the Centers for Disease Control and Prevention Behavioral Risk Factor Surveillance System Survey, Internet site http://www.cdc.gov/brfss/index.htm

1.145 Weight: Advised by Medical Professional to Lose Weight by Sex, 2000

"In the past 12 months, has a doctor, nurse, or other health professional given you advice about your weight?"

(percent of people aged 18 or older responding "yes, to lose weight," by state and sex, 2000)

	total	men	women
U.S. total	**11.7%**	**10.1%**	**12.9%**
Alabama	13.6	11.2	15.8
Alaska	10.0	8.7	11.5
Arizona	12.4	12.0	12.7
Arkansas	11.1	8.7	13.3
California	12.0	10.7	13.3
Colorado	9.2	9.3	9.2
Connecticut	13.4	12.5	14.2
Delaware	11.9	10.0	13.7
District of Columbia	15.4	12.2	18.1
Florida	11.9	10.6	13.1
Georgia	13.9	11.5	16.1
Hawaii	12.4	11.2	13.6
Idaho	8.9	6.4	11.4
Illinois	12.0	10.5	13.3
Indiana	10.8	8.8	12.7
Iowa	8.9	7.4	10.3
Kansas	11.0	10.9	11.0
Kentucky	13.5	11.8	15.0
Louisiana	11.0	7.9	13.7
Maine	11.8	10.9	12.7
Maryland	14.3	13.7	14.8
Massachusetts	13.6	13.1	14.0
Michigan	12.6	12.8	12.4
Minnesota	7.6	5.9	9.3
Mississippi	14.2	12.5	15.7
Missouri	10.4	10.0	10.6
Montana	9.4	7.1	11.6
Nebraska	9.5	8.1	10.9
Nevada	12.2	11.2	13.3
New Hampshire	11.7	11.5	12.0
New Jersey	13.7	13.2	14.1
New Mexico	9.6	7.9	11.2
New York	13.8	11.7	15.6
North Carolina	12.6	10.1	14.8
North Dakota	8.4	6.8	9.9
Ohio	9.3	9.2	9.5
Oklahoma	8.1	6.5	9.6
Oregon	11.3	8.6	13.9
Pennsylvania	12.5	11.7	13.2
Rhode Island	14.2	13.0	15.3
South Carolina	12.4	10.1	14.4
South Dakota	9.2	7.7	10.5
Tennessee	11.5	10.3	12.7
Texas	12.4	9.6	15.1
Utah	10.5	9.4	11.5
Vermont	11.0	10.2	11.7
Virginia	10.2	8.4	11.9
Washington	9.2	8.5	10.0
West Virginia	13.1	12.8	13.4
Wisconsin	9.0	8.4	9.5
Wyoming	9.4	8.6	10.2

Source: Compiled by New Strategist based on the Centers for Disease Control and Prevention Behavioral Risk Factor Surveillance System Survey, Internet site http://www.cdc.gov/brfss/index.htm

1.146 Women's Health: Currently Pregnant, 2000

"To your knowledge, are you now pregnant?"

(percent of women aged 18 to 49 responding "yes," by state, 2000)

	currently pregnant
U.S. total	**4.6%**
Alabama	4.5
Alaska	5.5
Arizona	7.0
Arkansas	3.6
California	5.1
Colorado	5.5
Connecticut	5.3
Delaware	4.3
District of Columbia	4.1
Florida	3.6
Georgia	5.5
Hawaii	4.6
Idaho	6.2
Illinois	5.4
Indiana	5.3
Iowa	4.5
Kansas	6.5
Kentucky	4.4
Louisiana	4.4
Maine	2.4
Maryland	5.0
Massachusetts	4.1
Michigan	5.2
Minnesota	4.0
Mississippi	5.5
Missouri	4.1
Montana	5.2
Nebraska	5.8
Nevada	2.3
New Hampshire	6.6
New Jersey	5.4
New Mexico	4.2
New York	4.0
North Carolina	3.8
North Dakota	3.4
Ohio	4.6
Oklahoma	3.6
Oregon	5.1
Pennsylvania	4.1
Rhode Island	4.7
South Carolina	5.5
South Dakota	4.8
Tennessee	5.3
Texas	5.3
Utah	7.2
Vermont	3.1
Virginia	4.6
Washington	4.3
West Virginia	2.4
Wisconsin	3.3
Wyoming	6.2

Source: Compiled by New Strategist based on the Centers for Disease Control and Prevention Behavioral Risk Factor Surveillance System Survey, Internet site http://www.cdc.gov/brfss/index.htm

1.147 Women's Health: Hysterectomy by Age, 2000

"Have you had a hysterectomy?"

(percent of women aged 18 or older responding "yes," by state and age, 2000)

	total	18 to 39	40 to 49	50 to 59	60 to 64	65 or older
U.S. total	**22.2%**	**3.2%**	**19.7%**	**35.7%**	**44.8%**	**44.4%**
Alabama	29.7	5.1	33.6	47.1	52.9	52.8
Alaska	15.9	2.3	17.9	30.5	50.4	43.5
Arizona	25.6	5.5	23.8	39.8	47.8	52.8
Arkansas	30.0	6.8	29.5	52.1	47.2	49.3
California	20.0	2.6	16.0	35.5	38.5	48.1
Colorado	23.8	3.2	19.9	40.5	45.8	56.5
Connecticut	17.2	2.9	13.7	29.7	37.5	32.1
Delaware	17.3	1.8	13.9	29.7	40.1	36.3
District of Columbia	18.1	2.3	15.3	28.1	29.2	44.5
Florida	24.0	3.6	20.6	32.3	44.1	43.5
Georgia	26.4	4.5	23.1	48.9	48.9	58.9
Hawaii	15.4	1.6	10.3	23.7	33.0	36.6
Idaho	28.6	5.8	26.3	43.5	58.4	57.3
Illinois	18.8	2.7	12.6	32.4	50.3	39.1
Indiana	23.5	3.9	24.6	39.0	48.5	44.1
Iowa	19.9	2.4	14.5	25.7	42.0	43.3
Kansas	25.9	4.5	23.9	41.6	45.8	51.0
Kentucky	26.1	4.3	27.0	44.9	53.3	46.0
Louisiana	29.9	6.0	31.1	53.3	64.1	53.4
Maine	20.1	2.2	18.6	30.1	43.1	40.7
Maryland	19.5	3.6	16.2	34.2	41.4	38.1
Massachusetts	16.3	2.3	12.1	26.4	34.2	40.7
Michigan	19.5	5.3	35.7	59.8	56.5	62.0
Minnesota	16.9	3.2	24.8	37.8	40.9	45.2
Mississippi	32.5	2.9	19.6	39.4	44.9	44.2
Missouri	24.1	3.1	15.1	31.8	44.3	42.4
Montana	23.2	2.9	19.6	39.4	44.9	44.2
Nebraska	20.4	3.1	15.1	31.8	44.3	42.4
Nevada	27.8	6.6	21.8	47.6	56.4	57.2
New Hampshire	14.4	2.2	14.4	22.1	20.4	34.8
New Jersey	15.8	3.2	12.8	20.8	33.8	33.9
New Mexico	21.9	3.9	21.1	33.9	49.8	47.3
New York	15.2	1.9	10.1	22.3	22.0	38.0
North Carolina	25.7	4.2	22.2	46.1	52.4	48.9
North Dakota	20.8	2.5	19.8	33.6	36.0	44.6
Ohio	22.6	2.8	18.7	40.5	55.4	41.2
Oklahoma	28.0	5.6	23.6	44.3	54.2	53.5
Oregon	23.5	2.6	18.2	40.9	41.6	48.7
Pennsylvania	20.5	2.8	12.2	32.7	47.9	40.6
Rhode Island	19.0	2.9	17.0	25.6	39.2	39.3
South Carolina	27.9	4.7	30.6	51.6	48.5	50.7
South Dakota	20.9	2.5	20.2	35.2	35.6	40.5
Tennessee	27.7	6.9	26.5	39.9	50.6	53.1
Texas	25.4	4.0	25.7	47.3	44.8	54.4
Utah	27.1	4.9	31.8	45.9	55.2	58.3
Vermont	15.2	2.3	14.8	27.8	23.3	31.8
Virginia	21.0	2.4	17.4	39.4	42.8	44.5
Washington	23.2	2.2	18.3	35.9	55.9	53.0
West Virginia	24.6	3.6	21.5	41.5	45.9	42.8
Wisconsin	18.2	3.9	12.8	28.7	37.8	38.0
Wyoming	28.7	8.0	28.1	41.0	55.0	55.2

Source: Compiled by New Strategist based on the Centers for Disease Control and Prevention Behavioral Risk Factor Surveillance System Survey. Internet site http://www.cdc.gov/brfss/index.htm

1.148   Women's Health: Hysterectomy by Education, 2000

"Have you had a hysterectomy?"

(percent of women aged 18 or older responding "yes," by state and educational attainment, 2000)

	total	less than high school	high school graduate	some college	college graduate
U.S. total	**22.2%**	**32.2%**	**25.9%**	**21.3%**	**15.5%**
Alabama	29.7	42.4	33.6	26.3	16.3
Alaska	15.9	33.2	14.1	17.4	12.1
Arizona	25.6	28.6	26.1	26.5	21.5
Arkansas	30.0	42.6	30.6	30.4	18.9
California	20.0	14.2	22.5	23.6	16.8
Colorado	23.8	18.6	29.8	24.4	20.2
Connecticut	17.2	32.2	19.5	14.9	12.7
Delaware	17.3	25.8	18.3	21.1	10.7
District of Columbia	18.1	18.8	23.8	21.8	12.7
Florida	24.0	28.7	27.6	21.5	19.8
Georgia	26.4	43.7	26.9	24.9	16.1
Hawaii	15.4	23.8	17.9	13.1	13.0
Idaho	28.6	40.9	31.5	29.0	17.6
Illinois	18.8	30.8	23.0	16.6	11.7
Indiana	23.5	35.6	26.8	21.8	13.8
Iowa	19.9	26.6	26.2	18.5	10.2
Kansas	25.9	40.9	28.8	24.4	18.7
Kentucky	26.1	37.5	27.7	23.8	14.0
Louisiana	29.9	40.1	32.3	27.6	19.6
Maine	20.1	35.4	22.7	18.7	11.7
Maryland	19.5	32.2	25.3	16.9	13.7
Massachusetts	16.3	31.1	21.2	15.7	9.1
Michigan	19.5	29.4	27.3	13.6	12.6
Minnesota	16.9	32.3	22.2	16.1	8.6
Mississippi	32.5	41.7	36.1	28.6	24.2
Missouri	24.1	38.8	28.6	19.4	15.1
Montana	23.2	36.2	26.2	19.9	19.4
Nebraska	20.4	28.6	25.4	18.9	11.6
Nevada	27.8	36.7	32.8	26.4	19.2
New Hampshire	14.4	22.3	16.0	15.6	9.0
New Jersey	15.8	19.9	20.0	15.8	9.6
New Mexico	21.9	22.0	25.7	21.2	19.2
New York	15.2	24.3	19.6	13.7	8.8
North Carolina	25.7	38.6	29.8	22.8	14.4
North Dakota	20.8	32.5	22.9	18.9	16.2
Ohio	22.6	39.8	22.5	22.2	15.9
Oklahoma	28.0	38.6	29.9	24.3	22.7
Oregon	23.5	21.1	28.0	25.6	16.6
Pennsylvania	20.5	28.5	25.3	16.8	12.9
Rhode Island	19.0	33.3	25.0	11.6	13.3
South Carolina	27.9	39.7	31.2	22.2	22.1
South Dakota	20.9	33.2	24.3	17.9	16.0
Tennessee	27.7	42.4	29.2	23.2	15.9
Texas	25.4	24.4	27.8	28.5	20.7
Utah	27.1	32.0	32.2	27.5	19.2
Vermont	15.2	24.6	18.9	15.1	9.3
Virginia	21.0	37.0	25.7	17.0	13.3
Washington	23.2	26.6	26.3	25.5	16.7
West Virginia	24.6	34.4	25.6	22.9	14.7
Wisconsin	18.2	22.9	23.8	17.7	8.2
Wyoming	28.7	45.6	33.0	26.7	19.5

Source: Compiled by New Strategist based on the Centers for Disease Control and Prevention Behavioral Risk Factor Surveillance System Survey. Internet site http://www.cdc.gov/brfss/index.htm

1.149 Women's Health: Hysterectomy by Household Income, 2000

"Have you had a hysterectomy?"

(percent of women aged 18 or older responding "yes," by state and household income, 2000)

	total	less than $15,000	$15,000 to $24,999	$25,000 to $34,999	$35,000 to $49,999	$50,000 or more
U.S. total	22.2%	27.1%	24.4%	22.2%	19.7%	16.1%
Alabama	29.7	38.2	29.6	29.8	21.9	22.8
Alaska	15.9	22.0	17.8	15.1	16.1	13.5
Arizona	25.6	24.6	23.5	18.0	26.0	22.8
Arkansas	30.0	35.2	27.5	31.0	27.0	28.2
California	20.0	18.5	22.9	20.7	21.2	16.8
Colorado	23.8	23.3	29.6	28.7	17.9	19.7
Connecticut	17.2	26.1	19.7	17.8	16.9	11.5
Delaware	17.3	23.4	23.3	15.8	14.1	12.2
District of Columbia	18.1	18.0	20.7	19.3	12.7	14.2
Florida	24.0	27.1	24.8	25.8	21.8	19.5
Georgia	26.4	34.2	26.4	27.4	24.4	20.0
Hawaii	15.4	15.8	21.7	14.1	14.2	13.6
Idaho	28.6	35.0	28.8	23.7	25.9	26.0
Illinois	18.8	29.2	20.5	22.1	16.8	13.0
Indiana	23.5	32.1	30.7	24.1	22.4	15.3
Iowa	19.9	25.2	26.7	22.2	14.2	12.7
Kansas	25.9	34.5	32.5	24.6	21.3	20.6
Kentucky	26.1	34.3	32.1	22.7	23.7	18.6
Louisiana	29.9	34.2	28.0	28.3	27.0	27.8
Maine	20.1	23.4	23.4	19.9	17.5	11.5
Maryland	19.5	26.9	23.2	22.2	18.6	15.2
Massachusetts	16.3	23.7	24.7	17.8	12.6	8.8
Michigan	19.5	28.7	24.1	20.5	16.9	14.1
Minnesota	16.9	29.0	23.3	17.8	14.5	10.6
Mississippi	32.5	39.7	28.4	29.3	27.1	29.3
Missouri	24.1	31.0	25.7	24.8	22.1	16.0
Montana	23.2	19.8	24.3	25.1	23.4	14.9
Nebraska	20.4	24.2	24.0	22.2	16.2	13.8
Nevada	27.8	37.7	38.9	29.3	24.5	20.3
New Hampshire	14.4	23.2	20.5	11.9	7.2	13.3
New Jersey	15.8	21.5	22.4	17.1	14.2	8.5
New Mexico	21.9	21.5	21.9	21.7	23.9	18.1
New York	15.2	24.2	17.9	19.3	13.2	9.5
North Carolina	25.7	37.8	28.9	24.1	25.7	15.0
North Dakota	20.8	24.5	22.7	14.8	19.6	17.7
Ohio	22.6	32.4	22.0	22.5	15.5	17.8
Oklahoma	28.0	31.4	27.1	30.3	24.8	22.1
Oregon	23.5	30.8	19.6	24.6	22.4	20.9
Pennsylvania	20.5	29.9	27.6	22.0	15.7	10.8
Rhode Island	19.0	24.1	21.2	21.6	14.3	11.0
South Carolina	27.9	32.4	32.7	24.3	20.4	25.0
South Dakota	20.9	23.7	20.6	20.7	16.3	16.3
Tennessee	27.7	32.8	31.3	25.8	21.0	18.4
Texas	25.4	23.6	24.6	25.9	25.4	22.7
Utah	27.1	33.2	30.2	18.9	23.7	26.9
Vermont	15.2	24.2	18.8	13.2	14.2	9.7
Virginia	21.0	27.2	27.0	26.5	14.7	17.9
Washington	23.2	23.6	28.9	23.5	22.5	18.9
West Virginia	24.6	30.4	28.2	22.4	19.8	15.5
Wisconsin	18.2	35.4	19.0	16.6	10.0	16.0
Wyoming	28.7	33.4	29.8	22.5	27.9	26.8

Source: Compiled by New Strategist based on the Centers for Disease Control and Prevention Behavioral Risk Factor Surveillance System Survey, Internet site http://www.cdc.gov/brfss/index.htm

1.150 Women's Health: Ever Had Clinical Breast Exam by Age, 2000

"Have you ever had a clinical breast exam?"

(percent of women aged 18 or older responding "yes," by state and age, 2000)

	total	18 to 39	40 to 49	50 to 59	60 to 64	65 or older
U.S. total	**89.7%**	**87.9%**	**94.1%**	**93.6%**	**91.2%**	**84.7%**
Alabama	89.9	89.1	94.5	94.9	89.9	82.8
Alaska	93.0	90.4	96.4	93.9	98.3	94.4
Arizona	80.2	76.7	81.7	83.8	88.1	80.1
Arkansas	90.2	90.3	94.2	92.7	89.8	85.3
California	84.9	81.1	89.1	90.3	88.5	83.7
Colorado	88.7	84.9	94.0	92.4	99.1	85.0
Connecticut	90.2	87.9	93.5	95.4	95.8	86.1
Delaware	89.8	86.9	95.8	91.9	89.6	88.9
District of Columbia	88.3	91.0	87.4	88.9	90.2	81.9
Florida	85.2	82.2	92.0	86.6	88.0	82.6
Georgia	89.5	89.7	90.7	92.2	92.2	84.3
Hawaii	84.7	80.1	87.3	90.8	92.0	83.8
Idaho	90.5	89.1	94.8	95.2	90.4	84.8
Illinois	85.5	81.3	92.2	93.8	94.1	78.7
Indiana	88.8	88.5	95.3	90.2	84.9	82.5
Iowa	91.1	90.1	95.5	95.0	93.8	86.3
Kansas	87.7	86.7	92.2	91.3	92.0	81.7
Kentucky	87.8	86.6	93.0	90.2	86.4	83.3
Louisiana	85.3	83.2	91.1	90.1	87.0	79.2
Maine	92.5	91.5	95.2	97.6	95.7	87.2
Maryland	90.5	89.2	92.6	93.7	91.7	87.7
Massachusetts	91.3	88.7	96.6	95.4	91.3	88.4
Michigan	89.8	88.6	97.1	93.9	85.4	82.2
Minnesota	92.4	91.4	96.2	95.7	95.4	87.4
Mississippi	87.9	87.0	90.8	91.2	91.3	84.7
Missouri	87.5	86.5	92.7	91.8	85.6	81.7
Montana	93.2	89.8	97.9	97.7	95.9	90.4
Nebraska	88.7	84.9	96.0	96.9	93.9	82.3
Nevada	88.2	88.0	93.7	86.6	92.5	81.5
New Hampshire	94.4	92.6	95.8	97.4	95.6	94.3
New Jersey	85.0	81.9	92.6	90.9	88.3	78.4
New Mexico	88.1	84.5	93.1	93.9	89.8	85.4
New York	86.9	83.6	91.3	91.8	90.8	83.4
North Carolina	91.5	90.5	95.4	95.9	92.6	85.8
North Dakota	90.2	87.2	93.7	97.1	97.2	87.5
Ohio	88.4	85.8	92.1	94.5	89.8	86.6
Oklahoma	89.9	87.6	93.2	93.9	92.7	87.9
Oregon	91.2	88.4	94.5	96.8	93.8	87.9
Pennsylvania	90.8	91.0	95.9	92.7	91.2	85.4
Rhode Island	90.8	89.6	94.9	94.1	89.5	87.7
South Carolina	88.8	88.4	90.6	91.0	91.0	85.9
South Dakota	91.4	90.0	96.6	96.7	90.6	86.7
Tennessee	86.4	86.1	92.9	90.2	83.0	78.5
Texas	83.7	80.7	86.3	91.7	84.9	81.6
Utah	90.6	86.0	95.4	93.5	97.3	91.8
Vermont	89.7	87.4	96.1	93.1	90.6	84.6
Virginia	87.8	85.6	96.1	90.7	85.5	80.9
Washington	93.3	90.8	98.0	95.9	96.8	90.3
West Virginia	89.9	88.6	95.0	95.2	89.7	84.2
Wisconsin	90.6	89.9	94.4	95.0	95.3	84.6
Wyoming	91.7	90.4	96.8	97.8	91.4	82.9

Source: Compiled by New Strategist based on the Centers for Disease Control and Prevention Behavioral Risk Factor (defined as having a body mass index of 25.0 or higher). Surveillance System Survey, Internet site http://www.cdc.gov/brfss/index.htm

1.151 Women's Health: Ever Had Clinical Breast Exam by Education, 2000

"Have you ever had a clinical breast exam?"

(percent of women aged 18 or older responding "yes," by state and educational attainment, 2000)

	total	less than high school	high school graduate	some college	college graduate
U.S. total	**89.7%**	**78.3%**	**87.5%**	**91.9%**	**94.4%**
Alabama	89.9	80.5	88.4	93.7	96.5
Alaska	93.0	82.1	91.1	93.1	97.2
Arizona	80.2	67.9	74.2	88.5	85.1
Arkansas	90.2	76.8	90.9	92.4	96.2
California	84.9	70.3	83.7	90.0	90.7
Colorado	88.7	62.1	86.1	94.0	93.5
Connecticut	90.2	81.5	89.3	89.8	94.0
Delaware	89.8	72.6	88.1	92.2	93.6
District of Columbia	88.3	73.6	87.4	92.4	91.0
Florida	85.2	72.8	83.5	88.8	89.4
Georgia	89.5	79.2	87.2	92.5	95.7
Hawaii	84.7	82.3	79.9	83.2	91.1
Idaho	90.5	78.5	89.1	92.0	95.9
Illinois	85.5	74.7	83.4	85.8	91.8
Indiana	88.8	74.9	87.0	94.3	91.9
Iowa	91.1	78.8	88.3	92.8	96.7
Kansas	87.7	76.2	81.7	91.9	94.0
Kentucky	87.8	79.8	87.9	90.6	92.2
Louisiana	85.3	77.9	83.6	88.2	91.0
Maine	92.5	84.9	93.0	93.1	94.4
Maryland	90.5	83.3	86.6	90.2	95.9
Massachusetts	91.3	84.1	89.1	92.3	94.2
Michigan	89.8	78.3	87.6	90.9	96.8
Minnesota	92.4	81.3	90.4	92.1	97.2
Mississippi	87.9	75.9	87.7	91.7	95.1
Missouri	87.5	76.9	86.1	90.8	90.8
Montana	93.2	81.6	90.8	97.0	95.3
Nebraska	88.7	63.6	88.0	93.2	93.2
Nevada	88.2	78.4	83.1	90.9	95.7
New Hampshire	94.4	86.0	92.3	95.5	97.9
New Jersey	85.0	71.2	82.7	85.8	93.0
New Mexico	88.1	73.1	86.1	92.0	96.0
New York	86.9	77.7	82.6	89.3	92.0
North Carolina	91.5	82.2	90.8	93.3	96.9
North Dakota	90.2	74.6	91.2	91.9	92.7
Ohio	88.4	78.0	85.7	92.8	91.7
Oklahoma	89.9	81.3	87.4	93.4	95.5
Oregon	91.2	76.6	88.3	94.4	96.5
Pennsylvania	90.8	85.4	89.1	92.6	94.4
Rhode Island	90.8	84.8	89.4	90.7	95.4
South Carolina	88.8	80.6	87.0	91.7	93.8
South Dakota	91.4	79.6	90.9	91.8	95.9
Tennessee	86.4	77.2	86.5	87.8	93.3
Texas	83.7	69.0	82.3	87.5	93.4
Utah	90.6	77.5	88.6	90.5	95.9
Vermont	89.7	76.1	87.4	90.4	94.7
Virginia	87.8	83.8	81.9	89.8	94.0
Washington	93.3	87.1	90.7	94.5	95.4
West Virginia	89.9	81.1	89.1	93.0	95.9
Wisconsin	90.6	78.1	89.3	92.8	95.0
Wyoming	91.7	82.1	86.7	95.2	97.2

Source: Compiled by New Strategist based on the Centers for Disease Control and Prevention Behavioral Risk Factor Surveillance System Survey, Internet site http://www.cdc.gov/brfss/index.htm

1.152 Women's Health: Ever Had Clinical Breast Exam by Household Income, 2000

"Have you ever had a clinical breast exam?"

(percent of women aged 18 or older responding "yes," by state and household income, 2000)

	total	less than $15,000	$15,000 to $24,999	$25,000 to $34,999	$35,000 to $49,999	$50,000 or more
U.S. total	**89.7%**	**80.6%**	**85.6%**	**90.5%**	**93.0%**	**95.3%**
Alabama	89.9	80.0	83.8	93.4	94.7	95.6
Alaska	93.0	86.2	92.3	95.0	96.6	95.4
Arizona	80.2	48.3	74.6	83.0	92.4	85.8
Arkansas	90.2	79.9	88.5	89.9	95.4	97.2
California	84.9	75.4	78.6	85.6	90.0	93.7
Colorado	88.7	72.3	80.1	88.0	93.4	96.3
Connecticut	90.2	85.7	84.7	93.8	91.1	94.9
Delaware	89.8	80.8	83.8	92.5	89.8	97.7
District of Columbia	88.3	78.8	83.9	91.4	89.3	94.5
Florida	85.2	77.0	80.6	85.7	91.7	93.1
Georgia	89.5	78.9	86.8	89.1	90.9	96.5
Hawaii	84.7	78.2	80.7	82.8	89.7	92.6
Idaho	90.5	77.7	87.9	93.6	95.8	95.6
Illinois	85.5	72.9	81.8	81.5	91.0	91.7
Indiana	88.8	76.1	85.9	86.1	93.6	96.7
Iowa	91.1	80.5	88.3	93.7	92.4	97.1
Kansas	87.7	74.5	85.3	90.5	90.1	95.1
Kentucky	87.8	79.1	88.2	90.3	90.5	94.4
Louisiana	85.3	76.3	83.4	87.5	93.0	93.0
Maine	92.5	86.9	90.7	95.6	97.4	94.3
Maryland	90.5	82.0	82.6	89.2	91.8	96.2
Massachusetts	91.3	86.9	86.8	91.4	92.2	96.1
Michigan	89.8	83.2	82.0	95.6	91.8	95.7
Minnesota	92.4	79.6	89.8	92.0	92.8	97.3
Mississippi	87.9	83.1	84.9	89.9	94.5	96.9
Missouri	87.5	80.2	84.6	86.0	90.6	94.8
Montana	93.2	92.6	89.0	95.8	92.7	99.2
Nebraska	88.7	78.7	81.8	91.8	94.6	98.5
Nevada	88.2	66.8	87.2	86.2	89.3	93.5
New Hampshire	94.4	95.7	94.1	89.6	98.1	95.9
New Jersey	85.0	74.3	80.2	78.7	85.5	94.1
New Mexico	88.1	82.2	86.9	91.0	93.5	95.2
New York	86.9	74.8	81.4	90.6	93.1	90.9
North Carolina	91.5	84.5	89.4	93.5	92.9	96.0
North Dakota	90.2	87.5	86.9	93.3	96.8	92.7
Ohio	88.4	74.6	87.5	82.2	92.1	94.4
Oklahoma	89.9	84.7	84.7	93.3	94.3	96.5
Oregon	91.2	87.3	85.9	90.4	94.9	97.5
Pennsylvania	90.8	83.3	88.8	88.2	96.6	95.7
Rhode Island	90.8	84.2	88.8	92.9	93.0	95.5
South Carolina	88.8	81.9	82.8	86.4	93.9	95.1
South Dakota	91.4	84.8	89.5	93.3	94.3	97.2
Tennessee	86.4	82.0	82.8	81.4	91.3	92.7
Texas	83.7	75.7	80.5	83.6	89.1	94.8
Utah	90.6	83.1	88.0	92.5	94.5	94.4
Vermont	89.7	84.1	86.7	90.3	94.7	93.7
Virginia	87.8	75.4	83.9	89.1	93.0	93.6
Washington	93.3	90.2	90.6	93.7	96.7	96.7
West Virginia	89.9	87.3	88.3	92.2	95.1	95.1
Wisconsin	90.6	84.4	82.5	90.6	98.1	94.2
Wyoming	91.7	83.3	90.8	92.0	95.6	96.6

Source: Compiled by New Strategist based on the Centers for Disease Control and Prevention Behavioral Risk Factor Surveillance System Survey, Internet site http://www.cdc.gov/brfss/index.htm

1.153 Women's Health: Clinical Breast Exam in Past Year, 2000

"How long has it been since your last breast exam?"

(percent of women aged 18 or older who have ever had a clinical breast exam responding "past year," by state, 2000)

	breast exam in past year
U.S. total	**77.5%**
Alabama	71.6
Alaska	78.7
Arizona	78.7
Arkansas	70.0
California	73.4
Colorado	75.0
Connecticut	83.5
Delaware	84.5
District of Columbia	82.7
Florida	77.2
Georgia	77.0
Hawaii	79.6
Idaho	67.4
Illinois	78.9
Indiana	74.7
Iowa	77.5
Kansas	77.4
Kentucky	78.9
Louisiana	80.5
Maine	82.0
Maryland	83.8
Massachusetts	83.6
Michigan	81.2
Minnesota	72.0
Mississippi	72.6
Missouri	78.5
Montana	76.4
Nebraska	79.7
Nevada	71.5
New Hampshire	79.6
New Jersey	80.9
New Mexico	74.0
New York	83.3
North Carolina	79.2
North Dakota	75.7
Ohio	76.2
Oklahoma	72.4
Oregon	71.1
Pennsylvania	77.6
Rhode Island	84.1
South Carolina	81.0
South Dakota	79.9
Tennessee	79.8
Texas	72.8
Utah	68.6
Vermont	79.3
Virginia	79.0
Washington	69.9
West Virginia	76.2
Wisconsin	76.5
Wyoming	68.9

Source: Compiled by New Strategist based on the Centers for Disease Control and Prevention Behavioral Risk Factor Surveillance System Survey, Internet site http://www.cdc.gov/brfss/index.htm

1.154 Women's Health: Ever Had a Mammogram by Age, 2000

"Have you ever had a mammogram?"

(percent of women aged 18 or older responding "yes," by state and age, 2000)

	total	18 to 39	40 to 49	50 to 59	60 to 64	65 or older
U.S. total	**62.2%**	**22.6%**	**82.6%**	**92.1%**	**91.2%**	**90.1%**
Alabama	65.1	27.4	85.2	90.7	89.9	90.4
Alaska	56.5	22.1	79.7	92.8	94.1	90.5
Arizona	62.8	25.5	80.5	89.9	96.5	94.5
Arkansas	62.1	23.9	80.0	89.4	91.3	85.5
California	60.1	18.3	84.2	94.3	97.3	94.3
Colorado	59.2	18.8	79.0	91.1	92.7	93.7
Connecticut	65.3	21.3	91.9	94.8	88.4	92.8
Delaware	66.8	29.0	88.2	95.0	96.6	94.3
District of Columbia	65.6	27.5	90.2	93.0	98.8	93.9
Florida	68.0	27.6	83.0	90.5	92.6	91.3
Georgia	62.1	28.1	80.2	90.6	96.3	90.1
Hawaii	63.2	22.0	84.5	91.5	94.4	91.1
Idaho	57.5	16.2	75.5	90.3	87.8	87.5
Illinois	61.3	22.5	82.5	91.7	90.4	88.0
Indiana	59.7	19.4	85.2	88.6	89.9	85.4
Iowa	62.0	19.4	82.1	93.8	93.7	85.1
Kansas	62.6	22.9	82.6	92.1	90.5	90.4
Kentucky	63.1	24.7	84.4	90.0	91.2	86.7
Louisiana	61.9	27.9	82.7	89.4	87.7	85.6
Maine	62.6	17.0	88.2	96.3	90.2	88.9
Maryland	64.3	25.2	85.8	94.3	92.8	93.2
Massachusetts	63.7	21.3	90.7	95.4	94.3	90.6
Michigan	64.2	23.3	86.9	94.4	95.7	92.1
Minnesota	61.0	22.7	79.2	92.1	94.6	89.9
Mississippi	59.3	25.6	75.0	88.7	84.7	88.0
Missouri	61.1	20.0	81.4	90.5	90.2	84.3
Montana	61.1	16.5	77.8	93.5	90.8	90.7
Nebraska	62.3	24.9	81.9	92.6	95.8	84.0
Nevada	64.3	26.9	82.6	96.1	87.6	91.9
New Hampshire	59.7	14.2	86.7	95.1	93.8	92.1
New Jersey	61.8	23.9	84.7	87.7	86.0	85.9
New Mexico	59.4	20.7	79.7	92.8	88.7	91.0
New York	63.9	21.9	88.6	94.8	92.6	87.6
North Carolina	64.5	27.3	84.9	92.5	94.2	89.4
North Dakota	60.6	19.7	82.4	94.4	88.0	89.2
Ohio	63.1	22.0	83.3	93.9	91.1	91.5
Oklahoma	58.3	19.5	74.6	86.1	85.6	85.8
Oregon	64.2	20.7	83.2	95.1	96.3	92.4
Pennsylvania	65.5	23.6	87.2	90.1	96.3	90.8
Rhode Island	66.6	26.4	89.4	94.6	93.7	92.0
South Carolina	64.8	27.9	82.3	96.8	92.9	91.9
South Dakota	60.2	17.9	80.1	91.9	86.2	89.8
Tennessee	62.9	23.5	85.2	92.1	85.4	88.4
Texas	59.7	25.6	80.4	91.5	83.3	85.3
Utah	54.8	16.4	80.9	90.2	91.2	88.2
Vermont	57.7	15.3	83.0	92.1	93.1	87.1
Virginia	63.1	26.4	84.3	90.6	91.2	91.1
Washington	61.5	19.4	83.0	93.7	91.1	92.0
West Virginia	63.8	25.3	81.7	90.6	87.9	86.5
Wisconsin	62.5	20.9	82.2	95.2	94.7	87.7
Wyoming	60.5	19.5	79.4	91.7	85.7	90.2

Source: Compiled by New Strategist based on the Centers for Disease Control and Prevention Behavioral Risk Factor Surveillance System Survey, Internet site http://www.cdc.gov/brfss/index.htm

1.155 Women's Health: Ever Had a Mammogram by Education, 2000

"Have you ever had a mammogram?"

(percent of women aged 18 or older responding "yes," by state and educational attainment, 2000)

	total	less than high school	high school graduate	some college	college graduate
U.S. total	**62.2%**	**65.9%**	**64.2%**	**59.2%**	**61.0%**
Alabama	65.1	71.3	61.2	65.0	66.2
Alaska	56.5	59.7	54.5	57.8	56.1
Arizona	62.8	66.8	62.1	61.9	62.5
Arkansas	62.1	67.3	63.1	59.7	59.9
California	60.1	53.1	58.0	64.2	62.0
Colorado	59.2	55.1	63.1	55.6	60.6
Connecticut	65.3	65.9	68.1	63.4	64.5
Delaware	66.8	66.9	68.5	62.0	69.0
District of Columbia	65.6	67.0	70.4	66.8	61.7
Florida	68.0	66.5	68.6	65.1	71.1
Georgia	62.1	65.9	61.1	61.7	60.9
Hawaii	63.2	78.5	59.1	60.6	65.6
Idaho	57.5	58.4	55.5	58.6	58.4
Illinois	61.3	71.4	62.9	57.4	59.6
Indiana	59.7	58.0	63.7	58.4	55.0
Iowa	62.0	64.0	69.6	55.6	59.3
Kansas	62.6	68.4	65.5	59.2	60.7
Kentucky	63.1	64.7	65.6	60.2	59.7
Louisiana	61.9	66.9	63.3	57.8	60.1
Maine	62.6	68.0	62.6	54.2	69.3
Maryland	64.3	66.4	68.7	62.1	61.6
Massachusetts	63.7	65.2	68.6	61.4	61.3
Michigan	64.2	64.3	70.5	58.3	62.8
Minnesota	61.0	75.9	66.6	56.9	56.8
Mississippi	59.3	60.6	64.1	56.6	54.2
Missouri	61.1	68.4	66.4	55.4	55.8
Montana	61.1	63.6	58.5	56.3	68.4
Nebraska	62.3	52.8	68.7	57.8	60.8
Nevada	64.3	67.2	61.6	63.1	68.7
New Hampshire	59.7	58.1	64.1	56.2	59.4
New Jersey	61.8	60.0	66.1	60.1	59.8
New Mexico	59.4	62.3	56.4	54.6	66.0
New York	63.9	64.9	65.1	60.7	65.0
North Carolina	64.5	73.2	65.3	59.2	63.3
North Dakota	60.6	65.4	64.8	55.5	60.2
Ohio	63.1	66.9	64.6	60.4	61.9
Oklahoma	58.3	57.6	56.1	59.5	60.7
Oregon	64.2	52.4	64.8	67.1	64.8
Pennsylvania	65.5	71.0	71.0	58.2	61.1
Rhode Island	66.6	65.9	72.3	60.4	67.0
South Carolina	64.8	75.3	66.5	57.8	63.1
South Dakota	60.2	66.8	64.6	57.7	54.9
Tennessee	62.9	68.7	63.7	61.7	56.3
Texas	59.7	54.4	61.4	59.0	63.0
Utah	54.8	46.5	59.9	52.3	54.7
Vermont	57.7	48.7	59.1	57.1	59.1
Virginia	63.1	66.3	61.8	60.5	65.8
Washington	61.5	53.3	60.5	63.7	61.5
West Virginia	63.8	70.4	64.4	59.3	62.4
Wisconsin	62.5	62.7	66.1	61.1	58.4
Wyoming	60.5	59.5	67.0	56.5	57.5

Source: Compiled by New Strategist based on the Centers for Disease Control and Prevention Behavioral Risk Factor Surveillance System Survey, Internet site http://www.cdc.gov/brfss/index.htm

1.156 Women's Health: Ever Had a Mammogram by Household Income, 2000

"Have you ever had a mammogram?"

(percent of women aged 18 or older responding "yes," by state and household income, 2000)

	total	less than $15,000	$15,000 to $24,999	$25,000 to $34,999	$35,000 to $49,999	$50,000 or more
U.S. total	**62.2%**	**60.0%**	**59.4%**	**58.0%**	**60.7%**	**65.1%**
Alabama	65.1	64.3	63.5	59.8	62.1	66.9
Alaska	56.5	55.4	50.4	46.8	55.7	62.6
Arizona	62.8	39.0	60.6	59.6	67.5	65.6
Arkansas	62.1	62.8	53.9	57.0	65.9	67.2
California	60.1	52.7	55.9	63.0	63.5	61.0
Colorado	59.2	60.0	54.7	62.1	52.9	60.0
Connecticut	65.3	63.5	63.3	61.1	61.0	65.3
Delaware	66.8	61.1	62.2	66.6	63.1	67.9
District of Columbia	65.6	67.1	61.6	61.3	68.3	64.3
Florida	68.0	68.6	66.4	65.9	63.0	71.7
Georgia	62.1	61.1	55.3	61.4	61.3	61.9
Hawaii	63.2	54.6	62.9	59.3	64.1	70.2
Idaho	57.5	52.2	54.5	53.2	55.8	66.4
Illinois	61.3	56.3	64.6	57.8	57.9	62.6
Indiana	59.7	52.7	58.6	54.7	61.9	60.4
Iowa	62.0	54.8	61.9	56.2	60.9	67.1
Kansas	62.6	61.1	59.8	56.7	57.3	69.9
Kentucky	63.1	59.1	62.5	57.3	60.0	68.1
Louisiana	61.9	60.4	57.8	57.1	62.6	66.6
Maine	62.6	57.9	60.6	54.1	58.3	69.3
Maryland	64.3	59.2	62.7	59.9	60.5	66.0
Massachusetts	63.7	63.0	65.0	62.3	62.4	62.6
Michigan	64.2	62.6	62.3	67.0	58.5	64.3
Minnesota	61.0	71.0	58.7	60.6	51.0	63.1
Mississippi	59.3	59.1	58.4	56.1	59.5	57.3
Missouri	61.1	53.1	59.2	58.3	64.6	59.4
Montana	61.1	48.5	54.3	53.7	65.5	65.4
Nebraska	62.3	53.1	58.2	60.6	58.3	69.9
Nevada	64.3	72.3	62.1	61.9	53.7	66.4
New Hampshire	59.7	68.0	59.6	52.6	52.6	64.7
New Jersey	61.8	66.1	62.3	59.3	57.2	62.4
New Mexico	59.4	54.4	55.0	57.1	62.2	65.4
New York	63.9	60.0	63.6	61.9	66.5	64.9
North Carolina	64.5	71.3	60.9	62.3	63.2	62.4
North Dakota	60.6	54.5	61.8	54.8	59.9	61.6
Ohio	63.1	67.6	62.9	55.7	55.6	61.9
Oklahoma	58.3	51.2	52.3	54.8	59.7	66.6
Oregon	64.2	61.3	58.0	64.6	62.7	69.0
Pennsylvania	65.5	65.1	66.8	59.7	62.7	63.9
Rhode Island	66.6	64.4	63.7	66.2	63.0	68.3
South Carolina	64.8	66.7	66.1	57.8	57.2	68.4
South Dakota	60.2	59.4	55.8	60.0	54.9	62.5
Tennessee	62.9	66.1	61.7	51.2	57.2	63.8
Texas	59.7	56.5	55.2	54.4	61.4	65.5
Utah	54.8	50.1	59.0	50.2	50.4	60.9
Vermont	57.7	56.0	52.9	51.4	57.9	61.5
Virginia	63.1	56.9	56.4	48.5	59.2	70.7
Washington	61.5	55.2	58.9	59.6	57.8	63.2
West Virginia	63.8	64.3	59.2	58.9	69.6	62.4
Wisconsin	62.5	66.3	53.1	56.4	61.8	66.1
Wyoming	60.5	58.1	53.6	53.4	60.9	67.1

Source: Compiled by New Strategist based on the Centers for Disease Control and Prevention Behavioral Risk Factor Surveillance System Survey, Internet site http://www.cdc.gov/brfss/index.htm

1.157 Women's Health: Mammogram in Past Year, 2000

"How long has it been since you had your last mammogram?"

(percent of women aged 18 or older who have ever had a mammogram responding "past year," by state, 2000)

	mammogram in past year
U.S. total	**69.1%**
Alabama	61.4
Alaska	65.9
Arizona	76.9
Arkansas	65.3
California	66.7
Colorado	66.3
Connecticut	76.2
Delaware	76.7
District of Columbia	71.2
Florida	71.8
Georgia	66.9
Hawaii	71.6
Idaho	58.3
Illinois	70.5
Indiana	69.1
Iowa	69.4
Kansas	67.4
Kentucky	69.4
Louisiana	73.1
Maine	71.9
Maryland	72.6
Massachusetts	76.7
Michigan	73.3
Minnesota	66.9
Mississippi	61.1
Missouri	69.2
Montana	68.5
Nebraska	70.8
Nevada	65.4
New Hampshire	74.1
New Jersey	75.6
New Mexico	66.2
New York	73.7
North Carolina	69.7
North Dakota	67.4
Ohio	71.7
Oklahoma	65.8
Oregon	65.4
Pennsylvania	68.3
Rhode Island	75.3
South Carolina	69.2
South Dakota	70.0
Tennessee	69.1
Texas	65.2
Utah	60.0
Vermont	70.4
Virginia	66.6
Washington	63.3
West Virginia	70.0
Wisconsin	66.7
Wyoming	61.2

Source: Compiled by New Strategist based on the Centers for Disease Control and Prevention Behavioral Risk Factor Surveillance System Survey, Internet site http://www.cdc.gov/brfss/index.htm

1.158 Women's Health: Ever Had Pap Smear by Age, 2000

"Have you ever had a Pap smear?"

(percent of women aged 18 or older responding "yes," by state and age, 2000)

	total	18 to 39	40 to 49	50 to 59	60 to 64	65 or older
U.S. total	**94.8%**	**93.7%**	**98.5%**	**98.0%**	**97.1%**	**92.3%**
Alabama	96.3	95.0	99.3	97.9	96.3	94.7
Alaska	97.5	95.9	99.9	99.7	94.1	97.0
Arizona	93.5	93.0	96.9	95.2	91.4	91.1
Arkansas	96.0	94.3	99.5	97.8	98.0	94.5
California	94.2	90.0	97.6	98.6	99.5	95.3
Colorado	95.8	92.8	99.8	100.0	98.3	94.7
Connecticut	93.9	91.4	98.0	98.6	96.8	90.8
Delaware	96.7	94.5	99.4	99.7	99.2	96.1
District of Columbia	94.7	91.9	97.7	96.7	97.6	95.5
Florida	93.9	91.3	97.7	95.8	97.1	92.4
Georgia	96.7	95.7	99.7	97.8	96.1	94.6
Hawaii	93.9	90.5	98.2	97.0	97.6	92.5
Idaho	95.0	92.5	98.4	98.7	95.6	93.5
Illinois	93.2	90.0	99.0	97.4	96.8	89.7
Indiana	94.1	92.9	99.1	96.2	94.9	89.6
Iowa	95.9	94.4	99.2	99.3	99.1	92.3
Kansas	96.2	95.4	99.1	97.7	98.0	93.8
Kentucky	93.0	94.6	96.6	94.9	91.9	85.1
Louisiana	93.9	93.0	98.6	96.7	94.5	89.0
Maine	94.5	94.6	98.5	96.6	91.0	90.2
Maryland	94.9	93.8	97.3	98.0	96.0	91.5
Massachusetts	93.7	93.2	98.3	96.4	98.2	87.7
Michigan	94.5	90.5	99.1	97.9	98.1	94.0
Minnesota	96.0	94.5	99.2	97.7	98.5	93.8
Mississippi	95.0	96.3	97.1	97.7	96.8	88.0
Missouri	95.7	94.7	98.8	99.3	97.5	91.8
Montana	97.1	94.8	100.0	99.4	99.3	96.1
Nebraska	93.0	91.8	98.1	98.4	94.5	86.8
Nevada	95.0	93.8	97.7	98.2	94.5	91.3
New Hampshire	96.8	94.7%	99.2%	98.6	100.0%	96.0
New Jersey	90.4	86.8	95.9	96.1	97.0	86.0
New Mexico	94.5	92.8	99.6	97.8	95.7	89.8
New York	92.9	91.1	96.7	98.3	94.4	88.2
North Carolina	96.4	95.4	99.0	99.1	97.9	93.3
North Dakota	94.2	93.3	98.3	99.6	93.3	89.1
Ohio	95.6	95.4	98.8	98.8	99.4	90.2
Oklahoma	96.2	94.0	98.4	98.3	98.4	96.4
Oregon	96.5	95.0	98.8	99.1	97.5	94.7
Pennsylvania	94.2	92.6	99.0	98.0	97.2	89.7
Rhode Island	94.0	91.4	98.3	97.7	96.6	91.5
South Carolina	95.9	94.9	98.3	97.2	94.2	94.7
South Dakota	96.4	95.1	98.9	98.7	98.7	94.7
Tennessee	93.6	94.0	95.6	95.8	94.1	88.8
Texas	92.9	89.6	96.2	97.7	96.4	91.9
Utah	94.3	90.1	98.2	98.1	98.3	96.5
Vermont	93.7	92.3	98.6	97.0	95.4	88.6
Virginia	94.2	92.6	92.5	98.4	98.6	94.6
Washington	96.5	93.8	99.7	99.3	98.9	95.6
West Virginia	95.3	94.2	98.5	99.1	97.9	91.2
Wisconsin	96.6	96.0	98.2	98.9	97.3	94.2
Wyoming	96.4	93.6	99.5	100.0	99.3	94.5

Source: Compiled by New Strategist based on the Centers for Disease Control and Prevention Behavioral Risk Factor Surveillance System Survey, Internet site http://www.cdc.gov/brfss/index.htm

1.159 Women's Health: Ever Had Pap Smear by Education, 2000

"Have you ever had a Pap smear?"

(percent of women aged 18 or older responding "yes," by state and educational attainment, 2000)

	total	less than high school	high school graduate	some college	college graduate
U.S. total	94.8%	90.1%	94.3%	95.5%	97.1%
Alabama	96.3	93.6	97.3	94.1	99.1
Alaska	97.5	98.6	97.7	95.6	99.0
Arizona	93.5	86.1	94.0	96.0	93.8
Arkansas	96.0	91.1	97.3	96.2	96.7
California	94.2	91.1	91.7	95.4	97.6
Colorado	95.8	94.8	95.4	94.1	97.9
Connecticut	93.9	87.9	94.2	93.7	95.7
Delaware	96.7	92.9	97.8	95.8	97.2
District of Columbia	94.7	88.5	93.1	98.2	95.6
Florida	93.9	90.1	93.7	93.3	96.5
Georgia	96.7	94.0	96.9	95.9	98.9
Hawaii	93.9	89.7	92.3	93.0	97.3
Idaho	95.0	92.7	94.3	95.0	97.5
Illinois	93.2	88.7	92.2	92.8	96.3
Indiana	94.1	88.7	93.2	96.7	95.3
Iowa	95.9	86.8	96.9	95.4	97.7
Kansas	96.2	93.9	93.4	97.3	99.1
Kentucky	93.0	90.3	92.7	94.0	95.2
Louisiana	93.9	90.6	94.7	93.9	95.8
Maine	94.5	92.1	92.3	94.8	98.5
Maryland	94.9	93.0	93.3	94.4	97.0
Massachusetts	93.7	90.1	91.8	93.7	96.2
Michigan	94.5	89.1	95.3	93.4	97.1
Minnesota	96.0	93.0	95.0	96.1	97.8
Mississippi	95.0	88.2	95.1	96.4	98.7
Missouri	95.7	89.7	96.3	96.9	96.3
Montana	97.1	89.5	96.6	98.1	99.2
Nebraska	93.0	80.7	92.2	95.4	95.9
Nevada	95.0	88.1	95.6	95.5	96.2
New Hampshire	96.8	90.0	96.5	97.1	98.7
New Jersey	90.4	79.8	90.5	90.6	94.7
New Mexico	94.5	89.1	93.7	95.9	97.7
New York	92.9	84.1	92.3	93.4	96.0
North Carolina	96.4	92.8	96.3	97.4	97.9
North Dakota	94.2	86.2	93.3	95.0	97.4
Ohio	95.6	92.1	95.7	96.4	95.4
Oklahoma	96.2	94.0	95.3	97.1	98.4
Oregon	96.5	95.3	95.4	96.5	98.2
Pennsylvania	94.2	86.7	94.3	94.8	96.7
Rhode Island	94.0	87.1	93.3	95.5	96.2
South Carolina	95.9	93.1	95.5	97.3	97.0
South Dakota	96.4	92.5	96.0	96.7	98.0
Tennessee	93.6	89.1	94.3	94.0	96.0
Texas	92.9	87.2	92.9	93.5	96.9
Utah	94.3	88.2	94.0	92.7	98.4
Vermont	93.7	90.2	92.7	92.1	97.1
Virginia	94.2	93.6	92.2	97.5	93.4
Washington	96.5	95.1	95.7	95.8	98.4
West Virginia	95.3	94.2	94.1	95.6	98.8
Wisconsin	96.6	94.6	95.8	97.2	97.9
Wyoming	96.4	95.0	94.9	97.0	98.2

Source: Compiled by New Strategist based on the Centers for Disease Control and Prevention Behavioral Risk Factor Surveillance System Survey, Internet site http://www.cdc.gov/brfss/index.htm

1.160 Women's Health: Ever Had Pap Smear by Household Income, 2000

"Have you ever had a Pap smear?"

(percent of women aged 18 or older responding "yes," by state and household income, 2000)

	total	less than $15,000	$15,000 to $24,999	$25,000 to $34,999	$35,000 to $49,999	$50,000 or more
U.S. total	**94.8%**	**90.9%**	**93.8%**	**96.1%**	**96.9%**	**97.9%**
Alabama	96.3	93.8	97.3	95.4	98.1	97.2
Alaska	97.5	97.7	97.3	97.3	99.4	97.9
Arizona	93.5	94.4	89.1	93.9	96.3	98.3
Arkansas	96.0	90.9	96.8	95.0	97.6	99.0
California	94.2	90.3	91.0	96.2	96.0	97.1
Colorado	95.8	93.9	92.7	96.8	96.2	99.2
Connecticut	93.9	87.3	92.7	93.5	96.4	96.7
Delaware	96.7	96.8	95.7	98.7	97.1	99.3
District of Columbia	94.7	90.9	93.5	96.5	93.8	97.7
Florida	93.9	89.0	92.6	95.8	96.9	97.7
Georgia	96.7	92.7	96.4	98.3	97.9	98.5
Hawaii	93.9	89.3	95.7	94.8	98.2	97.4
Idaho	95.0	87.6	95.8	97.2	97.1	98.2
Illinois	93.2	92.0	94.4	90.5	96.6	95.1
Indiana	94.1	84.4	94.7	94.2	95.9	98.1
Iowa	95.9	90.3	93.7	98.8	95.3	98.8
Kansas	96.2	88.5	95.9	98.4	97.6	98.8
Kentucky	93.0	86.9	94.2	94.3	95.3	97.5
Louisiana	93.9	91.5	93.3	97.4	95.9	97.0
Maine	94.5	95.6	93.9	90.7	97.2	98.0
Maryland	94.9	86.5	94.4	94.8	95.6	97.8
Massachusetts	93.7	90.3	91.7	94.7	96.4	96.9
Michigan	94.5	90.6	92.8	97.4	96.6	95.6
Minnesota	96.0	89.2	92.7	97.7	96.8	98.9
Mississippi	95.0	90.2	96.0	98.9	96.9	99.8
Missouri	95.7	91.5	94.0	96.3	98.4	99.2
Montana	97.1	97.6	98.2	97.2	95.0	100.0
Nebraska	93.0	80.1	88.8	96.0	97.0	99.5
Nevada	95.0	81.5	96.8	95.8	94.0	97.8
New Hampshire	96.8	95.1	98.0	96.6	97.6	97.9
New Jersey	90.4	84.2	86.9	86.8	92.2	95.3
New Mexico	94.5	92.0	93.1	96.8	97.3	97.8
New York	92.9	87.2	91.0	93.8	95.7	96.0
North Carolina	96.4	93.6	97.3	97.0	97.2	98.8
North Dakota	94.2	92.8	92.9	96.0	98.6	95.4
Ohio	95.6	93.9	92.0	97.9	95.2	98.2
Oklahoma	96.2	88.9	95.1	98.2	98.1	98.3
Oregon	96.5	94.4	97.1	94.2	98.0	98.6
Pennsylvania	94.2	89.2	93.1	93.7	98.6	97.9
Rhode Island	94.0	90.5	90.7	93.3	96.9	98.5
South Carolina	95.9	94.2	94.8	95.8	96.9	98.9
South Dakota	96.4	92.7	95.8	97.2	98.1	98.9
Tennessee	93.6	92.4	93.8	92.5	94.7	95.5
Texas	92.9	88.7	91.3	96.1	96.0	97.1
Utah	94.3	88.2	93.4	99.4	96.5	96.8
Vermont	93.7	89.5	94.1	94.3	95.9	96.4
Virginia	94.2	92.5	93.3	96.5	89.0	97.6
Washington	96.5	92.9	96.9	94.5	99.3	97.9
West Virginia	95.3	94.4	93.8	96.1	97.7	97.2
Wisconsin	96.6	98.3	92.6	97.7	97.2	99.3
Wyoming	96.4	94.1	95.9	97.3	98.3	97.9

Source: Compiled by New Strategist based on the Centers for Disease Control and Prevention Behavioral Risk Factor Surveillance System Survey. Internet site http://www.cdc.gov/brfss/index.htm

1.161 Women's Health: Pap Smear in Past Year, 2000

"How long has it been since your last Pap smear?"

(percent of women aged 18 or older who have ever had a Pap smear responding "past year," by state, 2000)

	Pap smear in past year
U.S. total	**70.5%**
Alabama	67.5
Alaska	76.2
Arizona	73.4
Arkansas	63.3
California	67.6
Colorado	68.9
Connecticut	76.3
Delaware	78.1
District of Columbia	76.8
Florida	69.7
Georgia	71.5
Hawaii	76.8
Idaho	59.5
Illinois	70.9
Indiana	65.5
Iowa	69.3
Kansas	67.3
Kentucky	72.9
Louisiana	77.1
Maine	72.9
Maryland	77.6
Massachusetts	77.4
Michigan	75.5
Minnesota	66.4
Mississippi	69.1
Missouri	69.9
Montana	69.4
Nebraska	73.2
Nevada	67.4
New Hampshire	74.3
New Jersey	74.0
New Mexico	67.2
New York	76.8
North Carolina	73.0
North Dakota	68.4
Ohio	70.8
Oklahoma	66.7
Oregon	62.8
Pennsylvania	70.3
Rhode Island	75.2
South Carolina	73.3
South Dakota	74.5
Tennessee	74.8
Texas	67.1
Utah	62.6
Vermont	73.3
Virginia	74.6
Washington	63.0
West Virginia	67.5
Wisconsin	68.3
Wyoming	59.5

Source: Compiled by New Strategist based on the Centers for Disease Control and Prevention Behavioral Risk Factor Surveillance System Survey, Internet site http://www.cdc.gov/brfss/index.htm

Part Two: Youth

Youth Risk Behavior Surveillance System

Youth Risk Behavior Surveillance System

This analysis and the tables in the following section appeared in
Centers for Disease Control and Prevention's Surveillance Summaries,
Morbidity and Mortality Weekly Report, *Volume 51, No. SS-4, June 28, 2002*

Jo Anne Grunbaum, Ed.D.[1]

Laura Kann, Ph.D.[1]

Steven A. Kinchen[1]

Barbara Williams, Ph.D.
Westat, Rockville, Maryland

James G. Ross, M.S.
ORC Macro, Calverton, Maryland

Richard Lowry, M.D., M.S.[1]

Lloyd Kolbe, Ph.D.[1]
[1] *Division of Adolescent and School Health*
National Center for Chronic Disease Prevention and Health Promotion

Introduction

In the United States, 70.6 percent of all deaths among youth and young adults aged 10–24 years result from only four causes: motor-vehicle crashes (31.4 percent), other unintentional injuries (12 percent), homicide (15.3 percent), and suicide (11.9 percent) (*1*). Substantial morbidity and social problems also result from the approximately 870,000 pregnancies that occur each year among women aged 15–19 years (*2*) and the estimated 3 million cases of sexually transmitted diseases (STDs) that occur each year among persons aged 10–19 years (*3*). Among adults aged 25 years or older, 64.6 percent of all deaths in the United States result from cardiovascular disease (41 percent) and cancer (23.6 percent) (*1*). Leading causes of mortality and morbidity among all age groups in the United States are related to the following categories of health behavior: behaviors that contribute to unintentional injuries and violence; tobacco use; alcohol and other drug use; sexual behaviors that contribute to unintended pregnancy and STDs, including human immunodeficiency virus (HIV) infection; unhealthy dietary behaviors; and physical inactivity. These behaviors are frequently interrelated and often are established during youth and extend into adulthood.

To monitor priority health-risk behaviors in each of these categories among youth and young adults, CDC developed the Youth Risk Behavior Surveillance System (YRBSS) (*4*). The YRBSS includes national, state, territorial, and local school-based surveys of students in grades 9–12. National surveys were conducted in 1991, 1993, 1995, 1997, 1999, and 2001. Comparable state and local surveys also were conducted.

This report summarizes results from the 2001 national school-based survey and trends during 1991–2001 in selected risk behaviors. Data from 34 state and 18 local school-based surveys also are included. The national survey and all of the state and local surveys except one were conducted during spring 2001. Hawaii conducted its survey during fall 2001.

METHODS

Sampling: National Youth Risk Behavior Survey

The 2001 national school-based YRBS employed a three-stage cluster sample design to produce a nationally representative sample of students in grades 9–12. The first-stage sampling frame contained 1,256 primary sampling units (PSUs), consisting of large counties or groups of smaller, adjacent counties. From the 1,256 PSUs, 57 were selected from 16 strata formed on the basis of the degree of urbanization and the percentage of black and Hispanic students in the PSU.[1] PSUs were selected with probability proportional to school enrollment size. At the second sampling stage, 199 schools were selected with probability proportional to school enrollment size. To enable separate analysis of data for black and Hispanic students, schools with substantial numbers of black and Hispanic students were sampled at higher rates than all other schools. The third stage of sampling consisted of randomly selecting one or two intact classes of a required subject (e.g., English or social studies) from grades 9–12 at each chosen school. All students in selected classes were eligible to participate in the survey.

A weighting factor was applied to each student record to adjust for nonresponse and for varying probabilities of selection, including those resulting from oversampling of black and Hispanic students. Numbers of students in other racial/ethnic populations (excluding white, black, and Hispanic students) were too low for meaningful analysis in this report. Weights were scaled so that 1) the weighted count of students was equal to the total sample size, and 2) the weighted proportions of students in each grade matched national population proportions.

National data are representative of students in grades 9–12 in public and private schools in the 50 states and the District of Columbia. SUDAAN was used to compute 95 percent confidence intervals, which were used to determine differences between subpopulations at the p<0.05 level (5). Differences between prevalence estimates were considered statistically significant if the 95 percent confidence intervals did not overlap. Secular trends were analyzed by using logistic regression analyses that controlled for sex, grade, and race/ethnicity and that simultaneously assessed linear and higher order (i.e., quadratic) time effects (6). Quadratic trends indicate a significant but nonlinear trend in the data. When the trend includes significant linear and quadratic components, the data demonstrate certain nonlinear variation (e.g., leveling off or change of direction) in addition to a linear trend. For the national YRBS, 13,627 questionnaires were completed in 150 schools. Of the 13,627 completed questionnaires, 26 failed quality control (a questionnaire that fails quality control has fewer than 20 valid items after editing) and were excluded from analyses for a total of 13,601 usable questionnaires. The school response rate was 75 percent, and the student response rate was 83 percent, resulting in an overall response rate of 63 percent. Additional information regarding the YRBS is available at http://www.cdc.gov/yrbs.

State and local surveys, by year of survey, number of states, and number of large cities—United States, Youth Risk Behavior Surveillance System, 1991–2001

year of survey	no. of states	no. of large cities
1991	26	11
1993	40	14
1995	40	17
1997	38	17
1999	41	17
2001	38	19

Sampling: State and Local Youth Risk Behavior Surveys

In 2001, each state and local school-based YRBS employed a two-stage cluster sample design to produce representative samples of students in grades 9–12 in its jurisdiction. In the majority of states and cities, schools were selected with probability proportional to school enrollment size. At the second sampling stage, intact classes of a required subject or intact classes during a required period (e.g., second period) were selected randomly. All students in selected classes were eligible to participate in the survey. Certain states and cities modified these procedures to meet their individual needs. For example, all schools, rather than a sample of schools, were selected to participate.

In 2001, the student sample sizes for the state and local YRBS ranged from 955 to 7,191. School response rates ranged from 42 percent to 100 percent; student response rates ranged from 48 percent to 96 percent; and overall response rates ranged from 41 percent to 90 percent. School response rate multiplied by student response rate produces an overall response rate for each site. For surveys from 22 states and 14 large cities, each with an overall response rate of greater than or equal to 60 percent and appropriate documentation, the data were weighted and are considered representative of students in grades 9–12 in that jurisdiction. For surveys from 12 states and 4 large cities that did not have an overall response rate of greater than or equal to 60 percent and appropriate documentation, the data were not weighted. Unweighted data from these 12 states and 4 large cities apply only to students participating in the survey. The Illinois survey excludes students from Chicago; the Louisiana survey excludes students from New Orleans; and the New York survey excludes students from New York City.

Body mass index (BMI) was calculated from self-reported height and weight and then applied to reference data from the National Health and Nutrition Examination Survey (7) to determine the percentage of students who were at risk for becoming overweight and who were overweight. At risk for becoming overweight was defined as a BMI greater than or equal to 85th percentile and greater than 95th percentile by age and sex. Overweight was defined as a BMI greater than or equal to 95th percentile by age and sex. A BMI greater than or equal to 95th percentile by age and sex among youth is approximately equivalent to a BMI greater than or equal to 30 among adults. For an adult, a BMI of 30 is approximately 30 pounds overweight.

Data Collection

Survey procedures for the national, state, and local surveys were designed to protect students' privacy by allowing for anonymous and voluntary participation. Students completed the self-administered questionnaire during one class period and recorded their responses directly on a computer-scanable booklet or answer sheet. The core questionnaire contained 87 multiple-choice questions. To meet individual needs, some states and large cities added or deleted some questions. Before the survey was administered, local parental permission procedures were followed.

RESULTS

Behaviors That Contribute to Unintentional Injuries

• **Seat Belt Use**. Nationwide, 14.1 percent of students had rarely or never worn seat belts when riding in a car driven by someone else (Figure 1). Male students (18.1 percent) were significantly more likely than female students (10.2 percent) to have rarely or never worn seat belts. This significant sex difference was identified for white and Hispanic students and for students in all of the grade subpopula-

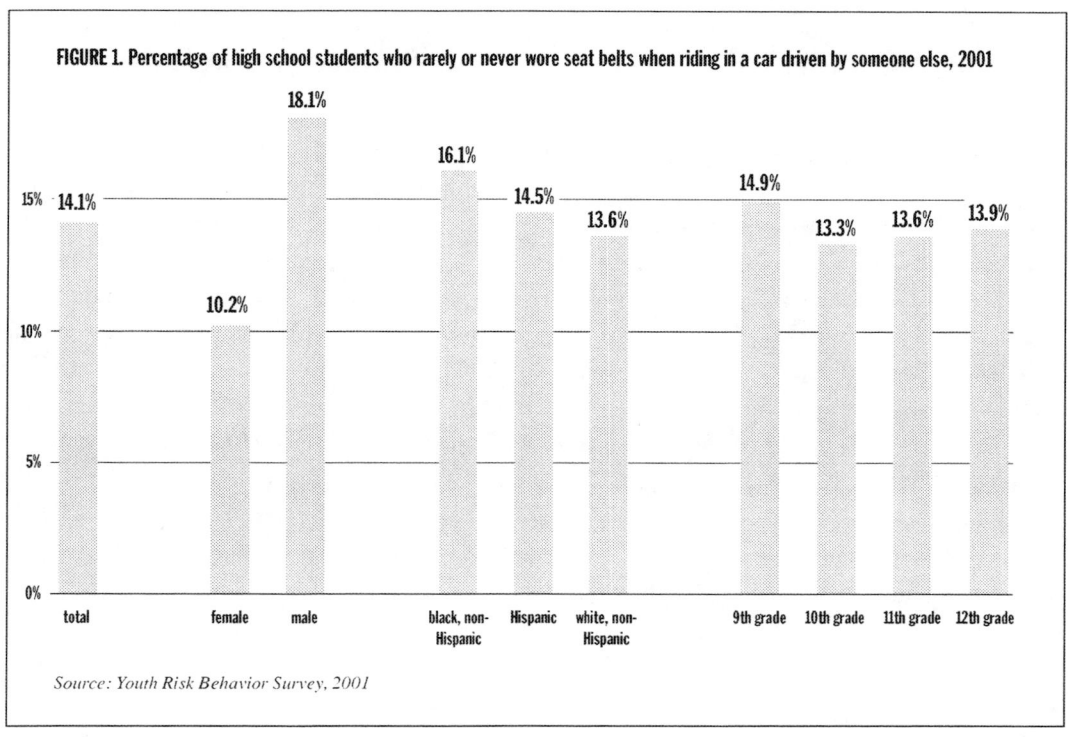

FIGURE 1. Percentage of high school students who rarely or never wore seat belts when riding in a car driven by someone else, 2001

Source: Youth Risk Behavior Survey, 2001

FIGURE 2. Percentage of high school students who rode with a driver who had been drinking alcohol one or more times during the 30 days preceding the survey, 2001

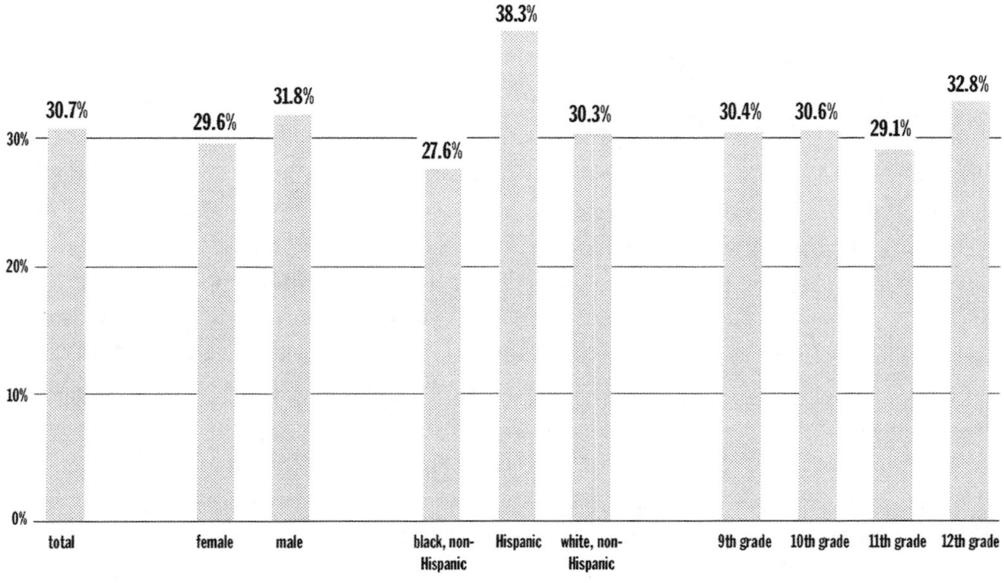

Source: Youth Risk Behavior Survey, 2001

tions. Prevalence of rarely or never wearing seat belts varied fourfold from 7.5 percent to 27.4 percent (median: 14.9 percent) across state surveys, and varied sixfold from 6.7 percent to 38.2 percent (median: 13.5 percent) across local surveys.

- **Motorcycle Helmet Use.** Nationwide, 25.3 percent of students had ridden a motorcycle during the 12 months preceding the survey. Of these students, 37.2 percent rarely or never wore a motorcycle helmet. Male students (40.9 percent) were significantly more likely than female students (30.1 percent) to have rarely or never worn a motorcycle helmet. This significant sex difference was identified for white students and students in grade 12. Overall, Hispanic students (55.3 percent) were significantly more likely than white students (33.6 percent) to report this behavior. This significant racial/ethnic difference was identified for both female and male students. Prevalence of rarely or never wearing a motorcycle helmet varied threefold from 19.5 percent to 66.1 percent (median: 40.3 percent) across state surveys and from 30.6 percent to 67.6 percent (median: 42.5 percent) across local surveys.

- **Bicycle Helmet Use.** Nationwide, 65.1 percent of students had ridden a bicycle during the 12 months preceding the survey. Of these students, 84.7 percent rarely or never wore a bicycle helmet. Overall, black students (90.7 percent) were significantly more likely than white students (83.6 percent) to have rarely or never worn a bicycle helmet. This significant racial/ethnic difference was identified for female students. Prevalence of rarely or never wearing a bicycle helmet ranged from 54.8 percent to 95.8 percent (median: 88.6 percent) across state surveys and from 70.1 percent to 94.4 percent (median: 87.9 percent) across local surveys.

- **Riding with a Driver Who Had Been Drinking Alcohol.** During the 30 days preceding the survey, 30.7 percent of students nationwide had ridden one or more times with a driver who had been drinking alcohol (Figure 2). Male students in grade 11 (32.8 percent) were significantly more likely than female students in grade 11 (25.4 percent) to report this behavior. Overall, Hispanic students (38.3 percent) were significantly more likely than white and black students (30.3 percent and 27.6 percent, respectively) to have ridden with a driver who had been drinking alcohol. This significant racial/ethnic difference was identified for female students. Prevalence of riding with a driver who had been drinking alcohol ranged from 17.1 percent to 43.5 percent (median: 31.8 percent) across state surveys and from 19.3 percent to 39.6 percent (median: 29.5 percent) across local surveys.

- **Driving After Drinking Alcohol.** During the 30 days preceding the survey, 13.3 percent of students nationwide had driven a car or other vehicle one or more times after drinking alcohol. Male students (17.2 percent) were significantly more likely than female students (9.5 percent) to have driven after drinking alcohol. This significant sex difference was identified for all the racial/ethnic subpopulations and for students in grades 9, 11, and 12. Overall, white students and Hispanic students (14.7 percent and 13 percent, respectively) were significantly more likely than black students (7.7 percent) to have driven after drinking alcohol. White and Hispanic female students (10.9 percent and 10.5 percent, respectively) were significantly more likely than black female students (3.3 percent), and white male students (18.6 percent) were significantly more likely than black male students (12.5 percent) to report this behavior. Overall, students in grade 10 (10.4 percent) were significantly more likely than students in grade 9 (6.6 percent) to have driven after drinking alcohol; students in grade 11 (16.7 percent) were significantly more likely than students in grades 9 and 10 (6.6 percent and 10.4 percent, respectively) to report this behavior; and students in grade 12 (22.1 percent) were significantly more likely than students in grades 9, 10, and 11 (6.6 percent, 10.4 percent, and 16.7 percent, respectively) to report this behavior. Prevalence of driving after drinking alcohol varied fourfold from 6.4 percent to 26.8 percent (median: 13 percent) across state surveys and varied fourfold across local surveys from 3.8 percent to 13.8 percent (median: 8 percent).

Behaviors That Contribute to Violence

• **Carrying a Weapon.** Nationwide, 17.4 percent of students had carried a weapon (e.g., a gun, knife, or club) on one or more of the 30 days preceding the survey. Male students (29.3 percent) were significantly more likely than female students (6.2 percent) to have carried a weapon. This significant sex difference was identified for all the racial/ethnic and grade subpopulations. Black female students (8.6 percent) were significantly more likely than white female students (5.1 percent) to have carried a weapon, and white male students (31.3 percent) were significantly more likely than black male students (22.4 percent) to have done so. Prevalence of carrying a weapon ranged from 10.6 percent to 22.9 percent (median: 16.2 percent) across state surveys and from 8.3 percent to 21.2 percent (median: 13.7 percent) across local surveys.

Nationwide, 5.7 percent of students had carried a gun on one or more of the 30 days preceding the survey. Male students (10.3 percent) were significantly more likely than female students (1.3 percent) to have carried a gun. This significant sex difference was identified for all the racial/ethnic and grade subpopulations. Prevalence of carrying a gun varied threefold from 2.9 percent to 10.1 percent (median: 5 percent), across state surveys and varied fivefold from 1.3 percent to 7.1 percent (median: 4.8 percent), across local surveys.

• **Physical Fighting.** Among students nationwide, 33.2 percent had been in a physical fight one or more times during the 12 months preceding the survey. Male students (43.1 percent) were significantly more likely than female students (23.9 percent) to have been in a physical fight. This significant sex difference was identified for all the racial/ethnic and grade subpopulations. Black and Hispanic female students (29.6 percent and 29.3 percent, respectively) were significantly more likely than white female students (21.7 percent) to report this behavior. Overall, students in grades 9 and 10 (39.5 percent and 34.7 percent, respectively) were significantly more likely than students in grades 11 and 12 (29.1 percent and 26.5 percent, respectively) to report this behavior. Across state surveys, prevalence of being in a physical fight ranged from 25.9 percent to 35.6 percent (median: 31.4 percent). Across local surveys, prevalence ranged from 30.3 percent to 43.4 percent (median: 34.6 percent).

Nationwide, 4 percent of students had been treated by a doctor or nurse for injuries sustained in a physical fight one or more times during the 12 months preceding the survey. Male students (5.2 percent) were significantly more likely than female students (2.9 percent) to have been injured in a physical fight. This significant sex difference was identified for white students and students in grades 9 and 12. Overall, black students (5.3 percent) were significantly more likely than white students (3.4 percent) to have been injured in a physical fight. This significant racial/ethnic difference was identified for female students. Across state surveys, prevalence of injurious physical fighting varied threefold from 2 percent to 6.4 percent (median: 3.5 percent). Across local surveys, prevalence ranged from 3.9 percent to 7.1 percent (median: 4.6 percent).

• **Dating Violence.** Nationwide, 9.5 percent of students had been hit, slapped, or physically hurt on purpose by their boyfriend or girlfriend one or more times during the 12 months preceding the survey. Prevalence of dating violence ranged from 6.9 percent to 18.1 percent (median: 10.3 percent) across state surveys and from 6 percent to 17.2 percent (median: 10.2 percent) across local surveys.

- **Forced Sexual Intercourse**. Nationwide, 7.7 percent of students had ever been forced to have sexual intercourse when they did not want to. Female students (10.3 percent) were significantly more likely than male students (5.1 percent) to have been forced to have sexual intercourse. This significant sex difference was identified for white and Hispanic students and students in grades 10, 11, and 12. Overall, black students (9.6 percent) were significantly more likely than white students (6.9 percent) to have been forced to have sexual intercourse. This significant racial/ethnic difference was identified for male students. Prevalence of forced sexual intercourse ranged from 5.4 percent to 12.1 percent (median: 8.5 percent) across state surveys and from 5.6 percent to 13.3 percent (median: 9.2 percent) across local surveys.

- **School-Related Violence**. Nationwide, 6.6 percent of students had missed one or more days of school during the 30 days preceding the survey because they felt unsafe at school or on their way to or from school. Overall, Hispanic and black students (10.2 percent and 9.8 percent, respectively) were significantly more likely than white students (5 percent) to have missed school because they felt unsafe. This significant racial/ethnic difference was identified for both male and female students. Overall, students in grade 9 (8.8 percent) were significantly more likely than students in grades 11 and 12 (5.9 percent and 4.4 percent, respectively) to report this behavior. Prevalence across state surveys varied sixfold from 3 percent to 16.9 percent (median: 7.3 percent). Prevalence across local surveys ranged from 6.6 percent to 17 percent (median: 11.4 percent).

Among students nationwide, 6.4 percent carried a weapon on school property on one or more of the 30 days preceding the survey. Male students (10.2 percent) were significantly more likely than female students (2.9 percent) to have carried a weapon on school property. This significant sex difference was identified for white and Hispanic students and students in all the grade subpopulations. Prevalence of carrying a weapon on school property varied fourfold from 2.4 percent to 10.3 percent (median: 6.2 percent) across state surveys and ranged from 4.1 percent to 9.3 percent (median: 5.5 percent) across local surveys.

Nationwide, 8.9 percent of students had been threatened or injured with a weapon on school property one or more times during the 12 months preceding the survey. Male students (11.5 percent) were significantly more likely than female students (6.5 percent) to have been threatened or injured with a weapon on school property. This significant sex difference was identified for white and black students and students in all the grade subpopulations. Overall, students in grade 9 (12.7 percent) were significantly more likely than students in grades 10, 11, and 12 (9.1 percent, 6.9 percent, and 5.3 percent, respectively) to have been threatened or injured with a weapon on school property, and students in grade 10 (9.1 percent) were significantly more likely than students in grade 12 (5.3 percent) to report this behavior. Prevalence of being threatened or injured with a weapon on school property ranged from 5.9 percent to 11.2 percent (median: 8.5 percent) across state surveys and from 7.9 percent to 14.8 percent (median: 9.8 percent) across local surveys.

Nationwide, 12.5 percent of students had been in a physical fight on school property one or more times during the 12 months preceding the survey. Male students (18 percent) were significantly more likely than female students (7.2 percent) to have been in a physical fight on school property. This significant sex difference was identified for all the racial/ethnic and grade subpopulations. Overall, black students (16.8 percent) were significantly more likely than white students (11.2 percent) to have been in a physical fight on school property. Black and Hispanic female students (12.7 percent and 11 percent, respectively) were significantly more likely than white female students (5.4 percent) to report this behavior. Overall, students in grades 9 and 10 (17.3 percent and 13.5 percent, respectively) were significantly more likely than students in grades 11 and 12 (9.4 percent and 7.5 percent, respectively) to have been in a physical fight on school property, and students in grade 9 (17.3 percent) were significantly more likely than students in grade 10 (13.5 percent) to report this behavior. Across state surveys, prevalence of having engaged in a physical fight on school property ranged from 8.8 percent to 14.2 percent (median: 11.8 percent). Across local surveys, prevalence ranged from 11.2 percent to 21.5 percent (median: 14 percent).

• **Sadness and Suicide Ideation and Attempts.** Nationwide, during the 12 months preceding the survey, 28.3 percent of students had felt so sad or hopeless almost every day for two or more weeks in a row that they stopped doing some usual activities. Overall, female students (34.5 percent) were significantly more likely than male students (21.6 percent) to have felt sad or hopeless almost every day for two or more weeks. This significant sex difference was identified for all the racial/ethnic and grade subpopulations. Overall, Hispanic students (34 percent) were significantly more likely than black and white students (28.8 percent and 26.5 percent, respectively) to have felt sad or hopeless almost every day for two or more weeks. Hispanic female students (42.3 percent) were significantly more likely than white female students (32.3 percent) and Hispanic male students (25.4 percent) were significantly more likely than white male students (20.5 percent) to report this behavior. Prevalence of feeling sad or hopeless ranged from 20.5 percent to 30.7 percent (median: 27.2 percent) across state surveys and from 24.2 percent to 35.3 percent (median: 31.1 percent) across local surveys.

During the 12 months preceding the survey, 19 percent of students had seriously considered attempting suicide. Female students (23.6 percent) were significantly more likely than male students (14.2 percent) to have considered attempting suicide. This significant sex difference was identified for

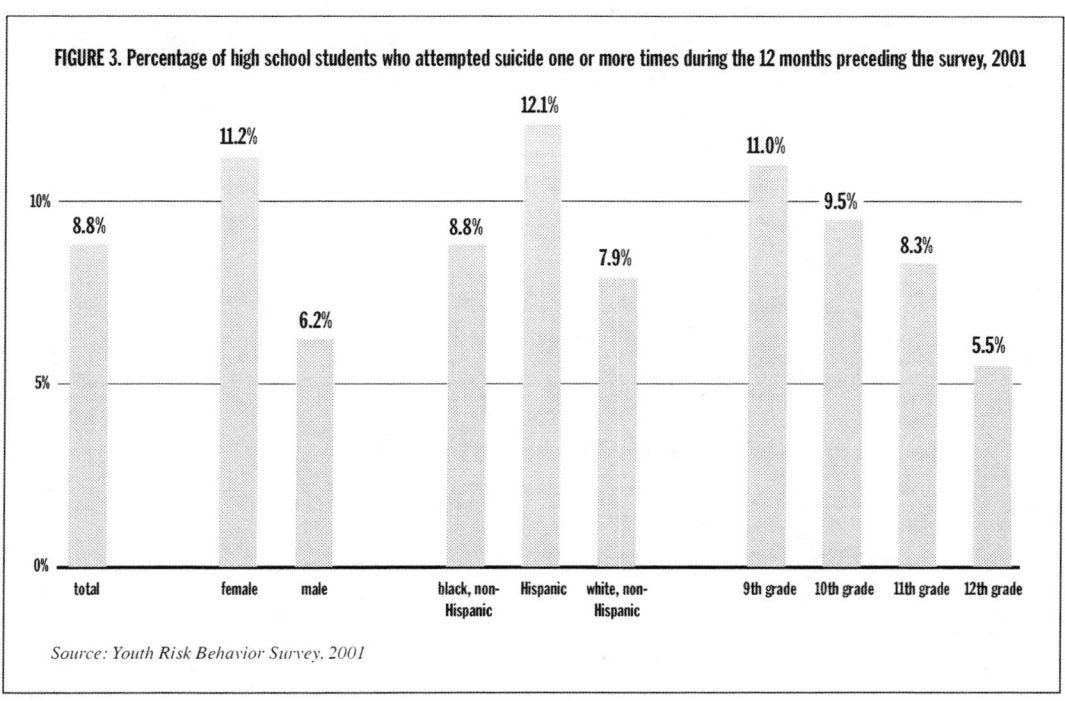

FIGURE 3. Percentage of high school students who attempted suicide one or more times during the 12 months preceding the survey, 2001

Source: Youth Risk Behavior Survey, 2001

all the racial/ethnic subpopulations and students in grades 9, 10, and 11. Overall, white and Hispanic students (19.7 percent and 19.4 percent, respectively) were significantly more likely than black students (13.3 percent) to have considered attempting suicide. Hispanic and white female students (26.5 percent and 24.2 percent, respectively) were significantly more likely than black female students (17.2 percent), and white male students (14.9 percent) were significantly more likely than black male students (9.2 percent) to have considered attempting suicide. Prevalence of seriously considering suicide ranged from 14.6 percent to 21.9 percent (median: 18.4 percent) across state surveys and from 10 percent to 21 percent (median: 16 percent) across local surveys. During the 12 months preceding the survey, 14.8 percent of students nationwide had made a specific plan to attempt suicide. Overall, female students (17.7 percent) were significantly more likely than male students (11.8 percent) to have made a suicide plan. This significant sex difference was identified for all the racial/ethnic subpopulations and students in grades 9, 10, and 11. Overall, white and Hispanic students (15.3 percent and 14.1 percent, respectively) were significantly more likely than black students (10.3 percent) to have made a suicide plan. White female students (18 percent) were significantly more likely than black female students (13 percent), and white male students (12.5 percent) were significantly more likely than black male students (7.5 percent) to have made a suicide plan. Overall, students in grade 9 (16 percent) were significantly more likely than students in grade 12 (12.2 percent) to have made a suicide plan. Prevalence of having made a suicide plan ranged from 11.3 percent to 17.7 percent (median: 13.9 percent) across state surveys and from 7.9 percent to 16.9 percent (median: 13.3 percent) across local surveys.

Nationwide, 8.8 percent of students had attempted suicide one or more times during the 12 months preceding the survey (Figure 3). Female students (11.2 percent) were significantly more likely than male students (6.2 percent) to have attempted suicide. This significant sex difference was identified for white and Hispanic students and students in grades 9, 10, and 11. Overall, Hispanic students (12.1 percent) were significantly more likely than black and white students (8.8 percent and 7.9 percent, respectively) to have attempted suicide. This significant racial/ethnic difference was identified for Hispanic female students. Overall, students in grades 9, 10, and 11 (11 percent, 9.5 percent, and 8.3 percent, respectively) were significantly more likely than students in grade 12 (5.5 percent) to have attempted suicide. The percentage of students attempting suicide ranged from 6.3 percent to 13.4 percent (median: 8.6 percent) across state surveys and from 7.4 percent to 13 percent (median: 10.4 percent) across local surveys.

Nationwide, 2.6 percent of students made a suicide attempt during the 12 months preceding the survey that resulted in an injury, poisoning, or overdose that had to be treated by a doctor or nurse. Overall, students in grades 9 and 10 (3.2 percent and 3 percent, respectively) were significantly more likely than students in grade 12 (1.6 percent) to have made a suicide attempt that required medical attention. Prevalence of injurious suicide attempts varied fourfold from 1.2 percent to 4.6 percent (median: 2.5 percent) across state surveys and varied threefold from 1.7 percent to 5.7 percent (median: 3.4 percent) across local surveys.

Tobacco Use

• **Cigarette Use**. Nationwide, 63.9 percent of students had ever tried cigarette smoking (even one or two puffs) (i.e., lifetime cigarette use). Male students (66.3 percent) were significantly more likely than female students (61.6 percent) to have ever tried cigarette smoking. Overall, Hispanic students

(69.3 percent) were significantly more likely than black students (58.3 percent) to have ever tried cigarette smoking. Hispanic female students (67.8 percent) were significantly more likely than black female students (56.7 percent), and Hispanic and white male students (70.9 percent and 67.4 percent, respectively) were significantly more likely than black male students (59.9 percent) to report this behavior. Overall, students in grades 11 and 12 (65.9 percent and 71.1 percent, respectively) were significantly more likely than students in grade 9 (58.4 percent) to have ever tried cigarette smoking, and students in grade 12 (71.1 percent) were significantly more likely than students in grade 10 (62.6 percent) to report this behavior. Prevalence of lifetime cigarette use ranged from 30.5 percent to 71.6 percent (median: 66 percent) across state surveys and from 48.9 percent to 68 percent (median: 58 percent) across local surveys.

One fifth of students (20 percent) nationwide had ever smoked one or more cigarettes every day for 30 days (i.e., lifetime daily cigarette use). Overall, white students (23.9 percent) were significantly more likely than Hispanic and black students (12.4 percent and 7.7 percent, respectively), and Hispanic students (12.4 percent) were significantly more likely than black students (7.7 percent) to report lifetime daily cigarette use. These significant racial/ethnic differences were identified for female students. White male students (24.7 percent) were significantly more likely than Hispanic and black male students (13.4 percent and 9 percent, respectively) to report lifetime daily cigarette use. Overall, students in grades 11 and 12 (22.1 percent and 26.9 percent, respectively) were significantly more likely than students in grade 9 (14.3 percent) to report lifetime daily cigarette use, and students in grade 12 (26.9 percent) were significantly more likely than students in grade 10 (19.1 percent) to report this behavior. Across state surveys, prevalence of lifetime daily cigarette use varied threefold from 8.5 percent to 25.6 percent (median: 19.5 percent). Across local surveys, prevalence varied threefold from 5.7 percent to 16.8 percent (median: 9.4 percent).

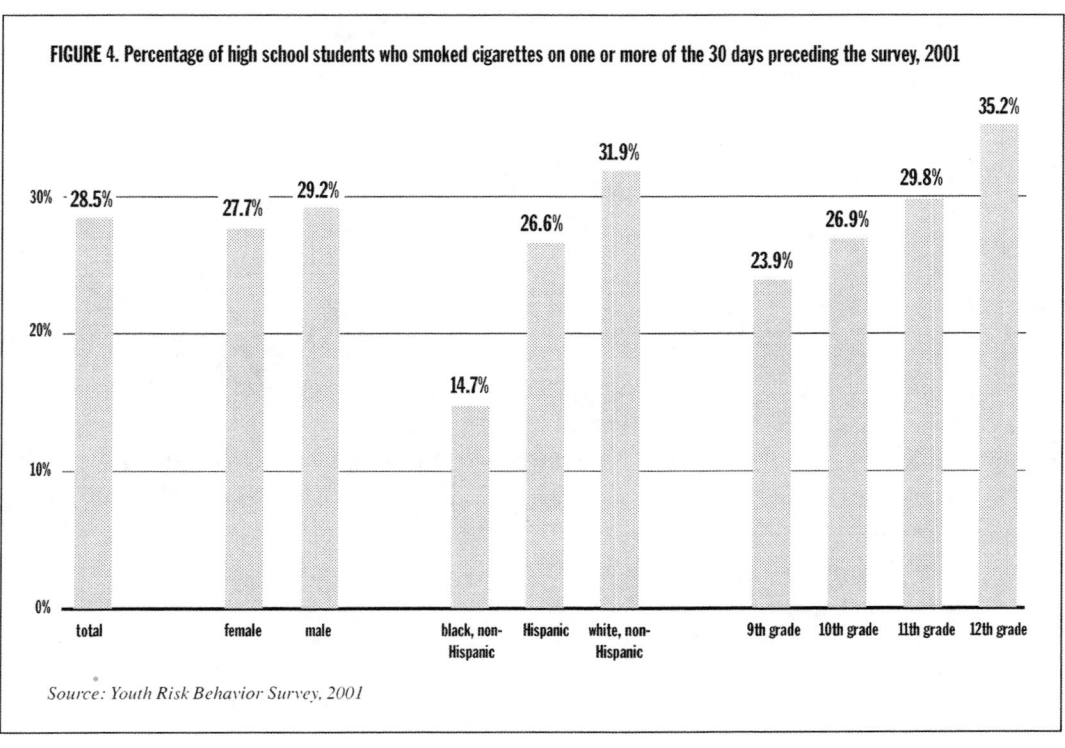

FIGURE 4. Percentage of high school students who smoked cigarettes on one or more of the 30 days preceding the survey, 2001

Source: Youth Risk Behavior Survey, 2001

Nationwide, 28.5 percent of students had smoked cigarettes on one or more of the 30 days preceding the survey (i.e., current cigarette use) (Figure 4). White and Hispanic students (31.9 percent and 26.6 percent, respectively) were significantly more likely than black students (14.7 percent) to report current cigarette use. This significant racial/ethnic difference was identified for both female and male students. Overall, students in grade 12 (35.2 percent) were significantly more likely than students in grades 9 and 10 (23.9 percent and 26.9 percent, respectively) to report current cigarette use. Across state surveys, prevalence of current cigarette use varied fourfold from 8.3 percent to 35.3 percent (median: 27.6 percent). Across local surveys, prevalence ranged from 11.9 percent to 24.7 percent (median: 17 percent).

Nationwide, 13.8 percent of students had smoked cigarettes on 20 or more of the 30 days preceding the survey (i.e., current frequent cigarette use). Overall, white students (17.2 percent) were significantly more likely than Hispanic and black students (7.3 percent and 4.6 percent, respectively) to report current frequent cigarette use. This significant racial/ethnic difference was identified for both female and male students. Overall, students in grades 11 and 12 (15.2 percent and 21 percent, respectively) were significantly more likely than students in grade 9 (8.9 percent) to report current frequent cigarette use, and students in grade 12 (21 percent) were significantly more likely than students in grade 10 (12.3 percent) to report this behavior. Prevalence of current frequent cigarette use varied fourfold from 4.2 percent to 18.8 percent (median: 14 percent) across state surveys and varied fourfold from 2.7 percent to 9.9 percent (median: 4.8 percent) across local surveys.

Nationwide, 4.1 percent of students who reported current cigarette use, smoked more than 10 cigarettes per day on the days they smoked. Overall, male students (5.2 percent) were significantly more likely than female students (3.1 percent) to smoke more than 10 cigarettes per day. This significant sex difference was identified for white students. Overall, white students (5.3 percent) were significantly more likely than Hispanic and black students (1.8 percent and 1.1 percent, respectively) to smoke more than 10 cigarettes per day. This significant racial/ethnic difference was identified for male students. White female students (4 percent) were significantly more likely than black female students (0.7 percent) to smoke more than 10 cigarettes per day. Overall, students in grades 11 and 12 (4.8 percent and 6.6 percent, respectively) were significantly more likely than students in grade 9 (2.2 percent) to smoke more than 10 cigarettes per day, and students in grade 12 (6.6 percent) were significantly more likely than students in grade 10 (3.6 percent) to report this behavior. Prevalence varied sevenfold from 1 percent to 7.3 percent (median: 3.7 percent) across state surveys and varied eightfold from 0.3 percent to 2.5 percent (median: 1.1 percent) across local surveys.

• **Smokeless Tobacco Use**. Nationwide, 8.2 percent of students had used smokeless tobacco (chewing tobacco, snuff, or dip) on one or more of the 30 days preceding the survey (i.e., current smokeless tobacco use). Overall, male students (14.8 percent) were significantly more likely than female students (1.9 percent) to report current smokeless tobacco use. This significant sex difference was identified for all the racial/ethnic and grade subpopulations. Overall, white and Hispanic students (10.3 percent and 4.1 percent, respectively) were significantly more likely than black students (1.8 percent) to report current smokeless tobacco use, and white students (10.3 percent) were significantly more likely than Hispanic students (4.1 percent) to do so. These significant racial/ethnic differences were identified for male students. White female students (2.1 percent) were significantly more likely than black female students (0.7 percent) to report current smokeless tobacco use. Prevalence of current smokeless tobacco use varied sixfold from 2.9 percent to 18.1 percent (median: 8.2 percent) across state surveys and from 1.1 percent to 6.4 percent (median: 3 percent) across local surveys.

- **Cigar Use**. Nationwide, 15.2 percent of students had smoked cigars, cigarillos, or little cigars on one or more of the 30 days preceding the survey (i.e., current cigar use). Overall, male students (22.1 percent) were significantly more likely than female students (8.5 percent) to report current cigar use. This significant sex difference was identified for all the racial/ethnic and grade subpopulations. White male students (23.8 percent) were significantly more likely than black male students (15.8 percent) to report current cigar use. Overall, students in grade 12 (18 percent) were significantly more likely than students in grade 9 (12.5 percent) to report current cigar use. Prevalence of current cigar use varied fivefold from 4.1 percent to 19.3 percent (median: 14.8 percent) across state surveys and varied three-fold from 5.1 percent to 16.3 percent (median: 12 percent) across local surveys.

- **Current Tobacco Use**. Nationwide, 33.9 percent of students had reported current cigarette use, current smokeless tobacco use, or current cigar use on one or more of the 30 days preceding the survey (i.e., current tobacco use). Male students (38.5 percent) were significantly more likely than female students (29.5 percent) to report current tobacco use. This significant sex difference was identified for white students and students in grades 11 and 12. Overall, white and Hispanic students (37.7 percent and 29.4 percent, respectively) were significantly more likely than black students (19.4 percent) to report current tobacco use, and white students (37.7 percent) were significantly more likely than Hispanic students (29.4 percent) to do so. White and Hispanic female students (32.3 percent and 27.2 percent, respectively) were significantly more likely than black female students (17.4 percent) to report current tobacco use, and white male students (43.4 percent) were significantly more likely than Hispanic and black male students (31.5 percent and 21.6 percent, respectively) to do so. Overall, students in grades 11 and 12 (36.1 percent and 41 percent, respectively) were significantly more likely than students in grade 9 (28.1 percent) to report current tobacco use, and students in grade 12 (41 percent) were significantly more likely than students in grade 10 (32.6 percent) to do so. Across state surveys, current tobacco use varied fourfold from 9.8 percent to 41.4 percent (median: 32.5 percent). Across local surveys, prevalence ranged from 14.7 percent to 27.1 percent (median: 19.1 percent).

- **Access to Cigarettes and Proof of Age**. Data regarding access to cigarettes are reported only for those students under age 18 years who reported current cigarette use. Nationwide, 19.1 percent of these students had purchased their cigarettes in a store or gas station during the 30 days preceding the survey. Male students (25.7 percent) were significantly more likely than female students (13.1 percent) to have done so. This significant sex difference was identified for white students and students in all of the grade subpopulations. Overall, students in grades 10, 11, and 12 (19.1 percent, 28.7 percent, and 23.6 percent, respectively) were significantly more likely than students in grade 9 (8.8 percent) to have purchased cigarettes in a store or gas station, and students in grade 11 (28.7 percent) were significantly more likely than students in grade 10 (19.1 percent) to have done so. State prevalence varied ninefold from 4.4 percent to 39.1 percent (median: 18.6 percent), and local prevalence varied three-fold from 14.2 percent to 46.4 percent (median: 26.9 percent). Approximately two thirds of students (67.2 percent) who purchased or attempted to purchase cigarettes in a store or gas station during the 30 days preceding the survey had not been asked to show proof of age. State prevalence ranged from 60 percent to 74.1 percent (median: 69.7 percent).

Alcohol and Other Drug Use

• **Alcohol Use**. Nationwide, 78.2 percent of students had had one or more drinks of alcohol during their lifetime (i.e., lifetime alcohol use). Overall, Hispanic and white students (80.8 percent and 80.1 percent, respectively) were significantly more likely than black students (69.1 percent) to report lifetime alcohol use. This significant racial/ethnic difference was identified for both female and male students. Overall, students in grades 11 and 12 (80.4 percent and 85.1 percent, respectively) were significantly more likely than students in grade 9 (73.1 percent) to report lifetime alcohol use, and students in grade 12 (85.1 percent) were significantly more likely than students in grade 10 (76.3 percent) to do so. Prevalence of lifetime alcohol use ranged from 40.6 percent to 83.4 percent (median: 78.9 percent) across state surveys and from 57.7 percent to 81.1 percent (median: 73.9 percent) across local surveys.

Nearly one half (47.1 percent) of students nationwide had had one or more drinks of alcohol on one or more of the 30 days preceding the survey (i.e., current alcohol use) (Figure 5). Male students in grade 11 (53.6 percent) were significantly more likely than female students in grade 11 (45.1 percent) to report current alcohol use. Overall, white and Hispanic students (50.4 percent and 49.2 percent, respectively) were significantly more likely than black students (32.7 percent) to report current alcohol use. This significant racial/ethnic difference was identified for female and male students. Overall, students in grades 11 and 12 (49.3 percent and 55.2 percent, respectively) were significantly more likely than students in grade 9 (41.1 percent) to report current alcohol use, and students in grade 12 (55.2 percent) were significantly more likely than students in grade 10 (45.2 percent) to report this behavior. Across state surveys, prevalence of current alcohol use varied threefold from 17.9 percent to 59.2 percent (median: 47.8 percent). Across local surveys, prevalence ranged from 28.3 percent to 45.4 percent (median: 39.8 percent).

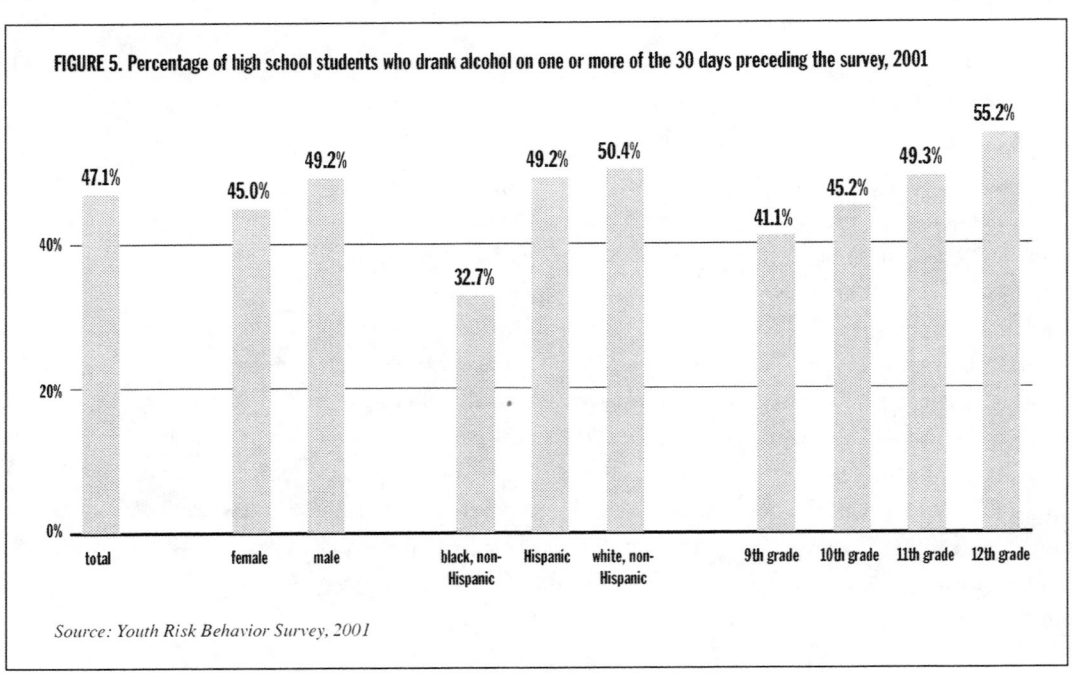

FIGURE 5. Percentage of high school students who drank alcohol on one or more of the 30 days preceding the survey, 2001

Source: Youth Risk Behavior Survey, 2001

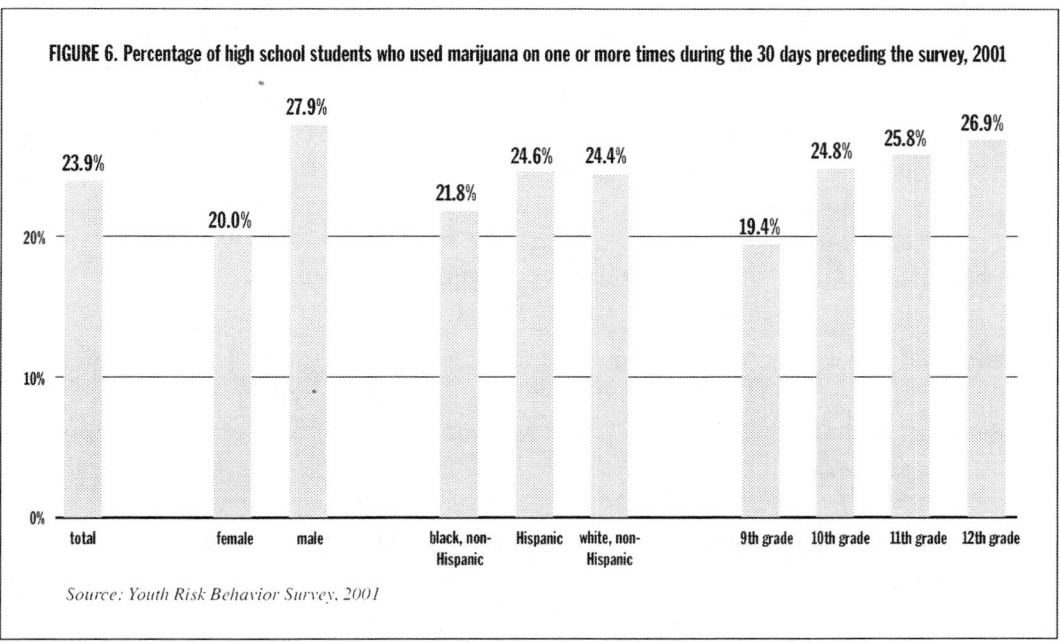

FIGURE 6. Percentage of high school students who used marijuana on one or more times during the 30 days preceding the survey, 2001

Source: Youth Risk Behavior Survey, 2001

Nationwide, 29.9 percent of students had had five or more drinks of alcohol on one or more occasions during the 30 days preceding the survey (i.e., episodic heavy drinking). Overall, male students (33.5 percent) were significantly more likely than female students (26.4 percent) to report episodic heavy drinking. This significant sex difference was identified for white and black students and students in grades 11 and 12. Overall, white and Hispanic students (34 percent and 30.1 percent, respectively) were significantly more likely than black students (11.1 percent) to report episodic heavy drinking. This significant racial/ethnic difference was identified for both female and male students. Overall, students in grades 11 and 12 (32.2 percent and 36.7 percent, respectively) were significantly more likely than students in grade 9 (24.5 percent) to report episodic heavy drinking, and students in grade 12 (36.7 percent) were significantly more likely than students in grade 10 (28.2 percent) to report this behavior. Prevalence of episodic heavy drinking varied fourfold from 10.9 percent to 41.5 percent (median: 30.3 percent) across state surveys and ranged from 10.6 percent to 26.1 percent (median: 19.9 percent) across local surveys.

• **Marijuana Use**. Nationwide, 42.4 percent of students had used marijuana during their lifetime (i.e., lifetime marijuana use). Overall, male students (46.5 percent) were significantly more likely than female students (38.4 percent) to report lifetime marijuana use. This significant sex difference was identified for white and Hispanic students and students in grades 9, 10, and 11. Overall, students in grades 10, 11, and 12 (41.7 percent, 47.2 percent, and 51.5 percent, respectively) were significantly more likely than students in grade 9 (32.7 percent) to report lifetime marijuana use, and students in grade 12 (51.5 percent) were significantly more likely than students in grade 10 (41.7 percent) to report this behavior. Prevalence of lifetime marijuana use ranged from 19.7 percent to 50.8 percent (median: 41.3 percent) across state surveys and from 29.7 percent to 49.7 percent (median: 40.6 percent) across local surveys.

Approximately one fourth (23.9 percent) of students had used marijuana one or more times during the 30 days preceding the survey (i.e., current marijuana use) (Figure 6). Overall, male students (27.9 percent) were significantly more likely than female students (20 percent) to report current marijuana use. This significant sex difference was identified for white and black students and all grade subpopulations. Overall, students in grades 10, 11, and 12 (24.8 percent, 25.8 percent, and 26.9 percent, respectively) were significantly more likely than students in grade 9 (19.4 percent) to report current marijuana use. Prevalence of current marijuana use varied threefold from 9.7 percent to 33.2 percent (median: 23.4 percent) across state surveys and ranged from 16.8 percent to 28.7 percent (median: 20.4 percent) across local surveys.

- **Cocaine Use**. Nationwide, 9.4 percent of students had used a form of cocaine (e.g., powder, crack—pellet-sized pieces of highly purified cocaine—or freebase—a process whereby cocaine is dissolved in ether or sodium and the precipitate filtered off) during their lifetime (i.e., lifetime cocaine use). Overall, Hispanic and white students (14.9 percent and 9.9 percent, respectively) were significantly more likely than black students (2.1 percent) to report lifetime cocaine use, and Hispanic students (14.9 percent) were significantly more likely than white students (9.9 percent) to report this behavior. These significant racial/ethnic differences were identified for male students. Hispanic and white female students (13.1 percent and 9.2 percent, respectively) were significantly more likely than black female students (1.3 percent) to report lifetime cocaine use. Overall, students in grade 12 (12.1 percent) were significantly more likely than students in grade 9 (7.2 percent) to report lifetime cocaine use. Prevalence of lifetime cocaine use varied threefold from 4.1 percent to 13 percent (median: 8.3 percent) across state surveys and varied fourfold from 2.6 percent to 10.4 percent (median: 6.3 percent) across local surveys.

Nationwide, 4.2 percent of students had used a form of cocaine one or more times during the 30 days preceding the survey (i.e., current cocaine use). Black male students (2.2 percent) were significantly more likely than black female students (0.4 percent) to report current cocaine use. Overall, Hispanic and white students (7.1 percent and 4.2 percent, respectively) were significantly more likely than black students (1.3 percent) to report current cocaine use, and Hispanic students (7.1 percent) were significantly more likely than white students (4.2 percent) to report this behavior. These significant racial/ethnic differences were identified for male students. Hispanic and white female students (5.9 percent and 3.9 percent, respectively) were significantly more likely than black female students (0.4 percent) to report current cocaine use. Prevalence of current cocaine use varied threefold from 2.1 percent to 6.3 percent (median: 3.7 percent) across state surveys and varied fivefold from 1.2 percent to 5.9 percent (median: 2.9 percent) across local surveys.

- **Inhalant Use**. Nationwide, 14.7 percent of students had sniffed glue, breathed the contents of aerosol spray cans, or inhaled any paints or sprays to get high during their lifetime (i.e., lifetime inhalant use). Overall, white and Hispanic students (16.3 percent and 15.2 percent, respectively) were significantly more likely than black students (5.8 percent) to report lifetime inhalant use. This significant racial/ethnic difference was identified for both female and male students. Across state surveys, prevalence of lifetime inhalant use ranged from 9.9 percent to 16.4 percent (median: 13.5 percent). Across local surveys, prevalence varied threefold from 6.1 percent to 17.2 percent (median: 8.7 percent).

Nationwide, 4.7 percent of students had used inhalants one or more times during the 30 days preceding the survey (i.e., current inhalant use). Overall, Hispanic and white students (5.5 percent and 4.9 percent, respectively) were significantly more likely than black students (2.6 percent) to report current inhalant use. White male students (5.4 percent) were significantly more likely than black male students (2.7 percent) to report current inhalant use. Overall, students in grades 9 and 10 (6.2 percent and 4.8 percent) were significantly more likely than students in grade 12 (2.9 percent) to report current inhalant use. Prevalence of current inhalant use ranged from 2.3 percent to 5.6 percent (median: 4.2 percent) across state surveys and varied threefold from 1.8 percent to 4.8 percent (median: 3.3 percent) across local surveys.

- **Heroin Use**. Nationwide, 3.1 percent of students had used heroin during their lifetime (i.e., lifetime heroin use). Overall, male students (3.8 percent) were significantly more likely than female students (2.5 percent) to report lifetime heroin use. This significant sex difference was identified for white and black students. Overall, white and Hispanic students (3.3 percent and 3.1 percent, respectively) were significantly more likely than black students (1.7 percent) to report lifetime heroin use. This significant racial/ethnic difference was identified for female students. Prevalence of heroin use varied threefold from 1.4 percent to 4.3 percent (median: 3 percent) across state surveys and varied fivefold from 0.9 percent to 4.6 percent (median: 2.9 percent) across local surveys.

- **Methamphetamine Use**. Nationwide, 9.8 percent of students had used methamphetamines during their lifetime (i.e., lifetime methamphetamine use). Overall, white and Hispanic students (11.4 percent and 9.1 percent, respectively) were significantly more likely than black students (2.1 percent) to report lifetime methamphetamine use. This significant racial/ethnic difference was identified for both female and male students. Lifetime methamphetamine use varied threefold from 5.3 percent to 15.6 percent (median: 7.9 percent) across state surveys and varied threefold from 2.8 percent to 8.6 percent (median: 5.2 percent) across local surveys.

- **Steroid Use**. Nationwide, 5 percent of students had used illegal steroids (i.e., without a doctor's prescription) during their lifetime (i.e., lifetime steroid use). Overall, male students (6 percent) were significantly more likely than female students (3.9 percent) to report lifetime steroid use. This significant sex difference was identified for white students and students in grade 12. Overall, white students (5.3 percent) were significantly more likely than black students (3.2 percent) to report lifetime steroid use. This significant racial/ethnic difference was identified for female students. Prevalence of lifetime illegal steroid use varied threefold from 2.6 percent to 6.9 percent (median: 5 percent) across state surveys and ranged from 2.3 percent to 5.7 percent (median: 4.5 percent) across local surveys.

- **Injection-Drug Use**. Nationwide, 2.3 percent of students had injected illegal drugs during their lifetime (i.e., lifetime injection-drug use).[2] Overall, male students (3.1 percent) were significantly more likely than female students (1.6 percent) to report lifetime injection-drug use. This significant sex difference was identified for white and black students and for students in grade 12. Prevalence varied sixfold from 1.1 percent to 6.9 percent (median: 2.3 percent) across state surveys and varied fourfold from 0.8 percent to 3.2 percent (median: 2.2 percent) across local surveys.

Age of Initiation of Risk Behavior

- **Cigarette Smoking**. Nationwide, 22.1 percent of students had smoked a whole cigarette before age 13 years. Male students (24.5 percent) were significantly more likely than female students (19.8 percent) to have smoked a whole cigarette before age 13 years. Overall, white and Hispanic students (23.6 percent and 22.6 percent, respectively) were significantly more likely than black students (14.2 percent) to have smoked a whole cigarette before age 13 years. This significant racial/ethnic difference was identified for both female and male students. Overall, students in grade 9 (26.2 percent) were significantly more likely than students in grades 11 and 12 (18.5 percent and 19 percent, respectively) to have smoked a whole cigarette before age 13 years. Across state surveys, prevalence ranged from 12.2 percent to 28.1 percent (median: 23 percent). Prevalence across local surveys ranged from 11.1 percent to 21.2 percent (median: 17.3 percent).

- **Alcohol Use**. Nationwide, 29.1 percent of students had first drunk alcohol (other than a few sips) before age 13 years. Overall, male students (34.2 percent) were significantly more likely than female students (24.2 percent) to have drunk alcohol before age 13 years. This significant sex difference was identified for all the racial/ethnic and grade subpopulations. Overall, Hispanic students (33.7 percent) were significantly more likely than white students (28.4 percent) to have drunk alcohol before age 13 years. Hispanic male students (40.8 percent) were significantly more likely than white and black male students (33.3 percent and 32.4 percent, respectively) to report this behavior. Overall, students in grades 9 and 10 (39.7 percent and 28.8 percent, respectively) were significantly more likely than students in grades 11 and 12 (23.4 percent and 21.2 percent) to have drunk alcohol before age 13 years, and students in grade 9 (39.7 percent) were significantly more likely than students in grade 10 (28.8 percent) to have done so. Prevalence ranged from 21.7 percent to 35.1 percent (median: 29.1 percent) across state surveys and from 25.6 percent to 34.7 percent (median: 30.3 percent) across local surveys.

- **Marijuana Use**. One tenth (10.2 percent) of students nationwide had tried marijuana before age 13 years. Overall, male students (13.2 percent) were significantly more likely than female students (7.5 percent) to have used marijuana before age 13 years. This significant sex difference was identified for all the racial/ethnic and grade subpopulations. Hispanic male students (16.5 percent) were significantly more likely than white male students (12 percent) to have tried marijuana before age 13 years. Overall, students in grades 9 and 10 (11.6 percent and 12.1 percent, respectively) were significantly more likely than students in grade 12 (7.8 percent) to have used marijuana before age 13 years, and students in grade 10 (12.1 percent) were significantly more likely than students in grade 11 (8.5 percent) to have done so. Prevalence varied fourfold from 4.5 percent to 17.8 percent (median: 11.1 percent) across state surveys. Across local surveys, prevalence ranged from 7.5 percent to 15.6 percent (median: 11.5 percent).

Tobacco, Alcohol, and Other Drug Use on School Property

Nationwide, 9.9 percent of students had smoked cigarettes on school property on one or more of the 30 days preceding the survey. Overall, male students (11.3 percent) were significantly more likely than female students (8.5 percent) to have smoked cigarettes on school property. This significant sex difference was identified for students in grade 9. Overall, white students (11.3 percent) were significantly more likely than Hispanic and black students (7.7 percent and 4.9 percent, respectively) to have smoked cigarettes on school property. This significant racial/ethnic difference was identified for male students. White and Hispanic female students (9.8 percent and 7.9 percent, respectively) were significantly more likely than black female students (2.8 percent) to report this behavior. Across state surveys, prevalence varied sixfold from 2.7 percent to 16 percent (median: 9.8 percent). Across local surveys, prevalence varied threefold from 3.5 percent to 11.1 percent (median: 6.3 percent).

Nationwide, 5 percent of students had used smokeless tobacco on school property on one or more of the 30 days preceding the survey. Overall, male students (9.4 percent) were significantly more likely than female students (0.7 percent) to have used smokeless tobacco on school property. This significant sex difference was identified for all the racial/ethnic and grade subpopulations. Overall, white and Hispanic students (6.2 percent and 2.7 percent, respectively) were significantly more likely than black students (1.1 percent) to have used smokeless tobacco on school property, and white students (6.2 percent) were significantly more likely than Hispanic students (2.7 percent) to have done so. White male students (11.9 percent) were significantly more likely than Hispanic and black male students (4.3 percent and 2 percent, respectively) to report this behavior. Prevalence varied 13-fold from 0.9 percent to 11.5 percent (median: 4.5 percent) across state surveys. Across local surveys, prevalence varied fivefold from 0.7 percent to 3.3 percent (median: 1.7 percent)

Nationwide, 4.9 percent of students had had one or more drinks of alcohol on school property on one or more of the 30 days preceding the survey. Overall, male students (6.1 percent) were significantly more likely than female students (3.8 percent) to have drunk alcohol on school property. This significant sex difference was identified for white and black students and students in grades 11 and 12. Overall, Hispanic students (7 percent) were significantly more likely than white students (4.2 percent) to have drunk alcohol on school property, and Hispanic female students (7.1 percent) were significantly more likely than white and black female students (3.2 percent and 3.1 percent, respectively) to have done so. Across state surveys, prevalence varied threefold from 2.4 percent to 8.3 percent (median: 4.9 percent). Prevalence across local surveys varied threefold from 3.2 percent to 9.2 percent (median: 6.3 percent).

Nationwide, 5.4 percent of students had used marijuana on school property one or more times during the 30 days preceding the survey. Overall, male students (8 percent) were significantly more likely than female students (2.9 percent) to have used marijuana on school property. This significant sex difference was identified for white and black students and students in all the grade subpopulations. Overall, Hispanic students (7.4 percent) were significantly more likely than white students (4.8

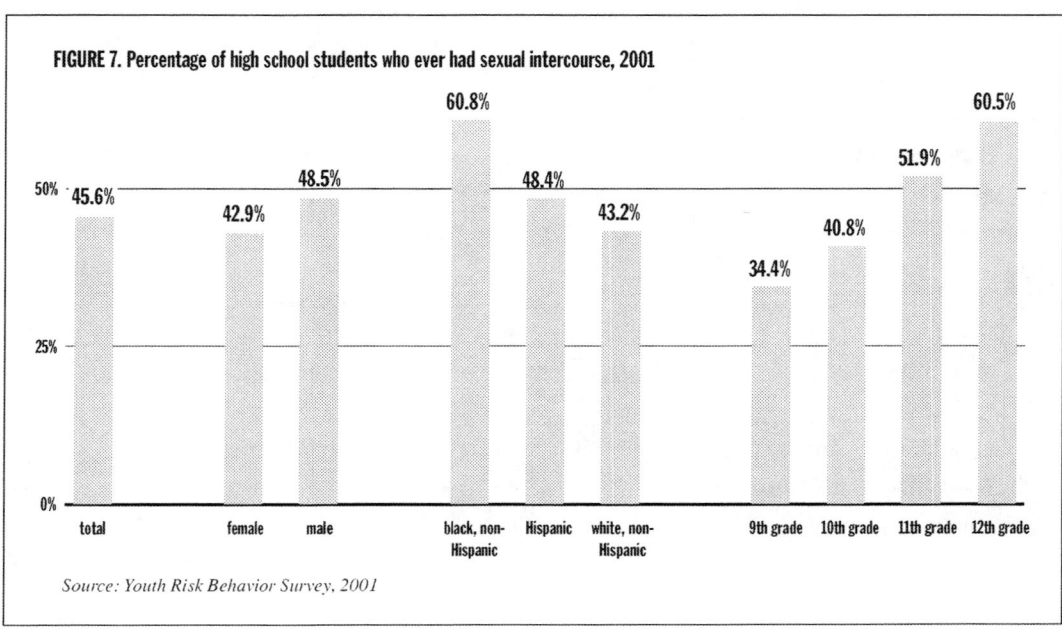

FIGURE 7. Percentage of high school students who ever had sexual intercourse, 2001

- total: 45.6%
- female: 42.9%
- male: 48.5%
- black, non-Hispanic: 60.8%
- Hispanic: 48.4%
- white, non-Hispanic: 43.2%
- 9th grade: 34.4%
- 10th grade: 40.8%
- 11th grade: 51.9%
- 12th grade: 60.5%

Source: Youth Risk Behavior Survey, 2001

percent) to have used marijuana on school property. Hispanic female students (5.8 percent) were significantly more likely than black and white female students (2.3 percent and 2.2 percent, respectively) to report this behavior. Across state surveys, prevalence varied fourfold from 2.5 percent to 10.9 percent (median: 5.2 percent). Prevalence across local surveys ranged from 5.1 percent to 10.3 percent (median: 6 percent).

Nationwide, 28.5 percent of students had been offered, sold, or given an illegal drug on school property during the 12 months preceding the survey. Overall, male students (34.6 percent) were significantly more likely than female students (22.7 percent) to have been offered, sold, or given an illegal drug on school property. This significant sex difference was identified for all the racial/ethnic and grade subpopulations. Overall, Hispanic students (34.2 percent) were significantly more likely than white and black students (28.3 percent and 21.9 percent, respectively) to have been offered, sold, or given an illegal drug on school property, and white students (28.3 percent) were significantly more likely than black students (21.9 percent) to report this behavior. Hispanic female students (28.7 percent) were significantly more likely than white and black female students (22.7 percent and 16.2 percent, respectively) to have been offered, sold, or given an illegal drug on school property, and white female students (22.7 percent) were significantly more likely than black female students (16.2 percent) to report this behavior. Hispanic male students (39.8 percent) were significantly more likely than black male students (27.9 percent) to have been offered, sold, or given an illegal drug on school property. Prevalence across state surveys ranged from 16.9 percent to 36 percent (median: 27.6 percent). Prevalence across local surveys varied threefold from 13.9 percent to 41.2 percent (median: 30.7 percent).

Sexual Behaviors That Contribute to Unintended Pregnancy and STDs, Including HIV Infection

• **Sexual Intercourse**. Nationwide, 45.6 percent of students had had sexual intercourse during their lifetime (Figure 7). Overall, male students (48.5 percent) were significantly more likely than female students (42.9 percent) to have had sexual intercourse. This significant sex difference was identified for black students and students in grade 9. Overall, black students (60.8 percent) were significantly more likely than Hispanic and white students (48.4 percent and 43.2 percent, respectively) to have had sexual intercourse. Black female students (53.4 percent) were significantly more likely than white female students (41.3 percent) to have had sexual intercourse. Black and Hispanic male students (68.8 percent and 53 percent, respectively) were significantly more likely than white male students (45.1 percent) to have had sexual intercourse, and black male students (68.8 percent) were significantly more likely than Hispanic male students (53 percent) to report this behavior. Overall, students in grades 11 and 12 (51.9 percent and 60.5 percent, respectively) were significantly more likely than students in grades 9 and 10 (34.4 percent and 40.8 percent, respectively) to have had sexual intercourse, and students in grade 12 (60.5 percent) were significantly more likely than students in grade 11 (51.9 percent) to report this behavior. Prevalence of lifetime sexual intercourse ranged from 32.7 percent to 60.6 percent (median: 44.3 percent) across state surveys and from 29.8 percent to 61.6 percent (median: 50.8 percent) across local surveys.

Nationwide, 6.6 percent of students had initiated sexual intercourse before age 13 years. Overall, male students (9.3 percent) were significantly more likely than female students (4 percent) to have initiated sexual intercourse before age 13 years. This significant sex difference was identified for all the racial/ethnic and grade subpopulations. Overall, black students (16.3 percent) were significantly more likely than Hispanic and white students (7.6 percent and 4.7 percent, respectively) to have initiated sexual intercourse before age 13 years. This significant racial/ethnic difference was identified for male students. Hispanic male students (11.4 percent) were significantly more likely than white male students (6.2 percent) to report this behavior. Black female students (7.6 percent) were significantly more likely than white female students (3.3 percent) to have initiated sexual intercourse before age 13 years. Overall, students in grades 9 and 10 (9.2 percent and 7.5 percent, respectively) were significantly more likely than students in grades 11 and 12 (4.6 percent and 3.6 percent, respectively) to have initiated sexual intercourse before age 13 years. Across state surveys, prevalence varied fivefold from 3.1 percent to 14 percent (median: 5.3 percent). Prevalence varied threefold from 5.2 percent to 17.2 percent (median: 10.9 percent) across local surveys.

Nationwide, 14.2 percent of students had had sexual intercourse during their lifetime with four or more sex partners. Male students (17.2 percent) were significantly more likely than female students (11.4 percent) to have had four or more sex partners. This significant sex difference was identified for black and Hispanic students and students in grades 9, 10, and 11. Overall, black students (26.6 percent) were significantly more likely than Hispanic and white students (14.9 percent and 12 percent, respectively) to report this behavior. Black female students (15.6 percent) were significantly more likely than Hispanic female students (9.5 percent) to have had four or more sex partners. Black male students (38.7 percent) were significantly more likely than Hispanic and white male students (20.6 percent and 12.8 percent, respectively) to have had four or more sex partners, and Hispanic male students (20.6 percent) were significantly more likely than white male students (12.8 percent) to report this behavior. Overall, students in grade 11 (15.2 percent) were significantly more likely than students in grade 9 (9.6 percent) to have had four or more sexual partners, and students in grade 12 (21.6 percent) were significantly more likely than students in grades 9, 10, and 11 (9.6 percent, 12.6 percent, and 15.2 percent, respectively) to report this behavior. Prevalence varied threefold from 8.4 percent to 25.5 percent (median: 13.2 percent) across state surveys. Across local surveys, prevalence varied threefold from 7.8 percent to 25.9 percent (median: 18.9 percent).

One third (33.4 percent) of students nationwide had had sexual intercourse during the three months preceding the survey (i.e., currently sexually active). Black male students (52.3 percent) were significantly more likely than black female students (39.5 percent) to be currently sexually active. Overall, black students (45.6 percent) were significantly more likely than Hispanic and white students (35.9 percent and 31.3 percent, respectively) to be currently sexually active. This significant racial/ethnic difference was identified for male students, and Hispanic male students (37.3 percent) were significantly more likely than white male students (30 percent) to report this behavior. Overall, students in grades 10, 11, and 12 (29.7 percent, 38.1 percent, and 47.9 percent, respectively) were significantly more likely than students in grade 9 (22.7 percent) to be currently sexually active; students in grades 11 and 12 (38.1 percent and 47.9 percent, respectively) were significantly more likely than students in grade 10 (29.7 percent) to report this behavior; and students in grade 12 (47.9 percent) were significantly more likely than students in grade 11 (38.1 percent) to report this behavior. Prevalence ranged from 23 percent to 44.9 percent (median: 33.3 percent) across state surveys. Across local surveys, prevalence ranged from 19.8 percent to 45.1 percent (median: 35.9 percent).

Nationwide, 86.1 percent of students had never had sexual intercourse, had sexual intercourse but not during the three months preceding the survey, or had used a condom the last time they had sexual intercourse during the three months preceding the survey (i.e., responsible sexual behavior). Overall, male students (88.5 percent) were significantly more likely than female students (83.9 percent) to have engaged in responsible sexual behavior. This significant sex difference was identified for white students and students in grades 10 and 12. Overall, students in grade 9 (92.8 percent) were significantly more likely than students in grades 10, 11, and 12 (88.3 percent, 84.5 percent, and 75.8 percent, respectively) to have engaged in responsible sexual behavior; students in grade 10 (88.3 percent) were significantly more likely than students in grades 11 and 12 (84.5 percent and 75.8 percent, respectively) to report this behavior; and students in grade 11 (84.5 percent) were significantly more likely than students in grade 12 (75.8 percent) to report this behavior. Prevalence of responsible sexual behavior ranged from 83.7 percent to 92.8 percent (median: 87.1 percent) across state surveys and from 83.4 percent to 92.8 percent (median: 89.1 percent) across local surveys.

- **Condom Use**. Among the 33.4 percent of currently sexually active students nationwide, 57.9 percent reported that either they or their partner had used a condom during last sexual intercourse. Overall, male students (65.1 percent) were significantly more likely than female students (51.3 percent) to report condom use. This significant sex difference was identified for white and black students and students in grades 10, 11, and 12. Overall, black students (67.1 percent) were significantly more likely than white and Hispanic students (56.8 percent and 53.5 percent, respectively) to report condom use. This significant racial/ethnic difference was identified for both female and male students. Overall, students in grades 9, 10, and 11 (67.5 percent, 60.1 percent, and 58.9 percent, respectively) were significantly more likely than students in grade 12 (49.3 percent) to report condom use, and students in grade 9 (67.5 percent) were significantly more likely than students in grade 11 (58.9 percent) to report condom use. Prevalence ranged from 45.5 percent to 68.3 percent (median: 59.2 percent) across state surveys and from 53.3 percent to 76.1 percent (median: 65.1 percent) across local surveys.

- **Birth Control Pill Use**. Among the 33.4 percent of currently sexually active students nationwide, 18.2 percent reported that either they or their partner had used birth control pills before last sexual intercourse. Overall, female students (21.1 percent) were significantly more likely than male students (14.9 percent) to report birth control pill use. This significant sex difference was identified for white students and students in grade 11. Overall, white students (23.4 percent) were significantly more likely than Hispanic and black students (9.6 percent and 7.9 percent, respectively) to report birth control pill use. This significant racial/ethnic difference was identified for both female and male students. Overall, students in grades 10, 11, and 12 (15.8 percent, 18.6 percent, and 26.3 percent, respectively) were significantly more likely than students in grade 9 (7.6 percent) to report birth control pill use, and students in grade 12 (26.3 percent) were significantly more likely than students in grades 10 and 11 (15.8 percent and 18.6 percent, respectively) to report this behavior. Prevalence varied threefold from 10.8 percent to 36.1 percent (median: 19.5 percent) across state surveys. Across local surveys, prevalence ranged from 6.4 percent to 16.7 percent (median: 9.4 percent).

- **Alcohol or Drug Use at Last Sexual Intercourse**. Among the 33.4 percent of currently sexually active students nationwide, 25.6 percent had used alcohol or drugs at last sexual intercourse. Male students (30.9 percent) were significantly more likely than female students (20.7 percent) to have used alcohol or drugs at last sexual intercourse. This significant sex difference was identified for white and black students and students in grades 10, 11, and 12. Overall, white and Hispanic students (27.8 percent and 24.1 percent, respectively) were significantly more likely than black students (17.8 percent) to have used alcohol or drugs at last sexual intercourse, and this significant racial/ethnic difference was identified for female students. Prevalence ranged from 20.2 percent to 33.5 percent (median: 24.9 percent) across state surveys and from 13.5 percent to 26.4 percent (median: 18.3 percent) across local surveys.

- **Pregnancy**. Nationwide, 4.7 percent of students reported that they had been pregnant or had gotten someone else pregnant. White female students (4 percent) were significantly more likely than white male students (2.5 percent) and female students in grade 12 (9.4 percent) were significantly more likely than male students in grade 12 (4.8 percent) to have been pregnant or to have gotten someone pregnant. Overall, black and Hispanic students (11.4 percent and 5.7 percent, respectively) were significantly more likely than white students (3.3 percent) to have been pregnant or to have gotten someone pregnant; black students (11.4 percent) were significantly more likely than Hispanic students (5.7 percent) to report this information. This significant racial/ethnic difference was identified for male students. Black female students (11.9 percent) were significantly more likely than Hispanic and white female students (6.2 percent and 4 percent, respectively) to have been pregnant. Overall, students in grade 12 (7.1 percent) were significantly more likely than students in grades 9, 10, and 11 (3.2 percent, 4.4 percent, and 4.8 percent, respectively) to have been pregnant or to have gotten someone pregnant. Prevalence varied threefold from 2.2 percent to 7.4 percent (median: 4.2 percent) across state surveys and varied fourfold from 2.3 percent to 10.3 percent (median: 6.3 percent) across local surveys.

- **HIV Education**. Nationwide, 89 percent of students reported being taught in school about acquired immunodeficiency syndrome (AIDS) or HIV infection. Overall, white students (91.1 percent) were significantly more likely than black and Hispanic students (86.1 percent and 80.5 percent, respectively) to have been taught about AIDS or HIV infection in school. This significant racial/ethnic difference was identified for male students. White female students (90.4 percent) were significantly more likely than Hispanic female students (81.4 percent) to have been taught about AIDS or HIV infection in school. Overall, students in grades 11 and 12 (90.5 percent and 90.2 percent, respectively) were significantly more likely than students in grade 9 (86.7 percent) to have been taught about AIDS or HIV infection in school. Across state surveys, prevalence ranged from 79.8 percent to 93.8 percent (median: 88.6 percent). Prevalence ranged from 81 percent to 91 percent (median: 86.7 percent) across local surveys.

Dietary Behaviors

- **Overweight**. Nationwide, 13.6 percent of students were at risk for becoming overweight. Overall, male students (15.5 percent) were significantly more likely than female students (11.7 percent) to be at risk for becoming overweight. This significant sex difference was identified for white students and students in grades 9 and 10. Overall, black and Hispanic students (17.8 percent and 16.3 percent, respectively) were significantly more likely than white students (12.5 percent) to be at risk for becoming overweight. This significant racial/ethnic difference was identified for female students. Overall, students in grade 9 (15.7 percent) were significantly more likely than students in grade 12 (11.8 percent) to be at risk for becoming overweight. Prevalence of being at risk for becoming overweight ranged from 8.4 percent to 15.9 percent (median: 14 percent) across state surveys and from 11.5 percent to 18.7 percent (median: 16.1 percent) across local surveys.

Nationwide, 10.5 percent of students were overweight (Figure 8). Overall, male students (14.2 percent) were significantly more likely than female students (6.9 percent) to be overweight. This significant sex difference was identified for white and Hispanic students and students in all grade subpopulations. Overall, black and Hispanic students (16 percent and 15.1 percent, respectively) were significantly more likely than white students (8.8 percent) to be overweight. This significant racial/ethnic difference was identified for both female and male students. Black female students (14.6 percent) were significantly more likely than Hispanic female students (8.8 percent) to be overweight. Across state surveys, prevalence of being overweight ranged from 6.1 percent to 14.2 percent (median: 10.4 percent). Across local surveys, prevalence ranged from 7.8 percent to 18 percent (median: 12.5 percent).

Nationwide, 29.2 percent of students thought they were overweight. Overall, female students (34.9 percent) were significantly more likely than male students (23.3 percent) to consider themselves overweight. This significant sex difference was identified for all the racial/ethnic and grade subpopulations. Overall, Hispanic students (34.8 percent) were significantly more likely than white and black students (29.2 percent and 25.7 percent, respectively) to consider themselves overweight, and white students (29.2 percent) were significantly more likely than black students (25.7 percent) to consider themselves overweight. This significant racial/ethnic difference was identified for male students. Hispanic female students (40.3 percent) were significantly more likely than black female students (32.3 percent) to consider themselves overweight. Across state surveys, prevalence ranged from 26.4 percent to 33.6 percent (median: 30.7 percent). Across local surveys, prevalence ranged from 18.7 percent to 32.9 percent (median: 28.5 percent).

Nationwide, 46 percent of students were trying to lose weight during the 30 days preceding the survey. Overall, female students (62.3 percent) were significantly more likely than male students (28.8 percent) to be trying to lose weight. This significant sex difference was identified for all the racial/

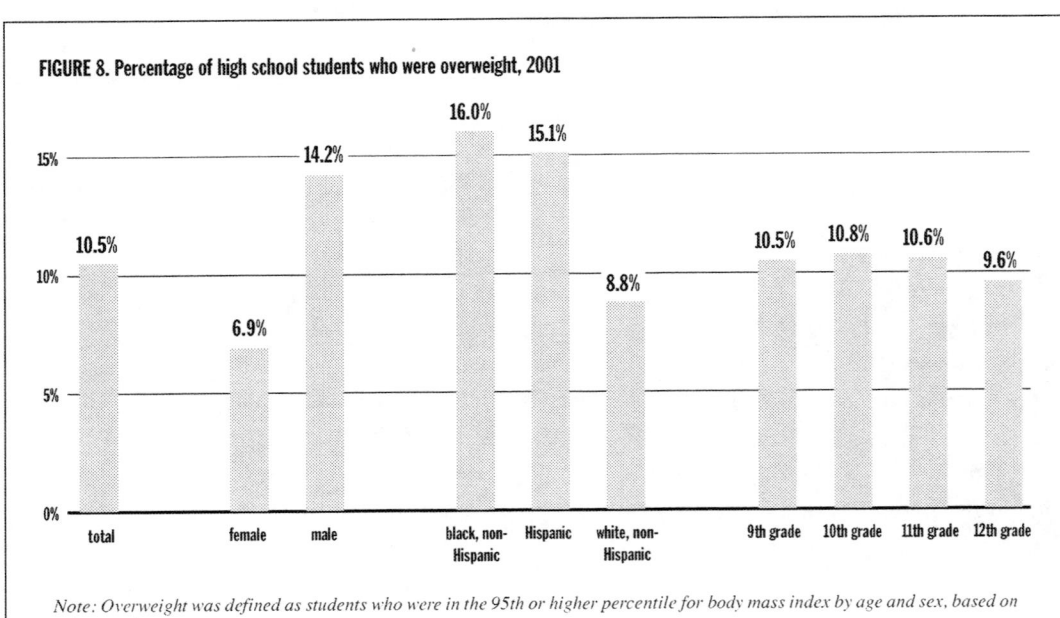

FIGURE 8. Percentage of high school students who were overweight, 2001

Note: Overweight was defined as students who were in the 95th or higher percentile for body mass index by age and sex, based on reference data.
Source: Youth Risk Behavior Survey, 2001

ethnic and grade subpopulations. Overall, Hispanic and white students (51.5 percent and 47.1 percent, respectively) were significantly more likely than black students (36.9 percent) to be trying to lose weight. This significant racial/ethnic difference was identified for female students. Hispanic male students (39.1 percent) were significantly more likely than white and black male students (27.9 percent and 23.6 percent, respectively) to report this. Prevalence ranged from 40.6 percent to 51.5 percent (median: 44.5 percent) across state surveys and from 34.7 percent to 50.1 percent (median: 41.5 percent) across local surveys.

- **Consumption of Fruits and Vegetables**. Nationwide, 21.4 percent of students had eaten five or more servings per day of fruits and vegetables during the seven days preceding the survey (Figure 9).[3] Overall, male students (23.3 percent) were significantly more likely than female students (19.7 percent) to have eaten five or more servings per day of fruits and vegetables. This significant sex difference was identified for black students. Overall, black students (24.5 percent) were significantly more likely than white students (20.2 percent) to have eaten five or more servings per day of fruits and vegetables, and this significant racial/ethnic difference was identified for male students. Prevalence ranged from 13.1 percent to 27.4 percent (median: 19.9 percent) across state surveys and from 14.9 percent to 29.5 percent (median: 21.6 percent) across local surveys.

- **Consumption of Milk**. Overall, 16.4 percent of students drank three or more glasses per day of milk during the seven days preceding the survey. Male students (22.3 percent) were significantly more likely than female students (10.9 percent) to have drunk three or more glasses per day of milk. This significant sex difference was identified for all the racial/ethnic and grade subpopulations. Overall, white students (18.1 percent) were significantly more likely than Hispanic and black students (13.8 percent and 12 percent, respectively) to have drunk three or more glasses per day of milk, and this significant racial/ethnic difference was identified for male students. White female students (12.1 percent) were significantly more likely than black female students (8.1 percent) to have drunk three or

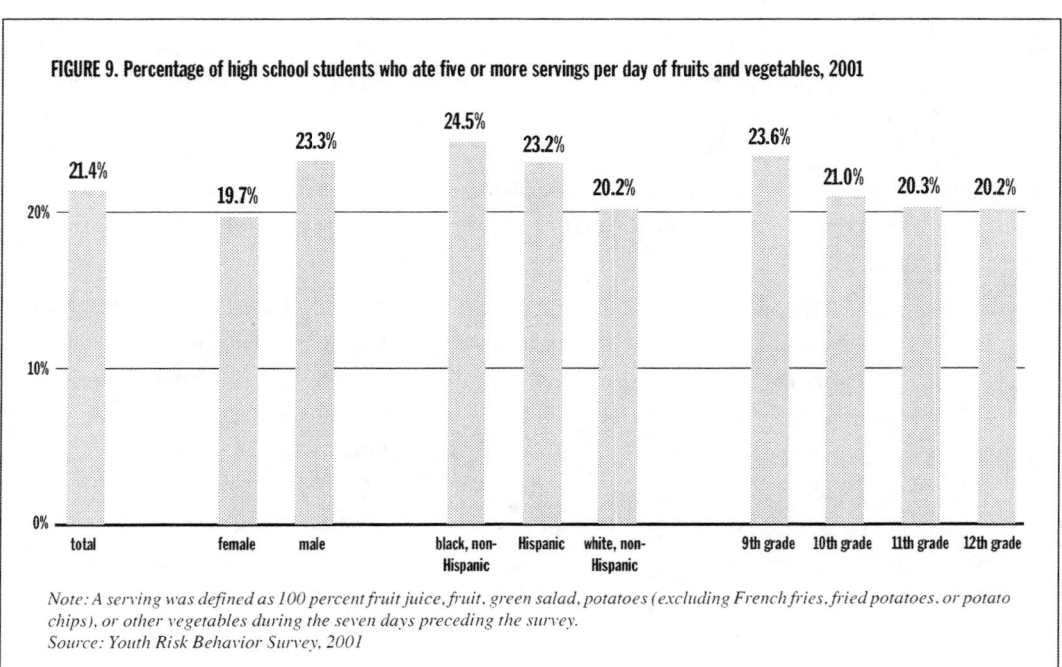

FIGURE 9. Percentage of high school students who ate five or more servings per day of fruits and vegetables, 2001

Note: A serving was defined as 100 percent fruit juice, fruit, green salad, potatoes (excluding French fries, fried potatoes, or potato chips), or other vegetables during the seven days preceding the survey.
Source: Youth Risk Behavior Survey, 2001

more glasses per day of milk. Across state surveys, prevalence varied threefold from 10.5 percent to 29.7 percent (median: 18.4 percent). Prevalence varied fourfold from 5 percent to 18.1 percent (median: 11.4 percent) across local surveys.

• **Attempted Weight Control**. Nationwide, 59.9 percent of students had exercised to lose weight or to avoid gaining weight during the 30 days preceding the survey. Overall, female students (68.4 percent) were significantly more likely than male students (51 percent) to have exercised to lose weight or to avoid gaining weight. This significant sex difference was identified for white and Hispanic students and students in all the grade subpopulations. Overall, white and Hispanic students (61.9 percent and 61.5 percent, respectively) were significantly more likely than black students (50.1 percent) to have exercised to lose weight or to avoid gaining weight. This significant racial/ethnic difference was identified for female students. White female students (72.5 percent) were significantly more likely than Hispanic female students (66.2 percent) to have exercised to lose weight or to avoid gaining weight, and Hispanic male students (56.8 percent) were significantly more likely than white and black male students (50.9 percent and 46.6 percent, respectively) to report this behavior. Overall, students in grade 9 (64.2 percent) were significantly more likely than students in grades 11 and 12 (56.3 percent and 57.2 percent, respectively) to have exercised to lose weight or to avoid gaining weight. Prevalence ranged from 53.2 percent to 64.5 percent (median: 59.3 percent) across state surveys and from 45.1 percent to 66.3 percent (median: 54.6 percent) across local surveys.

Nationwide, 43.8 percent of students had eaten less food, fewer calories, or foods low in fat to lose weight or to avoid gaining weight during the 30 days preceding the survey. Overall, female students (58.6 percent) were significantly more likely than male students (28.2 percent) to have eaten less food, fewer calories, or foods low in fat to lose weight or to avoid gaining weight. This significant sex difference was identified for all the racial/ethnic and grade subpopulations. Overall, white and Hispanic students (45.9 percent and 44.9 percent, respectively) were significantly more likely than black students (32.5 percent) to have eaten less food, fewer calories, or foods low in fat to lose weight or to avoid gaining weight. This significant racial/ethnic difference was identified for female students. White female students (63.1 percent) were significantly more likely than Hispanic female students (56.5 percent) to have eaten less food, fewer calories, or foods low in fat to lose weight or to avoid gaining weight, and Hispanic male students (32.7 percent) were significantly more likely than black male students (24.5 percent) to report this behavior. Across state surveys, prevalence ranged from 35.9 percent to 46.4 percent (median: 40.9 percent). Prevalence ranged from 29.5 percent to 42.4 percent (median: 37.5 percent) across local surveys.

Nationwide, 13.5 percent of students had gone without eating for 24 or more hours to lose weight or to avoid gaining weight. Overall, female students (19.1 percent) were significantly more likely than male students (7.6 percent) to have gone without eating for 24 or more hours to lose weight or to avoid gaining weight. This significant sex difference was identified for white and Hispanic students and all the grade subpopulations. Hispanic and white female students (23.1 percent and 19.7 percent, respectively) were significantly more likely than black female students (15.2 percent) to have gone without eating for 24 or more hours to lose weight or to avoid gaining weight. Overall, students in grade 9 (15.4 percent) were significantly more likely than students in grades 11 and 12 (11.5 percent and 11.5 percent, respectively) to report this behavior. Prevalence ranged from

10.3 percent to 16.2 percent (median: 13.5 percent) across state surveys and from 8.1 percent to 16.1 percent (median: 13.4 percent) across local surveys.

One tenth (9.2 percent) of students nationwide had taken diet pills, powders, or liquids without a doctor's advice to lose weight or to avoid gaining weight. Overall, female students (12.6 percent) were significantly more likely than male students (5.5 percent) to have taken diet pills, powders, or liquids without a doctor's advice to lose weight or to avoid gaining weight. This significant sex difference was identified for white and Hispanic students and all the grade subpopulations. Overall, Hispanic and white students (10.1 percent and 9.5 percent, respectively) were significantly more likely than black students (6 percent) to report this behavior. This significant racial/ethnic difference was identified for female students. Across state surveys, prevalence varied threefold from 4.9 percent to 13 percent (median: 8.5 percent). Prevalence varied threefold from 3.2 percent to 10.6 percent (median: 6.9 percent) across local surveys.

Nationwide, 5.4 percent of students had vomited or taken laxatives to lose weight or to avoid gaining weight. Overall, female students (7.8 percent) were significantly more likely than male students (2.9 percent) to have vomited or taken laxatives to lose weight or to avoid gaining weight. This significant sex difference was identified for white and Hispanic students and students in all the grade subpopulations. Overall, Hispanic students (7.2 percent) were significantly more likely than black students (4 percent) to report this behavior. Hispanic and white female students (10.8 percent and 8.2 percent, respectively) were significantly more likely than black female students (4.2 percent) to report this behavior. Prevalence ranged from 3.6 percent to 7.6 percent (median: 5.6 percent) across state surveys and varied threefold from 2.5 percent to 8.5 percent (median: 5.5 percent) across local surveys.

Physical Activity

• **Vigorous and Moderate Physical Activity**. Approximately two thirds (64.6 percent) of students nationwide had participated in activities that made them sweat and breathe hard for 20 or more minutes on three or more of the seven days preceding the survey (i.e., sufficient vigorous physical activity). Overall, male students (72.6 percent) were significantly more likely than female students (57 percent) to report sufficient vigorous physical activity. This significant sex difference was identified for all the racial/ethnic and grade subpopulations. Overall, white students (66.5 percent) were significantly more likely than Hispanic and black students (60.5 percent and 59.7 percent, respectively) to report sufficient vigorous physical activity. This significant racial/ethnic difference was identified for female students. White male students (73.7 percent) were significantly more likely than Hispanic male students (68.8 percent) to report sufficient vigorous physical activity. Overall, students in grades 9, 10, and 11 (71.9 percent, 67 percent, and 61.3 percent, respectively) were significantly more likely than students in grade 12 (55.5 percent) to report sufficient vigorous physical activity. Students in grades 9 and 10 (71.9 percent and 67 percent, respectively) were significantly more likely than students in grade 11 (61.3 percent) to report sufficient vigorous physical activity, and students in grade 9 (71.9 percent) were significantly more likely than students in grade 10 (67 percent) to report this behavior. Prevalence of sufficient vigorous physical activity ranged from 54.9 percent to 74.1 percent (median: 64.3 percent) across state surveys and from 40.7 percent to 65 percent (median: 54.9 percent) across local surveys.

One-fourth (25.5 percent) of students nationwide had participated in activities that did not make them sweat or breathe hard for 30 or more minutes on five or more of the seven days preceding the survey (i.e., sufficient moderate physical activity). Overall, male students (28.4 percent) were significantly more likely than female students (22.8 percent) to report sufficient moderate physical activity. This significant sex difference was identified for all the racial/ethnic subpopulations and students in grades 10 and 11. Overall, white students (27.3 percent) were significantly more likely than Hispanic and black students (22.1 percent and 20.1 percent, respectively) to report sufficient moderate physical activity. This significant racial/ethnic difference was identified for female students. White male students (29.8 percent) were significantly more likely than black male students (23.7 percent) to report sufficient moderate physical activity. Across state surveys, prevalence of sufficient moderate physical activity ranged from 19.2 percent to 31 percent (median: 25.4 percent). Across local surveys, prevalence ranged from 12.3 percent to 26.5 percent (median: 21.6 percent).

Nationwide, 31.2 percent of students had not participated in vigorous physical activity for 20 or more minutes on three or more of the seven days preceding the survey and had not participated in moderate physical activity for 30 or more minutes on five or more of the seven days preceding the survey (i.e., insufficient amount of physical activity). Overall, female students (37.9 percent) were significantly more likely than male students (24.2 percent) to report an insufficient amount of physical activity. This significant sex difference was identified for all the racial/ethnic and grade subpopulations. Overall, black and Hispanic students (36.4 percent and 35.4 percent, respectively) were significantly more likely than white students (29.3 percent) to report an insufficient amount of physical activity. This significant racial/ethnic difference was identified for female students. Overall, students in grades 10, 11, and 12 (29.6 percent, 34.4 percent, and 38.9 percent, respectively) were significantly more likely than students in grade 9 (24.3 percent) to report an insufficient amount of physical activ-

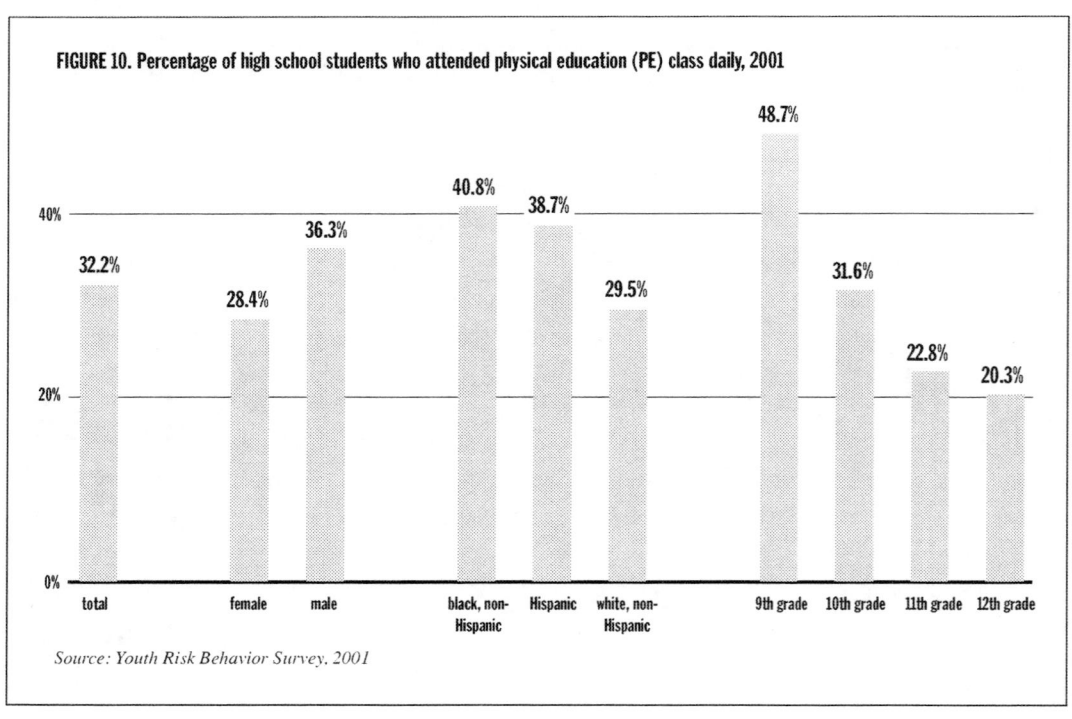

FIGURE 10. Percentage of high school students who attended physical education (PE) class daily, 2001

Source: Youth Risk Behavior Survey, 2001

ity. Students in grades 11 and 12 (34.4 percent and 38.9 percent, respectively) were significantly more likely than students in grade 10 (29.6 percent) to report this information. Prevalence of insufficient physical activity ranged from 22 percent to 41 percent (median: 31.2 percent) across state surveys and from 30.5 percent to 56.7 percent (median: 41.1 percent) across local surveys.

One-tenth (9.5 percent) of students nationwide had not participated in either vigorous physical activity for 20 or more minutes or moderate physical activity for 30 or more minutes on any of the seven days preceding the survey (i.e., no vigorous or moderate physical activity). Overall, female students (11.6 percent) were significantly more likely than male students (7.2 percent) to report no vigorous or moderate physical activity. This significant sex difference was identified for white and black students and students in grades 11 and 12. Overall, black and Hispanic students (12.9 percent and 11.2 percent, respectively) were significantly more likely than white students (8.2 percent) to report no vigorous or moderate physical activity. Black female students (16.9 percent) were significantly more likely than white female students (10.2 percent), and Hispanic male students (9.3 percent) were significantly more likely than white male students (6.2 percent), to report this information. Overall, students in grades 11 and 12 (11.1 percent and 12 percent, respectively) were significantly more likely than students in grades 9 and 10 (7.1 percent and 8.5 percent, respectively) to report no vigorous or moderate physical activity. Across state surveys, prevalence varied fourfold from 4.2 percent to 15.6 percent (median: 9.2 percent). Across local surveys, prevalence ranged from 10.1 percent to 25.3 percent (median: 13.1 percent).

• **Participation in Physical Education Class**. Nationwide, 51.7 percent of students were enrolled in a physical education (PE) class. Black male students (67.4 percent) were significantly more likely than white male students (52 percent) to be enrolled in a PE class. Overall, students in grades 9 and 10 (73.7 percent and 54.1 percent, respectively) were significantly more likely than students in grades 11 and 12 (39.1 percent and 31.3 percent, respectively) to be enrolled in a PE class, and students in grade 9 (73.7 percent) were significantly more likely than students in grade 10 (54.1 percent) to report this. Across state surveys, prevalence of being enrolled in a PE class varied fourfold from 22.1 percent to 93.6 percent (median: 47.1 percent). Across local surveys, prevalence varied threefold from 33.3 percent to 85.6 percent (median: 56 percent).

Approximately one third (32.2 percent) of students nationwide attended PE class daily (Figure 10). Male students in grade 11 (30 percent) were significantly more likely than female students in grade 11 (15.6 percent) to have attended PE class daily, and male students in grade 12 (26.1 percent) were significantly more likely than female students in grade 12 (14.7 percent) to report this behavior. Overall, students in grade 9 (48.7 percent) were significantly more likely than students in grades 10, 11, and 12 (31.6 percent, 22.8 percent, and 20.3 percent respectively) to have attended PE class daily, and students in grade 10 (31.6 percent) were significantly more likely than students in grade 12 (20.3 percent) to report this behavior. Across state surveys, prevalence varied 20-fold from 3.6 percent to 70.6 percent (median: 28.1 percent). Prevalence varied sixfold across local surveys from 10.3 percent to 57.1 percent (median: 23.8 percent).

Among the 51.7 percent of students enrolled in PE class, 83.4 percent exercised 20 or more minutes during an average PE class. Overall, male students (87.7 percent) were significantly more likely than female students (78.8 percent) to have exercised 20 or more minutes during an average PE class. This significant sex difference was identified for white and black students and students in grades

10, 11, and 12. Overall, white students (85.2 percent) were significantly more likely than black students (76.4 percent) to have exercised 20 or more minutes during an average PE class. This significant racial/ethnic difference was identified for both female and male students. Prevalence ranged from 71.9 percent to 91.5 percent (median: 83.6 percent) across state surveys and from 54.9 percent to 84.9 percent (median: 75.1 percent) across local surveys.

- **Participation on Sports Teams.** Nationwide, 55.2 percent of students had played on one or more sports teams during the 12 months preceding the survey. Overall, male students (60.9 percent) were significantly more likely than female students (49.9 percent) to have played on sports teams. This significant sex difference was identified for all the racial/ethnic and grade subpopulations. Overall, white students (57.4 percent) were significantly more likely than Hispanic students (48.8 percent) to have played on sports teams. White female students (53.3 percent) were significantly more likely than black and Hispanic female students (41.6 percent and 40.1 percent, respectively) to have played on sports teams. Overall, students in grades 9, 10, and 11 (59.9 percent, 56.2 percent, and 54.5 percent, respectively) were significantly more likely than students in grade 12 (48.5 percent) to have played on sports teams, and students in grade 9 (59.9 percent) were significantly more likely than students in grade 11 (54.5 percent) to report this behavior. Prevalence of having played on sports teams ranged from 49.3 percent to 68.3 percent (median: 58.6 percent) across state surveys and from 41.4 percent to 55.5 percent (median: 48 percent) across local surveys.

- **Strengthening Exercises.** Nationwide, 53.4 percent of students had done strengthening exercises (e.g., push-ups, sit-ups, and weightlifting) on three or more of the seven days preceding the survey. Overall, male students (62.8 percent) were significantly more likely than female students (44.5 percent) to have participated in strengthening activities. This significant sex difference was identified for all the racial/ethnic and grade subpopulations. Overall, white students (54.8 percent) were significantly more likely than black students (47.9 percent) to have participated in strengthening activities. This significant racial/ethnic difference was identified for female students. Overall, students in grade 9 (58.7 percent) were significantly more likely than students in grades 11 and 12 (51.1 percent and 48 percent, respectively) to have participated in strengthening activities, and students in grade 10 (53.9 percent) were significantly more likely than students in grade 12 (48 percent) to report this behavior. Across state surveys, prevalence ranged from 43.7 percent to 59.2 percent (median: 51.1 percent). Across local surveys, prevalence ranged from 34.1 percent to 52.4 percent (median: 44.2 percent).

- **Watching Television.** Nationwide, 38.3 percent of students had watched television three or more hours per day during an average school day. Overall, male students (41.8 percent) were significantly more likely than female students (35 percent) to have watched television for three or more hours per day. This significant sex difference was identified for white students and students in grade 9. Overall, black and Hispanic students (68.9 percent and 47.8 percent, respectively) were significantly more likely than white students (31 percent) to have watched television for three or more hours per day, and black students (68.9 percent) were significantly more likely than Hispanic students (47.8 percent) to report this behavior. This significant racial/ethnic difference was identified for both female and male students. Overall, students in grade 9 (45.3 percent) were significantly more likely than students in grades 11 and 12 (34.7 percent and 31.3 percent, respectively) to have watched television for three or more hours per day, and students in grade 10 (39.2 percent) were significantly more likely than students in grade 12 (31.3 percent) to report this behavior. Prevalence varied threefold from 17.7

percent to 54.7 percent (median: 32.4 percent) across state surveys and from 41.8 percent to 66.8 percent (median: 52.6 percent) across local surveys.

Trends during 1991–2001

During 1991–2001, significant decreases occurred in the percentage of students who never or rarely wore seatbelts (25.9 percent–14.1 percent), rode with a driver who had been drinking alcohol (39.9 percent–30.7 percent), participated in a physical fight (42.5 percent–33.2 percent), seriously considered suicide (29 percent–19 percent), and planned to attempt suicide (18.6 percent–14.8). The percentage of students who carried a weapon decreased significantly from 1991 to 1997 (26.1 percent–18.3 percent) and then remained constant from 1997 to 2001 (18.3 percent–17.4 percent). The percentage of students who reported lifetime and current marijuana use increased significantly from 1991 to 1997 (31.3 percent–47.1 percent and 14.7 percent–26.2 percent, respectively) and then decreased significantly from 1997 to 2001 (47.1 percent–42.4 percent and 26.2 percent–23.9 percent, respectively). The percentage of students who reported lifetime and current cocaine use increased significantly from 1991 to 2001 (5.9 percent–9.4 percent and 1.7 percent–4.2 percent, respectively).

During 1991–2001, the percentage of students who ever had sexual intercourse and had sexual intercourse with four or more partners decreased significantly (54.1 percent–45.6 percent and 18.7 percent–14.2 percent, respectively). During 1991–1999, the percentage of currently sexually active students who used a condom at last sexual intercourse increased significantly (46.2 percent–58 percent) and then leveled off by 2001 (58 percent–57.9 percent).

The percentage of students who reported current cigarette use and frequent cigarette use increased significantly from 1991 to 1997 (27.5 percent–36.4 percent and 12.7 percent–16.7 percent, respectively) and then decreased significantly from 1997 to 2001 (36.4 percent–28.5 percent and 16.7 percent–13.8 percent, respectively). During 1995–2001, current smokeless tobacco use decreased significantly (11.4 percent–8.2 percent), and from 1997 to 2001, current cigar use decreased significantly (22 percent–15.2 percent). While the percentage of students enrolled in PE class remained constant from 1991 to 2001 (48.9 percent–51.7 percent), the percentage of students enrolled in daily PE classes decreased significantly from 1991 to 1995 (41.6 percent–25.4 percent) and then increased significantly from 1995 to 2001 (25.4 percent–32.2 percent).

Discussion

Trend analysis of selected risk behaviors indicated increases and decreases in the risk for unintentional injuries and violence and decreases in the risk for HIV infection, other STDs, unintended pregnancy, and chronic diseases. Nonetheless, too many high school students nationwide continue to practice behaviors that place them at risk for serious acute and chronic health problems. Certain risk behaviors are more likely to be found among particular subpopulations of students. The association between race/ethnicity and certain risk behaviors might be attenuated by controlling for socioeconomic status (8). However, underlying causes (e.g., economic factors, education levels, or cultural influences) of subgroup differences could not be identified in this analysis. Additional research is needed to assess the effect of specific educational, socioeconomic, cultural, and racial/ethnic factors on the prevalence of health-risk behaviors among youth.

Considerable variation in prevalence of risk behaviors also occurs from state to state and from city to city. For example, across state surveys, a fivefold variation or greater was identified for the following risk behaviors:

- Feeling too unsafe to go to school;
- Smoking more than 10 cigarettes per day;
- Current smokeless tobacco use;
- Current cigar use;
- Purchasing cigarettes at a store or a gas station;
- Lifetime injection-drug use;
- Cigarette use on school property;
- Smokeless tobacco use on school property;
- Initiating sexual intercourse before age 13 years; and
- Attending PE class daily.

Across local surveys, a similar fivefold variation was identified for the following risk behaviors:

- Rarely or never wearing seatbelts;
- Carrying a gun;
- Smoking more than 10 cigarettes per day;
- Current smokeless tobacco use;
- Current cocaine use;
- Lifetime heroin use;
- Smokeless tobacco use on school property; and
- Attending PE class daily.

These variations might occur, in part, because of differences in state and local laws and policies, enforcement practices, access to illegal drugs, availability of effective interventions, prevailing behavioral norms, demographic characteristics of the population, and adult practices. However, further research is needed to obtain increased understanding of the effect of these factors on the prevalence of risk behaviors.

Limitations

The findings in this report are subject to several limitations. First, these data apply only to youth who attend school and, therefore, are not representative of all persons in this age group. Nationwide, approximately 5 percent of persons aged 16–17 years were not enrolled in a high school program and had not completed high school (9). Second, the extent of underreporting or overreporting of behaviors cannot be determined, although the survey questions demonstrate good test-retest reliability (10). Third, BMI is calculated based on self-reported height and weight and, therefore, tends to underestimate the prevalence of overweight and at risk for overweight. Fourth, unweighted state and local data represent only those students who participated in the survey and are not generalizable to the entire jurisdiction. Fifth, data are not available from all 50 states.

Use of YRBS Data

The national YRBS data are used routinely by CDC and other federal agencies. The following are examples of how CDC uses YRBS data:

- Assess trends in priority health-risk behaviors among high school students.

- Monitor progress toward 15 Healthy People 2010 health objectives and three Leading Health Indicators.

- Evaluate relevant components of CDC's Performance Plan in compliance with the Government Performance and Results Act (11).

- Evaluate the contribution of HIV prevention efforts in schools toward helping the nation reach HIV prevention objectives for youth.

State and local agencies and nongovernmental organizations use YRBS data to prioritize health education and health promotion goals, support curricula or program modifications, support legislation that promotes health, and seek funding for new initiatives. For example, in Washington, D.C., YRBS data were used as the basis for development and implementation of a teacher-training program entitled "What Every Teacher Needs to Know If Someone in School Has AIDS." The Missouri Department of Health's Adolescent Health Task Force developed objectives for the six health risk behavior categories measured in the YRBS and used the results from the YRBS as indicators of success. San Francisco used YRBS data to help determine how many hours of study would be devoted to certain topics in the classroom. Utah supplemented the health education core curriculum with an eating disorder prevention program after reviewing YRBS data. In Colorado, YRBS data were used to help pass the Comprehensive Health Education Act, which encouraged schools to provide comprehensive health education in a planned and sequential program of activities. The increased accessibility of the Internet has encouraged several states and local agencies to post YRBS data on their web sites. The Council of Chief State School Officers' website (http://www.ccsso.org) has links to several state YRBS reports. Continued support for the YRBSS will help monitor and ensure the effectiveness of these and other public health and school health programs for youth.

References

1. Anderson R.N. Deaths: leading causes for 1999. National Vital Statistics Report 2001; 49 (11): 1–88.

2. Ventura S.J., Mosher W.D., Curtin S.C., Abma J.C., Henshaw S. Trends in pregnancy rates for the United States, 1976–97: an update. National Vital Statistics Report 2001; 49 (4): 1–10.

3. Institute of Medicine, Committee on Prevention and Control of Sexually Transmitted Diseases. The hidden epidemic: confronting sexually transmitted diseases. Eng T.R., Butler W.T., eds. Washington, DC: National Academy Press, 1997.

4. Kolbe L.J., Kann L., Collins J.L. Overview of the Youth Risk Behavior Surveillance System. Public Health Report 1993; 108 (supplement 1): 2–10.

5. Research Triangle Institute. SUDAAN: software for the statistical analysis of correlated data, release 8.0 [user's manual]. Research Triangle Park, NC: Research Triangle Institute, 2001.

6. Hinkle D.E., Wiersma W., Jurs S.G. Applied statistics for the behavioral sciences. 2nd ed. Boston, MA: Houghton Mifflin, 1988: 383–9.

7. Kuczmarski R.J., Ogden C.L., Grummer-Strawn L.M., et al. CDC growth charts: United States. Washington, DC: US Department of Health and Human Services, CDC, National Center for Health Statistics. Advance data from vital and health statistics; December 4, 2000 (revised); publication no. 314.

8. Lowry R., Kann L., Collins J.L., Kolbe LJ. The effect of socioeconomic status on chronic disease risk behaviors among U.S. adolescents. JAMA 1996; 276: 792–7.

9. U.S. Department of Education. Dropout rates in the United States: 2000. Washington, DC: U.S. Department of Education, National Center for Educational Statistics, Office of Educational Research and Improvement, 2001; publication no. (NCES) 2002-114.

10. Brener N.D., Kann L., McManus T., Kinchen S.A., Sundberg E.C., Ross J.G. Reliability of the 1999 Youth Risk Behavior Survey Questionnaire. J Sch Health 2002 (in press).

11. CDC. FY 2002 performance plan. Atlanta GA: CDC, 2001.

Footnotes

1. In this report, black students refers to black or African-American, non-Hispanic students. Hispanic students refers to Hispanic or Latino students of any race. White students refers to white, non-Hispanic students.

2. Students were classified as injection-drug users only if they a) reported injecting-drug use not prescribed by a physician, and b) answered one or more times to any of the following questions: "During your life, how many times have you used any form of cocaine including powder, crack, or freebase?"; "During your life, how many times have you used heroin (also called smack, junk, or China white)?"; "During your life, how many times have you used methamphetamines (also called speed, crystal, crank, or ice)?"; and "During your life, how many times have you taken steroid pills or shots without a doctor's prescription?"

3. Fruits and vegetables include 100 percent fruit juice, fruit, green salad, potatoes (excluding French fries, fried potatoes, or potato chips), carrots, and other vegetables.

Results from the
2001 Youth Risk Behavior Surveillance System

2.1   Sample sizes and response rates: United States and selected U.S. sites, 2001

| | | response rate (percent) | | |
	sample size	school	student	overall
NATIONAL SURVEY	**13,601**	**75%**	**83%**	**63%**
STATE SURVEYS				
Weighted data				
Alabama	1,578	95	79	75
Arkansas	1,694	76	88	67
Delaware	2,915	97	77	75
Florida	4,237	94	76	71
Idaho	1,714	77	88	68
Maine	1,351	73	90	66
Massachusetts	4,204	96	80	77
Michigan	3,630	88	83	73
Mississippi	1,806	74	89	66
Missouri	1,650	81	87	71
Montana	2,755	89	80	71
Nevada	1,464	95	66	63
New Jersey	2,142	77	78	60
North Carolina	2,548	86	84	73
North Dakota	1,599	87	85	74
Rhode Island	1,392	84	75	63
South Dakota	1,614	88	83	73
Texas	7,067	80	79	63
Utah	1,071	97	69	67
Vermont	7,191	89	78	69
Wisconsin	2,120	83	78	65
Wyoming	2,770	90	78	70
Unweighted data				
Colorado	999	56	87	49
Hawaii	1,076	100	48	48
Illinois*	1,016	52	87	45
Indiana	1,183	76	73	55
Iowa	1,047	58	89	52
Kentucky	981	42	96	41
Louisiana*	1,106	60	83	50
Nebraska	1,856	52	95	50
New Hampshire	1,303	68	81	55
New York*	1,484	66	77	51
South Carolina	3,438	59	75	44
Tennessee	1,437	67	84	56

(continued)

(continued from previous page)

| | sample size | response rate (percent) | | |
		school	student	overall
LOCAL SURVEYS				
Weighted data				
Boston	1,543	96%	66%	63%
Chicago	955	95	68	64
Dallas	1,719	100	79	79
Ft. Lauderdale	2,112	96	83	79
Houston	1,632	94	68	64
Los Angeles	1,295	89	71	63
Miami	2,052	93	76	70
New York City	1,616	96	77	74
Orlando	1,561	100	84	84
Palm Beach	1,504	100	71	71
Philadelphia	1,037	89	68	61
San Bernardino	956	100	90	90
San Diego	1,814	100	79	79
San Francisco	1,431	100	63	63
Unweighted data				
Detroit	2,012	100	78	78
District of Columbia	1,469	77	68	52
Milwaukee	1,306	95	62	59
New Orleans	1,345	88	64	56

* Survey did not include students from one of the state's large school districts.
Source: Grunbaum, Jo Anne, et.al., Youth Risk Behavior Surveillance–United States, 2001, Mortality and Morbidity Weekly Report, *Vol. 51/SS-4, Centers for Disease Control and Prevention, June 28, 2002*

2.2 Percentage of high school students who rarely or never wore seat belts, motorcycle helmets, or bicycle helmets, by sex, race/ethnicity, and grade—United States, 2001

	rarely or never wore seatbelts when riding in a car driven by someone else			rarely or never wore motorcycle helmets among the 25% of students who rode motorcycles in the past 12 months			rarely or never wore bicycle helmets among the 65% of students who rode bicycles in the past 12 months		
	total	female	male	total	female	male	total	female	male
Total	**14.1**	**10.2**	**18.1**	**37.2**	**30.1**	**40.9**	**84.7**	**82.6**	**86.3**
	(±1.7)	(±1.5)	(±2.1)	(± 3.2)	(± 4.0)	(± 3.6)	(±2.9)	(±3.5)	(±2.8)
Race/ethnicity									
Black	16.1	12.2	20.3	44.6	32.1	51.1	90.7	90.4	90.9
	(±3.9)	(±3.3)	(±5.1)	(±10.5)	(± 9.2)	(±11.2)	(±2.3)	(±2.9)	(±3.4)
Hispanic	14.5	11.3	17.7	55.3	51.1	58	88.9	86.9	90.6
	(±2.7)	(±2.3)	(±3.8)	(± 7.9)	(±12.0)	(± 6.4)	(±2.9)	(±3.6)	(±3.1)
White	13.6	9.7	17.7	33.6	26.4	37.1	83.6	81.1	85.5
	(±2.1)	(±2.0)	(±2.5)	(± 3.4)	(± 4.3)	(± 3.7)	(±3.7)	(±4.4)	(±3.7)
Grade									
9	14.9	10.8	19.4	36.5	30	39.9	83.3	80.4	86
	(±2.4)	(±2.3)	(±3.1)	(± 5.4)	(± 7.7)	(± 5.7)	(±3.8)	(±5.2)	(±3.5)
10	13.3	10.3	16.6	34.7	30.2	36.9	83.5	81.5	85
	(±1.9)	(±2.2)	(±2.3)	(± 5.1)	(± 6.7)	(± 6.6)	(±4.3)	(±4.7)	(±4.7)
11	13.6	9.7	17.5	40.8	33.9	44	87.1	86.2	87.7
	(±2.0)	(±1.8)	(±2.9)	(± 4.6)	(± 8.2)	(± 5.9)	(±2.6)	(±3.6)	(±2.9)
12	13.9	9.4	18.6	36.1	25.7	42.3	86.3	85.1	87.1
	(±2.0)	(±2.5)	(±2.9)	(± 4.2)	(± 7.3)	(± 5.1)	(±3.4)	(±5.6)	(±3.2)

Note: Blacks and whites are non-Hispanic. Numbers in parentheses are plus or minus percentage points of the 95 percent confidence interval. Differences in percentages are considered statistically significant if the confidence intervals do not overlap.
Source: Grunbaum, Jo Anne, et al., Youth Risk Behavior Surveillance–United States, 2001, Mortality and Morbidity Weekly Report, Vol. 51/SS-4, Centers for Disease Control and Prevention, June 28, 2002

2.3 Percentage of high school students who rarely or never wore seat belts, motorcycle helmets, or bicycle helmets, by sex—selected U.S. sites, 2001

	rarely or never wore seatbelts when riding in a car driven by someone else			rarely or never wore motorcycle helmets among the 25% of students who rode motorcycles in the past 12 months			rarely or never wore bicycle helmets among the 65% of students who rode bicycles in the past 12 months		
	total	female	male	total	female	male	total	female	male
State surveys									
Weighted data									
Alabama	10.7	9.0	12.1	31.1	24.4	33.6	90.4	88.3	91.8
Arkansas	23.0	17.3	28.3	45.0	42.6	46.1	94.4	94.1	94.8
Delaware	14.9	9.7	20.3	31.8	19.6	39.6	82.4	79.0	85.3
Florida	15.6	12.7	18.3	39.9	32.0	44.0	88.4	86.6	89.6
Idaho	13.6	9.1	17.6	37.0	34.3	38.5	85.3	83.3	86.9
Maine	14.9	10.1	19.2	34.1	27.0	37.9	71.6	69.6	73.2
Massachusetts	20.7	15.6	25.5	19.5	14.2	21.8	78.5	74.6	81.3
Michigan	8.3	5.7	10.8	22.6	14.3	26.2	89.3	88.9	89.8
Mississippi	24.6	18.9	30.5	48.5	40.3	51.7	95.3	93.5	96.7
Missouri	19.1	13.5	24.6	34.7	19.4	41.4	89.8	88.5	90.9
Montana	19.8	13.3	25.6	44.2	37.9	47.0	85.1	84.1	85.8
Nevada	NA	NA	NA	NA	NA	NA	NA	NA	NA
New Jersey	15.0	10.1	19.7	27.7	15.9	33.1	86.9	84.3	89.0
North Carolina	9.5	6.0	12.9	34.9	26.8	39.3	87.1	88.4	86.3
North Dakota	20.7	11.7	28.8	52.0	51.2	52.4	95.5	95.3	96.0
Rhode Island	17.9	12.7	22.4	38.8	19.5	48.2	84.5	79.5	88.2
South Dakota	27.4	20.2	34.3	NA	NA	NA	93.1	93.7	92.6
Texas	10.4	7.7	12.9	47.1	44.8	48.2	92.4	91.6	93.0
Utah	7.5	4.5	10.4	40.8	34.3	44.5	84.5	85.3	83.9
Vermont	10.9	7.5	13.9	NA	NA	NA	54.8	51.7	57.1
Wisconsin	20.9	16.1	25.4	NA	NA	NA	88.4	88.6	88.3
Wyoming	20.0	13.5	26.1	44.9	40.4	46.5	86.2	83.9	88.1
Unweighted data									
Colorado	12.6	10.0	14.8	42.8	NA	43.2	83.3	83.4	83.1
Hawaii	7.6	6.3	8.9	56.9	NA	58.0	85.0	82.2	87.7
Illinois*	11.6	7.4	17.6	48.2	45.0	50.8	93.2	92.3	94.3
Indiana	13.3	9.3	17.6	42.1	40.5	42.6	93.3	93.3	93.4
Iowa	10.0	7.4	12.6	66.1	66.2	65.8	94.2	93.5	94.8
Kentucky	18.7	13.3	24.5	43.0	NA	50.0	91.9	92.1	91.7
Louisiana*	14.9	9.7	21.7	46.8	37.6	54.5	95.8	96.1	95.4
Nebraska	22.3	14.3	30.2	34.6	22.3	41.2	92.9	92.1	93.7
New Hampshire	13.3	8.5	18.3	20.3	15.1	24.0	NA	NA	NA
New York*	11.0	8.0	14.1	22.5	16.0	26.3	81.9	80.3	83.3
South Carolina	16.9	12.0	21.8	53.6	46.8	57.9	91.1	91.4	90.9
Tennessee	17.7	12.9	22.3	33.2	23.1	37.3	88.9	87.9	89.7

(continued)

(continued from previous page)

	rarely or never wore seatbelts when riding in a car driven by someone else			rarely or never wore motorcycle helmets among the 25% of students who rode motorcycles in the past 12 months			rarely or never wore bicycle helmets among the 65% of students who rode bicycles in the past 12 months		
	total	female	male	total	female	male	total	female	male
Local surveys									
Weighted data									
Boston	30.3	24.6	36.0	47.3	42.6	51.2	87.2	83.6	90.1
Chicago	34.0	28.0	40.4	67.6	NA	NA	92.6	92.6	93.5
Dallas	8.5	6.2	10.9	60.1	NA	61.3	91.9	88.4	94.6
Ft. Lauderdale	10.3	9.0	11.6	44.2	31.5	51.0	89.2	89.3	89.1
Houston	12.0	9.2	14.8	53.1	61.1	47.6	87.9	85.4	90.1
Los Angeles	6.7	7.4	6.1	42.5	NA	46.4	79.7	74.5	83.4
Miami	18.1	16.3	19.7	49.5	45.7	52.6	88.1	86.8	88.9
New York City	19.8	17.7	22.1	35.9	NA	40.4	88.0	89.0	87.2
Orlando	13.0	9.3	16.5	36.4	34.6	36.6	85.8	83.4	87.8
Palm Beach	16.4	14.1	18.4	34.2	31.3	35.4	86.3	85.9	86.4
Philadelphia	34.5	29.0	39.9	55.5	NA	58.8	90.9	87.9	94.1
San Bernardino	8.2	5.0	10.9	30.6	NA	34.7	81.3	77.5	84.1
San Diego	7.4	6.6	8.1	34.9	NA	36.9	72.1	70.2	73.2
San Francisco	8.7	8.1	9.3	33.6	NA	NA	70.1	67.5	72.0
Unweighted data									
Detroit	10.9	7.2	15.0	31.8	27.5	34.3	94.0	93.6	94.3
District of Columbia	14.1	10.1	18.2	34.4	NA	35.7	85.5	83.1	87.5
Milwaukee	38.2	31.1	46.1	NA	NA	NA	94.4	93.9	95.1
New Orleans	20.1	15.7	25.4	61.1	61.3	62.6	93.8	93.4	94.5

* Survey did not include students from one of the state's large school districts.
Note: NA means data not available.
Source: Grunbaum, Jo Anne, et al., Youth Risk Behavior Surveillance–United States, 2001, Mortality and Morbidity Weekly
Report, *Vol. 51/SS-4, Centers for Disease Control and Prevention, June 28, 2002*

2.4 Percentage of high school students who rode with a driver who had been drinking alcohol and who drove after drinking alcohol, by sex, race/ethnicity, and grade—United States, 2001

	rode with a driver who had been drinking alcohol in the past 30 days			drove after drinking alcohol in the past 30 days		
	total	female	male	total	female	male
Total	**30.7**	**29.6**	**31.8**	**13.3**	**9.5**	**17.2**
	(±2.0)	(±2.1)	(±2.3)	(±1.5)	(±1.4)	(±2.1)
Race/ethnicity						
Black	27.6	24.2	31.2	7.7	3.3	12.5
	(±3.3)	(±3.8)	(±4.8)	(±1.5)	(±1.2)	(±2.2)
Hispanic	38.3	39.3	37.1	13.1	10.5	15.8
	(±4.3)	(±5.0)	(±4.5)	(±2.0)	(±1.8)	(±3.2)
White	30.3	29.4	31.2	14.7	10.9	18.6
	(±2.2)	(±2.1)	(±2.6)	(±1.7)	(±1.8)	(±2.5)
Grade						
9	30.4	31.3	29.2	6.6	3.7	9.9
	(±2.4)	(±3.2)	(±2.6)	(±1.3)	(±1.4)	(±1.7)
10	30.6	29.9	31.5	10.4	8.4	12.5
	(±2.7)	(±2.9)	(±3.9)	(±2.2)	(±1.4)	(±3.7)
11	29.1	25.4	32.8	16.7	11.1	22.1
	(±2.8)	(±2.8)	(±3.4)	(±2.7)	(±2.4)	(±3.8)
12	32.8	31.3	34.5	22.1	17.3	27.2
	(±3.2)	(±4.0)	(±3.5)	(±2.7)	(±3.2)	(±3.2)

Note: Blacks and whites are non-Hispanic. Numbers in parentheses are plus or minus percentage points of the 95 percent confidence interval. Differences in percentages are considered statistically significant if the confidence intervals do not overlap.
Source: Grunbaum, Jo Anne, et al., Youth Risk Behavior Surveillance–United States, 2001, Mortality and Morbidity Weekly Report, *Vol. 51/SS-4, Centers for Disease Control and Prevention, June 28, 2002*

2.5 Percentage of high school students who rode with a driver who had been drinking alcohol and who drove after drinking alcohol, by sex—selected U.S. sites, 2001

	rode with a driver who had been drinking alcohol in the past 30 days			drove after drinking alcohol in the past 30 days		
	total	female	male	total	female	male
State surveys						
Weighted data						
Alabama	33.7	35.0	32.0	12.7	9.8	15.2
Arkansas	31.2	29.9	32.5	15.8	9.8	21.6
Delaware	29.2	26.7	32.0	12.1	8.6	15.9
Florida	31.5	30.3	32.5	12.9	10.6	14.9
Idaho	28.7	27.2	29.7	12.3	8.9	15.6
Maine	27.4	27.3	27.4	10.8	9.0	12.3
Massachusetts	30.5	28.7	32.3	12.2	7.8	16.6
Michigan	32.1	32.6	31.2	12.9	10.7	14.9
Mississippi	35.0	33.0	37.1	13.7	9.7	17.9
Missouri	32.6	30.3	34.8	15.9	13.0	18.7
Montana	39.3	39.0	39.5	21.8	19.6	23.8
Nevada	29.9	28.6	31.0	13.1	11.6	14.5
New Jersey	30.4	29.0	31.7	13.0	9.5	16.4
North Carolina	23.9	21.5	26.4	9.3	6.1	12.3
North Dakota	43.5	43.1	43.6	26.8	23.8	29.3
Rhode Island	32.3	29.5	34.7	15.5	9.1	21.6
South Dakota	38.1	37.6	38.7	21.9	19.1	24.5
Texas	39.7	39.9	39.6	16.3	12.1	20.3
Utah	17.1	12.1	21.6	6.4	3.4	9.3
Vermont	24.5	23.2	25.5	10.1	6.5	13.4
Wisconsin	36.3	37.3	35.3	17.0	16.2	17.7
Wyoming	35.9	35.1	36.6	20.2	15.5	24.6
Unweighted data						
Colorado	30.0	29.6	30.5	13.2	10.7	15.5
Hawaii	32.8	34.2	30.7	9.2	8.0	10.7
Illinois*	28.0	28.2	27.8	10.7	8.5	13.9
Indiana	27.0	26.4	27.2	10.2	7.2	13.6
Iowa	36.9	33.7	39.4	19.4	16.8	21.7
Kentucky	22.7	24.1	21.4	8.7	7.5	10.0
Louisiana*	37.1	37.8	35.9	14.8	11.7	19.0
Nebraska	43.5	43.3	43.7	24.8	20.5	29.1
New Hampshire	27.5	29.8	24.8	9.7	6.9	12.3
New York*	30.4	30.8	30.1	12.3	9.6	15.1
South Carolina	34.0	31.5	36.4	13.3	9.6	17.0
Tennessee	32.3	31.5	33.1	13.9	9.1	18.7

(continued)

(continued from previous page)

	rode with a driver who had been drinking alcohol in the past 30 days			drove after drinking alcohol in the past 30 days		
	total	female	male	total	female	male
Local surveys **Weighted data**						
Boston	25.2	25.8	24.6	5.5	4.0	7.0
Chicago	34.0	35.8	31.8	10.7	7.8	13.3
Dallas	39.6	39.5	39.6	11.4	8.4	14.7
Ft. Lauderdale	27.5	27.6	27.3	10.8	7.5	13.8
Houston	38.6	39.4	37.6	13.8	10.6	17.2
Los Angeles	29.4	29.6	28.7	7.6	5.1	9.8
Miami	26.7	25.2	28.4	8.8	6.0	11.7
New York City	20.7	20.3	21.0	4.5	2.6	6.4
Orlando	28.2	28.5	27.6	10.7	7.4	14.0
Palm Beach	34.5	33.1	36.0	13.6	9.8	17.5
Philadelphia	23.3	24.9	21.8	4.9	5.1	4.6
San Bernardino	34.8	33.4	35.9	10.4	8.1	12.5
San Diego	28.0	27.4	28.6	8.5	6.3	10.7
San Francisco	19.3	20.1	18.6	3.8	3.5	4.1
Unweighted data						
Detroit	34.2	35.3	32.6	6.7	5.4	7.8
District of Columbia	32.2	30.9	33.2	6.2	4.7	7.8
Milwaukee	29.7	30.4	28.9	7.2	5.5	9.1
New Orleans	32.4	31.5	33.5	7.3	6.1	8.4

Survey did not include students from one of the state's large school districts.
Source: Grunbaum, Jo Anne, et al., Youth Risk Behavior Surveillance–United States, 2001, Mortality and Morbidity Weekly Report, *Vol. 51/SS-4, Centers for Disease Control and Prevention, June 28, 2002"*

2.6 Percentage of high school students who carried a weapon or gun, by sex, race/ethnicity, and grade—United States, 2001

| | carried a weaon on at least one day during the past 30 days | | | carried a gun on at least one day during the past 30 days | | |
	total	female	male	total	female	male
Total	**17.4**	**6.2**	**29.3**	**5.7**	**1.3**	**10.3**
	(±1.9)	(±0.8)	(±3.3)	(±1.0)	(±0.3)	(±1.8)
Race/ethnicity						
Black	15.2	8.6	22.4	6.5	1.1	12.2
	(±2.4)	(±2.3)	(±3.6)	(±1.9)	(±0.6)	(±3.6)
Hispanic	16.5	7.4	26.0	4.8	1.6	8.0
	(±1.5)	(±1.6)	(±2.9)	(±1.1)	(±0.7)	(±2.0)
White	17.9	5.1	31.3	5.5	1.0	10.2
	(±2.6)	(±1.1)	(±4.3)	(±1.3)	(±0.5)	(±2.3)
Grade						
9	19.8	7.4	33.7	6.8	1.0	13.3
	(±2.8)	(±1.3)	(±4.3)	(±1.3)	(±0.6)	(±2.3)
10	16.7	5.4	28.4	4.9	1.0	9.0
	(±2.2)	(±1.2)	(±4.0)	(±0.8)	(±0.4)	(±1.6)
11	16.8	5.9	28.1	5.7	1.8	9.6
	(±2.5)	(±1.4)	(±4.2)	(±1.6)	(±1.1)	(±2.9)
12	15.1	5.3	25.6	4.7	1.2	8.3
	(±2.5)	(±1.7)	(±4.1)	(±1.3)	(±0.7)	(±2.2)

Note: Blacks and whites are non-Hispanic. Numbers in parentheses are plus or minus percentage points of the 95 percent confidence interval. Differences in percentages are considered statistically significant if the confidence intervals do not overlap.
Source: Grunbaum, Jo Anne, et al., Youth Risk Behavior Surveillance–United States, 2001, Mortality and Morbidity Weekly Report, *Vol. 51/SS-4, Centers for Disease Control and Prevention, June 28, 2002*

2.7 Percentage of high school students who carried a weapon or gun, by sex— selected U.S. sites, 2001

	carried a weaon on at least one day during the past 30 days			carried a gun on at least one day during the past 30 days		
	total	female	male	total	female	male
State surveys **Weighted data**						
Alabama	20.7	8.3	32.8	7.5	2.7	12.0
Arkansas	22.1	6.0	37.9	8.0	2.1	13.6
Delaware	14.5	4.7	24.8	4.8	0.8	9.0
Florida	16.4	6.5	25.8	5.7	1.9	9.2
Idaho	NA	NA	NA	NA	NA	NA
Maine	15.4	4.8	25.6	4.4	0.3	8.3
Massachusetts	13.2	4.2	22.0	3.1	0.6	5.6
Michigan	12.5	5.2	19.3	4.5	1.1	7.7
Mississippi	19.0	6.8	32.0	7.8	1.6	14.6
Missouri	20.2	6.6	33.6	8.8	1.7	15.7
Montana	21.4	5.5	36.5	9.0	1.4	16.1
Nevada	16.0	8.1	23.5	NA	NA	NA
New Jersey	13.1	5.5	20.7	4.8	1.4	8.2
North Carolina	18.3	7.5	29.1	NA	NA	NA
North Dakota	NA	NA	NA	NA	NA	NA
Rhode Island	11.3	3.1	19.5	4.6	0.8	8.3
South Dakota	NA	NA	NA	NA	NA	NA
Texas	17.9	6.4	29.1	5.2	1.4	9.0
Utah	16.8	5.7	27.5	6.0	1.4	10.5
Vermont	NA	NA	NA	NA	NA	NA
Wisconsin	13.3	5.4	21.0	4.8	1.3	8.3
Wyoming	22.9	8.0	37.3	10.1	2.6	17.2
Unweighted data						
Colorado	19.4	7.2	30.5	4.7	0.6	8.5
Hawaii	10.6	6.3	16.3	2.9	1.2	5.0
Illinois*	11.0	2.9	22.6	3.3	0.3	7.5
Indiana	13.9	3.0	26.7	4.5	0.9	8.4
Iowa	13.5	3.8	23.0	6.9	1.4	12.2
Kentucky	17.0	6.1	29.4	4.4	1.4	7.9
Louisiana*	14.9	7.0	25.6	6.3	2.1	12.1
Nebraska	15.7	2.8	28.5	6.5	0.7	12.4
New Hampshire	16.9	5.8	28.6	4.3	0.7	7.5
New York*	14.7	5.0	24.7	4.9	1.4	8.3
South Carolina	19.5	7.0	32.2	6.9	1.4	12.4
Tennessee	20.3	6.1	34.2	6.2	0.9	11.1

(continued)

(continued from previous page)

	carried a weaon on at least one day during the past 30 days			carried a gun on at least one day during the past 30 days		
	total	female	male	total	female	male
Local surveys						
Weighted data						
Boston	16.4	8.7	24.4	4.4	0.9	7.9
Chicago	21.2	16.4	26.4	6.8	1.7	12.2
Dallas	15.9	8.6	23.8	6.7	2.3	11.5
Ft. Lauderdale	10.9	3.7	18.2	2.8	0.6	4.8
Houston	15.7	7.9	23.8	6.1	2.0	10.4
Los Angeles	12.5	4.6	20.3	4.3	1.6	6.8
Miami	11.3	5.3	17.4	4.4	1.2	7.6
New York City	16.9	8.0	26.0	3.6	1.2	6.1
Orlando	12.4	4.5	20.5	4.8	1.5	8.1
Palm Beach	13.5	4.8	22.5	4.7	2.3	7.0
Philadelphia	12.7	7.5	18.0	4.8	1.2	8.5
San Bernardino	13.0	6.8	18.4	4.8	3.0	6.4
San Diego	12.3	5.2	19.5	3.1	0.8	5.2
San Francisco	8.3	4.2	12.3	1.3	0.2	2.3
Unweighted data						
Detroit	18.4	15.0	22.1	7.1	2.9	11.9
District of Columbia	20.3	13.9	26.5	5.7	2.0	9.4
Milwaukee	15.1	10.2	20.5	7.1	2.4	12.3
New Orleans	13.9	10.4	18.5	6.2	1.2	12.4

* Survey did not include students from one of the state's large school districts.
Note: NA means data not available.
Source: Grunbaum, Jo Anne, et al., Youth Risk Behavior Surveillance–United States, 2001, Mortality and Morbidity Weekly Report, Vol. 51/SS-4, Centers for Disease Control and Prevention, June 28, 2002

2.8 Percentage of high school students who engaged in violence or in behaviors resulting from violence, by sex, race/ethnicity, and grade—United States, 2001

	in a physical fight in the past 12 months			injured in physical fight seriously enough to be treated by doctor in the past 12 months			physically hurt by a boyfriend or girlfriend on purpose in the past 12 months			forced to have sexual intercourse		
	total	female	male	total	female	male	total	female	male	total	female	male
Total	**33.2**	**23.9**	**43.1**	**4.0**	**2.9**	**5.2**	**9.5**	**9.8**	**9.1**	**7.7**	**10.3**	**5.1**
	(±1.4)	(±1.9)	(±1.6)	(±0.4)	(±0.5)	(±0.7)	(±0.6)	(±0.9)	(±0.8)	(±0.9)	(±1.2)	(±1.3)
Race/ethnicity												
Black	36.5	29.6	43.9	5.3	4.8	5.8	11.2	11.7	10.7	9.6	10.6	8.5
	(±3.1)	(±3.8)	(±4.3)	(±0.8)	(±1.3)	(±1.2)	(±1.7)	(±1.9)	(±2.7)	(±1.2)	(±2.7)	(±2.1)
Hispanic	35.8	29.3	42.4	4.4	3.8	5.1	9.9	10.7	9.1	8.9	11.6	6.2
	(±1.8)	(±2.8)	(±2.4)	(±1.1)	(±1.2)	(±1.5)	(±1.4)	(±2.9)	(±1.8)	(±2.0)	(±1.9)	(±3.2)
White	32.2	21.7	43.1	3.4	2.1	4.8	9.1	9.4	8.9	6.9	9.8	3.8
	(±1.9)	(±2.4)	(±2.1)	(±0.5)	(±0.6)	(±0.8)	(±0.9)	(±1.1)	(±1.1)	(±1.1)	(±1.6)	(±0.9)
Grade												
9	39.5	30.3	50.0	4.5	2.8	6.5	8.5	9.2	7.7	7.3	8.6	5.9
	(±2.5)	(±3.2)	(±3.1)	(±0.7)	(±0.7)	(±1.2)	(±1.5)	(±2.0)	(±1.9)	(±1.6)	(±1.9)	(±2.7)
10	34.7	24.9	45.0	4.6	3.9	5.4	9.3	10.6	8.0	7.5	10.7	4.1
	(±2.7)	(±2.6)	(±4.0)	(±1.0)	(±1.2)	(±1.4)	(±1.3)	(±2.1)	(±1.7)	(±1.2)	(±1.9)	(±1.0)
11	29.1	20.3	38.0	3.1	2.6	3.7	9.5	9.4	9.6	7.1	9.9	4.3
	(±2.2)	(±1.9)	(±2.9)	(±0.8)	(±1.0)	(±1.2)	(±1.2)	(±1.7)	(±1.4)	(±1.1)	(±1.9)	(±1.1)
12	26.5	16.9	36.5	3.4	1.9	5.0	10.7	9.8	11.7	9.0	12.2	5.8
	(±2.0)	(±3.2)	(±2.3)	(±0.8)	(±0.8)	(±1.2)	(±1.3)	(±2.0)	(±2.4)	(±1.2)	(±2.3)	(±1.4)

Note: Blacks and whites are non-Hispanic. Numbers in parentheses are plus or minus percentage points of the 95 percent confidence interval. Differences in percentages are considered statistically significant if the confidence intervals do not overlap.
Source: Grunbaum, Jo Anne, et al., Youth Risk Behavior Surveillance—United States, 2001, Mortality and Morbidity Weekly Report, Vol. 51/SS-4, Centers for Disease Control and Prevention, June 28, 2002

2.9 Percentage of high school students who engaged in violence and in behaviors resulting from violence, by sex—selected U.S. sites, 2001

	in a physical fight in the past 12 months			injured in physical fight seriously enough to be treated by doctor in the past 12 months			physically hurt by a boyfriend or girlfriend on purpose in the past 12 months			forced to have sexual intercourse		
	total	female	male	total	female	male	total	female	male	total	female	male
State surveys												
Weighted data												
Alabama	30.3	22.5	37.4	3.6	2.1	4.7	13.9	13.2	14.1	10.4	12.9	7.6
Arkansas	31.2	22.9	39.3	2.9	1.7	4.1	10.0	9.3	10.7	9.7	13.2	6.4
Delaware	34.1	25.2	43.1	4.5	2.1	6.7	10.7	10.0	11.3	8.6	10.7	6.4
Florida	32.8	24.7	40.3	4.2	3.0	5.2	10.3	8.9	11.5	8.4	9.5	7.1
Idaho	28.7	19.1	37.3	3.1	1.5	4.7	9.8	7.6	11.8	7.8	10.5	5.2
Maine	30.9	22.4	38.7	3.9	2.5	5.1	12.0	10.7	13.2	7.8	10.3	5.2
Massachusetts	33.2	23.6	42.7	3.5	2.1	4.8	NA	NA	NA	NA	NA	NA
Michigan	33.8	25.2	41.8	3.8	2.2	5.0	11.8	11.7	11.8	9.5	12.0	7.0
Mississippi	31.8	23.4	40.6	3.2	2.2	4.1	10.1	10.2	10.1	10.4	12.6	8.1
Missouri	32.7	24.0	40.9	3.5	2.5	4.3	10.5	8.7	12.3	7.2	10.2	4.3
Montana	31.6	23.2	39.5	3.6	2.2	4.7	10.3	10.3	10.3	8.8	12.7	5.0
Nevada	35.6	25.7	44.9	NA	NA	NA	12.1	10.3	13.8	9.2	11.3	7.2
New Jersey	34.6	24.8	44.7	6.4	3.5	9.2	11.6	8.6	14.3	10.5	7.8	13.1
North Carolina	29.0	20.8	37.1	2.8	1.9	3.7	NA	NA	NA	NA	NA	NA
North Dakota	28.2	20.4	35.5	2.8	1.8	3.2	11.7	11.3	11.7	8.6	9.4	7.5
Rhode Island	31.4	21.3	41.0	5.9	3.5	8.1	9.2	7.4	10.7	7.7	8.2	7.0
South Dakota	30.8	22.3	38.9	2.4	1.0	3.6	9.3	10.2	8.5	8.0	10.9	5.1
Texas	32.6	23.0	41.6	3.7	2.1	5.3	9.8	10.8	8.7	8.1	11.5	4.8
Utah	27.9	19.3	36.2	3.7	2.0	5.3	9.5	7.9	11.0	NA	NA	NA
Vermont	26.5	17.8	34.7	3.3	2.0	4.4	7.3	6.3	8.3	NA	NA	NA
Wisconsin	31.4	26.1	36.5	NA	NA	NA	NA	NA	NA	NA	NA	NA
Wyoming	31.4	22.9	39.4	2.9	1.2	4.4	9.5	8.2	10.6	8.1	11.3	5.0

(continued)

(continued from previous page)

Unweighted data	in a physical fight in the past 12 months			injured in physical fight seriously enough to be treated by doctor in the past 12 months			physically hurt by a boyfriend or girlfriend on purpose in the past 12 months			forced to have sexual intercourse		
	total	female	male	total	female	male	total	female	male	total	female	male
Colorado	33.3	26.2	39.7	3.9	2.5	5.2	7.8	6.6	9.0	8.0	10.9	5.6
Hawaii	25.9	22.7	29.8	3.2	2.3	4.3	9.8	10.8	8.5	9.0	12.7	3.7
Illinois*	27.1	18.8	38.8	2.5	1.9	3.3	8.1	7.3	9.2	5.6	6.8	4.0
Indiana	28.1	19.8	37.6	2.7	3.0	2.4	11.4	11.6	11.1	NA	NA	NA
Iowa	31.5	19.9	42.2	2.8	1.8	3.6	7.4	6.4	8.3	5.9	7.4	4.6
Kentucky	28.4	20.9	36.6	2.7	1.8	3.7	11.7	11.2	12.5	8.3	8.6	8.0
Louisiana*	31.9	25.3	40.8	3.6	2.1	5.6	18.1	17.0	19.7	NA	NA	NA
Nebraska	27.3	19.9	34.5	2.0	1.2	2.8	6.9	6.1	7.8	5.4	7.5	3.4
New Hampshire	31.1	22.2	40.5	3.7	2.8	4.5	11.8	10.8	12.5	8.7	11.5	5.3
New York*	32.8	25.0	40.4	4.5	2.6	6.3	12.8	12.0	13.4	9.5	11.8	7.1
South Carolina	35.1	27.1	43.2	4.4	2.3	6.3	13.9	13.5	14.3	12.1	14.3	9.8
Tennessee	30.4	23.9	36.8	3.7	2.7	4.5	8.9	10.1	7.7	8.5	10.8	6.2

(continued)

(continued from previous page)

Local surveys Weighted data	in a physical fight in the past 12 months			injured in physical fight seriously enough to be treated by doctor in the past 12 months			physically hurt by a boyfriend or girlfriend on purpose in the past 12 months			forced to have sexual intercourse		
	total	female	male	total	female	male	total	female	male	total	female	male
Boston	33.3	27.4	39.7	4.6	4.0	5.2	NA	NA	NA	NA	NA	NA
Chicago	40.8	36.6	45.2	5.7	4.4	7.0	10.9	10.0	11.8	10.3	9.9	10.2
Dallas	41.0	32.8	49.8	3.9	1.9	6.0	10.4	10.8	10.0	10.5	12.9	8.0
Ft. Lauderdale	30.3	20.6	40.2	4.6	2.6	6.5	9.6	7.6	11.3	8.7	8.5	8.5
Houston	33.9	27.0	41.1	4.8	3.5	6.0	9.0	8.5	9.5	8.9	10.2	7.5
Los Angeles	35.0	26.6	43.2	4.5	2.9	5.7	8.5	7.9	9.1	8.1	8.7	7.3
Miami	32.7	24.7	40.4	4.3	2.3	6.1	9.6	8.3	10.8	6.3	7.1	5.4
New York City	40.5	33.6	47.7	4.5	2.9	6.1	6.0	5.9	5.9	5.6	6.7	4.4
Orlando	32.9	24.8	41.1	4.0	2.8	5.3	13.6	13.7	13.3	10.9	12.4	9.5
Palm Beach	33.5	22.4	44.6	5.3	3.4	7.3	8.9	6.0	11.7	8.1	8.1	8.2
Philadelphia	41.7	38.5	44.9	5.3	3.8	6.8	14.8	13.8	16.0	10.7	12.0	9.3
San Bernardino	34.3	26.2	41.8	4.4	1.3	7.2	13.0	12.6	13.4	11.6	12.9	10.3
San Diego	33.5	27.8	39.3	4.5	3.4	5.7	10.1	10.0	10.3	9.2	12.0	6.4
San Francisco	30.9	22.4	39.0	4.2	2.2	6.2	7.2	6.9	7.4	NA	NA	NA
Unweighted data												
Detroit	43.4	40.5	46.7	5.2	3.5	7.1	15.9	14.1	17.9	13.3	12.7	13.8
District of Columbia	37.4	34.0	41.2	5.8	5.8	5.5	17.2	17.1	17.0	12.6	13.9	11.0
Milwaukee	39.0	34.3	43.8	NA	NA	NA	NA	NA	NA	NA	NA	NA
New Orleans	43.4	39.0	49.1	7.1	5.9	8.6	11.2	11.1	10.7	6.7	6.4	7.1

* Survey did not include students from one of the state's large school districts.

Note: NA means data not available.

Source: Grunbaum, Jo Anne, et al., Youth Risk Behavior Surveillance—United States, 2001. Mortality and Morbidity Weekly Report, Vol. 51/SS-4, Centers for Disease Control and Prevention, June 28, 2002

2.10 Percentage of high school students who engaged in violence or in behaviors resulting from violence on school property, by sex, race/ethnicity, and grade—United States, 2001

	felt too unsafe to go to school in the past 30 days			carried a weapon on school property in the past 30 days			threatened or injured with a weapon on school property during past 12 months			engaged in a physical fight on school property during past 12 months		
	total	female	male	total	female	male	total	female	male	total	female	male
Total	**6.6**	**7.4**	**5.8**	**6.4**	**2.9**	**10.2**	**8.9**	**6.5**	**11.5**	**12.5**	**7.2**	**18.0**
	(±1.0)	(±1.3)	(±1.1)	(±1.0)	(±0.5)	(±1.7)	(±1.1)	(±1.0)	(±1.3)	(±1.0)	(±0.9)	(±1.5)
Race/ethnicity												
Black	9.8	10.0	9.6	6.3	4.2	8.4	9.3	6.7	11.9	16.8	12.7	21.3
	(±1.5)	(±2.3)	(±1.9)	(±1.8)	(±1.3)	(±3.0)	(±1.4)	(±1.6)	(±2.6)	(±2.5)	(±3.1)	(±3.2)
Hispanic	10.2	11.4	9.0	6.4	3.8	9.1	8.9	6.4	11.3	14.1	11.0	17.3
	(±1.3)	(±1.6)	(±1.6)	(±1.0)	(±1.5)	(±1.7)	(±2.1)	(±2.3)	(±2.8)	(±1.7)	(±1.9)	(±2.7)
White	5.0	5.6	4.2	6.1	2.3	10.0	8.5	6.0	11.1	11.2	5.4	17.2
	(±1.2)	(±1.3)	(±1.3)	(±1.2)	(±0.6)	(±2.1)	(±1.3)	(±1.2)	(±1.7)	(±1.2)	(±1.1)	(±1.8)
Grade												
9	8.8	9.6	8.0	6.7	2.9	10.7	12.7	10.0	15.7	17.3	10.2	25.1
	(±1.7)	(±2.1)	(±2.0)	(±1.3)	(±0.8)	(±2.2)	(±1.7)	(±1.9)	(±2.4)	(±1.5)	(±1.8)	(±2.5)
10	6.3	7.0	5.6	6.7	2.9	10.5	9.1	6.3	11.9	13.5	7.7	19.5
	(±1.3)	(±1.7)	(±1.6)	(±1.2)	(±0.9)	(±2.0)	(±1.5)	(±1.6)	(±1.8)	(±1.7)	(±1.4)	(±3.0)
11	5.9	6.8	5.0	6.1	2.9	9.5	6.9	4.7	9.1	9.4	5.1	13.8
	(±1.2)	(±1.8)	(±1.6)	(±1.4)	(±0.9)	(±2.6)	(±1.3)	(±1.3)	(±1.8)	(±1.4)	(±1.2)	(±2.1)
12	4.4	5.0	3.9	6.0	2.7	9.6	5.3	3.0	7.7	7.5	4.4	10.7
	(±0.7)	(±1.1)	(±1.2)	(±1.4)	(±1.1)	(±2.1)	(±1.0)	(±0.9)	(±1.8)	(±1.1)	(±1.3)	(±2.1)

Note: Blacks and whites are non-Hispanic. Numbers in parentheses are plus or minus percentage points of the 95 percent confidence interval. Differences in percentages are considered statistically significant if the confidence intervals do not overlap.
Source: Grunbaum, Jo Anne, et al., Youth Risk Behavior Surveillance–United States, 2001, Mortality and Morbidity Weekly Report, Vol. 51/SS-4, Centers for Disease Control and Prevention, June 28, 2002

2.11 Percentage of high school students who who engaged in violence or in behaviors resulting from violence on school property, by sex—selected U.S. sites, 2001

	felt too unsafe to go to school in the past 30 days			carried a weapon on school property in the past 30 days			threatened or injured with a weapon on school property during past 12 months			engaged in a physical fight on school property during past 12 months		
	total	female	male	total	female	male	total	female	male	total	female	male
State surveys												
Weighted data												
Alabama	7.4	6.8	7.7	7.4	4.7	9.9	7.1	5.7	8.2	11.6	6.7	16.1
Arkansas	7.6	9.0	6.2	7.9	1.8	13.8	9.4	7.0	11.8	12.7	8.4	16.9
Delaware	7.2	7.2	7.2	5.5	2.1	9.0	8.3	5.6	11.0	11.9	7.2	16.8
Florida	14.0	15.0	13.0	5.4	2.9	7.7	9.2	6.5	11.8	12.7	8.2	16.9
Idaho	5.1	5.3	4.6	10.3	4.2	15.9	8.0	5.7	9.9	12.8	6.7	18.0
Maine	9.4	8.5	10.0	5.2	2.0	8.1	8.7	5.9	11.3	11.3	6.8	15.4
Massachusetts	8.1	9.4	6.7	5.5	1.9	8.9	8.2	5.7	10.5	11.5	6.9	16.0
Michigan	7.2	7.5	6.7	4.9	2.4	7.3	9.0	6.8	10.9	11.4	6.9	15.7
Mississippi	6.9	6.4	7.5	6.5	2.9	10.3	8.1	5.8	10.6	12.1	7.2	17.2
Missouri	5.6	5.5	5.6	7.9	3.4	12.3	8.9	7.4	10.5	12.0	8.5	15.4
Montana	5.5	5.2	5.3	8.7	2.1	14.6	8.5	5.9	10.4	12.2	7.5	16.6
Nevada	16.9	20.0	13.9	6.9	4.2	9.5	8.8	5.0	12.5	13.0	7.9	17.9
New Jersey	9.4	9.2	9.7	6.8	3.0	10.5	11.2	7.0	15.2	13.2	7.8	18.7
North Carolina	9.2	9.1	9.4	4.8	2.4	7.3	7.6	5.4	9.7	10.7	7.0	14.4
North Dakota	3.0	3.2	2.4	6.4	2.2	10.2	8.9	6.1	11.2	11.1	5.1	16.6
Rhode Island	10.3	10.4	10.1	4.5	1.4	7.5	8.6	5.5	11.5	12.7	7.4	17.7
South Dakota	3.7	3.9	3.3	7.5	2.3	12.3	7.1	5.2	8.9	11.2	5.9	16.4
Texas	7.5	8.5	6.3	7.5	2.4	12.4	8.6	5.9	11.0	13.0	8.0	17.6
Utah	5.1	5.9	4.3	8.3	3.9	12.6	7.8	4.9	10.6	11.7	5.8	17.5
Vermont	4.1	3.5	4.5	8.6	2.8	13.9	6.2	3.8	8.1	12.8	6.8	18.3
Wisconsin	6.0	7.8	4.2	3.4	1.7	4.9	8.4	7.2	9.5	11.4	7.5	14.9
Wyoming	8.0	9.0	7.0	8.4	2.6	14.0	9.4	6.7	11.8	13.5	7.4	19.1

(continued)

(continued from previous page)

Unweighted data	felt too unsafe to go to school in the past 30 days			carried a weapon on school property in the past 30 days			threatened or injured with a weapon on school property during past 12 months			engaged in a physical fight on school property during past 12 months		
	total	female	male	total	female	male	total	female	male	total	female	male
Colorado	8.3	9.5	7.1	7.8	2.6	12.2	10.4	8.5	12.1	14.2	10.2	17.9
Hawaii	6.7	6.6	6.9	3.5	1.8	5.7	5.9	3.9	8.2	9.0	7.1	11.4
Illinois*	8.6	8.8	8.3	2.4	0.8	4.5	9.7	6.4	14.3	10.2	5.2	17.1
Indiana	7.0	8.1	5.3	4.3	1.1	7.8	7.6	5.2	10.1	8.8	4.9	13.1
Iowa	6.6	8.0	5.2	4.5	1.6	7.3	8.9	8.6	9.3	10.8	5.6	15.8
Kentucky	7.2	7.1	7.3	6.0	2.2	10.3	8.4	7.1	9.7	13.0	9.1	17.2
Louisiana*	8.9	9.4	8.2	4.1	2.1	6.8	8.0	4.3	12.5	9.8	7.1	13.5
Nebraska	4.3	4.7	4.0	4.7	0.8	8.4	7.1	4.8	9.4	8.8	3.7	13.7
New Hampshire	5.7	5.5	5.6	6.9	2.5	11.1	7.7	5.4	9.9	11.7	6.7	16.6
New York*	7.7	7.3	8.1	5.3	3.0	7.6	9.4	6.9	11.5	12.0	6.5	17.3
South Carolina	11.1	12.1	9.9	4.8	2.3	7.3	9.6	7.9	11.1	12.2	9.0	15.3
Tennessee	7.4	8.6	6.1	6.7	1.9	11.4	9.3	7.6	10.8	11.7	7.9	15.4

(continued)

(continued from previous page)

Local surveys	felt too unsafe to go to school in the past 30 days			carried a weapon on school property in the past 30 days			threatened or injured with a weapon on school property during past 12 months			engaged in a physical fight on school property during past 12 months		
	total	female	male	total	female	male	total	female	male	total	female	male
Weighted data												
Boston	9.8	10.0	9.4	7.9	4.2	11.5	8.8	5.9	11.6	11.2	8.9	13.6
Chicago	16.0	17.4	14.4	7.8	6.6	9.2	14.8	11.4	18.2	18.5	14.9	22.3
Dallas	8.5	9.0	7.9	5.7	3.9	7.6	9.2	5.7	12.8	15.1	10.3	20.2
Ft. Lauderdale	17.0	18.6	15.4	4.1	1.5	6.6	9.1	7.1	11.1	12.7	7.3	18.2
Houston	9.5	10.0	8.8	5.8	3.7	8.0	8.7	6.6	10.7	13.4	9.5	17.3
Los Angeles	14.4	16.8	11.9	5.4	2.5	8.3	10.4	6.5	14.0	14.0	9.1	18.5
Miami	11.4	12.2	10.8	4.4	2.0	7.0	8.7	6.2	11.1	14.8	9.4	20.1
New York City	10.6	11.2	10.2	7.3	3.0	11.8	9.5	6.4	12.5	15.8	12.7	19.0
Orlando	6.6	7.1	6.2	4.8	1.7	7.7	8.0	5.3	10.4	11.4	8.2	14.5
Palm Beach	14.6	13.6	15.4	5.0	2.4	7.5	10.5	5.9	15.0	11.9	7.0	16.7
Philadelphia	8.4	9.7	7.2	4.4	2.4	6.3	8.7	7.1	10.3	15.5	11.9	19.0
San Bernardino	16.6	17.4	15.7	5.9	3.5	8.0	11.9	9.5	14.0	11.8	6.5	16.6
San Diego	9.6	11.1	8.2	5.0	2.8	7.2	10.1	7.4	12.9	12.1	9.9	14.3
San Francisco	7.3	6.6	8.0	5.1	2.6	7.3	7.9	5.2	10.4	12.9	6.7	18.8
Unweighted data												
Detroit	13.8	14.0	13.7	8.6	6.9	10.4	11.9	9.4	14.5	18.0	15.5	20.7
District of Columbia	12.0	11.3	12.2	9.3	7.2	10.8	11.4	8.6	14.1	14.0	10.8	17.6
Milwaukee	14.0	14.5	13.3	5.6	4.0	7.3	13.6	12.0	15.4	15.1	13.1	16.9
New Orleans	11.4	11.1	11.2	4.9	4.5	5.4	10.9	11.2	10.2	21.5	18.3	25.7

* Survey did not include students from one of the state's large school districts.
Source: Grunbaum, Jo Anne, et al., Youth Risk Behavior Surveillance–United States, 2001. Mortality and Morbidity Weekly Report. *Vol. 51/SS-4. Centers for Disease Control and Prevention, June 28, 2002*

2.12 Percentage of high school students who felt sad or hopeless, who seriously considered attempting suicide, who made a suicide plan, or who attempted suicide, by sex, race/ethnicity, and grade——United States, 2001

	felt so sad or hopeless almost every day for two or more weeks that they stopped doing their usual activities			seriously considered attempting suicide in past 12 months			made a suicide plan in past 12 months			attempted suicide in past 12 months			suicide attempt required medical attention in past 12 months		
	total	female	male	total	female	male	total	female	male	total	female	male	total	female	male
Total	**28.3**	**34.5**	**21.6**	**19.0**	**23.6**	**14.2**	**14.8**	**17.7**	**11.8**	**8.8**	**11.2**	**6.2**	**2.6**	**3.1**	**2.1**
	(±1.3)	(±1.8)	(±1.2)	(±1.4)	(±1.8)	(±1.3)	(±1.1)	(±1.7)	(±0.9)	(±0.8)	(±1.0)	(±1.1)	(±0.4)	(±0.7)	(±0.4)
Race/ethnicity															
Black	28.8	36.3	20.9	13.3	17.2	9.2	10.3	13.0	7.5	8.8	9.8	7.5	3.4	3.1	3.6
	(±2.2)	(±3.4)	(±2.3)	(±1.5)	(±1.9)	(±2.2)	(±1.2)	(±2.4)	(±1.7)	(±1.2)	(±2.0)	(±2.0)	(±0.7)	(±0.9)	(±1.4)
Hispanic	34.0	42.3	25.4	19.4	26.5	12.2	14.1	17.8	10.5	12.1	15.9	8.0	3.4	4.2	2.5
	(±2.3)	(±3.3)	(±2.7)	(±2.8)	(±4.3)	(±2.3)	(±1.9)	(±2.6)	(±1.9)	(±1.6)	(±2.4)	(±1.6)	(±0.9)	(±1.4)	(±1.2)
White	26.5	32.3	20.5	19.7	24.2	14.9	15.3	18.0	12.5	7.9	10.3	5.3	2.3	2.9	1.7
	(±1.8)	(±2.9)	(±1.4)	(±1.8)	(±2.6)	(±1.6)	(±1.5)	(±2.4)	(±1.2)	(±1.0)	(±1.4)	(±1.3)	(±0.5)	(±0.9)	(±0.6)
Grade															
9	29.4	35.7	22.4	20.8	26.2	14.7	16.0	18.9	12.7	11.0	13.2	8.2	3.2	3.8	2.6
	(±2.2)	(±3.1)	(±3.0)	(±2.5)	(±2.4)	(±3.5)	(±1.7)	(±2.5)	(±2.6)	(±2.0)	(±2.3)	(±2.5)	(±0.9)	(±1.6)	(±1.0)
10	27.2	34.6	19.7	19.0	24.1	13.8	14.9	19.1	10.6	9.5	12.2	6.7	3.0	3.6	2.5
	(±2.1)	(±2.9)	(±2.1)	(±2.2)	(±3.5)	(±2.2)	(±1.8)	(±2.5)	(±1.9)	(±1.6)	(±2.3)	(±1.7)	(±0.7)	(±1.1)	(±0.9)
11	28.7	33.9	23.4	18.9	23.6	14.1	15.2	18.5	12.0	8.3	11.5	4.9	2.2	2.8	1.6
	(±1.6)	(±2.4)	(±1.8)	(±2.1)	(±3.1)	(±2.2)	(±1.7)	(±2.7)	(±1.5)	(±1.4)	(±2.2)	(±1.3)	(±0.7)	(±1.2)	(±0.7)
12	27.0	33.2	20.5	16.4	18.9	13.7	12.2	13.0	11.4	5.5	6.5	4.4	1.6	1.7	1.5
	(±2.6)	(±4.5)	(±1.9)	(±2.2)	(±4.2)	(±1.5)	(±1.9)	(±3.3)	(±1.4)	(±1.0)	(±1.7)	(±1.4)	(±0.5)	(±0.6)	(±0.7)

Note: Blacks and whites are non-Hispanic. Numbers in parentheses are plus or minus percentage points of the 95 percent confidence interval. Differences in percentages are considered statistically significant if the confidence intervals do not overlap.
Source: Grunbaum, Jo Anne, et al. Youth Risk Behavior Surveillance–United States, 2001, Mortality and Morbidity Weekly Report. Vol. 51/SS-4, Centers for Disease Control and Prevention. June 28, 2002

2.13 Percentage of high school students who felt sad or hopeless, who seriously considered attempting suicide, who made a suicide plan, or who attempted suicide, by sex—selected U.S. sites, 2001

	felt so sad or hopeless almost every day for two or more weeks that they stopped doing their usual activities			seriously considered attempting suicide in past 12 months			made a suicide plan in past 12 months			attempted suicide in past 12 months			suicide attempt required medical attention in past 12 months		
	total	female	male	total	female	male	total	female	male	total	female	male	total	female	male
State surveys															
Weighted data															
Alabama	27.6	33.6	21.8	15.6	17.6	13.2	12.0	14.3	9.6	7.8	10.2	5.2	2.2	2.3	2.2
Arkansas	29.7	37.4	22.3	19.6	23.9	15.4	14.2	17.8	10.7	8.8	11.6	5.9	2.2	2.6	1.8
Delaware	27.0	32.3	21.3	16.3	19.6	12.9	12.1	13.9	10.3	7.1	8.9	5.3	2.4	2.6	2.3
Florida	28.2	34.7	21.8	15.4	19.4	11.4	11.3	13.3	9.2	8.4	10.0	6.6	3.1	3.2	2.7
Idaho	26.4	33.1	19.7	16.7	20.1	13.4	14.1	15.9	12.2	8.1	10.5	5.5	2.2	2.5	1.9
Maine	26.7	34.1	19.6	18.6	24.9	12.5	16.5	20.3	12.8	9.2	11.6	6.7	4.6	4.6	4.7
Massachusetts	28.8	35.0	22.7	20.1	25.3	15.0	15.2	18.3	12.2	9.6	12.2	6.9	3.5	3.9	3.0
Michigan	27.3	32.9	21.8	18.1	23.1	13.1	14.8	18.2	11.4	10.2	11.7	8.4	3.5	3.3	3.5
Mississippi	29.1	33.1	24.8	14.6	17.4	11.6	11.7	14.1	9.0	6.3	8.5	3.8	1.8	2.2	1.4
Missouri	28.5	33.3	24.1	19.2	23.0	15.6	14.3	18.4	10.5	8.4	11.0	5.9	1.9	2.3	1.5
Montana	26.6	33.8	19.6	19.4	24.4	14.4	16.3	20.0	12.8	10.4	13.3	7.4	3.7	4.7	2.7
Nevada	29.7	35.5	24.2	19.6	25.5	14.0	16.4	20.9	12.2	10.8	13.2	8.3	3.8	4.4	3.3
New Jersey	30.7	35.9	25.3	17.3	19.7	14.8	13.0	12.7	13.4	8.4	8.2	8.7	2.4	1.8	3.1
North Carolina	29.3	38.0	20.8	18.1	21.8	14.3	NA	NA	NA	NA	NA	NA	NA	NA	NA
North Dakota	25.9	31.6	20.1	19.0	22.0	15.7	13.9	17.5	10.0	7.5	9.0	5.7	2.3	2.0	2.3
Rhode Island	25.7	30.9	20.5	16.5	19.5	13.7	12.4	15.6	9.2	8.1	10.3	5.9	4.4	4.7	4.0
South Dakota	23.1	30.2	16.3	19.3	23.9	14.8	17.7	21.0	14.6	13.1	14.7	11.4	NA	NA	NA
Texas	29.3	36.3	22.5	17.7	23.2	12.5	13.4	16.1	10.9	9.0	12.7	5.3	2.3	3.1	1.5
Utah	27.2	31.3	23.3	19.4	22.4	16.4	14.5	15.8	13.2	9.2	11.9	6.3	3.9	3.7	4.1
Vermont	NA	NA	NA	NA	NA	NA	13.4	16.8	10.2	6.8	9.5	4.1	2.3	2.7	1.7
Wisconsin	26.7	35.7	18.1	19.9	25.4	14.6	NA	NA	NA	8.6	11.3	5.8	2.5	3.2	1.8
Wyoming	26.2	33.1	20.0	18.5	22.6	14.6	14.2	16.5	12.1	7.4	10.0	4.9	2.4	3.3	1.6

(continued)

(continued from previous page)

	felt so sad or hopeless almost every day for two or more weeks that they stopped doing their usual activities			seriously considered attempting suicide in past 12 months			made a suicide plan in past 12 months			attempted suicide in past 12 months			suicide attempt required medical attention in past 12 months		
	total	female	male	total	female	male	total	female	male	total	female	male	total	female	male
Unweighted data															
Colorado	25.7	32.8	19.2	19.3	26.1	13.1	13.8	19.1	9.0	10.7	14.9	6.8	3.5	4.8	2.3
Hawaii	30.5	34.5	25.2	20.9	27.5	12.3	16.9	21.3	11.3	13.4	17.5	7.7	3.4	4.0	2.3
Illinois*	23.2	27.2	17.6	18.2	22.0	13.1	14.2	16.3	11.4	6.9	9.4	3.4	1.2	1.6	0.5
Indiana	26.1	31.7	19.7	18.4	22.6	13.3	16.2	18.6	13.5	8.6	11.2	5.2	2.9	3.5	1.9
Iowa	20.5	24.2	17.1	16.1	19.3	13.3	12.3	14.5	10.2	6.8	8.8	4.6	2.0	2.9	1.0
Kentucky	26.8	31.9	21.0	16.1	19.7	12.3	11.8	15.7	7.8	7.6	9.6	5.4	2.5	2.3	2.7
Louisiana*	27.5	32.1	21.3	14.9	16.8	12.2	13.8	15.7	10.9	8.7	8.5	9.2	3.4	3.1	3.8
Nebraska	21.8	26.3	17.2	17.7	22.0	13.4	12.7	16.0	9.5	6.3	8.7	3.9	1.5	2.0	0.9
New Hampshire	29.1	33.2	24.4	21.9	26.3	17.1	16.8	18.3	15.0	NA	NA	NA	NA	NA	NA
New York*	29.0	34.6	23.5	18.5	21.5	15.5	13.7	15.0	12.3	9.8	11.0	8.6	3.9	3.6	4.1
South Carolina	26.5	32.4	20.7	15.4	19.4	11.4	13.1	15.1	11.1	11.2	11.2	11.2	4.5	3.7	5.4
Tennessee	29.7	37.8	21.7	19.1	22.0	16.1	14.0	17.1	10.7	8.6	10.7	6.4	2.6	2.7	2.3

(continued)

(continued from previous page)

	felt so sad or hopeless almost every day for two or more weeks that they stopped doing their usual activities			seriously considered attempting suicide in past 12 months			made a suicide plan in past 12 months			attempted suicide in past 12 months			suicide attempt required medical attention in past 12 months		
	total	female	male	total	female	male	total	female	male	total	female	male	total	female	male
Local surveys															
Weighted data															
Boston	32.7	40.5	24.9	16.1	19.4	12.8	12.9	14.3	11.7	11.5	12.6	10.2	5.0	4.2	5.7
Chicago	34.1	42.6	25.2	17.3	22.0	12.0	15.3	19.6	10.3	11.8	15.6	6.9	2.7	2.6	2.5
Dallas	32.4	38.7	25.8	16.1	19.8	12.2	13.3	15.4	11.0	11.0	13.1	8.7	3.0	2.3	3.8
Ft. Lauderdale	29.0	36.3	21.5	13.9	18.1	9.4	11.0	13.1	8.8	7.6	8.3	6.3	3.2	1.5	4.7
Houston	30.2	35.9	24.3	14.5	18.6	10.4	11.7	14.2	9.3	10.2	12.4	7.8	2.8	3.7	1.9
Los Angeles	35.3	45.4	25.1	16.6	22.5	10.9	13.9	17.2	10.7	12.3	15.2	9.1	3.7	5.4	1.7
Miami	29.4	37.0	22.0	11.9	15.4	8.7	9.8	13.2	6.6	8.1	9.8	6.3	3.4	3.2	3.6
New York City	32.5	39.6	24.8	15.0	18.9	10.7	10.6	13.7	7.2	7.8	10.8	4.4	1.7	1.9	1.4
Orlando	29.6	34.7	24.0	17.6	20.9	14.2	13.8	16.6	10.8	10.9	11.9	9.5	3.5	2.7	4.2
Palm Beach	30.0	36.2	23.4	16.7	19.7	13.5	12.8	15.4	10.0	9.6	11.8	7.3	4.0	3.4	4.3
Philadelphia	32.2	39.0	25.7	16.6	19.8	13.5	15.3	16.3	13.9	12.0	13.5	10.3	3.1	2.7	3.6
San Bernardino	28.9	36.1	22.3	15.0	18.4	11.9	13.5	15.7	11.6	10.1	12.2	8.0	3.4	3.2	3.5
San Diego	32.6	41.0	24.1	21.0	26.1	16.1	16.9	22.1	11.9	10.5	14.5	6.3	3.5	3.5	3.6
San Francisco	28.6	32.8	24.5	14.0	17.7	10.4	13.2	15.9	10.5	7.4	8.3	6.4	2.5	2.4	2.7
Unweighted data															
Detroit	33.1	37.7	27.7	14.4	16.8	11.5	13.9	14.9	12.7	13.0	12.7	13.2	4.7	2.7	6.8
District of Columbia	28.6	29.4	27.4	16.5	19.0	13.7	14.2	14.4	14.0	12.3	14.5	9.4	5.7	5.5	5.7
Milwaukee	32.0	38.3	24.8	16.0	19.4	11.9	NA	NA	NA	10.3	12.7	7.4	4.2	4.1	4.3
New Orleans	24.2	28.8	17.6	10.0	12.0	6.9	7.9	8.9	6.0	9.6	10.3	7.9	3.6	3.3	3.3

* Survey did not include students from one of the state's large school districts.

Note: NA means data not available.

Source: Grunbaum, Jo Anne, et al., Youth Risk Behavior Surveillance–United States, 2001, Mortality and Morbidity Weekly Report. Vol. 51/SS-4. Centers for Disease Control and Prevention, June 28, 2002

2.14 Percentage of high school students who used tobacco, by sex, race/ethnicity, and grade—United States, 2001

	lifetime cigarette use (ever tried a cigarette, even a puff)			lifetime daily cigarette use (ever smoked one or more cigarettes a day for at least 30 days)			current cigarette use (smoked a cigarette on one or more of the past 30 days)			current frequent cigarette use (smoked a cigarette on 20 or more of the past 30 days)			smoked more than 10 cigarettes/day (on the days smoked during past 30 days)		
	total	female	male	total	female	male	total	female	male	total	female	male	total	female	male
Total	**63.9**	**61.6**	**66.3**	**20.0**	**19.2**	**20.9**	**28.5**	**27.7**	**29.2**	**13.8**	**12.9**	**14.9**	**4.1**	**3.1**	**5.2**
	(±2.1)	(±2.3)	(±2.3)	(±1.9)	(±1.9)	(±2.2)	(±2.0)	(±2.1)	(±2.6)	(±1.6)	(±1.6)	(±1.9)	(±0.8)	(±0.9)	(±1.0)
Race/ethnicity															
Black	58.3	56.7	59.9	7.7	6.5	9.0	14.7	13.3	16.3	4.6	3.1	6.2	1.1	0.7	1.5
	(±4.6)	(±5.9)	(±4.2)	(±1.9)	(±1.7)	(±3.2)	(±2.8)	(±3.4)	(±3.2)	(±1.7)	(±1.3)	(±2.7)	(±0.5)	(±0.4)	(±1.0)
Hispanic	69.3	67.8	70.9	12.4	11.5	13.4	26.6	26.0	27.2	7.3	5.9	8.8	1.8	1.7	1.9
	(±4.0)	(±3.9)	(±5.4)	(±2.4)	(±2.5)	(±3.4)	(±4.3)	(±3.7)	(±7.0)	(±1.8)	(±2.0)	(±2.7)	(±0.8)	(±1.3)	(±0.9)
White	64.8	62.2	67.4	23.9	23.2	24.7	31.9	31.2	32.7	17.2	16.2	18.1	5.3	4.0	6.6
	(±2.6)	(±2.9)	(±2.9)	(±2.3)	(±2.6)	(±2.6)	(±2.3)	(±2.5)	(±3.0)	(±1.9)	(±2.3)	(±2.2)	(±1.0)	(±1.3)	(±1.3)
Grade															
9	58.4	55.9	61.3	14.3	13.6	15.2	23.9	23.6	24.3	8.9	8.3	9.6	2.2	1.7	2.9
	(±3.8)	(±5.3)	(±3.4)	(±2.9)	(±3.2)	(±3.5)	(±2.9)	(±3.8)	(±3.1)	(±2.1)	(±2.3)	(±2.7)	(±0.9)	(±1.0)	(±1.1)
10	62.6	59.8	65.4	19.1	19.2	19.1	26.9	28.4	25.4	12.3	12.3	12.4	3.6	2.4	4.7
	(±3.5)	(±3.9)	(±4.3)	(±1.9)	(±3.0)	(±2.5)	(±3.2)	(±3.8)	(±3.5)	(±1.8)	(±2.0)	(±2.4)	(±1.2)	(±1.5)	(±1.4)
11	65.9	63.5	68.2	22.1	20.5	23.6	29.8	27.3	32.3	15.2	12.9	17.5	4.8	3.2	6.4
	(±2.8)	(±3.3)	(±3.7)	(±3.3)	(±3.2)	(±4.3)	(±3.7)	(±3.3)	(±5.0)	(±2.6)	(±2.2)	(±3.6)	(±1.3)	(±1.3)	(±2.1)
12	71.1	69.7	72.5	26.9	26.1	27.8	35.2	33.1	37.5	21.0	20.0	22.0	6.6	5.7	7.5
	(±3.9)	(±5.0)	(±3.4)	(±4.1)	(±4.3)	(±4.8)	(±4.1)	(±5.3)	(±4.6)	(±3.6)	(±4.3)	(±4.2)	(±1.6)	(±1.8)	(±2.4)

Note: Blacks and whites are non-Hispanic. Numbers in parentheses are plus or minus percentage points of the 95 percent confidence interval. Differences in percentages are considered statistically significant if the confidence intervals do not overlap.

Source: Grunbaum, Jo Anne, et al., Youth Risk Behavior Surveillance—United States, 2001, Mortality and Morbidity Weekly Report. Vol. 51/SS-4, Centers for Disease Control and Prevention. June 28, 2002

2.15 Percentage of high school students who used tobacco, by sex—selected U.S. sites, 2001

	lifetime cigarette use (ever tried a cigarette, even a puff)			lifetime daily cigarette use (ever smoked one or more cigarettes a day for at least 30 days)			current cigarette use (smoked a cigarette on one or more of the past 30 days)			current frequent cigarette use (smoked a cigarette on 20 or more of the past 30 days)			smoked more than 10 cigarettes/day (on the days smoked during past 30 days)		
	total	female	male	total	female	male	total	female	male	total	female	male	total	female	male
State surveys															
Weighted data															
Alabama	70.6	69.7	71.5	17.7	16.8	18.4	23.7	22.7	24.7	12.4	12.0	12.8	3.6	2.8	4.1
Arkansas	71.6	66.3	76.7	23.7	23.1	24.2	34.7	32.1	37.0	18.8	17.2	20.3	6.7	5.0	8.3
Delaware	65.5	65.8	65.0	18.7	18.4	18.9	24.2	23.4	24.7	12.8	12.2	13.6	3.8	2.2	5.5
Florida	57.4	57.5	57.1	13.7	14.9	12.4	21.5	22.9	19.9	9.3	9.7	8.9	2.9	2.6	3.1
Idaho	54.4	50.6	57.6	14.6	13.2	16.0	19.1	17.1	20.7	9.0	7.4	10.5	1.8	1.3	2.2
Maine	NA	NA	NA	NA	NA	NA	24.8	26.6	23.0	14.0	14.4	13.6	5.5	4.6	6.2
Massachusetts	61.9	62.4	61.5	19.5	19.9	19.1	26.0	27.0	25.0	13.2	13.5	12.8	4.3	3.2	5.4
Michigan	63.5	64.4	62.5	20.4	21.4	19.3	25.7	27.2	24.0	12.7	13.3	12.0	3.2	2.3	4.0
Mississippi	67.8	67.4	68.2	16.2	16.6	15.8	23.6	24.6	22.4	11.5	12.5	10.3	2.7	2.9	2.6
Missouri	68.5	68.7	68.4	23.4	24.0	22.9	30.3	30.4	30.1	18.0	17.7	18.3	5.5	4.4	6.6
Montana	66.5	66.5	66.2	23.2	24.8	21.4	28.5	31.8	25.4	14.9	16.4	13.5	3.7	3.5	3.9
Nevada	66.5	64.6	68.3	NA	NA	NA	25.2	25.8	24.6	11.3	12.8	9.9	2.7	2.1	3.2
New Jersey	63.0	63.3	62.7	19.6	19.0	20.0	29.4	28.9	29.7	14.9	13.8	15.7	3.9	2.0	5.7
North Carolina	NA	NA	NA	NA	NA	NA	27.8	27.2	28.4	14.5	13.8	15.2	3.8	3.3	4.3
North Dakota	67.9	66.8	68.7	NA	NA	NA	35.3	35.5	34.7	18.7	19.8	17.4	5.0	4.5	5.3
Rhode Island	60.2	62.2	57.9	18.5	19.0	17.8	24.8	25.6	24.1	14.2	13.1	15.1	4.8	3.1	6.1
South Dakota	67.4	63.3	71.4	25.4	26.0	24.8	33.1	34.4	31.6	17.3	17.4	17.1	3.6	2.8	4.3
Texas	66.1	63.5	68.5	16.0	15.4	16.5	28.4	24.9	31.8	10.4	8.9	11.8	2.0	1.1	2.9
Utah	30.5	26.8	34.1	8.5	8.9	8.1	8.3	9.6	7.1	4.2	5.1	3.3	1.0	0.5	1.4
Vermont	NA	NA	NA	NA	NA	NA	23.7	26.0	21.2	12.7	13.8	11.5	3.7	3.2	4.2
Wisconsin	64.0	65.6	62.4	24.9	29.2	20.8	32.6	36.7	28.6	16.4	18.7	14.2	4.0	2.8	5.3
Wyoming	64.6	62.4	66.6	20.7	22.4	19.3	28.4	29.6	27.0	13.6	15.3	12.2	3.4	3.5	3.3

(continued)

(continued from previous page)

	lifetime cigarette use (ever tried a cigarette, even a puff)			lifetime daily cigarette use (ever smoked one or more cigarettes a day for at least 30 days)			current cigarette use (smoked a cigarette on one or more of the past 30 days)			current frequent cigarette use (smoked a cigarette on 20 or more of the past 30 days)			smoked more than 10 cigarettes/ day (on the days smoked during past 30 days)		
	total	female	male	total	female	male	total	female	male	total	female	male	total	female	male
Unweighted data															
Colorado	66.3	67.2	65.6	19.2	21.0	17.6	26.7	29.3	24.3	12.5	12.7	12.3	1.8	1.1	2.4
Hawaii	55.0	56.7	52.6	13.2	14.3	11.5	15.0	18.0	11.0	6.1	6.3	5.7	1.3	1.2	1.4
Illinois*	56.4	53.7	60.1	16.1	16.7	15.4	25.3	26.6	23.5	12.0	11.7	12.4	3.1	2.3	4.2
Indiana	66.6	64.5	69.0	22.7	22.6	22.5	28.5	27.5	29.3	16.2	15.1	17.3	4.9	3.5	6.2
Iowa	61.9	57.9	65.5	19.1	19.4	19.0	29.7	29.5	29.7	14.1	14.6	13.8	4.3	3.7	4.9
Kentucky	68.3	66.5	70.1	25.6	26.4	24.8	33.0	34.1	32.0	18.8	18.3	19.4	7.3	5.2	9.6
Louisiana*	67.2	64.5	70.6	17.5	18.1	16.4	25.0	23.0	27.4	12.5	11.4	13.8	3.7	2.1	5.7
Nebraska	63.7	62.1	65.2	19.8	21.3	18.2	30.5	31.6	29.3	14.5	16.7	12.2	3.1	2.2	3.9
New Hampshire	NA	NA	NA	19.0	18.6	19.5	NA	NA	NA	NA	NA	NA	4.5	3.4	5.6
New York*	65.9	68.8	62.9	25.4	27.7	22.9	29.8	32.8	26.7	16.4	18.0	14.6	4.9	4.0	5.7
South Carolina	70.5	68.8	72.3	20.1	18.0	22.2	27.6	26.8	28.5	14.1	12.3	16.0	3.9	2.7	5.1
Tennessee	67.0	66.2	68.0	22.3	22.0	22.7	29.1	28.4	29.9	15.6	13.5	17.7	4.5	2.8	6.1

(continued)

(continued from previous page)

	lifetime cigarette use (ever tried a cigarette, even a puff)			lifetime daily cigarette use (ever smoked one or more cigarettes a day for at least 30 days)			current cigarette use (smoked a cigarette on one or more of the past 30 days)			current frequent cigarette use (smoked a cigarette on 20 or more of the past 30 days)			smoked more than 10 cigarettes/ day (on the days smoked during past 30 days)		
	total	female	male	total	female	male	total	female	male	total	female	male	total	female	male
Local surveys															
Weighted data															
Boston	57.1	57.5	56.8	9.1	8.4	9.7	15.4	15.1	15.6	4.9	4.2	5.4	1.5	1.3	1.7
Chicago	64.5	64.2	64.6	10.0	7.7	12.3	24.7	23.5	25.8	7.6	4.9	10.2	1.7	0.1	3.1
Dallas	68.0	64.2	72.1	8.5	6.8	10.4	17.8	15.8	20.0	3.6	2.5	4.8	0.7	0.4	1.0
Ft. Lauderdale	54.6	54.3	54.7	10.9	11.4	10.5	18.3	17.4	19.1	7.0	7.0	6.9	2.2	1.2	3.0
Houston	62.2	60.1	64.2	9.4	7.7	11.1	21.8	18.7	24.8	4.6	3.5	5.7	0.9	0.5	1.2
Los Angeles	60.0	58.7	61.0	6.7	6.2	7.3	14.5	13.6	15.2	2.7	2.4	3.1	0.3	NA	0.5
Miami	50.9	50.1	51.6	8.4	7.6	9.1	16.9	15.3	18.2	5.4	4.2	6.5	1.3	0.8	1.7
New York City	58.0	62.0	53.7	11.8	12.3	11.1	17.6	18.7	16.4	7.5	7.3	7.8	1.8	0.8	2.8
Orlando	58.1	54.2	62.2	13.0	11.7	14.1	17.8	15.4	20.1	8.8	7.2	10.2	2.5	1.7	3.1
Palm Beach	57.3	56.8	58.0	14.5	14.3	14.7	21.4	23.9	18.9	8.5	8.6	8.4	2.3	2.2	2.3
Philadelphia	62.6	64.1	61.0	NA	NA	NA	15.8	16.8	15.0	6.4	6.9	6.0	0.9	0.6	1.3
San Bernardino	57.6	56.3	58.7	8.2	7.9	8.5	12.0	11.2	12.7	3.4	3.3	3.4	0.9	0.3	1.5
San Diego	61.8	61.5	62.2	9.4	10.6	8.3	17.1	17.1	17.0	4.7	4.2	5.3	0.9	0.7	1.0
San Francisco	48.9	48.4	49.2	NA	NA	NA	13.3	13.8	12.8	3.7	2.5	4.8	0.4	0.1	0.7
Unweighted data															
Detroit	64.9	64.3	65.5	8.6	6.6	10.7	12.4	10.3	14.7	4.1	2.8	5.5	0.8	0.3	1.2
District of Columbia	56.7	55.2	58.1	9.6	8.3	11.2	13.1	11.1	15.5	3.2	3.0	3.4	0.9	0.6	1.3
Milwaukee	66.5	67.6	65.1	16.8	17.2	16.3	19.8	20.3	19.1	9.9	9.9	9.8	1.6	0.9	2.1
New Orleans	53.4	52.6	54.4	5.7	4.2	7.5	11.9	11.3	12.8	4.0	2.0	6.6	1.4	0.7	2.3

* Survey did not include students from one of the state's large school districts.
Note: NA means data not available.
Source: Grunbaum, Jo Anne, et al., Youth Risk Behavior Surveillance–United States, 2001, Mortality and Morbidity Weekly Report, Vol. 51/SS-4, Centers for Disease Control and Prevention, June 28, 2002

2.16 Percentage of high school students who used any tobacco product, smokeless tobacco products, or cigars, by sex, race/ethnicity, and grade—United States, 2001

	current tobacco use (used any kind of tobacco at least once during past 30 days)			current smokeless tobacco use (used chewing tobacco, snuff, or dip at least once during past 30 days)			current cigar use (used cigars, cigarillos, or little cigars at least once during past 30 days)		
	total	female	male	total	female	male	total	female	male
Total	**33.9**	**29.5**	**38.5**	**8.2**	**1.9**	**14.8**	**15.2**	**8.5**	**22.1**
	(±2.1)	(±2.1)	(±2.5)	(±1.5)	(±0.5)	(±2.9)	(±1.2)	(±1.3)	(±1.5)
Race/ethnicity									
Black	19.4	17.4	21.6	1.8	0.7	2.9	12.1	8.6	15.8
	(±3.0)	(±3.5)	(±3.9)	(±0.8)	(±0.7)	(±1.4)	(±2.6)	(±2.7)	(±3.1)
Hispanic	29.4	27.2	31.5	4.1	1.8	6.4	16.5	11.5	21.4
	(±4.0)	(±3.9)	(±6.2)	(±0.7)	(±0.8)	(±1.5)	(±2.5)	(±2.8)	(±3.8)
White	37.7	32.3	43.4	10.3	2.1	18.9	15.6	7.7	23.8
	(±2.2)	(±2.5)	(±2.8)	(±2.0)	(±0.6)	(±3.8)	(±1.4)	(±1.5)	(±1.9)
Grade									
9	28.1	25.6	30.7	6.6	1.5	12.2	12.5	8.4	16.9
	(±3.3)	(±4.1)	(±3.1)	(±1.8)	(±0.7)	(±3.2)	(±2.3)	(±2.6)	(±2.3)
10	32.6	30.5	34.9	8.7	2.3	15.2	14.4	9.3	19.6
	(±3.2)	(±3.6)	(±3.7)	(±1.7)	(±0.9)	(±3.2)	(±1.9)	(±2.1)	(±2.1)
11	36.1	29.0	43.4	9.0	1.7	16.5	16.8	8.3	25.3
	(±3.8)	(±3.4)	(±4.7)	(±2.1)	(±0.8)	(±4.0)	(±2.3)	(±1.7)	(±2.9)
12	41.0	34.3	48.2	8.7	1.6	16.0	18.0	7.9	28.6
	(±4.0)	(±5.2)	(±4.4)	(±2.0)	(±0.9)	(±3.8)	(±2.8)	(±2.4)	(±3.4)

Note: Blacks and whites are non-Hispanic. Numbers in parentheses are plus or minus percentage points of the 95 percent confidence interval. Differences in percentages are considered statistically significant if the confidence intervals do not overlap.
Source: Grunbaum, Jo Anne, et al., Youth Risk Behavior Surveillance–United States, 2001, Mortality and Morbidity Weekly Report, Vol. 51/SS-4, Centers for Disease Control and Prevention, June 28, 2002

2.17 Percentage of high school students who used any tobacco product, smokeless tobacco products, or cigars, by sex—selected U.S. sites, 2001

	current tobacco use (used any kind of tobacco at least once during past 30 days)			current smokeless tobacco use (used chewing tobacco, snuff, or dip at least once during past 30 days)			current cigar use (used cigars, cigarillos, or little cigars at least once during past 30 days)		
	total	female	male	total	female	male	total	female	male
State surveys									
Weighted data									
Alabama	30.5	26.1	34.9	9.8	2.0	17.4	15.9	11.4	20.1
Arkansas	41.4	33.5	49.0	13.5	1.7	24.9	19.3	10.6	27.7
Delaware	29.0	25.6	32.4	4.8	1.4	8.3	12.7	7.2	18.3
Florida	26.6	24.9	28.1	5.8	1.6	9.8	15.3	10.1	20.2
Idaho	23.4	18.0	28.3	8.3	1.9	14.3	11.1	4.1	17.6
Maine	29.2	28.0	30.1	6.2	3.1	8.9	12.0	7.0	16.6
Massachusetts	30.9	28.3	33.4	4.4	1.3	7.4	13.1	6.4	19.6
Michigan	29.9	29.1	30.6	7.7	3.3	11.9	14.9	8.4	20.9
Mississippi	29.6	26.9	32.3	8.2	1.6	15.2	15.7	10.3	21.2
Missouri	36.2	31.8	40.5	10.4	1.9	18.6	16.4	9.2	23.4
Montana	37.7	34.3	40.8	15.7	5.4	25.2	14.8	8.2	20.7
Nevada	NA	NA	NA	6.9	2.6	11.1	NA	NA	NA
New Jersey	33.0	30.4	35.6	7.1	1.6	12.7	15.6	7.4	23.8
North Carolina	NA	NA	NA	NA	NA	NA	NA	NA	NA
North Dakota	NA	NA	NA	13.2	3.5	22.4	NA	NA	NA
Rhode Island	29.2	26.9	31.5	3.9	1.5	6.1	14.0	6.3	21.5
South Dakota	39.8	35.2	44.3	15.1	5.6	24.3	14.3	9.1	19.2
Texas	32.7	26.6	38.7	8.8	1.7	15.5	15.6	9.2	21.7
Utah	9.8	10.0	9.5	3.8	0.8	6.7	4.1	2.1	6.0
Vermont	28.5	27.1	29.5	5.2	1.6	8.4	12.4	5.3	18.8
Wisconsin	39.5	39.9	39.1	9.1	3.7	14.2	17.3	10.6	23.4
Wyoming	38.4	32.8	43.7	18.1	6.9	28.6	16.5	8.4	24.1
Unweighted data									
Colorado	33.5	31.8	35.2	9.2	3.8	14.1	16.4	10.6	21.9
Hawaii	16.7	18.5	14.4	2.9	2.0	4.1	6.2	5.6	6.7
Illinois*	29.8	27.5	33.2	4.2	1.2	8.6	11.9	5.9	20.4
Indiana	32.4	29.0	36.3	6.5	1.4	12.5	14.2	7.1	22.1
Iowa	35.3	29.5	40.8	11.8	2.8	20.0	16.1	9.2	22.3
Kentucky	38.4	35.4	41.8	12.2	1.8	23.7	14.8	8.8	21.5
Louisiana*	30.1	25.0	36.9	8.5	2.0	17.1	17.6	10.0	27.3
Nebraska	35.2	32.1	38.3	9.8	2.7	16.8	14.6	8.7	20.4
New Hampshire	NA	NA	NA	5.6	1.8	9.4	13.4	5.3	21.7
New York*	32.9	33.8	32.1	5.9	2.9	9.0	14.3	8.0	20.4
South Carolina	33.0	29.2	37.1	8.1	1.3	14.8	17.6	10.5	24.5
Tennessee	37.0	32.4	41.9	12.0	1.7	22.0	16.9	11.3	22.3

(continued)

(continued from previous page)

	current tobacco use (used any kind of tobacco at least once during past 30 days)			current smokeless tobacco use (used chewing tobacco, snuff, or dip at least once during past 30 days)			current cigar use (used cigars, cigarillos, or little cigars at least once during past 30 days)		
	total	female	male	total	female	male	total	female	male
Local surveys									
Weighted data									
Boston	17.4	17.0	17.9	2.3	0.8	3.8	8.8	6.4	11.3
Chicago	27.1	24.4	29.6	2.6	1.5	3.6	14.1	9.6	18.1
Dallas	21.8	18.4	25.5	2.5	1.2	3.9	16.3	12.3	20.5
Ft. Lauderdale	21.8	19.5	24.0	3.0	0.7	5.0	13.1	8.7	17.2
Houston	23.6	19.7	27.6	3.5	1.3	5.7	12.2	9.1	15.3
Los Angeles	16.9	14.1	19.6	3.0	1.3	4.7	11.4	7.3	14.9
Miami	19.1	16.5	21.6	2.6	1.3	3.8	11.5	8.4	14.4
New York City	18.6	19.2	17.8	1.1	0.6	1.4	5.1	3.0	7.1
Orlando	23.0	18.0	28.0	4.6	1.5	7.5	14.8	9.2	20.3
Palm Beach	26.6	26.6	26.8	5.3	1.9	8.7	15.3	10.4	20.3
Philadelphia	18.1	17.5	18.7	2.2	1.0	3.5	7.3	5.3	9.0
San Bernardino	15.3	13.4	17.1	3.8	2.2	5.1	12.5	9.1	15.4
San Diego	20.0	19.6	20.6	2.5	1.2	3.8	11.9	10.2	13.6
San Francisco	NA	NA	NA	NA	NA	NA	8.7	8.3	9.1
Unweighted data									
Detroit	16.3	13.7	19.3	4.1	2.7	5.8	12.4	8.8	16.3
District of Columbia	17.0	14.5	19.7	6.4	3.9	8.8	10.2	7.6	12.7
Milwaukee	25.4	24.9	25.7	5.9	4.6	7.2	14.9	12.5	17.1
New Orleans	14.7	13.9	15.7	2.7	1.6	3.8	10.0	6.9	13.3

* *Survey did not include students from one of the state's large school districts.*
Note: NA means data not available.
Source: Grunbaum, Jo Anne, et al., Youth Risk Behavior Surveillance–United States, 2001, Mortality and Morbidity Weekly Report. *Vol. 51/SS-4, Centers for Disease Control and Prevention, June 28, 2002*

2.18 Percentage of high school students under age 18 who were current cigarette smokers and usually obtained their own cigarettes by purchasing them in a store or gas station and who purchased cigarettes without being asked to show proof of age, by sex, race/ethnicity, and grade—United States, 2001

	purchased cigarettes at a store or gas station in past 30 days			were not asked to show proof of age when purchasing cigarettes		
	total	female	male	total	female	male
Total	**19.1**	**13.1**	**25.7**	**67.2**	**72.9**	**64.0**
	(±2.2)	(± 2.5)	(±3.2)	(± 4.6)	(± 8.7)	(±5.8)
Race/ethnicity						
Black	24.1	19.9	27.8	NA	NA	NA
	(±8.5)	(±14.2)	(±7.3)	NA	NA	NA
Hispanic	16.7	13.5	20.2	71.4	NA	NA
	(±3.8)	(± 5.8)	(±4.6)	(±10.5)	NA	NA
White	19.2	12.4	26.7	65.1	73.2	60.9
	(±2.6)	(± 2.4)	(±4.2)	(± 6.1)	(±10.6)	(±7.0)
Grade						
9	8.8	4.7	13.3	NA	NA	NA
	(±2.5)	(± 2.8)	(±4.6)	NA	NA	NA
10	19.1	13.8	25.5	67.1	NA	NA
	(±2.8)	(± 3.6)	(±3.4)	(±10.4)	NA	NA
11	28.7	20.3	36.5	65.2	NA	58.1
	(±3.9)	(± 5.0)	(±6.0)	(± 6.6)	NA	(±7.3)
12	23.6	17.5	31.2	NA	NA	NA
	(±5.1)	(± 6.0)	(±7.7)	NA	NA	NA

Note: Blacks and whites are non-Hispanic. NA means data not available. Numbers in parentheses are plus or minus percentage points of the 95 percent confidence interval. Differences in percentages are considered statistically significant if the confidence intervals do not overlap.
Source: Grunbaum, Jo Anne, et al., Youth Risk Behavior Surveillance–United States, 2001, Mortality and Morbidity Weekly Report, *Vol. 51/SS-4, Centers for Disease Control and Prevention, June 28, 2002*

2.19 Percentage of high school students under age 18 who were current cigarette smokers and usually obtained their own cigarettes by purchasing them in a store or gas station and who purchased cigarettes without being asked to show proof of age, by sex—selected U.S. sites, 2001

	purchased cigarettes at a store or gas station in past 30 days			were not asked to show proof of age when purchasing cigarettes		
	total	female	male	total	female	male
State surveys						
Weighted data						
Alabama	22.4	19.4	25.7	NA	NA	NA
Arkansas	21.3	13.5	28.2	NA	NA	NA
Delaware	23.6	22.0	25.7	68.0	NA	NA
Florida	18.7	16.5	21.7	60.0	NA	NA
Idaho	6.8	2.8	10.2	NA	NA	NA
Maine	8.8	4.5	14.0	NA	NA	NA
Massachusetts	20.3	15.6	25.8	NA	NA	NA
Michigan	25.1	19.5	31.1	71.3	NA	NA
Mississippi	16.3	12.5	20.9	NA	NA	NA
Missouri	19.6	10.8	28.5	NA	NA	NA
Montana	11.7	4.8	20.6	NA	NA	NA
Nevada	12.7	13.2	12.1	NA	NA	NA
New Jersey	39.1	31.6	46.5	73.9	NA	70.4
North Carolina	NA	NA	NA	NA	NA	NA
North Dakota	15.1	10.3	20.1	NA	NA	NA
Rhode Island	28.4	20.9	38.0	NA	NA	NA
South Dakota	11.3	9.3	13.2	NA	NA	NA
Texas	18.6	13.4	22.7	74.1	NA	71.5
Utah	NA	NA	NA	NA	NA	NA
Vermont	NA	NA	NA	NA	NA	NA
Wisconsin	20.7	17.9	24.4	NA	NA	NA
Wyoming	11.8	10.3	13.7	NA	NA	NA
Unweighted data						
Colorado	14.0	12.8	14.6	NA	NA	NA
Hawaii	9.1	NA	NA	NA	NA	NA
Illinois*	19.8	13.3	NA	NA	NA	NA
Indiana	15.5	11.4	20.5	NA	NA	NA
Iowa	4.4	3.4	5.6	NA	NA	NA
Kentucky	18.6	14.0	25.0	NA	NA	NA
Louisiana*	20.0	11.2	NA	NA	NA	NA
Nebraska	9.8	7.5	12.5	NA	NA	NA
New Hampshire	14.7	9.8	21.0	NA	NA	NA
New York*	21.0	16.5	26.8	NA	NA	NA
South Carolina	20.8	15.0	27.0	68.2	NA	NA
Tennessee	21.6	15.9	28.1	NA	NA	NA

(continued)

(continued from previous page)

	purchased cigarettes at a store or gas station in past 30 days			were not asked to show proof of age when purchasing cigarettes		
	total	female	male	total	female	male
Local surveys						
Weighted data						
Boston	20.3	18.0	NA	NA	NA	NA
Chicago	31.0	NA	NA	NA	NA	NA
Dallas	19.3	10.2	28.0	NA	NA	NA
Ft. Lauderdale	24.3	22.5	26.8	NA	NA	NA
Houston	25.7	15.2	34.8	NA	NA	NA
Los Angeles	15.9	NA	NA	NA	NA	NA
Miami	26.9	25.9	28.0	NA	NA	NA
New York City	44.2	42.6	NA	NA	NA	NA
Orlando	27.3	20.3	33.4	NA	NA	NA
Palm Beach	21.1	16.2	27.5	NA	NA	NA
Philadelphia	46.4	NA	NA	NA	NA	NA
San Bernardino	NA	NA	NA	NA	NA	NA
San Diego	14.2	9.2	19.5	NA	NA	NA
San Francisco	28.9	NA	NA	NA	NA	NA
Unweighted data						
Detroit	34.5	NA	40.6	NA	NA	NA
District of Columbia	32.5	NA	NA	NA	NA	NA
Milwaukee	34.7	25.2	NA	NA	NA	NA
New Orleans	25.5	NA	NA	NA	NA	NA

* Survey did not include students from one of the state's large school districts.
Note: NA means data not available.
Source: Grunbaum, Jo Anne, et al., Youth Risk Behavior Surveillance–United States, 2001, Mortality and Morbidity Weekly Report, *Vol. 51/SS-4, Centers for Disease Control and Prevention, June 28, 2002*

2.20 Percentage of high school students who drank alcohol or used marijuana, by sex, race/ethnicity, and grade—United States, 2001

	lifetime alcohol use (ever had one or more drinks)			current alcohol use (drank alcohol in past 30 days)			five or more drinks of alcohol (on one or more occasions in past 30 days)			lifetime marijuana use (ever used marijuana)			current marijuana use (used marijuana in past 30 days)		
	total	female	male	total	female	male	total	female	male	total	female	male	total	female	male
Total	78.2	77.9	78.6	47.1	45.0	49.2	29.9	26.4	33.5	42.4	38.4	46.5	23.9	20.0	27.9
	(±1.7)	(±1.8)	(±1.9)	(±2.2)	(±2.2)	(±2.8)	(±2.0)	(±1.9)	(±2.9)	(±1.9)	(±2.1)	(±2.0)	(±1.5)	(±1.7)	(±1.6)
Race/ethnicity															
Black	69.1	69.7	68.4	32.7	30.6	35.0	11.1	7.5	15.1	40.2	34.3	46.7	21.8	16.0	28.2
	(±4.4)	(±5.5)	(±4.7)	(±4.6)	(±5.3)	(±4.9)	(±2.2)	(±2.0)	(±3.8)	(±5.8)	(±6.9)	(±5.9)	(±4.1)	(±3.9)	(±5.1)
Hispanic	80.8	80.1	81.6	49.2	48.8	49.5	30.1	28.7	31.4	44.7	39.7	50.0	24.6	22.4	26.8
	(±2.9)	(±3.3)	(±3.2)	(±3.0)	(±3.1)	(±4.1)	(±2.5)	(±2.8)	(±3.3)	(±2.3)	(±3.6)	(±3.5)	(±1.6)	(±3.1)	(±2.7)
White	80.1	79.6	80.7	50.4	48.3	52.6	34.0	30.5	37.7	42.8	39.2	46.4	24.4	20.6	28.4
	(±1.5)	(±1.9)	(±1.6)	(±2.2)	(±2.4)	(±3.1)	(±2.0)	(±2.1)	(±3.2)	(±2.2)	(±2.7)	(±2.3)	(±2.0)	(±2.4)	(±2.2)
Grade															
9	73.1	72.0	74.5	41.1	40.0	42.2	24.5	23.0	26.2	32.7	28.6	37.3	19.4	16.5	22.6
	(±2.9)	(±3.8)	(±3.7)	(±3.6)	(±4.0)	(±4.4)	(±2.8)	(±3.1)	(±4.2)	(±2.8)	(±3.5)	(±3.4)	(±2.4)	(±2.7)	(±2.9)
10	76.3	76.9	75.6	45.2	43.5	46.9	28.2	26.3	30.1	41.7	37.5	46.1	24.8	21.5	28.3
	(±1.6)	(±2.2)	(±2.3)	(±2.5)	(±3.1)	(±3.1)	(±2.6)	(±3.0)	(±3.5)	(±2.6)	(±2.6)	(±3.5)	(±2.2)	(±2.5)	(±3.3)
11	80.4	79.3	81.4	49.3	45.1	53.6	32.2	26.1	38.5	47.2	42.6	51.7	25.8	21.4	30.2
	(±3.2)	(±3.7)	(±3.6)	(±3.3)	(±3.0)	(±4.3)	(±3.4)	(±2.9)	(±4.6)	(±3.4)	(±3.4)	(±4.2)	(±2.6)	(±2.7)	(±3.2)
12	85.1	85.5	84.7	55.2	53.9	56.6	36.7	31.8	42.0	51.5	48.9	54.2	26.9	21.8	32.3
	(±1.9)	(±2.3)	(±2.6)	(±3.0)	(±4.3)	(±3.1)	(±3.7)	(±4.9)	(±4.2)	(±3.9)	(±5.4)	(±3.1)	(±3.5)	(±4.6)	(±3.3)

Note: Blacks and whites are non-Hispanic. Numbers in parentheses are plus or minus percentage points of the 95 percent confidence interval. Differences in percentages are considered statistically significant if the confidence intervals do not overlap.
Source: Grunbaum, Jo Anne, et al., Youth Risk Behavior Surveillance—United States, 2001. Mortality and Morbidity Weekly Report, Vol. 51/SS-4, Centers for Disease Control and Prevention, June 28, 2002

2.21 Percentage of high school students who drank alcohol or used marijuana, by sex—selected U.S. sites, 2001

	lifetime alcohol use (ever had one or more drinks)			current alcohol use (drank alcohol in past 30 days)			five or more drinks of alcohol (on one or more occasions in past 30 days)			lifetime marijuana use (ever used marijuana)			current marijuana use (used marijuana in past 30 days)		
	total	female	male	total	female	male	total	female	male	total	female	male	total	female	male
State surveys **Weighted data**															
Alabama	76.4	78.7	73.9	42.6	42.9	42.0	25.0	22.1	27.8	38.7	36.2	41.2	18.8	16.6	20.9
Arkansas	79.6	78.7	80.7	47.9	44.1	51.9	30.0	23.2	36.7	43.6	38.2	49.1	22.6	18.4	26.7
Delaware	77.6	78.2	77.2	46.4	45.0	47.8	27.3	23.3	31.4	46.9	42.5	51.5	26.3	21.8	30.7
Florida	74.5	75.1	74.1	45.0	45.5	44.6	24.8	23.3	26.3	40.2	36.3	44.0	23.1	20.0	26.0
Idaho	70.8	69.8	71.5	40.6	38.3	42.8	27.2	24.0	30.2	34.7	30.7	38.0	17.5	13.7	20.7
Maine	NA	NA	NA	47.8	49.6	45.8	31.5	29.1	33.9	NA	NA	NA	27.2	24.3	29.7
Massachusetts	81.2	81.7	80.7	53.0	51.7	54.3	32.7	28.9	36.4	50.4	47.1	53.7	30.9	27.3	34.5
Michigan	77.4	79.4	75.3	46.2	47.3	45.0	29.3	27.9	30.5	44.0	42.3	45.5	24.3	23.4	24.9
Mississippi	76.2	78.5	73.7	41.7	40.6	42.9	22.1	18.5	25.7	37.5	33.8	41.2	17.4	14.9	19.9
Missouri	80.1	80.6	79.6	47.6	46.1	49.2	34.1	31.5	36.8	43.3	40.6	45.8	24.4	21.9	26.8
Montana	82.9	82.8	82.6	54.1	52.5	55.7	41.4	39.3	43.5	46.7	45.7	47.5	27.1	25.5	28.7
Nevada	80.1	82.2	78.1	47.5	48.6	46.4	32.4	31.8	33.1	50.8	48.8	52.6	26.6	23.5	29.5
New Jersey	83.4	85.0	81.8	55.7	54.8	56.5	32.6	28.3	36.9	41.1	37.2	44.9	24.9	21.7	28.0
North Carolina	NA	NA	NA	38.2	35.9	40.5	20.7	18.7	22.8	40.3	38.2	42.3	20.8	17.8	23.9
North Dakota	NA	NA	NA	59.2	56.4	61.7	41.5	37.2	45.5	NA	NA	NA	22.0	18.4	25.1
Rhode Island	78.8	78.8	79.1	50.3	47.3	53.3	30.7	26.4	34.8	48.3	42.7	53.7	33.2	29.4	36.4
South Dakota	81.5	81.5	81.6	50.2	48.0	52.3	36.5	33.5	39.4	36.3	33.7	38.7	18.4	18.0	18.9
Texas	80.7	81.8	79.5	48.6	48.4	48.8	31.3	27.9	34.4	41.3	35.3	47.0	21.7	17.8	25.6
Utah	40.6	38.6	42.6	17.9	14.8	20.8	10.9	7.6	14.0	19.7	15.7	23.7	9.7	7.1	12.2
Vermont	NA	NA	NA	48.1	46.9	49.2	29.0	26.0	31.9	NA	NA	NA	30.3	26.3	34.0
Wisconsin	NA	NA	NA	54.1	54.4	53.8	34.2	30.9	37.4	42.7	41.0	44.3	25.1	22.2	27.7
Wyoming	82.3	81.5	83.2	51.3	48.6	54.0	38.1	33.5	42.5	41.0	38.5	43.3	20.4	16.9	23.7

(continued)

(continued from previous page)

Unweighted data	lifetime alcohol use (ever had one or more drinks)			current alcohol use (drank alcohol in past 30 days)			five or more drinks of alcohol (on one or more occasions in past 30 days)			lifetime marijuana use (ever used marijuana)			current marijuana use (used marijuana in past 30 days)		
	total	female	male	total	female	male	total	female	male	total	female	male	total	female	male
Colorado	79.7	79.3	80.1	50.9	52.9	49.5	34.3	34.8	34.0	48.9	45.5	52.1	30.2	27.0	33.3
Hawaii	67.2	69.3	64.5	34.2	34.6	33.8	18.8	16.8	21.4	38.8	38.0	39.6	20.5	18.4	23.2
Illinois*	73.9	74.6	73.0	43.0	45.3	39.8	28.4	29.1	27.7	36.9	33.2	42.2	20.0	18.8	21.9
Indiana	79.7	80.6	78.6	45.1	44.4	45.6	29.5	25.9	33.3	44.7	40.5	49.4	26.7	23.4	30.4
Iowa	81.3	79.7	82.6	52.3	50.8	53.6	37.0	32.8	40.6	33.9	30.5	36.8	16.5	13.2	19.5
Kentucky	72.7	73.6	71.8	40.7	39.6	41.9	28.3	24.9	32.3	40.5	36.7	45.1	20.4	17.1	24.2
Louisiana*	78.9	78.3	79.9	50.1	50.3	49.9	29.3	25.7	33.9	38.1	32.8	45.2	18.9	14.3	25.3
Nebraska	83.1	83.2	83.0	53.0	50.1	56.0	39.0	35.3	42.7	34.7	33.9	35.6	18.5	18.2	18.9
New Hampshire	78.9	80.4	77.3	52.5	52.9	51.9	32.1	30.7	33.7	44.6	42.4	47.1	28.4	25.4	31.6
New York*	83.4	87.2	79.5	54.0	56.3	51.5	34.7	33.2	36.0	46.7	45.1	48.2	26.7	24.4	28.9
South Carolina	74.4	75.4	73.3	44.0	42.3	45.7	24.7	22.1	27.3	41.3	35.8	47.0	23.9	20.0	27.8
Tennessee	74.6	74.3	75.1	44.2	43.3	45.2	27.3	24.7	29.8	47.0	42.7	51.4	23.8	20.5	26.8

(continued)

(continued from previous page)

	lifetime alcohol use (ever had one or more drinks)			current alcohol use (drank alcohol in past 30 days)			five or more drinks of alcohol (on one or more occasions in past 30 days)			lifetime marijuana use (ever used marijuana)			current marijuana use (used marijuana in past 30 days)		
	total	female	male	total	female	male	total	female	male	total	female	male	total	female	male
Local surveys															
Weighted data															
Boston	73.9	72.2	75.7	41.7	41.7	41.9	18.1	15.6	20.6	40.1	38.0	42.4	21.7	18.4	25.0
Chicago	74.5	76.0	73.0	42.3	42.2	42.3	21.4	19.6	23.0	49.3	44.9	53.7	28.7	22.9	34.7
Dallas	81.1	81.6	80.7	44.0	45.0	43.0	20.7	20.7	20.8	43.5	37.5	49.9	20.4	15.8	25.2
Ft. Lauderdale	73.9	75.3	72.3	43.9	44.7	43.2	21.1	19.4	22.5	40.8	35.7	45.6	21.8	18.5	24.9
Houston	75.2	78.9	71.3	43.9	44.7	43.1	25.4	24.1	26.9	40.7	32.9	48.9	20.4	15.9	25.2
Los Angeles	76.4	79.2	73.7	39.8	42.0	37.4	21.9	23.0	20.5	41.2	36.8	45.5	22.5	18.6	26.2
Miami	69.4	67.3	71.8	39.9	37.4	42.4	19.1	15.5	22.7	31.9	28.3	35.7	17.0	15.3	18.9
New York City	76.0	77.4	74.5	41.8	41.6	41.7	17.9	16.4	19.3	34.4	33.9	34.8	17.8	16.3	19.3
Orlando	69.9	70.4	69.4	39.4	38.0	40.9	20.7	17.9	23.5	37.8	33.8	41.8	20.2	15.8	24.6
Palm Beach	74.3	71.4	77.6	45.4	46.1	44.9	26.1	24.3	28.1	41.0	34.6	47.8	24.0	19.5	28.6
Philadelphia	70.3	74.3	66.0	31.6	34.1	28.8	13.6	14.0	13.4	42.7	41.9	43.2	21.4	21.8	21.2
San Bernardino	68.6	70.3	67.0	34.9	36.5	33.5	21.1	19.2	22.7	38.0	37.0	39.0	17.9	15.8	19.9
San Diego	76.5	77.4	75.6	41.0	42.6	39.3	24.3	25.3	23.3	41.8	39.5	44.1	22.5	20.8	24.3
San Francisco	57.7	59.9	55.6	29.1	29.6	28.6	13.2	12.4	14.0	33.6	33.9	33.2	18.3	17.7	18.9
Unweighted data															
Detroit	68.2	72.6	62.8	32.0	35.4	27.4	11.2	10.2	11.9	40.5	39.6	41.1	19.5	19.6	19.1
District of Columbia	58.9	59.9	57.6	28.3	27.4	29.1	10.6	10.3	10.9	36.5	34.0	39.2	20.2	16.6	23.8
Milwaukee	NA	NA	NA	36.3	36.3	36.1	19.0	18.3	19.7	49.7	47.7	51.7	23.7	22.1	25.1
New Orleans	65.9	70.3	59.5	35.7	39.4	30.4	12.6	12.4	12.4	29.7	27.5	32.0	16.8	14.9	18.8

* Survey did not include students from one of the state's large school districts.

Note: NA means data not available.

Source: Grunbaum, Jo Anne, et al., Youth Risk Behavior Surveillance–United States, 2001, Mortality and Morbidity Weekly Report, Vol. 51/SS-4, Centers for Disease Control and Prevention. June 28, 2002

2.22 Percentage of high school students who used cocaine or inhaled intoxicating substances, by sex, race/ethnicity, and grade—United States, 2001

	lifetime cocaine use (ever used cocaine)			current cocaine use (used cocaine in past 30 days)			lifetime inhalant use (ever used inhalants)			current inhalant use (used inhalants in past 30 days)		
	total	female	male	total	female	male	total	female	male	total	female	male
Total	9.4	8.4	10.3	4.2	3.7	4.7	14.7	14.9	14.5	4.7	4.2	5.1
	(±1.2)	(±1.3)	(±1.3)	(±0.7)	(±1.0)	(±0.7)	(±1.7)	(±2.0)	(±1.9)	(±0.8)	(±1.0)	(±0.9)
Race/ethnicity												
Black	2.1	1.3	2.9	1.3	0.4	2.2	5.8	6.4	5.3	2.6	2.6	2.7
	(±0.7)	(±0.7)	(±1.3)	(±0.5)	(±0.3)	(±1.0)	(±0.9)	(±1.4)	(±1.8)	(±0.7)	(±0.8)	(±1.4)
Hispanic	14.9	13.1	16.9	7.1	5.9	8.5	15.2	15.1	15.2	5.5	4.8	6.1
	(±3.0)	(±2.8)	(±4.2)	(±1.5)	(±1.6)	(±2.3)	(±1.8)	(±2.5)	(±2.6)	(±1.1)	(±1.6)	(±2.2)
White	9.9	9.2	10.5	4.2	3.9	4.5	16.3	16.5	16.2	4.9	4.5	5.4
	(±1.4)	(±1.6)	(±1.6)	(±0.9)	(±1.4)	(±0.8)	(±2.2)	(±2.5)	(±2.6)	(±1.1)	(±1.4)	(±1.3)
Grade												
9	7.2	7.1	7.3	3.7	3.6	3.7	17.4	19.1	15.5	6.2	6.4	6.0
	(±1.7)	(±2.1)	(±1.8)	(±1.1)	(±1.5)	(±1.1)	(±3.2)	(±3.7)	(±3.8)	(±2.1)	(±2.3)	(±2.7)
10	8.6	7.9	9.3	4.2	4.0	4.5	14.0	14.4	13.6	4.8	3.6	6.0
	(±1.5)	(±1.8)	(±1.9)	(±1.2)	(±1.8)	(±1.1)	(±2.4)	(±3.2)	(±2.3)	(±1.1)	(±1.2)	(±1.7)
11	10.4	8.7	12.1	4.4	3.4	5.3	13.8	12.9	14.8	4.0	3.5	4.4
	(±2.1)	(±2.0)	(±2.7)	(±1.1)	(±1.1)	(±1.6)	(±1.8)	(±2.5)	(±3.1)	(±0.8)	(±1.1)	(±1.5)
12	12.1	10.6	13.6	4.5	3.7	5.5	12.5	11.3	13.7	2.9	2.5	3.4
	(±2.1)	(±2.3)	(±2.4)	(±1.4)	(±1.7)	(±1.6)	(±1.9)	(±2.4)	(±3.1)	(±0.7)	(±0.9)	(±1.1)

Note: Cocaine use includes use of powder, crack or freebase. Inhalant use includes sniffed glue or breathing the contents of aerosol spray cans or any paints or sprays to get high. Blacks and whites are non-Hispanic. Numbers in parentheses are plus or minus percentage points of the 95 percent confidence interval. Differences in percentages are considered statistically significant if the confidence intervals do not overlap.

Source: Grunbaum, Jo Anne, et al., Youth Risk Behavior Surveillance—United States, 2001. Mortality and Morbidity Weekly Report, Vol. 51/SS-4, Centers for Disease Control and Prevention, June 28, 2002

2.23 Percentage of high school students who used cocaine or inhaled intoxicating substances, by sex—selected U.S. sites, 2001

	lifetime cocaine use (ever used cocaine)			current cocaine use (used cocaine in past 30 days)			lifetime inhalant use (ever used inhalants)			current inhalant use (used inhalants in past 30 days)		
	total	female	male	total	female	male	total	female	male	total	female	male
State surveys												
Weighted data												
Alabama	6.6	6.2	6.9	2.4	2.1	2.6	13.5	14.2	12.8	4.0	3.8	4.1
Arkansas	8.7	8.4	9.1	4.1	3.6	4.6	14.1	12.6	15.7	4.4	4.1	4.8
Delaware	6.3	5.8	6.8	2.4	1.7	3.0	10.5	8.7	12.4	3.2	1.8	4.6
Florida	8.3	7.8	8.6	4.0	3.1	4.7	12.0	11.2	12.6	4.4	3.8	4.8
Idaho	7.3	7.0	7.4	3.2	2.8	3.3	14.3	13.4	15.0	3.6	2.9	4.1
Maine	9.7	9.9	9.5	4.1	3.2	4.9	12.6	12.2	12.8	4.3	4.0	4.6
Massachusetts	8.3	6.8	9.7	NA	NA	NA	12.4	11.5	13.3	NA	NA	NA
Michigan	7.8	6.8	8.8	3.6	2.7	4.5	12.8	14.1	11.4	3.6	3.8	3.3
Mississippi	4.7	5.1	4.4	2.3	1.8	2.8	9.9	10.4	9.5	3.4	3.0	3.8
Missouri	8.6	8.2	9.1	3.4	2.3	4.5	12.7	12.3	13.1	3.6	3.4	3.7
Montana	9.4	9.2	9.5	4.0	3.3	4.4	15.0	14.7	15.1	4.2	3.4	5.0
Nevada	11.9	12.4	11.5	5.5	4.6	6.3	16.4	16.0	16.8	5.0	4.1	5.9
New Jersey	8.5	6.0	11.0	4.2	1.6	6.9	12.7	10.4	15.0	5.1	3.3	6.8
North Carolina	6.7	6.2	7.1	2.7	1.9	3.5	13.7	13.5	13.8	NA	NA	NA
North Dakota	9.3	7.1	11.0	NA	NA	NA	15.1	14.9	15.0	3.8	1.7	5.6
Rhode Island	9.9	7.8	11.8	5.5	3.6	7.2	11.8	8.9	14.6	4.7	2.3	6.9
South Dakota	7.6	7.3	7.6	3.1	2.5	3.3	15.2	14.8	15.4	4.2	2.8	5.5
Texas	13.0	11.7	14.3	6.3	5.4	7.1	13.9	13.4	14.3	4.5	3.8	5.1
Utah	4.1	3.5	4.7	2.7	1.9	3.4	12.2	10.6	13.7	5.1	4.2	5.9
Vermont	NA	NA	NA	4.1	2.9	5.1	NA	NA	NA	NA	NA	NA
Wisconsin	8.1	8.4	7.8	3.4	3.2	3.4	13.8	15.1	12.4	3.2	3.2	3.2
Wyoming	9.5	10.0	8.9	4.3	4.1	4.3	16.0	15.6	16.3	4.2	3.6	4.9

(continued)

(continued from previous page)

	lifetime cocaine use (ever used cocaine)			current cocaine use (used cocaine in past 30 days)			lifetime inhalant use (ever used inhalants)			current inhalant use (used inhalants in past 30 days)		
	total	female	male	total	female	male	total	female	male	total	female	male
Unweighted data												
Colorado	11.2	11.4	11.1	5.0	5.3	4.8	13.6	16.2	11.4	3.8	5.1	2.7
Hawaii	6.1	7.5	4.2	2.4	2.8	2.0	11.8	12.5	10.7	3.2	3.0	3.5
Illinois*	5.5	5.6	5.5	2.5	2.2	2.9	11.6	11.7	11.5	3.5	3.2	3.8
Indiana	8.2	6.6	9.7	3.6	2.1	5.3	15.5	12.4	18.8	4.2	3.4	4.9
Iowa	6.6	6.2	6.9	3.7	3.8	3.5	10.1	8.0	12.0	3.3	2.4	3.9
Kentucky	7.5	6.3	8.8	3.8	3.1	4.6	13.0	13.3	12.8	4.1	4.3	3.9
Louisiana*	8.8	6.6	11.9	3.8	1.5	7.0	14.2	13.9	14.2	4.7	3.9	5.5
Nebraska	5.3	4.8	5.6	2.1	1.4	2.7	10.7	11.2	10.2	2.3	2.2	2.5
New Hampshire	10.9	10.3	11.4	4.7	4.2	4.9	15.3	14.5	16.0	5.6	4.3	6.7
New York*	8.3	6.6	9.8	3.9	3.0	4.8	14.7	15.5	13.7	5.1	4.9	5.2
South Carolina	6.8	5.7	7.7	2.7	1.9	3.4	12.3	12.4	12.1	4.3	4.0	4.6
Tennessee	9.3	8.3	10.5	3.7	2.4	5.0	13.8	14.2	13.5	3.8	3.3	4.3

(continued)

(continued from previous page)

	lifetime cocaine use (ever used cocaine)			current cocaine use (used cocaine in past 30 days)			lifetime inhalant use (ever used inhalants)			current inhalant use (used inhalants in past 30 days)		
	total	female	male	total	female	male	total	female	male	total	female	male
Local surveys **Weighted data**												
Boston	3.6	2.6	4.5	NA	NA	NA	6.1	5.1	6.9	NA	NA	NA
Chicago	4.4	3.2	5.5	2.6	1.0	4.1	6.5	6.2	6.3	2.5	1.1	3.6
Dallas	10.4	9.4	11.4	5.2	4.8	5.5	11.3	11.9	10.6	3.4	3.8	2.9
Ft. Lauderdale	7.2	5.3	9.0	2.6	0.9	4.1	10.5	8.8	12.2	3.9	1.7	5.9
Houston	8.9	8.2	9.6	4.3	3.7	4.9	8.7	8.6	8.7	3.2	3.3	3.2
Los Angeles	10.1	10.4	9.5	5.9	6.2	5.8	17.2	17.5	17.0	4.6	4.7	4.6
Miami	8.1	7.3	8.9	4.0	2.0	6.0	7.7	6.8	8.7	2.6	2.0	3.3
New York City	2.6	2.6	2.5	1.2	1.1	1.3	7.5	7.6	7.2	2.2	2.5	1.9
Orlando	6.7	5.6	7.5	2.9	2.7	2.9	11.4	8.6	14.2	4.8	2.6	6.9
Palm Beach	8.4	7.5	9.3	4.5	3.3	5.5	11.2	8.9	13.3	4.2	3.1	5.2
Philadelphia	2.6	3.0	2.3	1.3	0.9	1.8	6.9	6.8	7.1	1.8	1.6	2.1
San Bernardino	8.6	7.1	10.1	3.6	3.4	3.8	11.6	10.6	12.5	3.8	3.3	4.2
San Diego	8.8	9.5	8.0	3.8	3.7	3.8	11.3	12.5	10.0	3.3	3.4	3.1
San Francisco	5.9	5.3	6.5	NA	NA	NA	NA	NA	NA	3.1	4.0	2.2
Unweighted data												
Detroit	3.3	1.8	5.0	2.2	1.2	3.2	6.5	5.0	8.1	2.8	2.5	3.0
District of Columbia	6.0	4.6	7.1	2.8	2.4	3.1	9.0	6.9	10.2	3.0	2.5	3.1
Milwaukee	6.0	4.2	7.9	3.0	1.9	3.9	7.1	7.3	6.8	3.7	2.7	4.8
New Orleans	3.2	2.0	4.0	2.3	1.3	2.7	7.0	7.1	6.2	3.3	3.0	3.1

* *Survey did not include students from one of the state's large school districts.*
Note: Cocaine use includes use of powder, crack or freebase. Inhalant use includes sniffed glue or breathing the contents of aerosol spray cans or any paints or sprays to get high. NA means data not available.
Source: Grunbaum, Jo Anne, et al., Youth Risk Behavior Surveillance–United States, 2001. Mortality and Morbidity Weekly Report. Vol. 51/SS-4. Centers for Disease Control and Prevention. June 28, 2002

2.24 Percentage of high school students who used heroin, methamphetamines, illegal steroids, or who injected illegal drugs, by sex, race/ethnicity, and grade—United States, 2001

	lifetime heroin use (ever used heroin)			lifetime methamphetamine use (ever used methamphetamines)			lifetime illegal steroid use (ever used illegal steroids)			lifetime illegal use of injecting drugs (ever used illegal injecting drugs)		
	total	female	male	total	female	male	total	female	male	total	female	male
Total	**3.1**	**2.5**	**3.8**	**9.8**	**9.2**	**10.5**	**5.0**	**3.9**	**6.0**	**2.3**	**1.6**	**3.1**
	(±0.4)	(±0.5)	(±0.5)	(±1.5)	(±1.8)	(±1.5)	(±0.5)	(±0.8)	(±0.6)	(±0.4)	(±0.4)	(±0.4)
Race/ethnicity												
Black	1.7	0.5	2.9	2.1	1.2	3.0	3.2	2.1	4.3	1.6	0.6	2.6
	(±0.6)	(±0.4)	(±1.2)	(±0.6)	(±0.7)	(±1.2)	(±0.8)	(±0.8)	(±1.5)	(±0.7)	(±0.6)	(±1.3)
Hispanic	3.1	3.0	3.2	9.1	8.8	9.4	4.2	3.1	5.4	2.5	2.2	2.8
	(±0.6)	(±1.1)	(±0.9)	(±1.9)	(±2.3)	(±2.2)	(±0.8)	(±1.1)	(±1.4)	(±0.7)	(±1.3)	(±0.8)
White	3.3	2.6	4.0	11.4	10.7	12.1	5.3	4.2	6.4	2.4	1.6	3.3
	(±0.5)	(±0.7)	(±0.7)	(±2.1)	(±2.3)	(±2.0)	(±0.8)	(±1.2)	(±0.9)	(±0.5)	(±0.6)	(±0.6)
Grade												
9	3.2	2.6	4.0	8.1	7.9	8.5	5.8	5.0	6.8	2.5	1.9	3.2
	(±0.8)	(±1.0)	(±1.1)	(±2.5)	(±2.4)	(±2.8)	(±1.3)	(±1.6)	(±1.8)	(±0.9)	(±0.9)	(±1.0)
10	3.3	2.6	4.0	9.7	8.9	10.5	4.9	3.9	6.0	2.6	1.7	3.5
	(±0.9)	(±1.3)	(±1.1)	(±1.6)	(±1.9)	(±1.8)	(±0.9)	(±1.0)	(±1.5)	(±0.7)	(±0.9)	(±1.0)
11	2.8	2.2	3.4	9.2	8.9	9.4	4.3	3.3	5.3	1.9	1.2	2.5
	(±0.6)	(±0.8)	(±1.1)	(±1.7)	(±1.8)	(±2.5)	(±0.9)	(±1.2)	(±1.3)	(±0.6)	(±0.7)	(±1.0)
12	3.0	2.1	3.9	12.8	11.5	14.2	4.3	2.9	5.8	2.1	1.0	3.1
	(±0.8)	(±1.0)	(±1.1)	(±2.7)	(±3.6)	(±2.3)	(±0.9)	(±1.3)	(±1.3)	(±0.6)	(±0.7)	(±1.0)

Note: Heroin use includes smack, junk, or China White. Methamphetamine use includes speed, crystal, crack, or ice. Illegal drug use includes drugs not prescribed by a physician. Blacks and whites are non-Hispanic. Numbers in parentheses are plus or minus percentage points of the 95 percent confidence interval. Differences in percentages are considered statistically significant if the confidence intervals do not overlap.
Source: Grunbaum, Jo Anne, et al., Youth Risk Behavior Surveillance—United States, 2001. Mortality and Morbidity Weekly Report. Vol. 51/SS-4, Centers for Disease Control and Prevention. June 28, 2002

2.25 Percentage of high school students who used heroin, methamphetamines, illegal steroids, or who injected illegal drugs, by sex—selected U.S. sites, 2001

	lifetime heroin use (ever used heroin)			lifetime methamphetamine use (ever used methamphetamines)			lifetime illegal steroid use (ever used illegal steroids)			lifetime illegal use of injecting drugs (ever used illegal injecting drugs)		
	total	female	male	total	female	male	total	female	male	total	female	male
State surveys **Weighted data**												
Alabama	2.5	1.1	3.7	7.4	7.9	6.9	4.8	3.5	5.9	1.9	1.5	2.1
Arkansas	3.0	2.7	3.3	11.8	11.6	12.0	6.9	5.1	8.8	2.3	2.1	2.5
Delaware	2.7	1.6	3.7	6.8	5.6	8.1	4.8	2.3	7.2	1.7	0.5	2.9
Florida	3.7	2.3	4.6	7.6	7.4	7.6	5.0	3.3	6.5	2.7	1.7	3.6
Idaho	3.0	2.0	3.7	7.2	7.0	7.2	3.6	2.0	4.9	2.0	1.5	2.5
Maine	3.9	2.5	5.2	8.4	9.0	7.7	5.5	3.1	7.7	2.5	1.6	3.3
Massachusetts	3.0	1.7	4.1	7.0	5.9	8.0	4.8	3.1	6.4	1.7	0.9	2.4
Michigan	3.3	1.8	4.5	8.2	7.6	8.7	4.3	2.8	5.4	2.4	1.4	3.3
Mississippi	2.3	1.4	3.3	5.5	6.1	5.0	4.4	3.1	5.8	1.8	0.8	2.7
Missouri	2.7	1.9	3.4	10.4	10.7	10.2	5.3	3.4	7.1	1.6	1.0	2.2
Montana	4.0	3.3	4.6	12.6	13.2	12.0	5.3	4.1	5.9	2.7	2.1	3.1
Nevada	NA	NA	NA	15.6	16.5	14.8	6.4	4.7	7.9	3.7	2.2	5.1
New Jersey	3.8	2.1	5.5	7.7	5.8	9.6	4.7	2.2	7.3	3.2	0.8	5.6
North Carolina	2.3	1.4	3.1	7.8	7.3	8.3	5.0	3.5	6.5	1.9	1.2	2.6
North Dakota	3.4	1.6	5.0	9.7	8.3	10.7	4.3	1.7	6.4	2.4	0.9	3.5
Rhode Island	4.0	1.9	5.9	8.6	5.6	11.4	5.4	2.1	8.3	3.5	1.0	5.6
South Dakota	NA	NA	NA	8.3	8.3	8.2	5.4	3.9	6.7	6.9	6.6	7.1
Texas	3.0	2.2	3.6	8.4	7.7	9.2	5.7	4.1	7.2	2.1	1.1	3.1
Utah	2.7	1.7	3.6	5.3	4.7	5.8	4.2	1.7	6.6	2.1	1.2	2.8
Vermont	3.4	2.5	4.1	7.8	7.0	8.4	5.1	4.4	5.7	2.6	1.9	3.2
Wisconsin	2.5	2.1	2.9	7.9	8.7	7.1	NA	NA	NA	NA	NA	NA
Wyoming	2.9	2.7	3.1	10.7	11.0	10.4	5.3	3.8	6.6	2.6	1.8	3.3

(continued)

(continued from previous page)

	lifetime heroin use (ever used heroin)			lifetime methamphetamine use (ever used methamphetamines)			lifetime illegal steroid use (ever used illegal steroids)			lifetime illegal use of injecting drugs (ever used illegal injecting drugs)		
	total	female	male	total	female	male	total	female	male	total	female	male
Unweighted data												
Colorado	3.3	2.8	3.8	10.9	10.8	10.9	4.7	3.8	5.6	2.3	2.3	2.3
Hawaii	2.5	1.8	3.2	6.5	7.1	5.8	2.8	2.5	3.2	2.0	1.5	2.8
Illinois*	2.2	1.5	3.1	5.6	5.6	5.7	3.2	2.0	4.8	1.3	0.5	2.4
Indiana	2.7	1.9	3.2	9.7	9.1	10.1	5.9	4.5	7.3	2.2	1.4	3.0
Iowa	2.7	1.6	3.5	6.5	5.6	7.3	4.3	2.6	6.0	2.3	2.0	2.6
Kentucky	2.4	2.0	2.8	9.7	8.8	10.7	5.5	3.9	7.4	2.7	2.0	3.3
Louisiana*	4.3	2.4	6.8	9.1	7.8	10.6	6.3	2.6	11.2	3.0	1.0	5.6
Nebraska	1.4	1.0	1.8	5.7	5.6	5.7	2.6	2.1	3.2	1.1	0.9	1.4
New Hampshire	4.0	3.3	4.4	NA	NA	NA	5.3	4.2	6.0	2.8	2.1	3.1
New York*	3.8	3.0	4.5	7.7	6.0	9.3	5.5	3.7	7.2	3.0	1.7	4.1
South Carolina	3.0	2.1	3.9	7.6	6.4	8.7	4.9	3.1	6.7	2.2	1.2	3.2
Tennessee	2.9	2.4	3.5	11.0	10.5	11.4	6.6	5.7	7.6	2.4	2.0	2.9

(continued)

(continued from previous page)

	lifetime heroin use (ever used heroin)			lifetime methamphetamine use (ever used methamphetamines)			lifetime illegal steroid use (ever used illegal steroids)			lifetime illegal use of injecting drugs (ever used illegal injecting drugs)		
	total	female	male	total	female	male	total	female	male	total	female	male
Local surveys **Weighted data**												
Boston	1.5	0.7	2.1	3.5	2.0	4.7	3.1	2.4	3.7	0.8	0.5	1.0
Chicago	2.5	0.7	4.0	2.8	1.4	3.6	5.2	3.8	6.0	2.2	0.4	3.6
Dallas	2.4	2.0	2.8	5.4	4.9	6.0	3.9	3.7	4.2	1.8	0.8	2.9
Ft. Lauderdale	3.3	1.4	4.9	5.6	4.5	6.3	4.5	2.1	6.6	2.9	1.0	4.5
Houston	3.0	2.3	3.6	6.0	5.2	6.8	5.7	5.1	6.4	2.3	1.4	3.2
Los Angeles	1.8	1.8	1.7	7.6	7.7	7.4	4.4	4.9	3.6	1.5	1.0	1.9
Miami	2.8	1.7	3.9	4.8	3.8	5.9	3.2	2.5	3.9	1.6	0.7	2.5
New York City	0.9	0.5	1.2	2.8	2.3	3.1	2.6	2.4	2.7	1.1	0.8	1.4
Orlando	3.7	2.3	4.8	7.3	6.0	8.4	4.8	3.7	5.7	2.2	0.7	3.4
Palm Beach	4.4	3.8	4.9	8.0	5.9	9.9	5.4	3.1	7.6	3.0	1.4	4.4
Philadelphia	2.6	1.5	3.7	4.6	3.9	5.1	4.1	3.9	4.4	1.3	1.2	1.5
San Bernardino	4.6	3.7	5.2	8.6	8.4	8.6	5.2	4.3	5.9	2.5	1.4	3.5
San Diego	2.9	2.0	3.8	8.4	9.1	7.7	5.2	5.3	5.1	1.8	1.4	2.1
San Francisco	1.7	1.4	2.0	4.6	4.9	4.3	2.3	2.5	2.2	1.6	0.9	2.2
Unweighted data												
Detroit	4.0	1.8	6.5	4.8	2.7	7.2	4.7	2.4	7.3	2.4	1.2	3.7
District of Columbia	4.6	3.2	5.7	6.6	4.5	8.4	4.2	2.8	4.7	3.2	1.6	4.3
Milwaukee	3.4	2.2	4.6	5.1	3.8	6.5	NA	NA	NA	NA	NA	NA
New Orleans	3.1	1.6	4.3	3.3	1.9	4.6	4.5	2.5	6.4	2.9	1.3	4.4

* Survey did not include students from one of the state's large school districts.

Note: Heroin use includes smack, junk, or China White. Methamphetamine use includes speed, crystal, crack, or ice. Illegal drug use includes drugs not prescribed by a physician. NA means data not available.

Source: Grunbaum, Jo Anne, et al., Youth Risk Behavior Surveillance–United States, 2001, Mortality and Morbidity Weekly Report. Vol. 51/SS-4, Centers for Disease Control and Prevention, June 28, 2002

2.26 Percentage of high school students who initiated drug-related behavior before age 13, by sex, race/ethnicity, and grade—United States, 2001

	smoked a whole cigarette before age 13			drank alcohol before age 13 (other than a few sips)			tried marijuana before age 13		
	total	female	male	total	female	male	total	female	male
Total	**22.1**	**19.8**	**24.5**	**29.1**	**24.2**	**34.2**	**10.2**	**7.5**	**13.2**
	(±1.8)	(±2.1)	(±2.0)	(±1.6)	(±1.8)	(±1.7)	(±1.2)	(±1.2)	(±1.5)
Race/ethnicity									
Black	14.2	12.4	16.1	28.2	24.3	32.4	11.4	6.5	16.7
	(±2.5)	(±2.6)	(±3.6)	(±2.9)	(±3.2)	(±3.5)	(±2.4)	(±1.6)	(±3.8)
Hispanic	22.6	20.6	24.8	33.7	27.1	40.8	12.9	9.6	16.5
	(±3.2)	(±3.9)	(±3.9)	(±2.6)	(±2.6)	(±3.9)	(±2.0)	(±2.1)	(±2.5)
White	23.6	21.2	26.3	28.4	23.6	33.3	9.5	7.1	12.0
	(±2.5)	(±2.8)	(±2.7)	(±2.2)	(±2.7)	(±2.3)	(±1.5)	(±1.5)	(±1.9)
Grade									
9	26.2	23.9	28.9	39.7	34.5	45.6	11.6	8.6	15.0
	(±2.9)	(±3.8)	(±2.9)	(±2.7)	(±3.4)	(±3.4)	(±1.8)	(±2.0)	(±2.4)
10	22.9	19.8	26.2	28.8	23.6	34.1	12.1	8.6	15.9
	(±3.0)	(±2.9)	(±4.2)	(±2.2)	(±2.4)	(±3.1)	(±1.6)	(±1.8)	(±1.9)
11	18.5	16.1	20.9	23.4	17.6	29.3	8.5	6.5	10.4
	(±2.2)	(±2.5)	(±2.7)	(±1.9)	(±2.4)	(±2.8)	(±1.4)	(±1.3)	(±2.1)
12	19.0	17.5	20.6	21.2	17.5	25.0	7.8	5.3	10.4
	(±2.8)	(±3.4)	(±3.4)	(±1.8)	(±2.2)	(±2.6)	(±1.7)	(±1.5)	(±2.4)

Note: Blacks and whites are non-Hispanic. Numbers in parentheses are plus or minus percentage points of the 95 percent confidence interval. Differences in percentages are considered statistically significant if the confidence intervals do not overlap.
Source: Grunbaum, Jo Anne, et al., Youth Risk Behavior Surveillance–United States, 2001, Mortality and Morbidity Weekly Report, *Vol. 51/SS-4, Centers for Disease Control and Prevention, June 28, 2002*

2.27 Percentage of high school students who initiated drug-related behavior before age 13, by sex—selected U.S. sites, 2001

	smoked a whole cigarette before age 13			drank alcohol before age 13 (other than a few sips)			tried marijuana before age 13		
	total	female	male	total	female	male	total	female	male
State surveys									
Weighted data									
Alabama	22.4	21.3	23.3	28.4	25.3	30.9	8.8	6.0	11.2
Arkansas	28.0	22.1	33.7	31.8	23.6	39.8	11.6	7.9	15.2
Delaware	23.8	21.7	26.1	28.8	23.4	34.4	12.2	6.6	18.0
Florida	19.9	19.5	20.3	30.7	26.5	34.8	11.3	8.4	14.1
Idaho	19.2	16.6	21.5	27.6	24.0	30.9	8.3	5.8	10.5
Maine	22.5	19.6	25.2	21.7	17.3	25.6	12.0	9.9	13.8
Massachusetts	19.3	17.8	20.9	27.9	23.5	32.1	11.9	9.2	14.5
Michigan	23.2	23.3	23.0	26.9	24.1	29.1	11.6	8.8	13.8
Mississippi	22.8	19.3	26.4	32.2	29.0	35.5	9.5	7.1	12.1
Missouri	25.7	22.8	28.5	30.0	25.5	34.3	12.4	8.4	16.3
Montana	25.0	23.3	26.2	35.1	28.9	40.8	12.3	10.3	13.9
Nevada	23.3	20.4	26.1	33.0	29.6	36.2	17.8	14.2	21.1
New Jersey	21.5	18.4	24.8	32.5	27.1	37.6	9.2	4.8	13.6
North Carolina	26.5	25.1	28.0	24.7	21.4	27.8	10.5	7.4	13.5
North Dakota	25.4	22.0	28.5	29.8	24.8	34.5	6.9	4.0	9.5
Rhode Island	22.3	21.6	22.4	29.7	24.7	34.6	12.8	8.2	17.2
South Dakota	25.8	19.7	31.7	31.6	25.5	37.2	8.8	6.2	11.2
Texas	21.3	16.6	25.7	29.4	24.0	34.6	11.0	6.9	15.0
Utah	12.2	10.0	14.4	NA	NA	NA	4.5	3.0	6.0
Vermont	21.5	20.9	21.7	26.0	21.8	29.7	12.2	9.0	15.1
Wisconsin	22.2	22.2	22.2	28.2	26.8	29.5	8.3	6.6	9.7
Wyoming	24.1	21.5	26.7	33.9	27.7	39.8	9.8	7.5	11.8
Unweighted data									
Colorado	25.8	27.0	25.0	33.8	28.9	38.7	15.6	14.5	16.8
Hawaii	19.2	20.5	17.3	26.4	24.5	28.4	11.8	11.2	12.5
Illinois*	16.3	14.8	18.4	22.9	19.0	28.2	6.6	4.2	10.1
Indiana	23.3	20.5	26.4	24.2	17.3	31.8	8.7	5.3	12.2
Iowa	19.9	17.3	22.6	27.2	21.4	32.8	6.4	5.0	7.9
Kentucky	28.1	24.5	31.9	28.0	21.8	35.1	11.7	7.6	16.4
Louisiana*	25.6	23.3	28.3	33.3	29.5	38.2	9.0	6.2	12.5
Nebraska	20.1	18.2	22.1	27.3	22.7	31.9	5.8	4.6	6.9
New Hampshire	22.7	20.6	24.7	28.3	23.3	33.6	12.1	9.8	14.4
New York*	24.3	23.8	24.9	29.9	26.0	33.9	9.8	5.9	13.7
South Carolina	26.1	21.8	30.6	31.8	26.9	36.6	11.9	7.3	16.6
Tennessee	25.8	22.7	29.0	29.1	23.5	34.6	12.2	8.5	15.8

(continued)

(continued from previous page)

	smoked a whole cigarette before age 13			drank alcohol before age 13 (other than a few sips)			tried marijuana before age 13		
	total	female	male	total	female	male	total	female	male
Local surveys									
Weighted data									
Boston	13.5	11.2	15.8	30.1	26.4	34.0	11.4	6.6	16.1
Chicago	21.0	16.6	25.5	32.4	28.5	36.7	15.6	9.6	21.7
Dallas	19.4	14.9	24.3	34.3	27.7	41.4	13.7	9.2	18.5
Ft. Lauderdale	15.9	15.0	16.8	27.6	23.7	31.9	8.9	5.0	12.6
Houston	20.4	15.0	26.0	31.0	26.8	35.3	12.9	8.6	17.5
Los Angeles	18.2	16.9	19.2	32.6	30.3	34.6	11.7	7.7	15.6
Miami	13.0	11.0	15.0	29.8	24.9	34.6	7.7	4.9	10.5
New York City	15.7	15.8	15.5	34.7	31.2	38.6	7.5	6.2	8.6
Orlando	19.2	17.4	20.8	30.9	27.2	34.8	11.9	8.5	15.2
Palm Beach	21.2	19.5	22.9	30.6	24.4	36.8	11.3	6.7	16.1
Philadelphia	17.7	18.8	16.5	32.4	28.7	36.0	10.6	7.4	13.9
San Bernardino	17.4	15.9	18.7	30.1	27.5	32.2	14.8	12.7	16.6
San Diego	16.7	16.3	17.1	30.1	26.2	34.0	13.5	11.4	15.8
San Francisco	11.1	9.8	12.2	25.6	22.3	28.8	8.0	6.5	9.3
Unweighted data									
Detroit	17.3	16.0	18.6	27.7	25.6	29.8	12.7	9.7	15.8
District of Columbia	15.3	12.7	17.9	25.6	22.3	29.2	10.5	6.5	14.6
Milwaukee	20.8	19.6	22.1	29.2	26.5	32.1	13.6	9.2	18.2
New Orleans	15.9	14.9	17.2	33.5	32.4	34.8	9.6	6.7	12.5

* Survey did not include students from one of the state's large school districts.
Note: NA means data not available.
Source: Grunbaum, Jo Anne, et al., Youth Risk Behavior Surveillance–United States, 2001, Mortality and Morbidity Weekly Report, Vol. 51/SS-4, Centers for Disease Control and Prevention, June 28, 2002

2.28 Percentage of high school students who engaged in drug-related behaviors on school property, by sex, race/ethnicity, and grade—United States, 2001

	cigarette use on school property in past 30 days			smokeless tobacco use on school property in past 30 days			alcohol use on school property in past 30 days			marijuana use on school property in past 30 days			offered, sold, or given an illegal drug on school property in past 30 days		
	total	female	male	total	female	male	total	female	male	total	female	male	total	female	male
Total	**9.9**	**8.5**	**11.3**	**5.0**	**0.7**	**9.4**	**4.9**	**3.8**	**6.1**	**5.4**	**2.9**	**8.0**	**28.5**	**22.7**	**34.6**
	(±1.2)	(±1.4)	(±1.3)	(±1.2)	(±0.3)	(±2.3)	(±0.5)	(±0.8)	(±0.8)	(±0.7)	(±0.6)	(±1.1)	(±2.0)	(±2.0)	(±2.4)
Race/ethnicity															
Black	4.9	2.8	7.2	1.1	0.3	2.0	5.3	3.1	7.5	6.1	2.3	10.2	21.9	16.2	27.9
	(±1.9)	(±1.7)	(±3.1)	(±0.6)	(±0.4)	(±1.1)	(±1.3)	(±1.1)	(±1.7)	(±1.2)	(±0.9)	(±2.2)	(±3.4)	(±3.1)	(±4.7)
Hispanic	7.7	7.9	7.5	2.7	1.0	4.3	7.0	7.1	6.9	7.4	5.8	9.0	34.2	28.7	39.8
	(±1.9)	(±2.9)	(±1.8)	(±0.6)	(±0.7)	(±1.5)	(±1.4)	(±1.7)	(±1.8)	(±1.1)	(±1.2)	(±2.0)	(±2.3)	(±2.6)	(±3.8)
White	11.3	9.8	12.8	6.2	0.7	11.9	4.2	3.2	5.3	4.8	2.2	7.4	28.3	22.7	34.2
	(±1.5)	(±1.8)	(±1.6)	(±1.7)	(±0.3)	(±3.2)	(±0.5)	(±0.9)	(±1.0)	(±0.9)	(±0.7)	(±1.3)	(±2.6)	(±2.6)	(±3.0)
Grade															
9	8.8	6.7	11.1	3.8	0.4	7.4	5.3	4.4	6.3	5.5	3.0	8.0	29.0	23.4	35.1
	(±1.7)	(±2.0)	(±2.0)	(±1.4)	(±0.3)	(±2.5)	(±0.9)	(±1.3)	(±1.2)	(±1.2)	(±1.1)	(±2.1)	(±3.1)	(±3.2)	(±4.6)
10	10.2	9.8	10.7	5.9	1.2	10.8	5.1	4.8	5.4	5.8	3.2	8.6	29.0	23.6	34.7
	(±1.6)	(±2.3)	(±1.8)	(±1.4)	(±0.7)	(±2.7)	(±0.9)	(±1.4)	(±1.2)	(±1.0)	(±0.9)	(±1.7)	(±2.7)	(±3.4)	(±3.3)
11	10.0	8.3	11.8	5.1	0.8	9.5	4.7	2.9	6.5	5.1	2.5	7.7	28.7	22.8	34.6
	(±1.8)	(±1.6)	(±2.5)	(±1.7)	(±0.5)	(±3.2)	(±0.9)	(±0.9)	(±1.5)	(±0.9)	(±0.9)	(±1.6)	(±2.7)	(±2.8)	(±3.6)
12	10.8	9.6	12.1	5.3	0.4	10.4	4.3	2.5	6.1	4.9	2.4	7.5	26.9	20.4	33.8
	(±2.5)	(±3.2)	(±2.5)	(±1.7)	(±0.3)	(±3.2)	(±0.9)	(±1.3)	(±1.6)	(±1.4)	(±1.0)	(±2.2)	(±2.6)	(±3.8)	(±3.4)

Note: Blacks and whites are non-Hispanic. Numbers in parentheses are plus or minus percentage points of the 95 percent confidence interval. Differences in percentages are considered statistically significant if the confidence intervals do not overlap.

Source: Grunbaum, Jo Anne, et al., Youth Risk Behavior Surveillance–United States, 2001. Mortality and Morbidity Weekly Report. Vol. 51/SS-4. Centers for Disease Control and Prevention. June 28, 2002

2.29   Percentage of high school students who engaged in drug-related behaviors on school property, by sex—selected U.S. sites, 2001

	cigarette use on school property in past 30 days			smokeless tobacco use on school property in past 30 days			alcohol use on school property in past 30 days			marijuana use on school property in past 30 days			offered, sold, or given an illegal drug on school property in past 30 days		
	total	female	male	total	female	male	total	female	male	total	female	male	total	female	male
State surveys															
Weighted data															
Alabama	6.7	5.8	7.5	6.1	0.9	10.9	3.3	2.4	4.1	3.0	1.6	4.2	24.3	22.4	26.1
Arkansas	11.0	8.2	13.7	8.6	0.8	16.1	5.5	2.9	8.1	4.1	2.1	6.1	21.1	16.2	25.8
Delaware	11.1	9.5	12.8	2.9	0.5	5.2	5.4	3.8	7.1	6.4	3.0	9.9	26.9	21.0	33.2
Florida	7.0	6.4	7.6	3.9	1.0	6.5	4.9	3.6	6.2	5.8	3.5	8.0	24.9	19.6	29.9
Idaho	5.4	3.0	7.5	4.6	0.9	8.2	4.2	3.0	5.3	4.7	2.0	6.9	23.2	16.8	28.7
Maine	8.7	8.5	9.0	3.0	1.2	4.7	5.0	3.7	6.3	6.9	4.9	8.6	32.4	26.5	37.8
Massachusetts	12.4	12.9	11.9	2.2	0.5	3.7	5.5	4.0	6.9	7.0	3.8	10.0	34.2	29.5	38.6
Michigan	9.1	9.4	8.8	4.0	1.2	6.5	4.9	4.0	5.6	5.6	4.0	7.1	35.6	32.6	38.2
Mississippi	6.6	5.9	7.3	5.6	0.9	10.5	5.0	3.6	6.3	3.3	1.2	5.6	18.7	13.6	23.9
Missouri	11.9	10.7	13.2	6.4	0.7	12.0	4.9	3.0	6.9	4.6	2.8	6.4	20.7	18.2	23.1
Montana	10.4	11.1	9.9	9.3	2.6	15.8	6.9	5.3	8.2	7.7	5.7	9.5	29.5	26.3	32.7
Nevada	10.3	10.5	10.2	4.0	1.2	6.7	8.1	7.5	8.7	7.7	4.9	10.4	35.7	31.8	39.4
New Jersey	14.8	13.4	16.1	4.5	0.6	8.3	5.0	2.9	6.9	5.2	2.3	8.1	28.8	22.0	35.5
North Carolina	11.2	9.9	12.5	NA	NA	NA	4.3	2.5	6.1	4.7	2.3	7.1	32.8	28.8	36.8
North Dakota	12.2	11.0	13.0	6.9	0.9	12.5	6.4	4.8	7.6	6.0	3.0	8.6	27.3	22.6	31.5
Rhode Island	14.0	14.2	13.7	3.0	1.1	4.7	8.3	5.0	11.4	10.9	7.6	13.9	30.9	25.4	36.3
South Dakota	13.9	14.5	13.0	7.9	2.3	13.3	7.5	5.9	9.1	5.4	5.1	5.4	26.7	23.7	29.5
Texas	7.4	5.3	9.5	5.4	0.7	9.7	5.9	4.9	6.7	5.4	3.5	7.1	28.2	23.3	32.8
Utah	2.7	3.2	2.3	2.3	0.5	4.1	4.0	2.7	5.2	2.6	1.5	3.6	22.5	17.9	26.7
Vermont	NA	NA	NA	NA	NA	NA	5.3	3.4	7.0	9.7	6.4	12.8	29.6	24.1	34.7
Wisconsin	9.8	10.6	9.1	NA	NA	NA	NA	NA	NA	NA	NA	NA	26.6	21.9	30.9
Wyoming	10.7	10.4	11.0	11.5	3.2	19.3	6.1	4.3	7.8	4.4	3.1	5.6	18.9	16.5	21.1

(continued)

(continued from previous page)

	cigarette use on school property in past 30 days			smokeless tobacco use on school property in past 30 days			alcohol use on school property in past 30 days			marijuana use on school property in past 30 days			offered, sold, or given an illegal drug on school property in past 30 days		
	total	female	male	total	female	male	total	female	male	total	female	male	total	female	male
Unweighted data															
Colorado	12.0	12.9	11.2	4.5	0.6	8.1	7.3	7.3	7.4	8.2	3.8	12.3	29.3	25.4	33.1
Hawaii	6.7	7.6	5.5	1.3	0.8	1.9	4.7	4.7	4.8	6.9	6.1	7.8	36.0	34.1	38.3
Illinois*	8.3	8.3	8.4	0.9	–	2.1	2.4	1.9	3.1	4.3	2.7	6.5	22.1	17.6	28.6
Indiana	9.7	7.9	11.6	3.2	0.6	6.2	2.4	1.8	3.2	3.3	1.9	4.9	30.4	24.7	37.0
Iowa	9.7	8.0	11.4	6.3	0.8	11.4	3.1	2.2	3.9	3.7	3.8	3.7	16.9	11.8	21.6
Kentucky	16.0	14.5	17.7	8.3	1.2	16.4	3.7	2.2	5.5	4.6	3.0	6.6	22.7	19.9	25.7
Louisiana*	7.2	5.4	9.8	5.0	1.1	9.9	4.5	2.8	6.9	3.0	1.2	5.5	24.5	20.6	29.5
Nebraska	10.7	12.1	9.3	5.1	1.0	9.2	3.2	2.6	3.8	2.5	1.8	3.3	17.0	14.0	20.1
New Hampshire	9.7	9.6	9.8	NA	NA	NA	4.4	1.9	6.8	6.9	4.2	9.6	32.9	27.8	38.5
New York*	13.7	13.1	14.4	3.6	1.5	5.6	4.7	4.1	5.3	6.3	4.2	8.4	34.3	28.9	39.9
South Carolina	9.2	7.6	10.9	4.0	0.6	7.3	5.3	3.3	7.2	3.9	1.9	6.0	28.4	23.3	33.5
Tennessee	9.7	8.1	11.3	7.2	0.3	13.8	3.9	2.6	5.3	3.7	2.1	5.3	27.9	22.5	33.2

(continued)

(continued from previous page)

	cigarette use on school property in past 30 days			smokeless tobacco use on school property in past 30 days			alcohol use on school property in past 30 days			marijuana use on school property in past 30 days			offered, sold, or given an illegal drug on school property in past 30 days		
	total	female	male	total	female	male	total	female	male	total	female	male	total	female	male
Local surveys **Weighted data**															
Boston	7.2	6.0	8.3	0.8	0.2	1.5	6.3	4.5	8.0	6.0	3.3	8.7	31.0	24.7	37.5
Chicago	11.1	9.3	12.8	1.5	–	2.8	8.7	7.8	9.5	10.3	4.8	15.9	28.2	18.9	37.7
Dallas	5.3	4.9	5.8	1.3	0.5	2.1	8.4	7.1	9.7	6.4	4.2	8.5	38.7	30.2	47.9
Ft. Lauderdale	7.2	6.2	8.2	2.5	0.6	4.0	4.0	2.3	5.5	6.3	2.5	9.7	27.0	22.1	32.1
Houston	6.0	4.8	7.3	2.2	0.6	3.7	6.8	7.5	6.2	5.2	3.3	7.1	31.4	27.1	35.7
Los Angeles	3.9	4.2	3.7	1.2	0.6	1.7	9.1	9.2	9.1	8.3	6.4	10.2	39.9	33.7	46.0
Miami	7.6	6.4	8.8	1.9	1.1	2.8	5.0	4.7	5.4	5.8	3.4	8.1	24.4	19.3	29.4
New York City	9.8	9.7	9.8	0.7	0.2	1.1	7.2	6.3	8.0	6.1	4.4	7.9	24.0	18.4	29.7
Orlando	6.0	5.0	6.8	2.6	1.0	4.0	5.5	4.1	6.7	5.7	4.2	7.1	30.4	23.4	37.3
Palm Beach	6.7	6.7	6.6	3.0	0.7	5.2	5.6	3.8	7.2	5.9	2.9	8.8	28.1	21.2	35.4
Philadelphia	8.1	8.8	7.4	1.3	0.2	2.5	3.2	2.0	4.2	5.9	5.8	6.1	33.9	29.5	38.4
San Bernardino	3.5	2.7	4.4	1.9	0.6	3.1	7.2	7.2	7.1	5.3	3.9	6.6	34.3	27.7	40.5
San Diego	4.4	4.4	4.6	1.3	0.5	2.2	9.2	9.2	9.2	7.1	5.3	9.0	41.2	35.1	47.5
San Francisco	6.6	6.3	6.7	NA	NA	NA	6.8	8.0	5.7	5.1	4.3	5.8	36.5	33.8	39.0
Unweighted data															
Detroit	4.6	3.1	6.2	2.4	1.2	3.7	5.9	5.9	5.7	6.1	4.4	8.0	32.1	29.5	35.0
District of Columbia	5.7	4.9	6.6	3.3	1.9	4.5	3.7	3.2	4.2	6.0	4.8	7.3	25.4	21.2	29.5
Milwaukee	10.2	10.3	9.7	NA	NA	NA	NA	NA	NA	NA	NA	NA	30.3	24.4	37.0
New Orleans	4.5	3.0	6.4	1.5	0.9	2.0	4.9	4.1	5.5	5.7	4.8	6.4	13.9	11.1	17.2

* Survey did not include students from one of the state's large school districts.

Note: NA means data not available.

Source: Grunbaum, Jo Anne, et al., Youth Risk Behavior Surveillance—United States, 2001. Mortality and Morbidity Weekly Report. Vol. 51/SS-4, Centers for Disease Control and Prevention, June 28, 2002

2.30 Percentage of high school students who engaged in sexual behaviors, by sex, race/ethnicity, and grade—United States, 2001

	ever had sexual intercourse			first sexual intercourse before age 13			four or more sex partners during lifetime			currently sexually active (sexual intercourse in past three months)			responsible sexual behavior*		
	total	female	male	total	female	male	total	female	male	total	female	male	total	female	male
Total	45.6	42.9	48.5	6.6	4.0	9.3	14.2	11.4	17.2	33.4	33.4	33.4	86.1	83.9	88.5
	(±2.3)	(±2.8)	(±2.7)	(±0.9)	(±0.9)	(±1.3)	(±1.2)	(±1.5)	(±1.6)	(±2.0)	(±2.5)	(±2.3)	(±1.1)	(±1.6)	(±1.3)
Race/ethnicity															
Black	60.8	53.4	68.8	16.3	7.6	25.7	26.6	15.6	38.7	45.6	39.5	52.3	85.2	84.8	85.9
	(±6.6)	(±5.1)	(±8.4)	(±2.6)	(±2.2)	(±5.0)	(±3.7)	(±3.6)	(±5.7)	(±5.4)	(±5.1)	(±7.2)	(±2.6)	(±2.8)	(±3.1)
Hispanic	48.4	44.0	53.0	7.6	4.1	11.4	14.9	9.5	20.6	35.9	34.5	37.3	83.6	82.1	85.2
	(±4.5)	(±5.0)	(±4.9)	(±2.0)	(±1.3)	(±3.6)	(±1.7)	(±2.0)	(±2.8)	(±3.2)	(±4.2)	(±3.6)	(±2.8)	(±3.3)	(±3.4)
White	43.2	41.3	45.1	4.7	3.3	6.2	12.0	11.1	12.8	31.3	32.3	30.0	86.6	84.2	89.3
	(±2.5)	(±3.2)	(±2.7)	(±1.1)	(±1.3)	(±1.2)	(±1.4)	(±1.8)	(±1.5)	(±2.2)	(±2.8)	(±2.3)	(±1.1)	(±1.7)	(±1.5)
Grade															
9	34.4	29.1	40.5	9.2	5.4	13.7	9.6	5.8	13.9	22.7	19.9	25.9	92.8	93.5	92.2
	(±3.6)	(±4.0)	(±4.6)	(±1.5)	(±1.3)	(±2.8)	(±1.6)	(±1.7)	(±2.3)	(±3.1)	(±3.4)	(±4.1)	(±1.2)	(±1.7)	(±1.8)
10	40.8	39.3	42.2	7.5	4.7	10.6	12.6	10.4	15.0	29.7	30.7	28.6	88.3	85.4	91.4
	(±3.0)	(±3.1)	(±4.1)	(±1.4)	(±1.7)	(±1.6)	(±1.8)	(±2.0)	(±2.4)	(±2.9)	(±2.9)	(±4.1)	(±1.8)	(±2.7)	(±1.7)
11	51.9	49.7	54.0	4.6	2.9	6.4	15.2	12.6	17.8	38.1	38.1	37.8	84.5	82.1	87.0
	(±2.9)	(±3.9)	(±3.6)	(±1.1)	(±1.2)	(±1.4)	(±1.5)	(±2.3)	(±2.4)	(±2.6)	(±3.6)	(±2.9)	(±1.8)	(±2.9)	(±2.0)
12	60.5	60.1	61.0	3.6	2.2	5.0	21.6	19.5	23.6	47.9	51.0	44.6	75.8	70.1	81.9
	(±4.0)	(±5.4)	(±4.3)	(±0.7)	(±0.8)	(±1.1)	(±2.4)	(±3.2)	(±3.6)	(±4.0)	(±5.4)	(±4.3)	(±2.2)	(±4.0)	(±2.5)

* Responsible sexual behavior includes those who have never had sex, those who have had sex but not in the past three months, and those who used a condom the last time they had sex.

Note: Blacks and whites are non-Hispanic. Numbers in parentheses are plus or minus percentage points of the 95 percent confidence interval. Differences in percentages are considered statistically significant if the confidence intervals do not overlap.

Source: Grunbaum, Jo Anne, et al., Youth Risk Behavior Surveillance–United States, 2001. Mortality and Morbidity Weekly Report. Vol. 51/SS-4, Centers for Disease Control and Prevention. June 28, 2002

2.31   Percentage of high school students who engaged in sexual behaviors, by sex—selected U.S. sites, 2001

	ever had sexual intercourse			first sexual intercourse before age 13			four or more sex partners during lifetime			currently sexually active (sexual intercourse in past three months)			responsible sexual behavior*		
	total	female	male	total	female	male	total	female	male	total	female	male	total	female	male
State surveys															
Weighted data															
Alabama	NA	NA	NA	NA	NA	NA	NA	NA	NA	NA	NA	NA	NA	NA	NA
Arkansas	55.5	53.3	57.8	9.8	5.2	14.3	20.5	15.7	25.1	40.2	40.6	39.9	85.8	84.0	87.6
Delaware	52.7	49.4	56.1	9.6	4.5	15.0	16.7	12.8	20.9	39.2	38.4	39.9	85.3	82.6	88.0
Florida	49.9	46.2	53.5	9.1	4.7	13.2	16.3	11.1	21.3	36.4	34.5	38.1	87.5	86.1	88.9
Idaho	36.2	35.3	36.8	4.7	3.0	6.4	NA	NA	NA	NA	NA	NA	NA	NA	NA
Maine	46.3	48.7	43.6	4.4	3.6	5.0	10.1	10.0	9.8	34.6	38.6	30.5	83.7	79.3	88.2
Massachusetts	44.3	42.3	46.3	5.3	2.5	8.0	12.0	9.4	14.6	32.5	33.1	31.9	86.6	85.3	87.9
Michigan	40.3	42.2	38.0	4.9	3.3	6.3	10.5	9.7	11.1	29.9	33.4	26.0	88.6	85.5	91.7
Mississippi	60.6	58.5	62.9	14.0	6.4	22.1	25.5	17.6	34.2	44.9	44.8	45.0	84.6	81.9	87.5
Missouri	50.9	49.6	52.2	6.5	3.0	10.0	17.0	14.7	19.3	38.8	38.9	38.7	85.2	83.1	87.2
Montana	43.9	43.7	43.9	5.3	3.5	7.0	13.8	13.2	14.4	30.7	32.0	29.3	87.3	83.8	90.8
Nevada	49.1	48.3	50.0	8.3	5.1	11.6	16.6	14.2	18.9	34.6	36.7	32.6	86.2	82.4	90.1
New Jersey	47.4	42.2	52.6	7.6	3.2	12.0	16.8	10.7	23.2	36.1	34.4	37.7	87.0	85.3	88.9
North Carolina	NA	NA	NA	NA	NA	NA	NA	NA	NA	NA	NA	NA	NA	NA	NA
North Dakota	42.0	40.9	43.0	4.4	2.2	6.3	12.1	12.2	11.6	30.8	31.0	30.4	87.6	86.4	89.0
Rhode Island	45.9	42.5	49.1	6.5	3.3	9.5	14.3	9.3	19.1	36.1	34.5	37.5	84.3	83.2	85.5
South Dakota	40.0	38.3	41.7	3.5	1.9	5.1	11.5	10.4	12.7	29.4	29.7	28.9	87.9	86.3	89.7
Texas	50.4	47.7	52.9	7.5	4.2	10.7	16.4	12.8	19.8	36.2	36.1	36.1	84.0	81.1	87.1
Utah	NA	NA	NA	NA	NA	NA	NA	NA	NA	NA	NA	NA	NA	NA	NA
Vermont	NA	NA	NA	5.0	3.6	6.3	10.3	9.4	11.1	29.1	30.4	27.7	88.4	86.1	90.6
Wisconsin	39.3	43.9	34.7	4.0	3.0	4.9	10.2	11.5	8.9	29.1	33.5	24.8	88.2	84.7	91.6
Wyoming	46.5	45.9	46.9	5.2	3.6	6.7	13.8	13.4	14.1	32.9	34.0	31.7	87.5	84.7	90.3

(continued)

(continued from previous page)

Unweighted data	ever had sexual intercourse			first sexual intercourse before age 13			four or more sex partners during lifetime			currently sexually active (sexual intercourse in past three months)			responsible sexual behavior		
	total	female	male	total	female	male	total	female	male	total	female	male	total	female	male
Colorado	42.3	39.9	44.3	6.0	3.9	7.8	12.7	10.0	15.3	29.1	29.9	28.2	90.4	87.8	93.0
Hawaii	33.6	35.5	30.8	4.8	3.5	6.0	8.4	8.7	7.7	23.2	24.5	21.4	87.7	85.2	90.8
Illinois*	32.7	30.8	35.5	3.6	1.7	6.4	8.4	5.1	13.2	23.0	22.8	23.2	92.8	92.7	92.9
Indiana	43.8	44.2	43.3	NA	NA	NA	NA	NA	NA	NA	NA	NA	NA	NA	NA
Iowa	42.9	41.5	43.9	4.1	3.2	5.1	12.3	11.1	13.6	33.7	33.7	33.3	86.4	84.0	88.8
Kentucky	47.1	45.5	48.8	7.0	3.2	11.5	13.8	11.0	17.1	35.4	34.3	36.5	84.6	83.2	86.2
Louisiana*	NA	NA	NA	NA	NA	NA	NA	NA	NA	NA	NA	NA	NA	NA	NA
Nebraska	42.5	43.6	41.1	3.1	2.3	3.9	11.2	11.7	10.6	30.1	33.1	26.9	87.8	84.7	91.0
New Hampshire	38.8	38.1	39.3	4.7	2.5	6.7	9.8	8.6	10.8	28.4	30.4	26.1	88.0	87.2	89.1
New York*	40.8	40.1	41.3	5.9	4.6	7.1	10.9	9.2	12.5	31.3	32.6	29.8	88.2	85.9	90.5
South Carolina	55.0	50.3	60.0	13.6	6.7	20.8	21.7	15.9	27.8	39.7	37.7	41.7	86.3	84.8	87.9
Tennessee	51.3	48.7	53.8	9.0	5.9	12.2	16.3	12.4	20.2	36.2	36.9	35.5	84.6	82.1	87.1

(continued)

(continued from previous page)

	ever had sexual intercourse			first sexual intercourse before age 13			four or more sex partners during lifetime			currently sexually active (sexual intercourse in past three months)			responsible sexual behavior**		
	total	female	male	total	female	male	total	female	male	total	female	male	total	female	male
Local surveys															
Weighted data															
Boston	51.6	46.0	57.8	13.1	3.7	23.3	21.0	11.8	30.9	36.5	33.9	39.4	90.0	89.7	90.2
Chicago	58.1	48.3	68.2	17.2	6.2	28.6	22.5	9.2	36.4	40.9	37.9	43.8	87.9	86.8	89.4
Dallas	56.8	51.4	62.8	12.2	5.9	19.3	20.6	13.3	28.8	38.8	37.7	40.0	83.4	81.3	85.8
Ft. Lauderdale	47.3	41.2	53.8	8.8	3.0	14.9	15.1	8.7	21.9	33.5	30.8	36.2	91.1	90.7	91.8
Houston	49.5	42.9	56.3	9.8	4.6	15.3	16.2	9.1	24.0	35.9	32.9	39.1	87.6	85.7	89.7
Los Angeles	40.0	34.2	45.7	6.3	3.2	9.4	9.2	5.5	13.1	24.9	22.7	26.8	88.6	87.6	89.8
Miami	50.8	43.6	57.8	9.1	3.3	15.0	17.1	9.0	25.4	35.3	32.8	37.6	89.1	87.1	91.4
New York City	50.9	45.6	56.6	12.3	5.5	19.5	18.9	10.1	28.4	36.6	34.5	38.9	89.5	87.5	91.6
Orlando	NA	NA	NA	NA	NA	NA	NA	NA	NA	NA	NA	NA	NA	NA	NA
Palm Beach	47.3	40.5	54.6	9.5	3.9	15.2	14.6	10.1	19.2	32.1	29.6	34.7	89.3	89.0	89.7
Philadelphia	61.6	60.1	63.3	17.1	8.9	25.9	25.9	18.0	34.8	42.1	41.8	42.8	85.3	83.6	86.9
San Bernardino	39.0	35.2	43.0	6.7	2.0	11.5	11.3	6.7	16.0	25.2	23.5	27.0	91.2	89.6	92.9
San Diego	38.2	34.4	42.3	5.6	2.7	8.6	11.2	9.0	13.5	26.6	27.0	26.3	90.4	90.0	90.8
San Francisco	29.8	28.6	30.9	5.2	2.8	7.4	7.8	5.0	10.5	19.8	20.6	19.1	92.8	91.2	94.5
Unweighted data															
Detroit	61.4	55.2	69.3	15.5	7.3	25.9	25.4	16.4	37.1	45.1	42.3	48.7	84.1	82.7	85.9
District of Columbia	61.6	53.5	71.7	16.6	6.8	28.7	23.8	18.8	29.9	41.1	39.3	43.4	89.1	86.4	92.5
Milwaukee	57.0	53.3	61.1	10.9	5.1	17.6	20.6	14.0	28.0	42.3	40.6	44.2	84.8	81.2	89.0
New Orleans	45.7	34.5	61.9	13.7	4.0	27.6	19.7	8.1	36.5	32.5	25.1	43.1	92.3	91.4	93.6

* Survey did not include students from one of the state's large school districts.
** Responsible sexual behavior includes those who have never had sex, those who have had sex but not in the past three months, and those who used a condom the last time they had sex.
Note: NA means data not available.
Source: Grunbaum, Jo Anne, et al., Youth Risk Behavior Surveillance–United States, 2001, Mortality and Morbidity Weekly Report. Vol. 51/SS-4. Centers for Disease Control and Prevention, June 28, 2002

2.32 Percentage of high school students who used a condom during or birth control pill before last sexual intercourse; used alcohol or drugs at last sexual intercourse; were ever pregnant or got someone pregnant; or were taught about AIDS/HIV in school, by sex, race/ethnicity, and grade—United States, 2001

	condom use during last sexual intercourse (among sexually active students)			birth control use before last sexual intercourse (among sexually active students)			alcohol or drug use at last sexual intercourse (among sexually active students)			have been pregnant or gotten someone pregnant			taught about AIDS/HIV in school		
	total	female	male	total	female	male	total	female	male	total	female	male	total	female	male
Total	57.9	51.3	65.1	18.2	21.1	14.9	25.6	20.7	30.9	4.7	5.4	4.0	89.0	89.0	89.1
	(±2.2)	(±3.4)	(±2.7)	(±1.7)	(±2.7)	(±1.9)	(±1.7)	(±2.7)	(±2.9)	(±0.5)	(±0.7)	(±0.8)	(±1.3)	(±1.8)	(±1.1)
Race/ethnicity															
Black	67.1	60.7	72.7	7.9	7.8	7.8	17.8	10.4	24.2	11.4	11.9	10.8	86.1	88.0	84.0
	(±3.5)	(±5.0)	(±4.6)	(±2.6)	(±3.7)	(±3.4)	(±2.6)	(±4.1)	(±6.1)	(±2.2)	(±2.8)	(±3.1)	(±2.4)	(±2.6)	(±2.9)
Hispanic	53.5	47.6	59.1	9.6	10.4	8.7	24.1	21.9	26.2	5.7	6.2	5.0	80.5	81.4	79.5
	(±5.1)	(±5.7)	(±6.5)	(±3.3)	(±4.4)	(±3.5)	(±2.8)	(±4.4)	(±4.1)	(±1.0)	(±1.5)	(±1.7)	(±4.1)	(±5.4)	(±3.4)
White	56.8	51.0	63.8	23.4	26.7	19.3	27.8	22.9	33.6	3.3	4.0	2.5	91.1	90.4	91.9
	(±3.0)	(±4.3)	(±4.0)	(±2.3)	(±3.2)	(±3.2)	(±2.2)	(±3.1)	(±3.3)	(±0.5)	(±0.9)	(±0.6)	(±1.4)	(±2.1)	(±1.2)
Grade															
9	67.5	66.6	68.9	7.6	9.2	5.6	24.0	24.5	23.8	3.2	2.6	3.9	86.7	86.3	87.3
	(±3.3)	(±5.1)	(±4.4)	(±2.8)	(±5.3)	(±2.9)	(±4.4)	(±6.1)	(±6.4)	(±1.0)	(±0.8)	(±1.7)	(±1.7)	(±2.5)	(±1.7)
10	60.1	52.2	69.3	15.8	18.2	12.8	27.7	20.8	35.7	4.4	5.0	3.8	89.8	90.2	89.4
	(±4.5)	(±6.7)	(±5.0)	(±2.6)	(±4.5)	(±3.3)	(±3.1)	(±4.1)	(±7.2)	(±0.7)	(±1.3)	(±0.8)	(±1.9)	(±2.5)	(±2.1)
11	58.9	52.7	65.3	18.6	22.4	14.8	24.7	18.4	31.3	4.8	5.9	3.6	90.5	90.5	90.5
	(±4.0)	(±6.0)	(±5.1)	(±3.0)	(±4.5)	(±2.8)	(±2.9)	(±3.7)	(±4.0)	(±0.8)	(±1.3)	(±1.1)	(±1.7)	(±2.2)	(±2.0)
12	49.3	41.2	59.2	26.3	28.9	23.1	25.4	19.9	32.0	7.1	9.4	4.8	90.2	90.0	90.4
	(±3.1)	(±5.3)	(±4.9)	(±3.5)	(±4.6)	(±5.3)	(±2.6)	(±4.1)	(±3.6)	(±1.3)	(±2.2)	(±1.3)	(±1.5)	(±2.8)	(±1.6)

Note: Blacks and whites are non-Hispanic. Numbers in parentheses are plus or minus percentage points of the 95 percent confidence interval. Differences in percentages are considered statistically significant if the confidence intervals do not overlap.
Source: Grunbaum, Jo Anne, et al., Youth Risk Behavior Surveillance–United States, 2001, Mortality and Morbidity Weekly Report. Vol. 51/SS-4, Centers for Disease Control and Prevention. June 28, 2002

2.33 Percentage of high school students who used a condom during or birth control pills before last sexual intercourse; used alcohol or drugs at last sexual intercourse; were ever pregnant or got someone pregnant; or were taught about AIDS/HIV in school, by sex—selected U.S. sites, 2001

	condom use during last sexual intercourse (among sexually active students)			birth control use before last sexual intercourse (among sexually active students)			alcohol or drug use at last sexual intercourse (among sexually active students)			have been pregnant or gotten someone pregnant			taught about AIDS/HIV in school		
	total	female	male	total	female	male	total	female	male	total	female	male	total	female	male
State surveys															
Weighted data															
Alabama	NA	NA	NA	NA	NA	NA	NA	NA	NA	NA	NA	NA	87.8	90.0	85.7
Arkansas	64.5	60.6	68.6	15.4	21.0	9.6	24.3	17.7	30.8	5.7	6.7	4.7	86.2	87.3	85.3
Delaware	62.2	54.6	69.8	20.1	24.4	15.7	22.1	16.4	27.7	6.4	7.0	5.8	91.2	92.7	89.7
Florida	65.1	59.3	70.3	13.4	17.1	9.5	24.0	18.1	29.6	5.7	6.2	5.2	88.7	90.8	87.0
Idaho	NA	NA	NA	NA	NA	NA	NA	NA	NA	NA	NA	NA	85.3	84.7	86.3
Maine	52.2	45.8	60.4	36.1	40.5	30.4	24.6	20.5	29.6	NA	NA	NA	93.5	95.3	91.8
Massachusetts	58.1	54.9	61.6	23.1	28.1	18.0	22.7	16.9	28.8	4.9	6.0	3.8	93.8	95.1	92.6
Michigan	61.0	56.2	67.3	21.7	25.6	16.8	23.7	19.9	28.3	2.9	3.2	2.7	88.6	88.9	88.7
Mississippi	65.3	59.1	71.7	12.8	17.2	8.1	21.9	15.2	28.8	5.9	6.6	5.2	85.3	85.9	84.8
Missouri	61.5	56.4	66.5	21.2	27.9	14.2	25.5	20.0	30.7	5.1	6.8	3.4	85.5	86.7	84.3
Montana	57.5	48.7	67.3	23.1	27.0	18.8	32.0	28.2	36.7	4.2	5.0	3.2	90.2	91.4	89.5
Nevada	59.1	51.2	68.5	17.3	21.0	12.9	24.4	19.9	29.7	5.8	6.1	5.5	86.5	85.4	87.6
New Jersey	63.7	57.0	70.0	12.9	16.1	9.2	26.6	15.7	36.9	6.3	5.7	7.0	90.7	92.9	88.5
North Carolina	NA	NA	NA	NA	NA	NA	NA	NA	NA	NA	NA	NA	91.1	92.0	90.2
North Dakota	59.1	55.8	63.2	25.7	31.9	19.7	33.5	28.6	38.9	3.1	3.2	2.7	89.4	92.4	86.4
Rhode Island	56.1	50.8	61.1	17.4	19.9	15.3	27.3	16.7	36.6	6.2	5.2	7.0	90.4	91.2	89.7
South Dakota	58.3	53.8	63.3	18.7	22.5	14.5	28.5	26.8	30.4	3.8	3.6	3.9	87.0	88.7	85.2
Texas	55.4	47.1	63.7	10.8	14.2	7.4	26.6	21.3	31.5	7.4	9.7	5.2	82.9	82.9	82.8
Utah	NA	NA	NA	NA	NA	NA	NA	NA	NA	NA	NA	NA	88.6	90.2	87.2
Vermont	59.5	54.0	65.3	30.7	37.1	23.5	28.0	21.9	34.4	2.9	3.1	2.6	NA	NA	NA
Wisconsin	59.2	53.9	65.9	25.6	29.5	20.5	25.7	21.7	30.8	3.9	5.6	2.2	92.0	92.1	92.0
Wyoming	61.8	54.8	69.2	25.7	31.8	19.0	30.2	22.1	38.3	4.1	5.1	3.1	89.9	90.7	89.4

(continued)

(continued from previous page)

Unweighted data

	condom use during last sexual intercourse (among sexually active students)			birth control use before last sexual intercourse (among sexually active students)			alcohol or drug use at last sexual intercourse (among sexually active students)			have been pregnant or gotten someone pregnant			taught about AIDS/HIV in school		
	total	female	male	total	female	male	total	female	male	total	female	male	total	female	male
Colorado	66.7	58.5	74.8	16.9	21.2	12.8	31.7	26.8	36.9	4.0	5.1	3.1	82.3	82.5	82.2
Hawaii	45.5	39.0	NA	17.2	16.8	NA	21.6	20.3	NA	3.5	4.0	2.6	87.0	88.3	85.4
Illinois*	68.3	67.7	NA	17.5	18.8	NA	27.8	26.1	NA	2.4	2.0	2.9	91.2	93.4	88.0
Indiana	NA	NA	NA	NA	NA	NA	NA	NA	NA	NA	NA	NA	90.0	89.5	90.8
Iowa	59.3	52.4	65.9	25.4	29.7	20.4	25.2	20.8	29.0	2.2	3.2	1.3	89.6	90.8	88.7
Kentucky	55.8	50.3	61.7	21.6	20.7	22.3	20.2	18.7	21.5	5.2	6.1	4.3	85.3	86.6	83.7
Louisiana*	NA	NA	NA	NA	NA	NA	NA	NA	NA	NA	NA	NA	79.8	81.1	78.3
Nebraska	59.2	53.5	66.2	23.4	24.8	21.4	30.0	26.6	34.2	2.6	3.3	1.8	84.6	85.0	84.2
New Hampshire	56.8	57.0	57.3	28.3	33.3	22.0	21.1	17.9	24.7	3.1	3.3	2.8	89.4	89.5	90.0
New York*	61.9	56.3	67.9	19.0	20.7	17.3	23.6	22.4	24.7	3.8	3.9	3.7	91.0	92.8	89.1
South Carolina	64.9	59.3	70.5	12.9	17.2	8.7	24.4	18.5	30.1	5.6	6.1	5.1	88.2	90.6	85.8
Tennessee	57.1	51.2	63.3	17.2	19.0	14.9	21.8	16.9	27.0	6.0	7.5	4.3	87.8	89.2	86.6

(continued)

(continued from previous page)

	condom use during last sexual intercourse (among sexually active students)			birth control use before last sexual intercourse (among sexually active students)			alcohol or drug use at last sexual intercourse (among sexually active students)			have been pregnant or gotten someone pregnant			taught about AIDS/HIV in school		
	total	female	male	total	female	male	total	female	male	total	female	male	total	female	male
Local surveys															
Weighted data															
Boston	72.0	69.3	74.5	12.8	13.3	12.1	17.4	14.8	19.5	7.8	8.9	6.8	84.3	84.7	84.2
Chicago	70.0	64.4	75.4	12.4	14.6	10.4	23.7	16.0	30.0	9.6	9.1	9.8	86.9	87.2	86.7
Dallas	56.6	49.8	63.7	6.8	6.9	6.6	20.9	16.9	25.1	8.0	9.2	6.7	83.0	85.3	80.5
Ft. Lauderdale	73.1	69.2	76.9	13.4	16.1	10.3	22.6	15.5	29.5	4.0	3.6	4.4	87.5	90.1	85.2
Houston	65.1	56.1	73.3	7.7	9.1	6.5	23.7	19.2	28.0	6.3	6.1	6.4	81.2	82.0	80.3
Los Angeles	53.3	44.0	61.2	6.7	7.3	6.2	18.6	12.2	23.4	4.0	5.0	2.9	82.4	83.5	81.6
Miami	68.8	60.0	76.8	6.9	7.6	5.5	18.3	13.3	23.0	7.0	8.0	6.1	83.1	84.4	81.9
New York City	71.0	63.1	78.3	7.0	9.8	4.4	16.9	10.2	23.4	5.0	5.9	3.8	87.6	87.9	87.2
Orlando	NA	NA	NA	NA	NA	NA	NA	NA	NA	NA	NA	NA	89.5	90.3	88.9
Palm Beach	66.1	61.9	69.8	14.6	16.9	12.5	24.3	17.9	29.6	4.2	4.4	3.9	86.7	85.2	88.4
Philadelphia	64.3	60.0	68.8	11.3	16.4	5.8	13.5	14.8	12.2	10.1	11.6	8.6	89.2	91.6	86.8
San Bernardino	63.8	55.3	NA	12.1	11.8	NA	26.4	21.4	NA	3.4	4.4	2.4	85.1	87.9	82.5
San Diego	62.7	61.6	63.7	16.7	19.1	14.2	24.1	18.4	30.0	4.7	4.4	5.1	89.4	90.7	88.0
San Francisco	62.9	56.2	70.0	9.2	10.6	7.7	15.2	14.0	16.5	2.3	3.0	1.5	90.0	90.4	89.6
Unweighted data															
Detroit	63.6	58.4	69.8	9.4	10.5	8.3	14.7	10.4	18.8	10.3	12.9	7.1	81.0	83.4	78.6
District of Columbia	72.9	64.8	82.2	8.4	11.0	5.1	15.9	12.2	19.7	9.7	12.7	6.3	91.0	93.0	88.8
Milwaukee	63.5	52.9	74.7	10.9	13.4	8.4	16.6	12.6	20.7	9.1	11.3	6.5	86.8	86.9	86.8
New Orleans	76.1	65.5	85.1	6.4	7.6	4.5	15.7	9.1	19.8	6.0	5.4	6.5	82.9	87.4	77.7

* Survey did not include students from one of the state's large school districts.

Note: NA means data not available.

Source: Grunbaum, Jo Anne, et al., Youth Risk Behavior Surveillance–United States, 2001, Mortality and Morbidity Weekly Report. Vol. 51/SS-4, Centers for Disease Control and Prevention. June 28, 2002

2.34 Percentage of high school students who were at risk for becoming overweight, were overweight, thought of themselves as overweight, or were trying to lose weight, by sex, race/ethnicity, and grade——United States, 2001

	at risk for becoming overweight			overweight			thought they were overweight			were trying to lose weight		
	total	female	male	total	female	male	total	female	male	total	female	male
Total	**13.6**	**11.7**	**15.5**	**10.5**	**6.9**	**14.2**	**29.2**	**34.9**	**23.3**	**46.0**	**62.3**	**28.8**
	(±0.8)	(±1.1)	(±1.3)	(±1.0)	(±0.9)	(±1.3)	(±1.2)	(±1.4)	(±1.5)	(±1.6)	(±1.7)	(±2.0)
Race/ethnicity												
Black	17.8	16.7	19.0	16.0	14.6	17.5	25.7	32.3	18.7	36.9	49.4	23.6
	(±2.7)	(±2.7)	(±3.6)	(±2.4)	(±3.3)	(±2.3)	(±1.9)	(±3.0)	(±2.3)	(±2.2)	(±3.0)	(±2.4)
Hispanic	16.3	16.3	16.3	15.1	8.8	21.3	34.8	40.3	29.1	51.5	63.4	39.1
	(±1.9)	(±2.6)	(±2.2)	(±2.8)	(±2.3)	(±3.9)	(±2.9)	(±3.8)	(±3.6)	(±3.0)	(±3.5)	(±3.5)
White	12.5	10.2	14.9	8.8	5.3	12.4	29.2	34.7	23.4	47.1	65.4	27.9
	(±1.1)	(±1.2)	(±1.7)	(±1.0)	(±0.9)	(±1.4)	(±1.3)	(±1.8)	(±1.8)	(±1.8)	(±1.9)	(±2.3)
Grade												
9	15.7	12.3	19.5	10.5	7.7	13.6	28.8	33.4	23.7	47.8	62.1	31.8
	(±1.7)	(±2.2)	(±2.8)	(±1.8)	(±1.7)	(±2.3)	(±2.1)	(±2.4)	(±2.9)	(±2.3)	(±2.8)	(±3.2)
10	13.6	11.3	15.9	10.8	6.6	15.2	29.8	35.6	23.9	45.7	62.1	28.6
	(±1.6)	(±1.7)	(±2.3)	(±1.6)	(±1.9)	(±2.4)	(±1.7)	(±2.3)	(±3.0)	(±1.8)	(±2.0)	(±3.3)
11	12.6	12.2	12.9	10.6	6.7	14.7	29.0	35.2	22.7	44.7	62.1	26.9
	(±1.4)	(±1.8)	(±2.4)	(±1.5)	(±1.3)	(±2.4)	(±2.6)	(±3.2)	(±2.6)	(±2.4)	(±2.7)	(±2.3)
12	11.8	11.0	12.7	9.6	6.3	13.2	29.1	35.9	22.2	45.3	63.1	26.8
	(±1.3)	(±1.6)	(±2.7)	(±1.8)	(±1.8)	(±2.7)	(±2.3)	(±3.8)	(±2.8)	(±4.6)	(±4.6)	(±4.2)

Note: Students at risk of becoming overweight were between the 85th and 95th percentile for body mass index, by age and sex, based on reference data. Students who were overweight were at or above the 95th percentile for body mass index, by age and sex, based on reference data. Blacks and whites are non-Hispanic. Numbers in parentheses are plus or minus percentage points of the 95 percent confidence interval. Differences in percentages are considered statistically significant if the confidence intervals do not overlap.

Source: Grunbaum, Jo Anne, et al., Youth Risk Behavior Surveillance–United States, 2001. Mortality and Morbidity Weekly Report. Vol. 51/SS-4. Centers for Disease Control and Prevention. June 28, 2002

2.35   Percentage of high school students who were at risk for becoming overweight, were overweight, thought of themselves as overweight, or were trying to lose weight, by sex—selected U.S. sites, 2001

State surveys Weighted data	at risk for becoming overweight			overweight			thought they were overweight			were trying to lose weight		
	total	female	male	total	female	male	total	female	male	total	female	male
Alabama	15.2	15.0	15.3	12.3	7.6	16.9	30.1	38.2	22.2	42.0	56.8	27.6
Arkansas	15.9	15.4	16.4	13.8	8.7	18.7	33.5	39.2	28.1	46.7	62.1	32.0
Delaware	15.0	14.7	15.3	10.8	8.9	12.9	30.2	35.7	24.2	43.8	58.6	28.1
Florida	14.3	13.2	15.2	10.4	6.8	13.6	28.7	33.6	24.1	42.2	57.1	28.0
Idaho	10.7	8.5	12.7	7.2	4.5	9.7	32.0	42.6	22.0	41.9	62.9	22.4
Maine	14.5	12.5	16.3	10.4	5.5	14.8	32.8	40.0	25.9	43.8	60.2	28.1
Massachusetts	15.0	13.2	16.6	10.0	6.3	13.5	33.4	40.0	26.9	46.9	62.8	31.3
Michigan	13.3	11.9	14.6	10.7	7.2	14.0	30.7	36.6	25.1	45.8	61.6	30.2
Mississippi	15.4	14.4	16.4	14.0	9.9	18.4	26.4	32.1	20.6	40.7	57.0	23.9
Missouri	15.0	12.8	17.0	12.8	8.5	17.0	31.9	37.7	26.4	47.8	63.4	32.7
Montana	11.4	10.5	12.1	6.1	3.7	8.3	30.1	41.0	20.0	42.0	61.4	23.5
Nevada	NA	NA	NA	NA	NA	NA	29.5	34.2	24.9	47.5	61.6	33.8
New Jersey	14.6	13.7	15.6	10.1	6.1	14.0	28.8	34.9	22.6	46.4	65.3	27.6
North Carolina	14.3	13.1	15.5	12.9	9.0	16.6	29.2	34.4	24.1	42.8	58.7	27.2
North Dakota	12.2	10.1	14.1	9.2	4.2	13.8	31.9	42.0	22.4	47.5	68.7	27.2
Rhode Island	14.2	13.2	15.2	9.2	3.5	14.8	30.8	36.5	25.1	42.0	58.5	25.7
South Dakota	12.7	11.9	13.5	7.6	4.7	10.7	30.9	40.0	22.2	46.3	66.8	26.4
Texas	14.8	14.4	15.1	14.2	8.7	19.4	31.2	37.3	25.4	47.5	62.8	32.9
Utah	8.4	9.0	7.9	6.2	2.6	9.6	28.7	39.6	18.4	44.1	65.0	24.3
Vermont	12.2	11.2	13.1	9.7	5.1	14.0	30.0	36.5	23.9	41.1	58.2	24.8
Wisconsin	14.3	13.9	14.6	9.6	5.6	13.3	32.4	40.2	24.9	43.3	60.6	26.6
Wyoming	10.8	9.4	12.1	6.6	3.7	9.3	27.5	35.6	19.8	41.7	63.4	21.5

(continued)

(continued from previous page)

Unweighted data	at risk for becoming overweight			overweight			thought they were overweight			were trying to lose weight		
	total	female	male	total	female	male	total	female	male	total	female	male
Colorado	8.6	7.6	9.5	7.1	2.5	11.1	26.9	34.4	20.2	40.6	59.7	23.4
Hawaii	11.9	10.2	13.9	12.1	8.3	16.6	33.4	36.4	29.5	47.9	56.6	36.9
Illinois*	12.9	12.0	14.3	9.5	5.4	15.3	32.5	36.7	26.5	47.4	63.1	25.1
Indiana	13.1	10.5	16.0	11.4	8.0	15.2	33.6	38.2	28.3	47.9	61.8	31.5
Iowa	14.0	13.2	14.8	9.8	6.7	12.8	31.9	40.5	23.6	47.9	66.1	30.9
Kentucky	15.2	12.9	17.6	12.3	8.9	16.0	33.0	36.8	28.6	51.5	64.0	37.5
Louisiana*	11.4	12.4	10.2	13.0	9.8	17.0	28.0	31.8	22.8	45.9	61.7	25.1
Nebraska	11.3	10.2	12.4	9.0	5.6	12.2	30.3	37.3	23.5	44.9	65.2	24.7
New Hampshire	14.1	11.2	17.1	8.6	5.3	12.0	31.4	38.8	23.5	43.9	62.0	24.6
New York*	13.8	13.1	14.6	10.6	4.5	16.1	32.6	38.1	27.2	48.4	64.3	32.2
South Carolina	14.3	14.1	14.4	12.9	9.4	16.3	26.4	33.2	19.6	41.7	56.5	26.9
Tennessee	14.0	11.6	16.4	13.2	10.1	16.3	30.1	37.0	23.4	43.9	61.0	27.4

(continued)

(continued from previous page)

	at risk for becoming overweight			overweight			thought they were overweight			were trying to lose weight		
	total	female	male	total	female	male	total	female	male	total	female	male
Local surveys												
Weighted data												
Boston	17.0	18.0	16.0	12.4	9.9	14.8	28.4	34.1	22.5	41.0	51.8	29.9
Chicago	18.7	22.6	14.6	12.7	10.1	15.5	28.6	34.3	22.8	43.6	52.8	34.2
Dallas	17.6	20.1	15.0	16.1	12.6	19.8	32.9	38.9	26.5	47.2	58.3	35.5
Ft. Lauderdale	12.3	12.0	12.5	8.9	5.5	12.2	26.2	31.3	21.3	41.1	54.1	28.0
Houston	16.5	16.1	17.0	12.6	9.9	15.4	28.8	33.2	24.3	45.7	57.1	33.9
Los Angeles	16.5	17.8	15.4	12.4	9.5	15.0	31.4	41.9	21.3	49.7	64.9	34.9
Miami	15.7	17.3	14.2	9.6	6.2	12.7	26.7	31.1	22.8	42.7	54.2	31.8
New York City	15.4	16.0	14.8	11.5	8.8	14.3	27.8	34.5	20.7	39.7	52.3	26.2
Orlando	14.0	14.0	14.0	11.3	6.8	15.8	28.8	32.8	24.7	41.3	52.9	29.4
Palm Beach	12.9	13.4	12.3	8.8	5.8	11.6	26.5	30.9	22.1	41.2	55.9	26.1
Philadelphia	17.1	20.6	13.7	15.2	11.8	18.6	27.6	31.9	22.9	41.8	52.4	31.1
San Bernardino	14.8	16.1	13.6	14.3	7.6	20.6	30.8	33.6	28.2	50.1	59.4	41.3
San Diego	14.2	13.1	15.3	7.8	4.5	10.8	29.3	35.0	23.7	45.6	59.4	31.9
San Francisco	11.5	12.1	11.0	10.6	5.9	14.8	32.1	39.2	25.2	44.1	57.5	30.9
Unweighted data												
Detroit	18.5	21.5	15.2	18.0	16.3	19.9	29.1	34.3	22.9	40.4	48.6	30.8
District of Columbia	15.0	16.6	13.3	14.6	13.1	16.1	22.7	30.8	14.2	34.7	42.9	25.1
Milwaukee	18.1	20.7	15.2	13.1	11.8	14.6	27.0	34.4	18.9	40.6	51.1	28.9
New Orleans	16.6	17.9	14.8	13.4	12.7	14.3	18.7	23.7	12.2	35.1	45.2	21.8

* Survey did not include students from one of the state's large school districts.

Note: Students at risk of becoming overweight were between the 85th and 95th percentile for body mass index, by age and sex, based on reference data. Students who were overweight were at or above the 95th percentile for body mass index, by age and sex, based on reference data. NA means data not available.

Source: Grunbaum, Jo Anne, et al., Youth Risk Behavior Surveillance–United States, 2001. Mortality and Morbidity Weekly Report, Vol. 51/SS-4. Centers for Disease Control and Prevention. June 28, 2002

2.36 Percentage of high school students who had eaten five or more servings per day of fruits and vegetables or who had drunk three or more glasses of milk per day, by sex, race/ethnicity, and grade—United States, 2001

	ate five or more servings of fruits and vegetables per day for past seven days			drank three or more glasses of milk per day for past seven days		
	total	female	male	total	female	male
Total	**21.4**	**19.7**	**23.3**	**16.4**	**10.9**	**22.3**
	(±1.3)	(±1.6)	(±1.9)	(±1.3)	(±1.2)	(±1.6)
Race/ethnicity						
Black	24.5	20.8	28.5	12.0	8.1	16.1
	(±1.8)	(±1.6)	(±2.9)	(±2.1)	(±2.2)	(±3.1)
Hispanic	23.2	22.3	23.9	13.8	9.2	18.7
	(±2.3)	(±3.6)	(±2.5)	(±1.6)	(±1.5)	(±2.4)
White	20.2	18.9	21.6	18.1	12.1	24.4
	(±1.5)	(±2.2)	(±2.2)	(±1.6)	(±1.6)	(±1.9)
Grade						
9	23.6	21.5	25.8	18.5	12.9	24.9
	(±1.9)	(±2.3)	(±2.7)	(±2.5)	(±2.4)	(±3.3)
10	21.0	18.9	23.3	16.6	10.8	22.5
	(±2.0)	(±2.3)	(±2.4)	(±1.6)	(±1.9)	(±2.6)
11	20.3	18.0	22.8	15.3	9.3	21.4
	(±1.9)	(±2.7)	(±3.2)	(±1.9)	(±1.7)	(±3.0)
12	20.2	19.9	20.6	14.4	9.7	19.3
	(±2.2)	(±2.4)	(±3.0)	(±1.8)	(±1.8)	(±2.5)

Note: A serving of fruit or vegetable includes drinking 100 percent fruit juice, eating fruit, green salad, potatoes (excluding french fries, fried ptatoes, or potato crisps), carrots, or other vegetables. Blacks and whites are non-Hispanic. Numbers in parentheses are plus or minus percentage points of the 95 percent confidence interval. Differences in percentages are considered statistically significant if the confidence intervals do not overlap.
Source: Grunbaum, Jo Anne, et al., Youth Risk Behavior Surveillance–United States, 2001, Mortality and Morbidity Weekly Report, *Vol. 51/SS-4, Centers for Disease Control and Prevention, June 28, 2002*

2.37 Percentage of high school students who had eaten five or more servings per day of fruits and vegetables or who had drunk three or more glasses of milk per day, by sex—selected U.S. sites, 2001

	ate five or more servings of fruits and vegetables per day for past seven days			drank three or more glasses of milk per day for past seven days		
	total	female	male	total	female	male
State surveys						
Weighted data						
Alabama	13.1	12.2	14.0	10.5	6.6	14.1
Arkansas	19.9	17.9	21.8	14.6	8.5	20.4
Delaware	24.9	23.1	27.0	16.1	11.2	21.3
Florida	20.3	17.8	22.6	14.3	9.6	18.9
Idaho	18.1	18.8	17.5	26.2	18.3	33.7
Maine	25.0	24.7	25.4	22.7	16.4	28.8
Massachusetts	NA	NA	NA	18.0	12.7	23.2
Michigan	20.6	19.3	22.0	20.4	14.4	26.5
Mississippi	20.8	17.8	23.8	12.8	6.4	19.5
Missouri	18.7	16.0	21.3	20.2	12.9	27.4
Montana	19.4	18.5	19.9	25.5	18.8	31.8
Nevada	NA	NA	NA	16.5	10.3	22.5
New Jersey	25.9	22.9	29.0	12.4	7.1	17.6
North Carolina	17.8	16.3	19.2	12.5	7.3	17.7
North Dakota	18.1	16.1	20.0	28.9	21.0	36.6
Rhode Island	27.4	22.9	31.9	23.1	15.2	30.9
South Dakota	15.9	13.1	18.7	24.7	16.8	32.5
Texas	19.9	17.3	22.4	14.3	8.1	20.4
Utah	22.9	20.4	25.1	25.9	20.2	31.3
Vermont	26.4	24.7	27.7	26.0	18.1	33.4
Wisconsin	NA	NA	NA	NA	NA	NA
Wyoming	21.0	17.3	24.6	25.0	18.0	31.8
Unweighted data						
Colorado	22.0	21.0	23.0	18.7	13.9	23.3
Hawaii	16.4	15.5	17.7	12.0	7.5	17.9
Illinois*	24.8	24.1	25.9	23.0	15.4	33.8
Indiana	16.2	13.1	19.8	17.4	11.9	24.0
Iowa	18.9	14.7	22.4	29.7	21.0	38.2
Kentucky	19.2	13.8	25.2	18.3	11.0	26.7
Louisiana*	16.9	14.0	21.0	11.7	7.7	17.1
Nebraska	18.2	15.8	20.6	23.2	15.7	30.7
New Hampshire	NA	NA	NA	24.0	18.7	30.1
New York*	20.7	19.4	21.9	18.4	14.6	22.4
South Carolina	17.3	15.8	18.8	10.6	6.2	14.9
Tennessee	20.2	16.7	23.7	14.8	8.8	20.9

(continued)

(continued from previous page)

	ate five or more servings of fruits and vegetables per day for past seven days			drank three or more glasses of milk per day for past seven days		
	total	female	male	total	female	male
Local surveys						
Weighted data						
Boston	NA	NA	NA	11.3	7.5	15.3
Chicago	29.5	28.0	30.8	18.1	11.4	24.6
Dallas	14.9	14.4	15.5	9.8	5.4	14.5
Ft. Lauderdale	22.6	20.3	24.7	12.3	8.0	16.4
Houston	24.3	21.7	27.3	9.8	6.3	13.5
Los Angeles	21.6	19.6	23.7	12.4	6.3	18.2
Miami	23.5	20.4	26.6	11.4	8.2	14.5
New York City	24.1	21.8	26.6	11.7	7.0	16.9
Orlando	19.7	17.8	21.6	13.3	9.7	17.1
Palm Beach	23.3	22.5	23.9	11.2	6.4	16.1
Philadelphia	15.5	16.3	14.4	9.2	7.3	10.7
San Bernardino	20.8	17.3	23.9	12.0	8.5	15.2
San Diego	20.1	18.6	21.6	12.4	8.5	16.4
San Francisco	NA	NA	NA	8.7	6.0	11.4
Unweighted data						
Detroit	18.7	18.4	19.1	9.2	8.1	10.4
District of Columbia	18.5	19.5	17.5	5.0	4.5	5.7
Milwaukee	NA	NA	NA	NA	NA	NA
New Orleans	26.7	25.0	28.3	16.1	12.3	21.3

* *Survey did not include students from one of the state's large school districts.*
Note: A serving of fruit or vegetable includes drinking 100 percent fruit juice, eating fruit, green salad, potatoes (excluding french fries, fried potatoes, or potato crisps), carrots, or other vegetables. NA means data not available.
Source: Grunbaum, Jo Anne, et al., Youth Risk Behavior Surveillance–United States, 2001, Mortality and Morbidity Weekly Report, *Vol. 51/SS-4, Centers for Disease Control and Prevention, June 28, 2002*

2.38 Percentage of high school students who engaged in behaviors associated with weight control, by sex, race/ethnicity, and grade—United States, 2001

	exercised to lose weight or to avoid gaining weight in past 30 days			ate less food, fewer calories, or foods low in fat to lose weight or to avoid gaining weight in past 30 days			went without eating for at least 24 hours to lose weight or to avoid gaining weight in past 30 days			took diet pills, powders, or liquids without a doctor's advice to lose weight or avoid gaining weight in past 30 days			vomited or took a laxative to lose weight or to avoid gaining weight in past 30 days		
	total	female	male	total	female	male	total	female	male	total	female	male	total	female	male
Total	59.9	68.4	51.0	43.8	58.6	28.2	13.5	19.1	7.6	9.2	12.6	5.5	5.4	7.8	2.9
	(±1.5)	(±1.7)	(±1.9)	(±1.8)	(±2.0)	(±1.7)	(±1.1)	(±1.5)	(±0.9)	(±1.0)	(±1.5)	(±0.6)	(±0.6)	(±0.9)	(±0.7)
Race/ethnicity															
Black	50.1	53.4	46.6	32.5	40.2	24.5	12.8	15.2	10.3	6.0	7.5	4.4	4.0	4.2	3.8
	(±3.1)	(±2.8)	(±5.8)	(±2.2)	(±2.6)	(±2.9)	(±1.8)	(±2.3)	(±2.5)	(±1.4)	(±2.6)	(±1.0)	(±1.1)	(±1.4)	(±1.3)
Hispanic	61.5	66.2	56.8	44.9	56.5	32.7	15.7	23.1	8.2	10.1	13.5	6.7	7.2	10.8	3.4
	(±1.9)	(±3.1)	(±2.9)	(±2.5)	(±3.8)	(±2.9)	(±1.4)	(±2.9)	(±1.5)	(±1.4)	(±2.2)	(±1.3)	(±1.2)	(±2.3)	(±1.3)
White	61.9	72.5	50.9	45.9	63.1	27.6	13.4	19.7	6.7	9.5	13.6	5.2	5.3	8.2	2.3
	(±1.6)	(±1.8)	(±2.5)	(±2.0)	(±2.1)	(±2.2)	(±1.5)	(±2.1)	(±1.1)	(±1.1)	(±1.9)	(±0.7)	(±0.8)	(±1.2)	(±0.8)
Grade															
9	64.2	71.5	56.1	44.0	57.0	29.4	15.4	21.1	9.2	8.2	10.1	6.1	6.1	8.5	3.4
	(±2.7)	(±3.2)	(±3.1)	(±2.3)	(±2.9)	(±3.3)	(±1.9)	(±2.6)	(±2.4)	(±1.2)	(±1.8)	(±1.3)	(±1.0)	(±1.6)	(±1.6)
10	60.4	68.4	52.1	44.5	60.1	28.2	14.5	21.2	7.6	9.3	13.1	5.2	6.0	8.5	3.4
	(±2.3)	(±2.4)	(±3.2)	(±2.7)	(±3.0)	(±3.3)	(±1.8)	(±2.6)	(±1.6)	(±1.4)	(±2.6)	(±0.9)	(±1.0)	(±1.4)	(±1.2)
11	56.3	65.8	46.8	41.6	56.1	26.6	11.5	16.3	6.5	8.9	12.2	5.5	4.4	6.6	2.2
	(±2.2)	(±2.6)	(±2.7)	(±2.7)	(±3.3)	(±2.5)	(±1.4)	(±2.0)	(±1.5)	(±1.2)	(±2.1)	(±1.1)	(±0.8)	(±1.2)	(±0.8)
12	57.2	66.9	47.1	45.2	61.5	28.1	11.5	16.4	6.4	10.6	15.9	5.1	4.7	7.0	2.3
	(±3.5)	(±4.2)	(±3.3)	(±3.4)	(±4.0)	(±2.9)	(±1.8)	(±2.8)	(±1.7)	(±1.7)	(±2.5)	(±1.6)	(±1.1)	(±1.9)	(±1.0)

Note: Blacks and whites are non-Hispanic. Numbers in parentheses are plus or minus percentage points of the 95 percent confidence interval. Differences in percentages are considered statistically significant if the confidence intervals do not overlap.
Source: Grunbaum, Jo Anne, et al., Youth Risk Behavior Surveillance–United States, 2001, Mortality and Morbidity Weekly Report. Vol. 51/SS-4, Centers for Disease Control and Prevention. June 28, 2002

2.39 Percentage of high school students who engaged in behaviors associated with weight control, by sex—selected U.S. sites, 2001

	exercised to lose weight or to avoid gaining weight in past 30 days			ate less food, fewer calories, or foods low in fat to lose weight or to avoid gaining weight in past 30 days			went without eating for at least 24 hours to lose weight or to avoid gaining weight in past 30 days			took diet pills, powders, or liquids without a doctor's advice to lose weight or avoid gaining weight in past 30 days			vomited or took a laxative to lose weight or to avoid gaining weight in past 30 days		
	total	female	male	total	female	male	total	female	male	total	female	male	total	female	male
State surveys															
Weighted data															
Alabama	54.3	63.4	45.4	37.2	50.7	24.0	13.0	18.2	7.6	10.1	14.3	5.6	4.8	5.6	3.8
Arkansas	59.7	66.1	53.5	42.9	57.9	28.6	15.1	22.2	8.3	11.7	16.8	6.9	5.3	9.3	1.4
Delaware	57.5	63.0	51.6	39.3	49.6	28.4	13.1	16.7	9.2	6.1	6.9	5.0	3.6	4.7	2.4
Florida	55.3	64.2	46.9	39.6	52.9	26.7	12.3	17.9	6.7	8.7	11.1	6.1	4.9	6.6	3.0
Idaho	58.9	72.5	46.1	38.7	58.1	20.6	10.3	16.4	4.5	6.7	10.2	3.3	5.8	8.4	3.3
Maine	60.4	71.1	50.4	39.9	56.2	24.4	12.7	18.5	7.0	5.9	8.3	3.5	6.2	8.2	4.2
Massachusetts	NA	NA	NA	NA	NA	NA	13.7	19.9	7.7	8.1	10.6	5.5	6.1	8.3	3.8
Michigan	61.4	70.6	52.1	42.6	57.1	28.4	14.3	19.0	9.6	9.7	12.3	7.0	7.6	9.4	5.6
Mississippi	53.2	60.5	45.5	38.7	52.6	24.2	14.7	19.5	9.6	9.9	12.8	6.8	5.3	6.7	3.7
Missouri	59.6	70.5	49.2	42.9	57.4	28.6	14.8	20.8	9.1	8.7	12.9	4.8	4.1	5.6	2.6
Montana	60.1	74.7	46.2	39.3	58.5	21.2	13.9	19.9	7.8	7.2	9.9	4.3	5.4	7.6	3.1
Nevada	60.6	69.1	52.4	39.9	54.2	26.2	14.6	20.9	8.6	12.0	15.2	8.9	7.1	10.0	4.3
New Jersey	58.9	67.3	50.7	44.7	59.0	30.3	12.0	15.3	8.8	11.1	14.3	7.9	5.2	6.1	4.2
North Carolina	58.1	67.7	48.7	NA	NA	NA	NA	NA	NA	8.2	10.9	5.4	5.6	6.4	4.8
North Dakota	60.8	77.0	45.3	41.5	61.0	22.8	12.3	19.3	5.6	8.5	12.0	4.9	6.1	9.8	2.5
Rhode Island	55.6	63.8	47.7	40.0	55.6	24.8	11.5	16.3	7.0	5.7	7.2	4.2	4.7	6.5	2.8
South Dakota	55.9	69.6	42.8	39.2	58.1	21.0	13.4	19.1	7.9	8.6	12.2	5.0	6.3	8.7	4.0
Texas	59.6	67.3	52.2	43.1	57.9	28.9	13.9	20.4	7.8	9.4	12.8	6.1	5.8	8.8	2.8
Utah	60.1	76.9	43.9	40.4	57.4	24.1	10.9	16.0	5.9	9.2	12.6	5.9	5.5	6.7	4.4
Vermont	NA	NA	NA	NA	NA	NA	NA	NA	NA	4.9	7.8	2.1	5.6	9.3	2.0
Wisconsin	NA	NA	NA	NA	NA	NA	NA	NA	NA	NA	NA	NA	NA	NA	NA
Wyoming	59.3	71.9	47.4	39.7	56.6	23.7	13.5	19.2	8.2	7.8	10.7	5.0	4.8	7.1	2.6

(continued)

(continued from previous page)

Unweighted data	exercised to lose weight or to avoid gaining weight in past 30 days			ate less food, fewer calories, or foods low in fat to lose weight or to avoid gaining weight in past 30 days			went without eating for at least 24 hours to lose weight or to avoid gaining weight in past 30 days			took diet pills, powders, or liquids without a doctor's advice to lose weight or avoid gaining weight in past 30 days			vomited or took a laxative to lose weight or to avoid gaining weight in past 30 days		
	total	female	male	total	female	male	total	female	male	total	female	male	total	female	male
Colorado	56.9	72.3	43.1	35.9	54.0	19.8	12.7	19.1	6.9	8.5	13.0	4.4	4.3	6.6	2.3
Hawaii	64.5	68.1	60.1	38.4	46.2	28.2	13.1	16.7	8.3	7.2	8.1	6.0	4.3	5.6	2.4
Illinois*	64.2	75.0	49.2	46.3	58.8	28.3	12.6	16.9	6.4	8.3	10.2	5.7	4.6	5.9	2.9
Indiana	59.3	68.2	48.8	44.5	59.4	26.8	13.5	18.6	7.1	9.7	12.2	6.6	6.7	8.7	4.2
Iowa	63.3	75.6	51.9	42.3	58.4	27.4	14.8	19.5	10.3	8.0	10.6	5.3	4.4	7.4	1.7
Kentucky	61.9	69.8	53.2	46.4	60.1	31.4	16.2	20.6	11.0	12.0	16.1	7.0	5.7	7.3	3.7
Louisiana*	59.2	66.6	49.5	41.4	53.8	24.7	15.9	20.4	9.9	13.0	14.7	10.8	6.3	6.4	6.0
Nebraska	59.6	72.3	46.9	43.1	61.2	25.1	12.4	17.5	7.3	7.2	11.2	3.2	4.5	7.3	1.7
New Hampshire	58.4	69.2	46.8	42.8	59.4	24.8	14.3	17.8	10.4	6.6	8.2	4.6	5.9	7.3	4.1
New York*	62.3	72.8	51.7	44.6	60.7	28.5	13.4	18.8	7.9	9.6	12.0	7.0	6.0	8.6	3.3
South Carolina	58.8	65.6	51.9	37.9	51.4	24.2	13.6	18.3	8.8	7.9	9.8	5.8	5.8	7.1	4.4
Tennessee	57.4	69.1	45.7	42.2	58.8	26.3	14.0	21.2	7.1	10.6	14.6	6.5	5.6	7.1	4.0

(continued)

(continued from previous page)

	exercised to lose weight or to avoid gaining weight in past 30 days			ate less food, fewer calories, or foods low in fat to lose weight or to avoid gaining weight in past 30 days			went without eating for at least 24 hours to lose weight or to avoid gaining weight in past 30 days			took diet pills, powders, or liquids without a doctor's advice to lose weight or avoid gaining weight in past 30 days			vomited or took a laxative to lose weight or to avoid gaining weight in past 30 days		
	total	female	male	total	female	male	total	female	male	total	female	male	total	female	male
Local surveys															
Weighted data															
Boston	NA	NA	NA	NA	NA	NA	14.8	19.4	10.1	6.3	6.8	5.6	5.5	6.6	4.4
Chicago	56.8	57.6	55.9	37.2	44.7	29.3	15.0	17.9	11.8	6.5	7.1	5.7	4.6	3.9	4.6
Dallas	61.3	65.7	56.6	38.7	48.8	27.8	12.2	16.8	7.2	9.1	12.3	5.6	6.1	8.6	3.5
Ft. Lauderdale	54.2	60.3	47.8	38.8	51.9	25.0	12.5	15.8	8.7	8.0	9.7	5.8	4.4	6.1	2.5
Houston	58.1	63.7	52.5	41.8	53.5	29.7	13.6	17.8	9.2	8.6	9.5	7.6	4.6	5.7	3.6
Los Angeles	66.3	69.6	63.4	42.4	54.0	31.0	10.6	14.8	6.5	5.6	6.6	4.5	6.7	10.2	3.2
Miami	55.2	59.6	51.4	40.0	51.1	29.3	12.4	15.0	10.1	6.9	7.6	6.3	4.6	5.2	3.9
New York City	50.3	53.8	46.7	33.4	43.8	22.5	10.2	15.1	4.9	5.5	6.8	4.1	2.5	3.5	1.3
Orlando	55.1	60.5	49.7	37.9	46.6	29.0	12.1	15.0	9.0	8.7	8.9	8.2	5.6	6.3	4.6
Palm Beach	53.9	59.5	48.1	40.0	50.7	28.8	14.1	19.7	8.3	6.6	7.6	5.3	5.6	6.8	4.2
Philadelphia	50.9	52.1	49.5	34.7	39.2	30.0	13.4	12.6	14.1	6.6	5.6	7.7	4.5	6.0	2.6
San Bernardino	62.7	63.6	61.9	40.7	46.0	35.9	15.9	17.3	14.5	10.6	12.6	8.8	6.7	6.6	6.6
San Diego	58.9	64.3	53.6	37.2	49.4	24.9	11.1	15.2	6.9	8.1	9.9	6.3	5.6	7.3	3.8
San Francisco	46.5	53.1	40.1	32.3	43.2	21.6	8.1	10.6	5.6	3.2	4.9	1.5	2.9	4.2	1.5
Unweighted data															
Detroit	52.8	55.0	50.2	34.3	39.8	27.7	16.1	17.4	14.3	10.0	9.6	10.7	8.5	6.5	10.9
District of Columbia	48.3	48.0	48.7	29.5	33.8	24.0	14.8	15.3	13.7	8.2	6.8	8.4	7.3	6.3	7.7
Milwaukee	NA	NA	NA	NA	NA	NA	NA	NA	NA	NA	NA	NA	NA	NA	NA
New Orleans	45.1	46.8	43.1	34.2	39.7	26.5	15.1	17.8	10.8	6.1	5.7	5.9	4.9	5.4	3.7

* Survey did not include students from one of the state's large school districts.

Note: NA means data not available.

Source: Grunbaum, Jo Anne, et al., Youth Risk Behavior Surveillance–United States, 2001, Mortality and Morbidity Weekly Report. Vol. 51/SS-4, Centers for Disease Control and Prevention. June 28, 2002

2.40 Percentage of high school students who participated in sufficient vigorous physical activity, sufficient moderate physical activity, insufficient physical activity, and no vigorous or moderate physical activity, by sex, race/ethnicity, and grade—United States, 2001

	participated in sufficient vigorous physical activity			participated in sufficient moderate physical activity			participated in an insufficient amount of physical activity			no vigorous or moderate physical activity		
	total	female	male	total	female	male	total	female	male	total	female	male
Total	64.6 (±1.5)	57.0 (±2.4)	72.6 (±1.7)	25.5 (±1.2)	22.8 (±1.5)	28.4 (±1.5)	31.2 (±1.5)	37.9 (±2.3)	24.2 (±1.5)	9.5 (±0.7)	11.6 (±1.3)	7.2 (±0.8)
Race/ethnicity												
Black	59.7 (±3.9)	47.8 (±5.1)	72.4 (±3.1)	20.1 (±2.5)	16.5 (±4.4)	23.7 (±2.2)	36.4 (±3.9)	46.7 (±5.7)	25.4 (±2.8)	12.9 (±1.7)	16.9 (±2.2)	8.4 (±1.5)
Hispanic	60.5 (±2.5)	52.4 (±3.9)	68.8 (±2.7)	22.1 (±1.9)	18.5 (±2.0)	25.9 (±3.6)	35.4 (±2.8)	43.0 (±4.3)	27.7 (±3.1)	11.2 (±1.3)	13.0 (±2.0)	9.3 (±2.0)
White	66.5 (±1.8)	59.8 (±2.9)	73.7 (±2.1)	27.3 (±1.4)	24.7 (±1.7)	29.8 (±1.8)	29.3 (±1.7)	35.3 (±2.7)	22.9 (±1.8)	8.2 (±0.9)	10.2 (±1.6)	6.2 (±0.9)
Grade												
9	71.9 (±2.7)	67.3 (±3.7)	77.1 (±3.2)	27.2 (±2.2)	25.9 (±2.9)	28.6 (±2.8)	24.3 (±2.7)	28.1 (±3.7)	20.1 (±3.2)	7.1 (±1.2)	8.1 (±1.8)	5.8 (±1.8)
10	67.0 (±1.9)	60.1 (±3.6)	74.0 (±2.4)	24.5 (±1.6)	21.0 (±2.1)	28.1 (±2.6)	29.6 (±1.8)	35.6 (±3.4)	23.6 (±2.2)	8.5 (±1.1)	10.0 (±1.8)	7.0 (±1.5)
11	61.3 (±2.5)	50.8 (±3.3)	72.2 (±3.1)	25.8 (±1.6)	21.7 (±1.9)	29.9 (±2.9)	34.4 (±2.3)	44.2 (±3.2)	24.4 (±2.6)	11.1 (±1.4)	14.4 (±2.1)	7.8 (±1.4)
12	55.5 (±3.2)	45.4 (±3.0)	66.1 (±5.1)	24.5 (±2.3)	22.0 (±3.2)	26.9 (±3.1)	38.9 (±2.8)	47.9 (±2.4)	29.5 (±4.2)	12.0 (±1.8)	15.2 (±2.4)	8.7 (±2.5)

Note: Sufficient vigorous physical activity: activities that made the student sweat and breathe hard for 20 or more minutes on at least three of the seven days preceding the survey. Sufficient moderate physical activity: activities that did not make the student sweat or breathe hard for 30 or more minutes on at least five of the seven days preceding the survey. Insufficient physical activity: Did not participate in vigorous activities and did not participate in moderate physical activities. No vigorous or moderate physical activity: Did not participte in either vigorous physical activity for 20 or more minutes or moderate physical activity for 30 or more minutes on any of the seven days preceding the survey. Blacks and whites are non-Hispanic. Numbers in parentheses are plus or minus percentage points of the 95 percent confidence interval. Differences in percentages are considered statistically significant if the confidence intervals do not overlap.

Source: Grunbaum, Jo Anne, et al., Youth Risk Behavior Surveillance–United States, 2001. Mortality and Morbidity Weekly Report, Vol. 51/SS-4. Centers for Disease Control and Prevention, June 28, 2002

2.41 Percentage of high school students who participated in sufficient vigorous physical activity, sufficient moderate physical activity, insufficient physical activity, and no vigorous or moderate physical activity, by sex—selected U.S. sites, 2001

	participated in sufficient vigorous physical activity			participated in sufficient moderate physical activity			participated in an insufficient amount of physical activity			no vigorous or moderate physical activity		
	total	female	male	total	female	male	total	female	male	total	female	male
State surveys												
Weighted data												
Alabama	58.4	48.0	69.0	20.2	16.7	23.7	38.4	48.3	28.2	11.3	13.5	8.9
Arkansas	61.5	51.7	70.8	23.3	20.8	25.8	33.9	42.7	25.5	11.1	13.9	8.5
Delaware	62.5	54.1	71.3	25.4	23.4	27.4	32.6	40.0	24.8	11.4	15.4	7.3
Florida	58.8	48.8	68.4	22.0	17.1	26.7	37.0	46.6	27.7	12.3	14.7	10.0
Idaho	67.1	59.4	74.6	29.3	26.8	31.7	27.9	34.5	21.3	7.9	9.1	6.5
Maine	65.9	60.5	71.3	29.1	28.2	29.8	29.5	34.3	24.7	6.4	7.4	5.4
Massachusetts	62.8	57.1	68.6	25.1	22.4	27.8	33.3	38.2	28.3	9.2	9.9	8.5
Michigan	64.5	57.4	71.7	26.9	24.0	29.8	31.2	37.0	25.3	9.6	11.1	8.2
Mississippi	54.9	42.7	67.9	19.8	16.0	23.9	40.9	51.9	29.0	15.6	20.3	10.6
Missouri	64.7	56.7	72.4	24.2	19.7	28.6	30.8	38.9	23.0	8.6	10.4	6.9
Montana	67.6	62.6	72.4	31.0	28.5	33.5	27.8	31.7	24.1	7.0	8.0	6.2
Nevada	66.3	56.9	75.4	27.9	24.9	30.8	29.0	37.2	21.1	7.8	9.6	6.0
New Jersey	65.6	56.2	75.1	28.5	24.7	32.1	29.7	37.7	21.6	8.9	10.2	7.5
North Carolina	64.0	54.9	73.1	23.5	20.3	26.6	31.9	39.8	24.0	10.5	13.7	7.3
North Dakota	60.4	54.0	66.9	25.7	22.3	28.9	34.1	40.3	27.8	8.3	9.6	7.1
Rhode Island	66.1	58.1	74.4	29.2	26.4	32.3	29.5	36.0	22.7	10.0	11.2	8.8
South Dakota	58.0	51.8	64.0	24.8	21.9	27.8	37.0	43.1	31.2	11.9	14.0	9.9
Texas	61.8	52.6	70.5	22.0	18.8	25.1	34.3	42.7	26.4	10.8	12.9	8.8
Utah	67.1	61.8	72.0	29.5	26.5	32.3	28.5	33.3	23.9	4.2	2.8	5.5
Vermont	67.2	60.7	73.4	28.2	25.7	30.6	28.2	33.6	23.0	8.3	9.1	7.5
Wisconsin	64.9	57.5	71.9	27.6	25.4	29.7	30.1	36.7	23.7	8.4	9.8	7.1
Wyoming	69.0	61.6	76.3	30.0	27.4	32.5	26.4	32.9	20.0	7.6	9.0	6.2

(continued)

(continued from previous page)

	participated in sufficient vigorous physical activity			participated in sufficient moderate physical activity			participated in an insufficient amount of physical activity			no vigorous or moderate physical activity		
	total	female	male	total	female	male	total	female	male	total	female	male
Unweighted data												
Colorado	70.2	63.6	76.6	26.2	23.3	28.8	26.4	32.8	20.4	6.7	7.1	5.8
Hawaii	55.8	47.9	66.3	19.2	14.9	24.8	40.7	48.5	30.1	12.0	15.9	6.8
Illinois*	74.1	72.8	76.0	28.5	27.4	30.2	22.0	22.8	20.9	4.6	3.6	5.8
Indiana	61.5	55.6	68.8	24.4	20.2	29.6	33.6	39.7	25.9	10.0	13.4	5.8
Iowa	74.1	70.8	77.0	29.3	27.6	30.9	22.0	25.4	19.1	4.6	5.4	3.9
Kentucky	59.8	51.7	68.9	20.3	17.3	23.4	36.3	43.6	28.2	11.2	12.4	10.1
Louisiana*	55.4	50.2	62.1	19.4	19.0	20.1	41.0	45.3	35.1	11.4	12.7	9.6
Nebraska	68.3	59.3	77.1	27.7	23.5	31.9	26.3	34.1	18.6	6.5	7.8	5.2
New Hampshire	62.2	59.2	65.9	NA	NA	NA	NA	NA	NA	NA	NA	NA
New York*	65.8	60.8	70.8	23.9	20.5	27.4	30.0	34.8	25.1	7.0	7.0	7.2
South Carolina	59.4	51.0	67.9	21.2	17.1	25.4	36.7	44.4	29.0	10.6	13.0	8.1
Tennessee	61.2	51.4	70.8	25.4	21.5	29.4	33.3	41.9	24.8	9.5	11.4	7.5

(continued)

(continued from previous page)

	participated in sufficient vigorous physical activity			participated in sufficient moderate physical activity			participated in an insufficient amount of physical activity			no vigorous or moderate physical activity		
	total	female	male	total	female	male	total	female	male	total	female	male
Local surveys												
Weighted data												
Boston	49.8	39.8	60.3	17.3	17.1	17.5	46.2	54.4	37.5	14.7	18.2	11.0
Chicago	63.5	55.5	71.8	25.5	23.6	27.1	30.5	37.7	23.1	11.7	13.9	9.5
Dallas	54.9	45.2	65.2	16.5	14.4	18.7	41.2	49.3	32.6	11.1	14.0	8.1
Ft. Lauderdale	56.9	43.7	70.2	18.0	15.0	21.1	39.5	51.4	27.5	12.4	15.6	9.1
Houston	55.2	47.5	63.3	18.3	16.7	20.1	41.1	48.5	33.4	13.2	16.2	10.1
Los Angeles	62.1	56.6	67.7	19.0	17.6	20.4	34.5	38.2	30.7	11.2	12.8	9.5
Miami	54.5	44.2	64.6	19.1	16.2	21.8	41.4	50.3	32.6	15.8	19.1	12.6
New York City	59.5	49.5	70.2	25.1	23.8	26.5	33.1	40.7	24.9	10.8	13.0	8.2
Orlando	56.5	47.1	66.3	26.5	24.4	28.9	36.5	44.3	28.0	11.4	14.8	7.5
Palm Beach	54.8	42.2	67.6	23.4	17.7	29.0	39.6	51.5	27.6	13.1	17.5	8.6
Philadelphia	52.7	45.1	60.5	22.4	18.9	25.8	42.1	49.5	34.3	16.1	19.0	13.0
San Bernardino	57.0	56.8	57.2	23.9	25.4	22.6	37.5	36.5	38.4	11.5	11.1	11.9
San Diego	65.0	57.8	72.3	25.7	23.7	27.6	31.4	37.0	25.6	10.1	11.2	9.0
San Francisco	NA	NA	NA	22.1	20.8	23.3	NA	NA	NA	NA	NA	NA
Unweighted data												
Detroit	48.8	41.5	57.5	21.1	19.9	22.0	45.9	51.8	39.2	18.0	21.8	13.5
District of Columbia	40.7	35.5	47.0	12.3	9.6	15.4	56.7	61.5	50.8	25.3	28.8	21.1
Milwaukee	49.5	41.4	58.6	23.6	18.9	28.9	45.7	54.0	36.3	15.6	21.6	8.6
New Orleans	47.4	42.4	54.8	18.6	16.7	21.5	47.7	52.3	40.8	20.4	22.4	17.7

Survey did not include students from one of the state's large school districts.

Note: Sufficient vigorous physical activity: activities that made the student sweat and breathe hard for 20 or more minutes on at least three of the seven days preceding the survey. Sufficient moderate physical activity: activities that did not make the student sweat or breathe hard for 30 or more minutes on at least five of the seven days preceding the survey. Insufficient physical activity: did not participate in vigorous activities and did not participate in moderate physical activities. No vigorous or moderate physical activity: did not participate in either vigorous physical activity for 20 or more minutes or moderate physical activity for 30 or more minutes on any of the seven days preceding the survey. NA means data not available.

Source: Grunbaum, Jo Anne, et al., Youth Risk Behavior Surveillance–United States, 2001. Mortality and Morbidity Weekly Report, Vol. 51/SS-4, Centers for Disease Control and Prevention, June 28, 2002

2.42 Percentage of high school students who were enrolled in a physical education class, attended PE class daily, spent 20 or more minutes exercising during an average PE class, or played on one or more sports teams, by sex, race/ethnicity, and grade—United States, 2001

	enrolled in PE class			attended PE class daily			exercised 20 or more minutes during an average PE class (among students enrolled in PE)			played on one or more sport teams in past 12 months		
	total	female	male	total	female	male	total	female	male	total	female	male
Total	**51.7**	**48.0**	**55.6**	**32.2**	**28.4**	**36.3**	**83.4**	**78.8**	**87.7**	**55.2**	**49.9**	**60.9**
	(±4.6)	(±6.0)	(±3.9)	(±4.9)	(±5.1)	(±5.4)	(±2.1)	(±2.6)	(±2.0)	(±1.9)	(±2.4)	(±2.3)
Race/ethnicity												
Black	60.5	54.0	67.4	40.8	35.6	46.3	76.4	71.0	81.0	52.7	41.6	64.4
	(±9.3)	(±10.7)	(±8.1)	(±11.4)	(±12.6)	(±10.4)	(±3.7)	(±4.2)	(±4.1)	(±3.8)	(±3.6)	(±4.6)
Hispanic	58.4	55.3	61.6	38.7	35.7	41.9	81.9	79.2	84.6	48.8	40.1	57.8
	(±7.2)	(±9.3)	(±5.9)	(±6.2)	(±7.6)	(±6.2)	(±4.0)	(±4.9)	(±3.9)	(±3.1)	(±3.9)	(±3.2)
White	48.3	44.9	52.0	29.5	25.6	33.8	85.2	79.7	90.3	57.4	53.3	61.7
	(±4.5)	(±5.9)	(±4.0)	(±5.2)	(±5.3)	(±5.8)	(±2.3)	(±3.3)	(±2.3)	(±2.7)	(±3.1)	(±3.0)
Grade												
9	73.7	73.4	74.0	48.7	49.3	48.2	81.7	78.9	85.0	59.9	56.7	63.5
	(±5.7)	(±7.0)	(±5.1)	(±7.4)	(±9.1)	(±7.4)	(±2.8)	(±3.9)	(±2.9)	(±2.8)	(±3.5)	(±3.1)
10	54.1	49.9	58.4	31.6	26.1	37.4	84.3	80.3	87.7	56.2	50.8	61.6
	(±6.0)	(±7.4)	(±5.8)	(±6.1)	(±6.1)	(±7.2)	(±2.7)	(±3.6)	(±2.9)	(±3.1)	(±4.3)	(±3.8)
11	39.1	31.6	46.7	22.8	15.6	30.0	85.9	79.1	90.6	54.5	47.7	61.5
	(±7.2)	(±8.8)	(±6.9)	(±4.7)	(±4.0)	(±5.7)	(±3.5)	(±4.5)	(±3.0)	(±2.4)	(±3.9)	(±2.9)
12	31.3	26.0	36.9	20.3	14.7	26.1	84.2	75.0	91.2	48.5	41.4	55.9
	(±5.4)	(±6.6)	(±5.9)	(±5.1)	(±4.5)	(±6.4)	(±3.5)	(±5.8)	(±3.3)	(±3.5)	(±3.7)	(±4.3)

Note: Blacks and whites are non-Hispanic. Numbers in parentheses are plus or minus percentage points of the 95 percent confidence interval. Differences in percentages are considered statistically significant if the confidence intervals do not overlap.

Source: Grunbaum, Jo Anne, et al., Youth Risk Behavior Surveillance–United States, 2001. Mortality and Morbidity Weekly Report. Vol. 51/SS-4, Centers for Disease Control and Prevention, June 28, 2002

2.43 Percentage of high school students who were enrolled in physical education class, attended PE class daily, spent 20 or more minutes exercising during an average PE class, or played on one or more sports teams, by sex—selected U.S. sites, 2001

State surveys Weighted data	enrolled in PE class			attended PE class daily			exercised 20 or more minutes during an average PE class (among students enrolled in PE)			played on one or more sport teams in past 12 months		
	total	female	male	total	female	male	total	female	male	total	female	male
Alabama	39.2	28.8	49.9	31.8	23.1	40.8	83.4	72.9	90.0	52.5	44.0	60.8
Arkansas	36.5	34.6	38.4	30.2	29.1	31.4	84.6	83.7	85.4	54.1	47.8	60.1
Delaware	42.1	40.6	43.4	32.0	31.0	32.8	81.0	77.5	84.5	56.0	50.2	62.0
Florida	41.6	33.7	49.3	25.4	20.8	29.8	80.8	73.5	85.8	49.6	44.1	54.8
Idaho	43.1	37.2	48.6	30.4	26.3	34.5	90.4	89.1	91.5	61.8	57.3	65.9
Maine	41.9	41.8	42.0	4.8	4.3	5.3	90.1	92.4	88.0	59.6	58.7	60.6
Massachusetts	68.0	66.5	69.5	17.7	16.9	18.6	NA	NA	NA	53.8	49.9	57.7
Michigan	44.1	38.0	50.0	29.4	25.9	32.7	83.2	80.8	85.2	60.8	56.8	64.5
Mississippi	31.7	17.8	47.3	22.7	12.5	33.9	82.0	65.9	88.6	54.8	44.8	65.2
Missouri	55.9	49.3	62.2	30.0	26.1	33.9	85.4	81.1	88.5	52.7	47.9	57.2
Montana	52.3	48.3	55.6	31.3	28.2	34.5	83.3	80.0	85.9	60.1	58.9	61.4
Nevada	NA	NA	NA	NA	NA	NA	NA	NA	NA	NA	NA	NA
New Jersey	92.4	92.5	92.4	66.5	66.9	66.0	71.9	64.5	79.7	59.0	52.7	65.4
North Carolina	47.1	37.8	56.5	34.4	28.2	40.6	88.9	86.3	90.8	NA	NA	NA
North Dakota	48.0	43.4	52.2	31.6	29.5	33.7	NA	NA	NA	61.6	59.6	63.6
Rhode Island	88.1	88.3	87.9	15.6	14.7	16.2	77.8	73.4	82.1	56.0	50.2	62.0
South Dakota	22.1	17.0	27.2	12.0	9.5	14.6	83.1	82.1	84.2	63.7	60.1	67.3
Texas	48.0	44.1	51.7	32.9	29.7	36.0	85.8	82.3	88.6	56.7	49.7	63.5
Utah	59.0	56.2	61.7	23.7	24.1	23.4	88.8	88.6	88.9	58.4	54.0	62.6
Vermont	49.1	45.3	52.6	27.7	24.8	30.4	86.6	85.0	88.1	NA	NA	NA
Wisconsin	NA	NA	NA	NA	NA	NA	79.6	74.4	84.3	60.0	54.4	65.4
Wyoming	58.2	50.0	66.0	30.9	27.8	34.0	87.1	83.8	89.4	63.8	59.3	68.3

(continued)

(continued from previous page)

Unweighted data	enrolled in PE class			attended PE class daily			exercised 20 or more minutes during an average PE class (among students enrolled in PE)			played on one or more sport teams in past 12 months		
	total	female	male	total	female	male	total	female	male	total	female	male
Colorado	50.9	44.4	56.8	24.4	22.7	26.1	91.5	89.8	92.7	63.3	62.6	63.7
Hawaii	41.5	35.0	49.9	10.1	8.5	12.3	86.6	85.1	88.5	49.3	45.7	54.2
Illinois*	82.0	82.7	81.3	70.6	72.4	68.3	80.8	79.1	83.4	66.8	65.4	68.9
Indiana	38.0	31.3	46.0	26.4	23.1	30.4	89.6	88.7	90.3	55.9	49.8	63.1
Iowa	80.0	76.0	84.0	14.0	12.8	14.6	76.6	73.6	79.5	68.3	67.3	69.5
Kentucky	29.0	21.7	36.9	19.2	14.7	23.9	78.2	NA	81.9	56.1	51.7	61.2
Louisiana*	58.1	52.0	66.1	46.5	42.0	52.7	72.9	70.3	75.9	52.6	45.6	61.9
Nebraska	43.0	33.6	52.4	40.0	31.8	48.0	91.5	90.3	92.3	67.6	62.9	72.2
New Hampshire	NA	NA	NA	NA	NA	NA	85.1	85.0	85.8	60.7	59.9	61.6
New York*	93.6	94.9	92.4	3.6	3.1	4.1	73.8	70.3	77.7	58.8	56.8	60.7
South Carolina	45.9	37.6	54.6	28.1	23.4	33.0	83.6	80.1	86.1	NA	NA	NA
Tennessee	41.6	37.2	45.8	25.6	19.8	31.3	84.2	78.6	89.5	50.8	43.9	57.2

(continued)

(continued from previous page)

	enrolled in PE class			attended PE class daily			exercised 20 or more minutes during an average PE class (among students enrolled in PE)			played on one or more sport teams in past 12 months		
	total	female	male	total	female	male	total	female	male	total	female	male
Local surveys												
Weighted data												
Boston	56.5	53.4	59.7	11.0	7.9	14.3	NA	NA	NA	45.2	36.2	54.5
Chicago	70.5	67.7	73.5	57.1	55.3	58.9	80.7	78.3	83.0	54.1	44.2	64.5
Dallas	46.4	41.3	52.0	10.3	7.7	13.1	79.2	75.3	82.5	48.0	39.7	56.9
Ft. Lauderdale	44.2	34.0	54.6	23.7	17.7	30.0	79.6	73.4	83.4	48.0	39.7	56.1
Houston	49.8	44.2	55.6	17.1	12.7	21.8	75.8	68.4	82.2	47.5	39.0	56.3
Los Angeles	66.6	63.8	69.6	55.1	56.1	54.5	78.9	71.4	86.0	50.4	47.4	53.4
Miami	41.3	34.0	48.8	15.4	11.0	20.0	78.3	73.2	82.3	43.8	34.8	52.7
New York City	85.6	85.3	86.2	45.6	48.0	43.4	71.1	66.1	76.7	44.6	36.1	53.5
Orlando	33.3	25.1	42.3	16.5	10.1	23.6	82.5	76.5	86.1	48.0	40.6	55.6
Palm Beach	55.2	49.3	61.7	21.1	20.6	21.8	73.8	65.1	81.0	46.3	38.9	53.7
Philadelphia	52.6	52.0	53.5	23.8	23.9	23.7	67.5	60.1	75.7	48.5	40.0	57.6
San Bernardino	60.6	58.7	62.6	50.8	52.2	49.6	74.3	68.1	80.4	52.5	43.0	61.5
San Diego	63.7	59.2	68.1	40.9	37.5	44.2	84.9	81.8	87.6	55.5	47.9	63.5
San Francisco	56.0	53.4	58.7	34.3	30.8	37.7	NA	NA	NA	44.5	39.2	49.8
Unweighted data												
Detroit	41.5	36.4	48.1	28.3	27.1	29.8	66.0	60.7	71.5	44.2	37.6	52.3
District of Columbia	60.2	59.8	60.6	14.3	15.2	13.4	69.1	66.8	72.6	41.4	33.3	51.0
Milwaukee	NA	NA	NA	NA	NA	NA	74.5	68.3	80.4	53.9	41.5	67.7
New Orleans	78.2	78.0	78.5	49.1	49.5	49.1	54.9	43.4	71.4	48.9	41.9	58.6

* Survey did not include students from one of the state's large school districts.

Note: NA means data not available.

Source: Grunbaum, Jo Anne, et al., Youth Risk Behavior Surveillance–United States, 2001. Mortality and Morbidity Weekly Report. Vol. 51/SS-4, Centers for Disease Control and Prevention, June 28, 2002

2.44 Percentage of high school students who participated in strengthening activities, or who watched three or more hours of television per day during an average school day, by sex, race/ethnicity, and grade—United States, 2001

	participated in strengthening exercises on three of past seven days			watched three or more hours of TV per day during an average school day		
	total	female	male	total	female	male
Total	**53.4**	**44.5**	**62.8**	**38.3**	**35.0**	**41.8**
	(±1.7)	(±2.6)	(±1.9)	(±2.3)	(±3.0)	(±1.9)
Race/ethnicity						
Black	47.9	35.4	61.1	68.9	68.6	69.1
	(±3.6)	(±4.2)	(±2.9)	(±3.5)	(±4.6)	(±4.5)
Hispanic	51.2	42.3	60.3	47.8	46.0	49.7
	(±2.9)	(±3.5)	(±3.7)	(±3.5)	(±3.6)	(±4.5)
White	54.8	46.7	63.4	31.0	26.5	35.7
	(±2.0)	(±3.2)	(±2.5)	(±2.0)	(±2.7)	(±1.8)
Grade						
9	58.7	52.6	65.6	45.3	39.6	51.4
	(±3.3)	(±4.8)	(±3.2)	(±4.5)	(±5.5)	(±4.3)
10	53.9	44.7	63.4	39.2	36.2	42.3
	(±1.7)	(±3.4)	(±2.2)	(±2.7)	(±4.2)	(±3.4)
11	51.1	39.7	63.0	34.7	32.5	36.8
	(±2.7)	(±3.7)	(±3.8)	(±2.5)	(±3.2)	(±2.6)
12	48.0	37.9	58.4	31.3	29.2	33.5
	(±2.6)	(±2.7)	(±4.4)	(±2.7)	(±3.3)	(±3.7)

Note: Strengthening activities include push-ups or weightlifting. Blacks and whites are non-Hispanic. Numbers in parentheses are plus or minus percentage points of the 95 percent confidence interval. Differences in percentages are considered statistically significant if the confidence intervals do not overlap.
Source: Grunbaum, Jo Anne, et al., Youth Risk Behavior Surveillance–United States, 2001. Mortality and Morbidity Weekly Report, *Vol. 51/SS-4, Centers for Disease Control and Prevention, June 28, 2002*

2.45 Percentage of high school students who participated in strengthening activities, or who watched three or more hours of television per day during an average school day, by sex— selected U.S. sites, 2001

	participated in strengthening exercises on three of past seven days			watched three or more hours of TV per day during an average school day		
	total	female	male	total	female	male
State surveys						
Weighted data						
Alabama	43.7	33.8	53.7	46.1	44.8	47.3
Arkansas	49.9	38.2	61.0	42.9	38.4	47.3
Delaware	50.5	41.5	60.1	40.7	35.9	45.8
Florida	46.5	35.3	57.3	44.9	42.2	47.5
Idaho	56.1	48.4	63.5	24.1	19.1	28.6
Maine	47.5	41.0	53.9	24.4	21.0	27.6
Massachusetts	46.7	39.5	53.8	30.4	25.4	35.4
Michigan	52.2	44.8	59.6	30.5	29.5	31.5
Mississippi	47.2	34.3	61.0	54.7	52.7	56.7
Missouri	57.0	47.2	66.3	38.1	32.2	43.5
Montana	58.3	52.9	63.2	23.5	20.7	26.0
Nevada	NA	NA	NA	NA	NA	NA
New Jersey	53.6	46.3	61.2	40.7	37.2	44.2
North Carolina	NA	NA	NA	NA	NA	NA
North Dakota	NA	NA	NA	26.3	20.4	31.6
Rhode Island	51.1	41.2	61.0	34.1	30.2	37.5
South Dakota	51.6	43.2	59.8	24.8	23.7	25.7
Texas	51.9	42.9	60.6	44.4	39.6	49.0
Utah	54.4	50.4	58.2	17.7	15.6	19.7
Vermont	NA	NA	NA	NA	NA	NA
Wisconsin	NA	NA	NA	NA	NA	NA
Wyoming	56.2	49.3	62.9	24.7	19.1	29.8
Unweighted data						
Colorado	59.2	50.4	67.3	29.2	23.8	34.2
Hawaii	47.2	38.2	59.2	42.2	38.9	46.7
Illinois*	59.2	56.9	62.7	29.0	25.9	33.7
Indiana	49.0	41.6	57.9	33.4	32.5	34.5
Iowa	53.6	46.4	60.1	24.9	20.0	29.3
Kentucky	46.7	38.6	55.8	34.4	30.3	38.7
Louisiana*	44.2	37.5	53.3	45.8	44.0	48.4
Nebraska	58.4	48.8	67.8	25.7	21.7	29.8
New Hampshire	51.4	43.9	60.1	27.3	23.2	31.7
New York*	50.3	45.4	55.2	31.5	30.1	33.1
South Carolina	48.8	37.8	59.8	48.2	48.2	48.1
Tennessee	50.6	38.7	62.3	44.6	41.3	47.9

(continued)

(continued from previous page)

	participated in strengthening exercises on three of past seven days			watched three or more hours of TV per day during an average school day		
	total	female	male	total	female	male
Local surveys						
Weighted data						
Boston	36.5	27.8	45.7	47.8	44.5	51.2
Chicago	51.0	41.2	61.3	58.6	57.6	59.3
Dallas	44.2	35.0	54.0	55.4	56.6	54.1
Ft. Lauderdale	42.7	30.0	55.6	49.6	47.3	52.2
Houston	50.7	41.5	60.2	58.9	57.4	60.4
Los Angeles	51.7	43.6	59.9	44.6	44.5	44.5
Miami	43.7	31.0	56.1	53.5	52.0	55.2
New York City	50.3	40.7	60.8	59.0	55.4	63.0
Orlando	45.6	32.3	59.6	44.9	43.6	46.5
Palm Beach	46.2	32.5	60.0	45.6	46.1	45.0
Philadelphia	36.2	30.3	42.3	56.7	57.0	56.5
San Bernardino	46.6	38.8	53.9	44.3	46.7	42.2
San Diego	52.4	44.9	60.2	41.8	41.8	41.9
San Francisco	42.6	32.6	52.4	45.0	43.2	46.7
Unweighted data						
Detroit	36.4	27.6	46.7	59.3	60.6	57.6
District of Columbia	34.1	28.5	40.7	52.6	55.2	50.6
Milwaukee	NA	NA	NA	NA	NA	NA
New Orleans	40.9	30.0	56.1	66.8	67.1	66.9

* Survey did not include students from one of the state's large school districts.
Note: Strengthening activities include push-ups or weightlifting. NA means data not available.
Source: Grunbaum, Jo Anne, et al., Youth Risk Behavior Surveillance–United States, 2001, Mortality and Morbidity Weekly Report, *Vol. 51/SS-4, Centers for Disease Control and Prevention, June 28, 2002*

Trends from the Youth Risk Behavior Surveillance System

The Youth Risk Behavior Surveillance System allows researchers to examine trends in the behavior of the nation's teenagers over time. The following tables show national, state, and local area trends in teen behavior since 1991, the earliest year for which survey data are available. For some geographic areas, 1993 or 1995 are the earliest years for which data are available. Trend tables are not shown for geographic areas participating in the 2001 survey that do not also have data available for 1995 or earlier years.

3.1 United States: 1991 and 2001

(responses to the Youth Risk Behavior Surveillance System Survey questions, and direction of change at the 95 percent confidence level, United States, 1991 and 2001)

		2001	1991	direction of change
1.	Of students who rode a motorcycle during the past 12 months, the percentage who never or rarely wore a motorcycle helmet	37.2	42.9	no change
2.	Of students who rode a bicycle during the past 12 months, the percentage who never or rarely wore a bicycle helmet	84.7	96.2	decreased
3.	Percentage of students who never or rarely wear a seat belt when riding in a car driven by someone else	14.1	25.9	decreased
4.	Percentage of students who during the past 30 days rode one or more times in a car or other vehicle driven by someone who had been drinking alcohol	30.7	39.9	decreased
5.	Percentage of students who during the past 30 days drove a car or other vehicle one or more times when they had been drinking alcohol	13.3	16.7	decreased
6.	Percentage of students who carried a weapon such as a gun, knife, or club on one or more of the past 30 days	17.4	26.1	decreased
7.	Percentage of students who were in a physical fight one or more times during the past 12 months	33.2	42.5	decreased
8.	Percentage of students who were injured in a physical fight one or more times during the past 12 months and had to be treated by a doctor or nurse	4.0	4.4	no change
9.	Percentage of students who seriously considered attempting suicide during the past 12 months	19.0	29.0	decreased
10.	Percentage of students who made a plan about how they would attempt suicide during the past 12 months	14.8	18.6	decreased
11.	Percentage of students who actually attempted suicide one or more times during the past 12 months	8.8	7.3	increased
12.	Percentage of students whose attempted suicide during the past 12 months resulted in an injury, poisoning, or overdose that had to be treated by a doctor or nurse	2.6	1.7	increased
13.	Percentage of students who ever tried cigarette smoking, even one or two puffs	63.9	70.1	decreased
14.	Percentage of students who smoked a whole cigarette for the first time before age 13	22.1	23.8	no change
15.	Percentage of students who smoked cigarettes on one or more of the past 30 days	28.5	27.5	no change
16.	Percentage of students who smoked two or more cigarettes per day on the days they smoked during the past 30 days	19.4	19.2	no change
17.	Percentage of students who had at least one drink of alcohol on one or more days during their life	78.2	81.6	decreased
18.	Percentage of students who had their first drink of alcohol other than a few sips before age 13	29.1	32.7	decreased
19.	Percentage of students who had at least one drink of alcohol on one or more of the past 30 days	47.1	50.8	decreased
20.	Percentage of students who had five or more drinks of alcohol in a row, that is, within a couple of hours, on one or more of the past 30 days	29.9	31.3	no change
21.	Percentage of students who used marijuana one or more times during their life	42.4	31.3	increased
22.	Percentage of students who tried marijuana for the first time before age 13	10.2	7.4	increased

(continued)

(continued from previous page)

		2001	1991	direction of change*
23.	Percentage of students who used marijuana one or more times during the past 30 days	23.9	14.7	increased
24.	Percentage of students who used any form of cocaine, including powder, crack, or freebase one or more times during their life	9.4	5.9	increased
25.	Percentage of students who used any form of cocaine, including powder, crack, or freebase one or more times during the past 30 days	4.2	1.7	increased
26.	Percentage of students who took steroid pills or shots without a doctor's prescription one or more times during their life	5.0	2.7	increased
27.	Percentage of students who had sexual intercourse	45.6	54.1	decreased
28.	Percentage of students who had sexual intercourse for the first time before age 13	6.6	10.2	decreased
29.	Percentage of students who had sexual intercourse with four or more people during their life	14.2	18.7	decreased
30.	Percentage of students who had sexual intercourse with one or more people during the past three months	33.4	37.5	decreased
31.	Of students who had sexual intercourse during the past three months, the percentage who drank alcohol or used drugs before last sexual intercourse	25.6	21.6	increased
32.	Of students who had sexual intercourse during the past three months, the percentage who used a condom during last sexual intercourse	57.9	46.2	increased
33.	Percentage of students who had been pregnant or gotten someone pregnant one or more times	4.7	6.0	no change
34.	Percentage of students who described themselves as slightly or very overweight	29.2	31.8	decreased
35.	Percentage of students who were trying to lose weight	46.0	41.8	increased
36.	Percentage of students who did exercises to strengthen or tone their muscles on three or more of the past seven days	53.4	47.8	increased
37.	Percentage of students who attended physical education (PE) class one or more days during an average school week	51.7	48.9	no change
38.	Percentage of students who had ever been taught about AIDS or HIV infection in school	89.0	83.3	increased
39.	Percentage of students who smoked cigarettes on 20 or more of the past 30 days	13.8	12.7	no change
40.	Percentage of students who smoked more than 10 cigarettes per day on the days that they smoked during the past 30 days	4.1	4.9	no change
41.	Percentage of students who have ever had sexual intercourse but have not had sexual intercourse during the past three months	26.7	30.7	decreased
42.	Percentage of students who attended physical education (PE) class daily	32.2	41.6	decreased
43.	Percentage of students who have never had sexual intercourse, who have had sexual intercourse but not during the past three months, or who used a condom the last time they had sexual intercourse during the past three months	86.1	80.0	increased

* Change over time is statistically significant for p< 0.05.
Source: Centers for Disease Control and Prevention, Youth Risk Behavior Surveillance System, http://www.cdc.gov/nccdphp/dash/ yrbs/index.htm

3.2 Alabama, 1991 and 2001

(responses to the Youth Risk Behavior Surveillance System Survey questions, and direction of change at the 95 percent confidence level, Alabama, 1991 and 2001)

		2001	1991	direction of change*
1.	Of students who rode a motorcycle during the past 12 months, the percentage who never or rarely wore a motorcycle helmet	31.1	38.8	decreased
2.	Of students who rode a bicycle during the past 12 months, the percentage who never or rarely wore a bicycle helmet	90.4	97.5	decreased
3.	Percentage of students who never or rarely wear a seat belt when riding in a car driven by someone else	10.7	39.1	decreased
4.	Percentage of students who during the past 30 days rode one or more times in a car or other vehicle driven by someone who had been drinking alcohol	33.7	42.7	decreased
5.	Percentage of students who during the past 30 days drove a car or other vehicle one or more times when they had been drinking alcohol	12.7	18.3	decreased
6.	Percentage of students who carried a weapon such as a gun, knife, or club on one or more of the past 30 days	20.7	33.1	decreased
7.	Percentage of students who were in a physical fight one or more times during the past 12 months	30.3	37.8	decreased
8.	Percentage of students who were injured in a physical fight one or more times during the past 12 months and had to be treated by a doctor or nurse	3.6	3.3	no change
9.	Percentage of students who ever tried cigarette smoking, even one or two puffs	70.6	74.2	no change
10.	Percentage of students who smoked a whole cigarette for the first time before age 13	22.4	28.2	decreased
11.	Percentage of students who smoked cigarettes on one or more of the past 30 days	23.7	27.8	no change
12.	Percentage of students who smoked two or more cigarettes per day on the days they smoked during the past 30 days	17.7	20.4	no change
13.	Percentage of students who had at least one drink of alcohol on one or more days during their life	76.4	78.4	no change
14.	Percentage of students who had their first drink of alcohol other than a few sips before age 13	28.4	33.8	decreased
15.	Percentage of students who had at least one drink of alcohol on one or more of the past 30 days	42.6	46.8	no change
16.	Percentage of students who had five or more drinks of alcohol in a row, that is, within a couple of hours, on one or more of the past 30 days	25.0	30.3	decreased
17.	Percentage of students who used marijuana one or more times during their life	38.7	25.0	increased
18.	Percentage of students who tried marijuana for the first time before age 13	8.8	6.6	no change
19.	Percentage of students who used marijuana one or more times during the past 30 days	18.8	9.6	increased
20.	Percentage of students who used any form of cocaine, including powder, crack, or freebase one or more times during their life	6.6	3.8	increased
21.	Percentage of students who used any form of cocaine, including powder, crack, or freebase one or more times during the past 30 days	2.4	1.7	no change
22.	Percentage of students who took steroid pills or shots without a doctor's prescription one or more times during their life	4.8	4.2	no change
23.	Percentage of students who described themselves as slightly or very overweight	30.1	26.4	no change
24.	Percentage of students who were trying to lose weight	42.0	36.4	increased
25.	Percentage of students who did exercises to strengthen or tone their muscles on three or more of the past seven days	43.7	44.0	no change

(continued)

(continued from previous page)

		2001	1991	direction of change*
26.	Percentage of students who attended physical education (PE) class one or more days during an average school week	39.2	51.9	decreased
27.	Percentage of students who had ever been taught about AIDS or HIV infection in school	87.8	82.7	increased
28.	Percentage of students who smoked cigarettes on 20 or more of the past 30 days	12.4	13.3	no change
29.	Percentage of students who smoked more than 10 cigarettes per day on the days that they smoked during the past 30 days	3.6	4.6	no change
30.	Percentage of students who attended physical education (PE) class daily	31.8	45.8	decreased

* Change over time is statistically significant for p< 0.05.
Source: Centers for Disease Control and Prevention, Youth Risk Behavior Surveillance System, http://www.cdc.gov/nccdphp/dash/ yrbs/index.htm

3.3 Arkansas, 1995 and 2001

(responses to the Youth Risk Behavior Surveillance System Survey questions, and direction of change at the 95 percent confidence level, Arkansas, 1995 and 2001)

		2001	1995	direction of change
1.	Of students who rode a motorcycle during the past 12 months, the percentage who never or rarely wore a motorcycle helmet	45.0	40.0	no change
2.	Of students who rode a bicycle during the past 12 months, the percentage who never or rarely wore a bicycle helmet	94.4	96.9	decreased
3.	Percentage of students who never or rarely wear a seat belt when riding in a car driven by someone else	23.0	26.2	no change
4.	Percentage of students who during the past 30 days rode one or more times in a car or other vehicle driven by someone who had been drinking alcohol	31.2	41.9	decreased
5.	Percentage of students who during the past 30 days drove a car or other vehicle one or more times when they had been drinking alcohol	15.8	18.0	no change
6.	Percentage of students who carried a weapon such as a gun, knife, or club on one or more of the past 30 days	22.1	26.1	decreased
7.	Percentage of students who carried a gun on one or more of the past 30 days	8.0	11.0	decreased
8.	Percentage of students who carried a weapon such as a gun, knife, or club on school property on one or more of the past 30 days	7.9	11.0	decreased
9.	Percentage of students who did not go to school on one or more of the past 30 days because they felt unsafe at school or on their way to or from school	7.6	5.4	no change
10.	Percentage of students who had been threatened or injured with a weapon on school property one or more times during the past 12 months	9.4	8.7	no change
11.	Percentage of students who were in a physical fight one or more times during the past 12 months	31.2	37.8	decreased
12.	Percentage of students who were injured in a physical fight one or more times during the past 12 months and had to be treated by a doctor or nurse	2.9	4.1	no change
13.	Percentage of students who were in a physical fight on school property one or more times during the past 12 months	12.7	17.0	decreased
14.	Percentage of students who seriously considered attempting suicide during the past 12 months	19.6	24.0	decreased
15.	Percentage of students who made a plan about how they would attempt suicide during the past 12 months	14.2	17.8	decreased
16.	Percentage of students who actually attempted suicide one or more times during the past 12 months	8.8	8.8	no change
17.	Percentage of students whose attempted suicide during the past 12 months resulted in an injury, poisoning, or overdose that had to be treated by a doctor or nurse	2.2	2.7	no change
18.	Percentage of students who ever tried cigarette smoking, even one or two puffs	71.6	74.4	no change
19.	Percentage of students who smoked a whole cigarette for the first time before age 13	28.0	29.0	no change
20.	Percentage of students who smoked cigarettes on one or more of the past 30 days	34.7	37.2	no change
21.	Percentage of students who smoked two or more cigarettes per day on the days they smoked during the past 30 days	25.9	26.7	no change
22.	Percentage of students who smoked cigarettes on school property on one or more of the past 30 days	11.0	13.9	no change
23.	Percentage of students who used chewing tobacco or snuff on one or more of the past 30 days	13.5	12.7	no change
24.	Percentage of students who used chewing tobacco or snuff on school property on one or more of the past 30 days	8.6	7.6	no change

(continued)

(continued from previous page)

	2001	1995	direction of change*
25. Percentage of students who had at least one drink of alcohol on one or more days during their life	79.6	79.3	no change
26. Percentage of students who had their first drink of alcohol other than a few sips before age 13	31.8	37.8	decreased
27. Percentage of students who had at least one drink of alcohol on one or more of the past 30 days	47.9	51.5	no change
28. Percentage of students who had five or more drinks of alcohol in a row, that is, within a couple of hours, on one or more of the past 30 days	30.0	32.2	no change
29. Percentage of students who had at least one drink of alcohol on school property on one or more of the past 30 days	5.5	5.7	no change
30. Percentage of students who used marijuana one or more times during their life	43.6	38.8	no change
31. Percentage of students who tried marijuana for the first time before age 13	11.6	7.4	increased
32. Percentage of students who used marijuana one or more times during the past 30 days	22.6	22.8	no change
33. Percentage of students who used marijuana on school property one or more times during the past 30 days	4.1	5.4	no change
34. Percentage of students who used any form of cocaine, including powder, crack, or freebase one or more times during their life	8.7	6.6	no change
35. Percentage of students who used any form of cocaine, including powder, crack, or freebase one or more times during the past 30 days	4.1	3.4	no change
36. Percentage of students who sniffed glue, breathed the contents of aerosol spray cans, or inhaled any paints or sprays to get high one or more times during their life	14.1	21.4	decreased
37. Percentage of students who took steroid pills or shots without a doctor's prescription one or more times during their life	6.9	4.9	increased
38. Percentage of students who used a needle to inject any illegal drug into their body one or more times during their life	2.3	2.2	no change
39. Percentage of students who were offered, sold, or given an illegal drug on school property by someone during the past 12 months	21.1	26.7	decreased
40. Percentage of students who had sexual intercourse	55.5	61.5	no change
41. Percentage of students who had sexual intercourse for the first time before age 13	9.8	13.7	decreased
42. Percentage of students who had sexual intercourse with four or more people during their life	20.5	25.8	decreased
43. Percentage of students who had sexual intercourse with one or more people during the past three months	40.2	44.9	no change
44. Of students who had sexual intercourse during the past three months, the percentage who drank alcohol or used drugs before last sexual intercourse	24.3	21.1	no change
45. Of students who had sexual intercourse during the past three months, the percentage who used a condom during last sexual intercourse	64.5	57.5	no change
46. Percentage of students who had been pregnant or gotten someone pregnant one or more times	5.7	7.1	no change
47. Percentage of students who described themselves as slightly or very overweight	33.5	27.4	increased
48. Percentage of students who were trying to lose weight	46.7	39.1	increased
49. Percentage of students who exercised to lose weight or to keep from gaining weight during the past 30 days	59.7	48.5	increased
50. Percentage of students who vomited or took laxatives to lose weight or to keep from gaining weight during the past 30 days	5.3	4.6	no change
51. Percentage of students who exercised or participated in physical activities for at least 20 minutes that made them sweat and breathe hard on three or more of the past seven days	61.5	58.6	no change

(continued)

(continued from previous page)

		2001	1991	direction of change[*]
52.	Percentage of students who did exercises to strengthen or tone their muscles on three or more of the past seven days	49.9	42.3	increased
53.	Percentage of students who attended physical education (PE) class one or more days during an average school week	36.5	32.4	no change
54.	Percentage of students who had ever been taught about AIDS or HIV infection in school	86.2	86.8	no change
55.	Percentage of students who smoked cigarettes on 20 or more of the past 30 days	18.8	18.3	no change
56.	Percentage of students who smoked more than 10 cigarettes per day on the days that they smoked during the past 30 days	6.7	7.1	no change
57.	Percentage of students who have ever had sexual intercourse but have not had sexual intercourse during the past three months	27.4	26.9	no change
58.	Percentage of students who attended physical education (PE) class daily	30.2	28.4	no change
59.	Percentage of students who have never had sexual intercourse, who have had sexual intercourse but not during the past three months, or who used a condom the last time they had sexual intercourse during the past three months	85.8	81.0	increased

* Change over time is statistically significant for p< 0.05.
Source: Centers for Disease Control and Prevention, Youth Risk Behavior Surveillance System. http://www.cdc.gov/nccdphp/dash/yrbs/index.htm

3.4 Idaho, 1991 and 2001

(responses to the Youth Risk Behavior Surveillance System Survey questions, and direction of change at the 95 percent confidence level, Idaho, 1991 and 2001)

		2001	1991	direction of change
1.	Of students who rode a motorcycle during the past 12 months, the percentage who never or rarely wore a motorcycle helmet	37.0	42.0	no change
2.	Of students who rode a bicycle during the past 12 months, the percentage who never or rarely wore a bicycle helmet	85.3	95.6	decreased
3.	Percentage of students who never or rarely wear a seat belt when riding in a car driven by someone else	13.6	32.9	decreased
4.	Percentage of students who during the past 30 days rode one or more times in a car or other vehicle driven by someone who had been drinking alcohol	28.7	35.3	decreased
5.	Percentage of students who during the past 30 days drove a car or other vehicle one or more times when they had been drinking alcohol	12.3	16.3	no change
6.	Percentage of students who were in a physical fight one or more times during the past 12 months	28.7	43.5	decreased
7.	Percentage of students who were injured in a physical fight one or more times during the past 12 months and had to be treated by a doctor or nurse	3.1	4.7	no change
8.	Percentage of students who seriously considered attempting suicide during the past 12 months	16.7	27.0	decreased
9.	Percentage of students who ever tried cigarette smoking, even one or two puffs	54.4	61.1	decreased
10.	Percentage of students who smoked a whole cigarette for the first time before age 13	19.2	24.5	decreased
11.	Percentage of students who smoked cigarettes on one or more of the past 30 days	19.1	23.3	no change
12.	Percentage of students who smoked two or more cigarettes per day on the days they smoked during the past 30 days	11.1	17.6	decreased
13.	Percentage of students who had at least one drink of alcohol on one or more days during their life	70.8	69.4	no change
14.	Percentage of students who had their first drink of alcohol other than a few sips before age 13	27.6	36.8	decreased
15.	Percentage of students who had at least one drink of alcohol on one or more of the past 30 days	40.6	42.2	no change
16.	Percentage of students who had five or more drinks of alcohol in a row, that is, within a couple of hours, on one or more of the past 30 days	27.2	29.9	no change
17.	Percentage of students who used marijuana one or more times during their life	34.7	25.3	increased
18.	Percentage of students who tried marijuana for the first time before age 13	8.3	8.2	no change
19.	Percentage of students who used marijuana one or more times during the past 30 days	17.5	10.2	increased
20.	Percentage of students who used any form of cocaine, including powder, crack, or freebase one or more times during their life	7.3	6.8	no change
21.	Percentage of students who took steroid pills or shots without a doctor's prescription one or more times during their life	3.6	3.7	no change
22.	Percentage of students who described themselves as slightly or very overweight	32.0	31.5	no change
23.	Percentage of students who were trying to lose weight	41.9	42.3	no change
24.	Percentage of students who did exercises to strengthen or tone their muscles on three or more of the past seven days	56.1	55.1	no change
25.	Percentage of students who attended physical education (PE) class one or more days during an average school week	43.1	45.5	no change

(continued)

(continued from previous page)

		2001	1991	direction of change*
26.	Percentage of students who had ever been taught about AIDS or HIV infection in school	85.3	73.8	increased
27.	Percentage of students who smoked cigarettes on 20 or more of the past 30 days	9.0	12.9	decreased
28.	Percentage of students who smoked more than 10 cigarettes per day on the days that they smoked during the past 30 days	1.8	4.4	decreased
29.	Percentage of students who attended physical education (PE) class daily	30.4	40.3	decreased

* Change over time is statistically significant for p< 0.05.
Source: Centers for Disease Control and Prevention, Youth Risk Behavior Surveillance System, http://www.cdc.gov/nccdphp/dash/yrbs/index.htm

3.5 Maine, 1995 and 2001

(responses to the Youth Risk Behavior Surveillance System Survey questions, and direction of change at the 95 percent confidence level, Maine, 1995 and 2001)

		2001	1995	direction of change*
1.	Of students who rode a motorcycle during the past 12 months, the percentage who never or rarely wore a motorcycle helmet	34.1	40.3	no change
2.	Of students who rode a bicycle during the past 12 months, the percentage who never or rarely wore a bicycle helmet	71.6	84.4	decreased
3.	Percentage of students who never or rarely wear a seat belt when riding in a car driven by someone else	14.9	21.3	decreased
4.	Percentage of students who during the past 30 days rode one or more times in a car or other vehicle driven by someone who had been drinking alcohol	27.4	34.2	decreased
5.	Percentage of students who during the past 30 days drove a car or other vehicle one or more times when they had been drinking alcohol	10.8	13.9	no change
6.	Percentage of students who carried a weapon such as a gun, knife, or club on one or more of the past 30 days	15.4	19.5	no change
7.	Percentage of students who carried a gun on one or more of the past 30 days	4.4	6.7	no change
8.	Percentage of students who carried a weapon such as a gun, knife, or club on school property on one or more of the past 30 days	5.2	9.9	decreased
9.	Percentage of students who did not go to school on one or more of the past 30 days because they felt unsafe at school or on their way to or from school	9.4	3.3	no change
10.	Percentage of students who had been threatened or injured with a weapon on school property one or more times during the past 12 months	8.7	6.6	no change
11.	Percentage of students who were in a physical fight one or more times during the past 12 months	30.9	33.0	no change
12.	Percentage of students who were injured in a physical fight one or more times during the past 12 months and had to be treated by a doctor or nurse	3.9	2.5	no change
13.	Percentage of students who were in a physical fight on school property one or more times during the past 12 months	11.3	14.2	no change
14.	Percentage of students who seriously considered attempting suicide during the past 12 months	18.6	25.1	decreased
15.	Percentage of students who made a plan about how they would attempt suicide during the past 12 months	16.5	18.5	no change
16.	Percentage of students who actually attempted suicide one or more times during the past 12 months	9.2	8.0	no change
17.	Percentage of students whose attempted suicide during the past 12 months resulted in an injury, poisoning, or overdose that had to be treated by a doctor or nurse	4.6	2.7	increased
18.	Percentage of students who smoked cigarettes on one or more of the past 30 days	24.8	37.8	decreased
19.	Percentage of students who smoked cigarettes on school property on one or more of the past 30 days	8.7	19.2	decreased
20.	Percentage of students who used chewing tobacco or snuff on one or more of the past 30 days	6.2	9.0	no change
21.	Percentage of students who used chewing tobacco or snuff on school property on one or more of the past 30 days	3.0	4.2	no change
22.	Percentage of students who had at least one drink of alcohol on one or more of the past 30 days	47.8	52.3	no change
23.	Percentage of students who had five or more drinks of alcohol in a row, that is, within a couple of hours, on one or more of the past 30 days	31.5	30.9	no change

(continued)

(continued from previous page)

		2001	1995	direction of change*
24.	Percentage of students who had at least one drink of alcohol on school property on one or more of the past 30 days	5.0	4.9	no change
25.	Percentage of students who used marijuana one or more times during the past 30 days	27.2	28.4	no change
26.	Percentage of students who used marijuana on school property one or more times during the past 30 days	6.9	8.3	no change
27.	Percentage of students who sniffed glue, breathed the contents of aerosol spray cans, or inhaled any paints or sprays to get high one or more times during their life	12.6	19.8	decreased
28.	Percentage of students who took steroid pills or shots without a doctor's prescription one or more times during their life	5.5	3.9	increased
29.	Percentage of students who used a needle to inject any illegal drug into their body one or more times during their life	2.5	1.5	increased
30.	Percentage of students who were offered, sold, or given an illegal drug on school property by someone during the past 12 months	32.4	36.0	no change
31.	Percentage of students who had sexual intercourse	46.3	49.0	no change
32.	Percentage of students who had sexual intercourse for the first time before age 13	4.4	4.3	no change
33.	Percentage of students who had sexual intercourse with four or more people during their life	10.1	12.8	no change
34.	Percentage of students who had sexual intercourse with one or more people during the past three months	34.6	35.0	no change
35.	Of students who had sexual intercourse during the past three months, the percentage who drank alcohol or used drugs before last sexual intercourse	24.6	24.1	no change
36.	Of students who had sexual intercourse during the past three months, the percentage who used a condom during last sexual intercourse	52.2	46.9	no change
37.	Percentage of students who described themselves as slightly or very overweight	32.8	31.1	no change
38.	Percentage of students who were trying to lose weight	43.8	42.5	no change
39.	Percentage of students who exercised to lose weight or to keep from gaining weight during the past 30 days	60.4	52.7	increased
40.	Percentage of students who vomited or took laxatives to lose weight or to keep from gaining weight during the past 30 days	6.2	5.1	no change
41.	Percentage of students who exercised or participated in physical activities for at least 20 minutes that made them sweat and breathe hard on three or more of the past seven days	65.9	63.1	no change
42.	Percentage of students who did exercises to strengthen or tone their muscles on three or more of the past seven days	47.5	44.5	no change
43.	Percentage of students who attended physical education (PE) class one or more days during an average school week	41.9	52.2	no change
44.	Percentage of students who had ever been taught about AIDS or HIV infection in school	93.5	92.5	no change
45.	Percentage of students who smoked cigarettes on 20 or more of the past 30 days	14.0	20.4	no change
46.	Percentage of students who have ever had sexual intercourse but have not had sexual intercourse during the past three months	24.7	28.7	no change
47.	Percentage of students who attended physical education (PE) class daily	4.8	10.3	no change
48.	Percentage of students who have never had sexual intercourse, who have had sexual intercourse but not during the past three months, or who used a condom the last time they had sexual intercourse during the past three months	83.7	81.7	no change

* Change over time is statistically significant for p< 0.05.
Source: Centers for Disease Control and Prevention, Youth Risk Behavior Surveillance System, http://www.cdc.gov/nccdphp/dash/yrbs/index.htm

3.6 Massachusetts, 1993 and 2001

(responses to the Youth Risk Behavior Surveillance System Survey questions, and direction of change at the 95 percent confidence level, Massachusetts, 1993 and 2001)

		2001	1993	direction of change[*]
1.	Of students who rode a motorcycle during the past 12 months, the percentage who never or rarely wore a motorcycle helmet	19.5	22.8	no change
2.	Of students who rode a bicycle during the past 12 months, the percentage who never or rarely wore a bicycle helmet	78.5	94.1	decreased
3.	Percentage of students who never or rarely wear a seat belt when riding in a car driven by someone else	20.7	41.0	decreased
4.	Percentage of students who during the past 30 days rode one or more times in a car or other vehicle driven by someone who had been drinking alcohol	30.5	32.5	no change
5.	Percentage of students who during the past 30 days drove a car or other vehicle one or more times when they had been drinking alcohol	12.2	11.5	no change
6.	Percentage of students who carried a weapon such as a gun, knife, or club on one or more of the past 30 days	13.2	20.3	decreased
7.	Percentage of students who carried a gun on one or more of the past 30 days	3.1	6.3	decreased
8.	Percentage of students who carried a weapon such as a gun, knife, or club on school property on one or more of the past 30 days	5.5	10.1	decreased
9.	Percentage of students who did not go to school on one or more of the past 30 days because they felt unsafe at school or on their way to or from school	8.1	5.3	no change
10.	Percentage of students who had been threatened or injured with a weapon on school property one or more times during the past 12 months	8.2	9.0	no change
11.	Percentage of students who were in a physical fight one or more times during the past 12 months	33.2	41.6	decreased
12.	Percentage of students who were injured in a physical fight one or more times during the past 12 months and had to be treated by a doctor or nurse	3.5	4.3	no change
13.	Percentage of students who were in a physical fight on school property one or more times during the past 12 months	11.5	15.4	decreased
14.	Percentage of students who seriously considered attempting suicide during the past 12 months	20.1	24.3	decreased
15.	Percentage of students who made a plan about how they would attempt suicide during the past 12 months	15.2	19.8	decreased
16.	Percentage of students who actually attempted suicide one or more times during the past 12 months	9.6	10.3	no change
17.	Percentage of students whose attempted suicide during the past 12 months resulted in an injury, poisoning, or overdose that had to be treated by a doctor or nurse	3.5	3.4	no change
18.	Percentage of students who ever tried cigarette smoking, even one or two puffs	61.9	67.8	decreased
19.	Percentage of students who smoked a whole cigarette for the first time before age 13	19.3	24.4	decreased
20.	Percentage of students who smoked cigarettes on one or more of the past 30 days	26.0	30.2	no change
21.	Percentage of students who smoked two or more cigarettes per day on the days they smoked during the past 30 days	16.9	21.8	decreased
22.	Percentage of students who smoked cigarettes on school property on one or more of the past 30 days	12.4	17.7	decreased
23.	Percentage of students who had at least one drink of alcohol on one or more days during their life	81.2	76.3	increased
24.	Percentage of students who had their first drink of alcohol other than a few sips before age 13	27.9	31.0	decreased
25.	Percentage of students who had at least one drink of alcohol on one or more of the past 30 days	53.0	47.4	increased

(continued)

(continued from previous page)

	2001	1993	direction of change[*]
26. Percentage of students who had five or more drinks of alcohol in a row, that is, within a couple of hours, on one or more of the past 30 days	32.7	27.5	increased
27. Percentage of students who had at least one drink of alcohol on school property on one or more of the past 30 days	5.5	5.4	no change
28. Percentage of students who used marijuana one or more times during their life	50.4	33.6	increased
29. Percentage of students who tried marijuana for the first time before age 13	11.9	6.8	increased
30. Percentage of students who used marijuana one or more times during the past 30 days	30.9	20.1	increased
31. Percentage of students who used marijuana on school property one or more times during the past 30 days	7.0	6.8	no change
32. Percentage of students who used any form of cocaine, including powder, crack, or freebase one or more times during their life	8.3	5.8	increased
33. Percentage of students who took steroid pills or shots without a doctor's prescription one or more times during their life	4.8	3.7	no change
34. Percentage of students who were offered, sold, or given an illegal drug on school property by someone during the past 12 months	34.2	31.4	no change
35. Percentage of students who had sexual intercourse	44.3	48.7	no change
36. Percentage of students who had sexual intercourse for the first time before age 13	5.3	8.3	decreased
37. Percentage of students who had sexual intercourse with four or more people during their life	12.0	14.5	no change
38. Percentage of students who had sexual intercourse with one or more people during the past three months	32.5	33.4	no change
39. Of students who had sexual intercourse during the past three months, the percentage who drank alcohol or used drugs before last sexual intercourse	22.7	21.6	no change
40. Of students who had sexual intercourse during the past three months, the percentage who used a condom during last sexual intercourse	58.1	51.8	increased
41. Percentage of students who had been pregnant or gotten someone pregnant one or more times	4.9	6.2	no change
42. Percentage of students who described themselves as slightly or very overweight	33.4	32.1	no change
43. Percentage of students who were trying to lose weight	46.9	41.2	increased
44. Percentage of students who exercised or participated in physical activities for at least 20 minutes that made them sweat and breathe hard on three or more of the past seven days	62.8	64.5	no change
45. Percentage of students who did exercises to strengthen or tone their muscles on three or more of the past seven days	46.7	47.4	no change
46. Percentage of students who attended physical education (PE) class one or more days during an average school week	68.0	80.2	decreased
47. Percentage of students who had ever been taught about AIDS or HIV infection in school	93.8	90.1	increased
48. Percentage of students who smoked cigarettes on 20 or more of the past 30 days	13.2	15.5	no change
49. Percentage of students who smoked more than 10 cigarettes per day on the days that they smoked during the past 30 days	4.3	6.2	decreased
50. Percentage of students who have ever had sexual intercourse but have not had sexual intercourse during the past three months	26.9	31.0	no change
51. Percentage of students who attended physical education (PE) class daily	17.7	11.7	no change
52. Percentage of students who have never had sexual intercourse, who have had sexual intercourse but not during the past three months, or who used a condom the last time they had sexual intercourse during the past three months	86.6	84.1	no change

* *Change over time is statistically significant for p< 0.05.*
Source: Centers for Disease Control and Prevention, Youth Risk Behavior Surveillance System, http://www.cdc.gov/nccdphp/dash/yrbs/index.htm

3.7 Mississippi, 1993 and 2001

(responses to the Youth Risk Behavior Surveillance System Survey questions, and direction of change at the 95 percent confidence level, Mississippi, 1993 and 2001)

		2001	1993	direction of change[*]
1.	Of students who rode a motorcycle during the past 12 months, the percentage who never or rarely wore a motorcycle helmet	48.5	56.0	no change
2.	Of students who rode a bicycle during the past 12 months, the percentage who never or rarely wore a bicycle helmet	95.3	98.0	decreased
3.	Percentage of students who never or rarely wear a seat belt when riding in a car driven by someone else	24.6	32.5	decreased
4.	Percentage of students who during the past 30 days rode one or more times in a car or other vehicle driven by someone who had been drinking alcohol	35.0	42.6	decreased
5.	Percentage of students who during the past 30 days drove a car or other vehicle one or more times when they had been drinking alcohol	13.7	19.7	decreased
6.	Percentage of students who carried a weapon such as a gun, knife, or club on one or more of the past 30 days	19.0	28.1	decreased
7.	Percentage of students who carried a gun on one or more of the past 30 days	7.8	11.9	decreased
8.	Percentage of students who carried a weapon such as a gun, knife, or club on school property on one or more of the past 30 days	6.5	13.5	decreased
9.	Percentage of students who did not go to school on one or more of the past 30 days because they felt unsafe at school or on their way to or from school	6.9	6.4	no change
10.	Percentage of students who had been threatened or injured with a weapon on school property one or more times during the past 12 months	8.1	8.2	no change
11.	Percentage of students who were in a physical fight one or more times during the past 12 months	31.8	39.3	decreased
12.	Percentage of students who were injured in a physical fight one or more times during the past 12 months and had to be treated by a doctor or nurse	3.2	3.1	no change
13.	Percentage of students who were in a physical fight on school property one or more times during the past 12 months	12.1	17.0	decreased
14.	Percentage of students who seriously considered attempting suicide during the past 12 months	14.6	24.8	decreased
15.	Percentage of students who made a plan about how they would attempt suicide during the past 12 months	11.7	18.4	decreased
16.	Percentage of students who actually attempted suicide one or more times during the past 12 months	6.3	9.8	decreased
17.	Percentage of students whose attempted suicide during the past 12 months resulted in an injury, poisoning, or overdose that had to be treated by a doctor or nurse	1.8	1.9	no change
18.	Percentage of students who ever tried cigarette smoking, even one or two puffs	67.8	75.9	decreased
19.	Percentage of students who smoked a whole cigarette for the first time before age 13	22.8	27.5	no change
20.	Percentage of students who smoked cigarettes on one or more of the past 30 days	23.6	27.6	no change
21.	Percentage of students who smoked two or more cigarettes per day on the days they smoked during the past 30 days	16.8	20.3	no change
22.	Percentage of students who smoked cigarettes on school property on one or more of the past 30 days	6.6	9.1	no change
23.	Percentage of students who had at least one drink of alcohol on one or more days during their life	76.2	78.2	no change
24.	Percentage of students who had their first drink of alcohol other than a few sips before age 13	32.2	34.0	no change
25.	Percentage of students who had at least one drink of alcohol on one or more of the past 30 days	41.7	47.0	decreased

(continued)

(continued from previous page)

	2001	1993	direction of change*
26. Percentage of students who had five or more drinks of alcohol in a row, that is, within a couple of hours, on one or more of the past 30 days	22.1	26.6	no change
27. Percentage of students who had at least one drink of alcohol on school property on one or more of the past 30 days	5.0	6.2	no change
28. Percentage of students who used marijuana one or more times during their life	37.5	20.8	increased
29. Percentage of students who tried marijuana for the first time before age 13	9.5	4.0	increased
30. Percentage of students who used marijuana one or more times during the past 30 days	17.4	8.8	increased
31. Percentage of students who used marijuana on school property one or more times during the past 30 days	3.3	1.8	no change
32. Percentage of students who used any form of cocaine, including powder, crack, or freebase one or more times during their life	4.7	2.0	increased
33. Percentage of students who used any form of cocaine, including powder, crack, or freebase one or more times during the past 30 days	2.3	0.7	increased
34. Percentage of students who took steroid pills or shots without a doctor's prescription one or more times during their life	4.4	1.8	increased
35. Percentage of students who were offered, sold, or given an illegal drug on school property by someone during the past 12 months	18.7	15.8	no change
36. Percentage of students who had sexual intercourse	60.6	69.0	decreased
37. Percentage of students who had sexual intercourse for the first time before age 13	14.0	18.6	no change
38. Percentage of students who had sexual intercourse with four or more people during their life	25.5	28.1	no change
39. Percentage of students who had sexual intercourse with one or more people during the past three months	44.9	50.4	no change
40. Of students who had sexual intercourse during the past three months, the percentage who drank alcohol or used drugs before last sexual intercourse	21.9	17.4	no change
41. Of students who had sexual intercourse during the past three months, the percentage who used a condom during last sexual intercourse	65.3	55.7	increased
42. Percentage of students who had been pregnant or gotten someone pregnant one or more times	5.9	9.2	no change
43. Percentage of students who described themselves as slightly or very overweight	26.4	31.9	decreased
44. Percentage of students who were trying to lose weight	40.7	38.1	no change
45. Percentage of students who exercised or participated in physical activities for at least 20 minutes that made them sweat and breathe hard on three or more of the past seven days	54.9	56.2	no change
46. Percentage of students who did exercises to strengthen or tone their muscles on three or more of the past seven days	47.2	39.3	increased
47. Percentage of students who attended physical education (PE) class one or more days during an average school week	31.7	21.6	increased
48. Percentage of students who had ever been taught about AIDS or HIV infection in school	85.3	75.1	increased
49. Percentage of students who smoked cigarettes on 20 or more of the past 30 days	11.5	13.6	no change
50. Percentage of students who smoked more than 10 cigarettes per day on the days that they smoked during the past 30 days	2.7	4.3	no change
51. Percentage of students who have ever had sexual intercourse but have not had sexual intercourse during the past three months	25.6	26.7	no change
52. Percentage of students who attended physical education (PE) class daily	22.7	17.9	no change
53. Percentage of students who have never had sexual intercourse, who have had sexual intercourse but not during the past three months, or who used a condom the last time they had sexual intercourse during the past three months	84.6	77.8	increased

* *Change over time is statistically significant for p< 0.05.*
Source: Centers for Disease Control and Prevention, Youth Risk Behavior Surveillance System, http://www.cdc.gov/nccdphp/dash/yrbs/index.htm

3.8 Missouri, 1995 and 2001

(responses to the Youth Risk Behavior Surveillance System Survey questions, and direction of change at the 95 percent confidence level, Missouri, 1995 and 2001)

		2001	1995	direction of change[*]
1.	Of students who rode a motorcycle during the past 12 months, the percentage who never or rarely wore a motorcycle helmet	34.7	43.6	no change
2.	Of students who rode a bicycle during the past 12 months, the percentage who never or rarely wore a bicycle helmet	89.8	96.0	decreased
3.	Percentage of students who never or rarely wear a seat belt when riding in a car driven by someone else	19.1	31.0	decreased
4.	Percentage of students who during the past 30 days rode one or more times in a car or other vehicle driven by someone who had been drinking alcohol	32.6	45.2	decreased
5.	Percentage of students who during the past 30 days drove a car or other vehicle one or more times when they had been drinking alcohol	15.9	21.4	decreased
6.	Percentage of students who carried a weapon such as a gun, knife, or club on one or more of the past 30 days	20.2	25.9	decreased
7.	Percentage of students who carried a gun on one or more of the past 30 days	8.8	12.0	no change
8.	Percentage of students who carried a weapon such as a gun, knife, or club on school property on one or more of the past 30 days	7.9	13.3	decreased
9.	Percentage of students who did not go to school on one or more of the past 30 days because they felt unsafe at school or on their way to or from school	5.6	4.1	no change
10.	Percentage of students who had been threatened or injured with a weapon on school property one or more times during the past 12 months	8.9	8.4	no change
11.	Percentage of students who were in a physical fight one or more times during the past 12 months	32.7	36.6	decreased
12.	Percentage of students who were injured in a physical fight one or more times during the past 12 months and had to be treated by a doctor or nurse	3.5	4.5	no change
13.	Percentage of students who were in a physical fight on school property one or more times during the past 12 months	12.0	15.4	decreased
14.	Percentage of students who seriously considered attempting suicide during the past 12 months	19.2	24.5	decreased
15.	Percentage of students who made a plan about how they would attempt suicide during the past 12 months	14.3	19.6	decreased
16.	Percentage of students who actually attempted suicide one or more times during the past 12 months	8.4	9.0	no change
17.	Percentage of students whose attempted suicide during the past 12 months resulted in an injury, poisoning, or overdose that had to be treated by a doctor or nurse	1.9	3.3	decreased
18.	Percentage of students who ever tried cigarette smoking, even one or two puffs	68.5	75.0	decreased
19.	Percentage of students who smoked a whole cigarette for the first time before age 13	25.7	32.2	decreased
20.	Percentage of students who smoked cigarettes on one or more of the past 30 days	30.3	39.8	decreased
21.	Percentage of students who smoked two or more cigarettes per day on the days they smoked during the past 30 days	24.3	30.1	decreased
22.	Percentage of students who smoked cigarettes on school property on one or more of the past 30 days	11.9	16.0	decreased
23.	Percentage of students who used chewing tobacco or snuff on one or more of the past 30 days	10.4	16.0	decreased
24.	Percentage of students who used chewing tobacco or snuff on school property on one or more of the past 30 days	6.4	9.5	no change

(continued)

	2001	1995	direction of change[*]
25. Percentage of students who had at least one drink of alcohol on one or more days during their life	80.1	82.7	no change
26. Percentage of students who had their first drink of alcohol other than a few sips before age 13	30.0	39.9	decreased
27. Percentage of students who had at least one drink of alcohol on one or more of the past 30 days	47.6	55.7	decreased
28. Percentage of students who had five or more drinks of alcohol in a row, that is, within a couple of hours, on one or more of the past 30 days	34.1	39.9	no change
29. Percentage of students who had at least one drink of alcohol on school property on one or more of the past 30 days	4.9	7.2	no change
30. Percentage of students who used marijuana one or more times during their life	43.3	36.3	increased
31. Percentage of students who tried marijuana for the first time before age 13	12.4	8.2	increased
32. Percentage of students who used marijuana one or more times during the past 30 days	24.4	21.8	no change
33. Percentage of students who used marijuana on school property one or more times during the past 30 days	4.6	6.3	no change
34. Percentage of students who used any form of cocaine, including powder, crack, or freebase one or more times during their life	8.6	7.4	no change
35. Percentage of students who used any form of cocaine, including powder, crack, or freebase one or more times during the past 30 days	3.4	4.2	no change
36. Percentage of students who sniffed glue, breathed the contents of aerosol spray cans, or inhaled any paints or sprays to get high one or more times during their life	12.7	20.0	decreased
37. Percentage of students who took steroid pills or shots without a doctor's prescription one or more times during their life	5.3	4.7	no change
38. Percentage of students who used a needle to inject any illegal drug into their body one or more times during their life	1.6	2.9	decreased
39. Percentage of students who were offered, sold, or given an illegal drug on school property by someone during the past 12 months	20.7	26.1	decreased
40. Percentage of students who had sexual intercourse	50.9	53.7	no change
41. Percentage of students who had sexual intercourse for the first time before age 13	6.5	8.9	no change
42. Percentage of students who had sexual intercourse with four or more people during their life	17.0	19.2	no change
43. Percentage of students who had sexual intercourse with one or more people during the past three months	38.8	39.1	no change
44. Of students who had sexual intercourse during the past three months, the percentage who drank alcohol or used drugs before last sexual intercourse	25.5	29.1	no change
45. Of students who had sexual intercourse during the past three months, the percentage who used a condom during last sexual intercourse	61.5	52.1	increased
46. Percentage of students who had been pregnant or gotten someone pregnant one or more times	5.1	6.2	no change
47. Percentage of students who described themselves as slightly or very overweight	31.9	30.7	no change
48. Percentage of students who were trying to lose weight	47.8	42.6	increased
49. Percentage of students who exercised to lose weight or to keep from gaining weight during the past 30 days	59.6	50.7	increased
50. Percentage of students who vomited or took laxatives to lose weight or to keep from gaining weight during the past 30 days	4.1	5.7	decreased
51. Percentage of students who exercised or participated in physical activities for at least 20 minutes that made them sweat and breathe hard on three or more of the past seven days	64.7	62.7	no change

(continued)

(continued from previous page)

	2001	1995	direction of change[*]
52. Percentage of students who did exercises to strengthen or tone their muscles on three or more of the past seven days	57.0	49.9	increased
53. Percentage of students who attended physical education (PE) class one or more days during an average school week	55.9	46.7	increased
54. Percentage of students who had ever been taught about AIDS or HIV infection in school	85.5	86.1	no change
55. Percentage of students who smoked cigarettes on 20 or more of the past 30 days	18.0	20.9	no change
56. Percentage of students who smoked more than 10 cigarettes per day on the days that they smoked during the past 30 days	5.5	8.6	decreased
57. Percentage of students who have ever had sexual intercourse but have not had sexual intercourse during the past three months	23.7	27.1	no change
58. Percentage of students who attended physical education (PE) class daily	30.0	33.9	no change
59. Percentage of students who have never had sexual intercourse, who have had sexual intercourse but not during the past three months, or who used a condom the last time they had sexual intercourse during the past three months	85.2	81.4	increased

* Change over time is statistically significant for p< 0.05.
Source: Centers for Disease Control and Prevention, Youth Risk Behavior Surveillance System. http://www.cdc.gov/nccdphp/dash/yrbs/index.htm

3.9 Montana, 1993 and 2001

(responses to the Youth Risk Behavior Surveillance System Survey questions, and direction of change at the 95 percent confidence level, Montana, 1993 and 2001)

		2001	1993	direction of change*
1.	Of students who rode a motorcycle during the past 12 months, the percentage who never or rarely wore a motorcycle helmet	44.2	51.0	decreased
2.	Of students who rode a bicycle during the past 12 months, the percentage who never or rarely wore a bicycle helmet	85.1	94.5	decreased
3.	Percentage of students who never or rarely wear a seat belt when riding in a car driven by someone else	19.8	30.0	decreased
4.	Percentage of students who during the past 30 days rode one or more times in a car or other vehicle driven by someone who had been drinking alcohol	39.3	45.9	decreased
5.	Percentage of students who during the past 30 days drove a car or other vehicle one or more times when they had been drinking alcohol	21.8	24.1	no change
6.	Percentage of students who carried a weapon such as a gun, knife, or club on one or more of the past 30 days	21.4	25.6	decreased
7.	Percentage of students who carried a gun on one or more of the past 30 days	9.0	12.3	decreased
8.	Percentage of students who carried a weapon such as a gun, knife, or club on school property on one or more of the past 30 days	8.7	13.7	decreased
9.	Percentage of students who did not go to school on one or more of the past 30 days because they felt unsafe at school or on their way to or from school	5.5	2.5	increased
10.	Percentage of students who had been threatened or injured with a weapon on school property one or more times during the past 12 months	8.5	6.7	no change
11.	Percentage of students who were in a physical fight one or more times during the past 12 months	31.6	41.9	decreased
12.	Percentage of students who were injured in a physical fight one or more times during the past 12 months and had to be treated by a doctor or nurse	3.6	3.1	no change
13.	Percentage of students who were in a physical fight on school property one or more times during the past 12 months	12.2	17.2	decreased
14.	Percentage of students who seriously considered attempting suicide during the past 12 months	19.4	25.1	decreased
15.	Percentage of students who made a plan about how they would attempt suicide during the past 12 months	16.3	20.8	decreased
16.	Percentage of students who actually attempted suicide one or more times during the past 12 months	10.4	8.9	no change
17.	Percentage of students whose attempted suicide during the past 12 months resulted in an injury, poisoning, or overdose that had to be treated by a doctor or nurse	3.7	3.1	no change
18.	Percentage of students who ever tried cigarette smoking, even one or two puffs	66.5	69.7	no change
19.	Percentage of students who smoked a whole cigarette for the first time before age 13	25.0	26.7	no change
20.	Percentage of students who smoked cigarettes on one or more of the past 30 days	28.5	30.7	no change
21.	Percentage of students who smoked two or more cigarettes per day on the days they smoked during the past 30 days	20.2	19.5	no change
22.	Percentage of students who smoked cigarettes on school property on one or more of the past 30 days	10.4	11.9	no change
23.	Percentage of students who had at least one drink of alcohol on one or more days during their life	82.9	83.2	no change
24.	Percentage of students who had their first drink of alcohol other than a few sips before age 13	35.1	40.0	decreased

(continued)

(continued from previous page)

	2001	1993	direction of change[*]
25. Percentage of students who had at least one drink of alcohol on one or more of the past 30 days	54.1	55.7	no change
26. Percentage of students who had five or more drinks of alcohol in a row, that is, within a couple of hours, on one or more of the past 30 days	41.4	41.4	no change
27. Percentage of students who had at least one drink of alcohol on school property on one or more of the past 30 days	6.9	8.8	no change
28. Percentage of students who used marijuana one or more times during their life	46.7	26.8	increased
29. Percentage of students who tried marijuana for the first time before age 13	12.3	7.6	increased
30. Percentage of students who used marijuana one or more times during the past 30 days	27.1	13.6	increased
31. Percentage of students who used marijuana on school property one or more times during the past 30 days	7.7	5.1	increased
32. Percentage of students who used any form of cocaine, including powder, crack, or freebase one or more times during their life	9.4	5.1	increased
33. Percentage of students who used any form of cocaine, including powder, crack, or freebase one or more times during the past 30 days	4.0	2.2	increased
34. Percentage of students who took steroid pills or shots without a doctor's prescription one or more times during their life	5.3	4.1	no change
35. Percentage of students who were offered, sold, or given an illegal drug on school property by someone during the past 12 months	29.5	22.0	increased
36. Percentage of students who had sexual intercourse	43.9	51.0	decreased
37. Percentage of students who had sexual intercourse for the first time before age 13	5.3	8.5	decreased
38. Percentage of students who had sexual intercourse with four or more people during their life	13.8	17.9	decreased
39. Percentage of students who had sexual intercourse with one or more people during the past three months	30.7	33.7	no change
40. Of students who had sexual intercourse during the past three months, the percentage who drank alcohol or used drugs before last sexual intercourse	32.0	34.7	no change
41. Of students who had sexual intercourse during the past three months, the percentage who used a condom during last sexual intercourse	57.5	51.5	no change
42. Percentage of students who had been pregnant or gotten someone pregnant one or more times	4.2	5.1	no change
43. Percentage of students who described themselves as slightly or very overweight	30.1	34.7	decreased
44. Percentage of students who were trying to lose weight	42.0	41.6	no change
45. Percentage of students who exercised or participated in physical activities for at least 20 minutes that made them sweat and breathe hard on three or more of the past seven days	67.6	67.8	no change
46. Percentage of students who did exercises to strengthen or tone their muscles on three or more of the past seven days	58.3	55.4	no change
47. Percentage of students who attended physical education (PE) class one or more days during an average school week	52.3	53.5	no change
48. Percentage of students who had ever been taught about AIDS or HIV infection in school	90.2	91.6	no change
49. Percentage of students who smoked cigarettes on 20 or more of the past 30 days	14.9	12.7	no change
50. Percentage of students who smoked more than 10 cigarettes per day on the days that they smoked during the past 30 days	3.7	4.0	no change
51. Percentage of students who have ever had sexual intercourse but have not had sexual intercourse during the past three months	30.2	34.2	no change

(continued)

(continued from previous page)

	2001	1993	direction of change*
52. Percentage of students who attended physical education (PE) class daily	31.3	38.3	no change
53. Percentage of students who have never had sexual intercourse, who have had sexual intercourse but not during the past three months, or who used a condom the last time they had sexual intercourse during the past three months	87.3	83.9	increased

* Change over time is statistically significant for p< 0.05.

Source: Centers for Disease Control and Prevention, Youth Risk Behavior Surveillance System, http://www.cdc.gov/nccdphp/dash/ yrbs/index.htm

3.10 Nevada, 1993 and 2001

(responses to the Youth Risk Behavior Surveillance System Survey questions, and direction of change at the 95 percent confidence level. Nevada, 1993 and 2001)

		2001	1993	direction of change*
1.	Percentage of students who during the past 30 days rode one or more times in a car or other vehicle driven by someone who had been drinking alcohol	29.9	35.2	decreased
2.	Percentage of students who during the past 30 days drove a car or other vehicle one or more times when they had been drinking alcohol	13.1	12.1	no change
3.	Percentage of students who carried a weapon such as a gun, knife, or club on one or more of the past 30 days	16.0	24.4	decreased
4.	Percentage of students who carried a weapon such as a gun, knife, or club on school property on one or more of the past 30 days	6.9	12.0	decreased
5.	Percentage of students who did not go to school on one or more of the past 30 days because they felt unsafe at school or on their way to or from school	16.9	7.8	increased
6.	Percentage of students who had been threatened or injured with a weapon on school property one or more times during the past 12 months	8.8	10.3	no change
7.	Percentage of students who were in a physical fight one or more times during the past 12 months	35.6	42.1	decreased
8.	Percentage of students who were in a physical fight on school property one or more times during the past 12 months	13.0	20.1	decreased
9.	Percentage of students who seriously considered attempting suicide during the past 12 months	19.6	26.8	decreased
10.	Percentage of students who made a plan about how they would attempt suicide during the past 12 months	16.4	21.2	decreased
11.	Percentage of students who actually attempted suicide one or more times during the past 12 months	10.8	11.5	no change
12.	Percentage of students whose attempted suicide during the past 12 months resulted in an injury, poisoning, or overdose that had to be treated by a doctor or nurse	3.8	3.3	no change
13.	Percentage of students who ever tried cigarette smoking, even one or two puffs	66.5	68.2	no change
14.	Percentage of students who smoked a whole cigarette for the first time before age 13	23.3	28.2	decreased
15.	Percentage of students who smoked cigarettes on one or more of the past 30 days	25.2	29.9	no change
16.	Percentage of students who smoked two or more cigarettes per day on the days they smoked during the past 30 days	15.9	20.8	decreased
17.	Percentage of students who smoked cigarettes on school property on one or more of the past 30 days	10.3	15.1	decreased
18.	Percentage of students who had at least one drink of alcohol on one or more days during their life	80.1	77.3	no change
19.	Percentage of students who had their first drink of alcohol other than a few sips before age 13	33.0	37.6	no change
20.	Percentage of students who had at least one drink of alcohol on one or more of the past 30 days	47.5	49.2	no change
21.	Percentage of students who had five or more drinks of alcohol in a row, that is, within a couple of hours, on one or more of the past 30 days	32.4	31.8	no change
22.	Percentage of students who had at least one drink of alcohol on school property on one or more of the past 30 days	8.1	6.2	no change
23.	Percentage of students who used marijuana one or more times during their life	50.8	35.9	increased
24.	Percentage of students who tried marijuana for the first time before age 13	17.8	8.9	increased

(continued)

(continued from previous page)

		2001	1993	direction of change*
25.	Percentage of students who used marijuana one or more times during the past 30 days	26.6	19.4	increased
26.	Percentage of students who used marijuana on school property one or more times during the past 30 days	7.7	7.8	no change
27.	Percentage of students who used any form of cocaine, including powder, crack, or freebase one or more times during their life	11.9	8.1	increased
28.	Percentage of students who used any form of cocaine, including powder, crack, or freebase one or more times during the past 30 days	5.5	3.7	no change
29.	Percentage of students who took steroid pills or shots without a doctor's prescription one or more times during their life	6.4	2.7	increased
30.	Percentage of students who were offered, sold, or given an illegal drug on school property by someone during the past 12 months	35.7	29.8	increased
31.	Percentage of students who had sexual intercourse	49.1	58.4	decreased
32.	Percentage of students who had sexual intercourse for the first time before age 13	8.3	9.7	no change
33.	Percentage of students who had sexual intercourse with four or more people during their life	16.6	23.0	decreased
34.	Percentage of students who had sexual intercourse with one or more people during the past three months	34.6	39.7	no change
35.	Of students who had sexual intercourse during the past three months, the percentage who drank alcohol or used drugs before last sexual intercourse	24.4	23.8	no change
36.	Of students who had sexual intercourse during the past three months, the percentage who used a condom during last sexual intercourse	59.1	50.3	increased
37.	Percentage of students who had been pregnant or gotten someone pregnant one or more times	5.8	9.7	decreased
38.	Percentage of students who described themselves as slightly or very overweight	29.5	31.3	no change
39.	Percentage of students who were trying to lose weight	47.5	39.8	increased
40.	Percentage of students who exercised or participated in physical activities for at least 20 minutes that made them sweat and breathe hard on three or more of the past seven days	66.3	68.3	no change
41.	Percentage of students who had ever been taught about AIDS or HIV infection in school	86.5	82.0	increased
42.	Percentage of students who smoked cigarettes on 20 or more of the past 30 days	11.3	14.0	no change
43.	Percentage of students who smoked more than 10 cigarettes per day on the days that they smoked during the past 30 days	2.7	3.5	no change
44.	Percentage of students who have ever had sexual intercourse but have not had sexual intercourse during the past three months	29.3	32.0	no change
45.	Percentage of students who have never had sexual intercourse, who have had sexual intercourse but not during the past three months, or who used a condom the last time they had sexual intercourse during the past three months	86.2	80.4	increased

* Change over time is statistically significant for p< 0.05.
Source: Centers for Disease Control and Prevention, Youth Risk Behavior Surveillance System, http://www.cdc.gov/nccdphp/dash/yrbs/index.htm

3.11 North Carolina, 1993 and 2001

(responses to the Youth Risk Behavior Surveillance System Survey questions, and direction of change at the 95 percent confidence level, North Carolina, 1993 and 2001)

		2001	1993	direction of change*
1.	Of students who rode a motorcycle during the past 12 months, the percentage who never or rarely wore a motorcycle helmet	34.9	39.4	no change
2.	Of students who rode a bicycle during the past 12 months, the percentage who never or rarely wore a bicycle helmet	87.1	95.6	decreased
3.	Percentage of students who never or rarely wear a seat belt when riding in a car driven by someone else	9.5	15.2	decreased
4.	Percentage of students who during the past 30 days rode one or more times in a car or other vehicle driven by someone who had been drinking alcohol	23.9	33.3	decreased
5.	Percentage of students who during the past 30 days drove a car or other vehicle one or more times when they had been drinking alcohol	9.3	12.7	decreased
6.	Percentage of students who carried a weapon such as a gun, knife, or club on one or more of the past 30 days	18.3	26.8	decreased
7.	Percentage of students who carried a weapon such as a gun, knife, or club on school property on one or more of the past 30 days	4.8	13.9	decreased
8.	Percentage of students who did not go to school on one or more of the past 30 days because they felt unsafe at school or on their way to or from school	9.2	5.3	increased
9.	Percentage of students who had been threatened or injured with a weapon on school property one or more times during the past 12 months	7.6	9.5	no change
10.	Percentage of students who were in a physical fight one or more times during the past 12 months	29.0	37.8	decreased
11.	Percentage of students who were injured in a physical fight one or more times during the past 12 months and had to be treated by a doctor or nurse	2.8	3.7	no change
12.	Percentage of students who were in a physical fight on school property one or more times during the past 12 months	10.7	14.5	decreased
13.	Percentage of students who seriously considered attempting suicide during the past 12 months	18.1	24.2	decreased
14.	Percentage of students who smoked a whole cigarette for the first time before age 13	26.5	29.8	no change
15.	Percentage of students who smoked cigarettes on one or more of the past 30 days	27.8	29.3	no change
16.	Percentage of students who smoked two or more cigarettes per day on the days they smoked during the past 30 days	19.1	20.0	no change
17.	Percentage of students who smoked cigarettes on school property on one or more of the past 30 days	11.2	14.9	decreased
18.	Percentage of students who had their first drink of alcohol other than a few sips before age 13	24.7	30.4	decreased
19.	Percentage of students who had at least one drink of alcohol on one or more of the past 30 days	38.2	43.7	decreased
20.	Percentage of students who had five or more drinks of alcohol in a row, that is, within a couple of hours, on one or more of the past 30 days	20.7	23.0	no change
21.	Percentage of students who had at least one drink of alcohol on school property on one or more of the past 30 days	4.3	5.4	no change
22.	Percentage of students who used marijuana one or more times during their life	40.3	29.0	increased
23.	Percentage of students who tried marijuana for the first time before age 13	10.5	7.1	increased
24.	Percentage of students who used marijuana one or more times during the past 30 days	20.8	14.8	increased

(continued)

(continued from previous page)

	2001	1993	direction of change*
25. Percentage of students who used marijuana on school property one or more times during the past 30 days	4.7	4.8	no change
26. Percentage of students who used any form of cocaine, including powder, crack, or freebase one or more times during their life	6.7	4.4	increased
27. Percentage of students who used any form of cocaine, including powder, crack, or freebase one or more times during the past 30 days	2.7	2.1	no change
28. Percentage of students who took steroid pills or shots without a doctor's prescription one or more times during their life	5.0	3.6	increased
29. Percentage of students who were offered, sold, or given an illegal drug on school property by someone during the past 12 months	32.8	28.9	increased
30. Percentage of students who described themselves as slightly or very overweight	29.2	33.4	decreased
31. Percentage of students who were trying to lose weight	42.8	39.8	increased
32. Percentage of students who exercised or participated in physical activities for at least 20 minutes that made them sweat and breathe hard on three or more of the past seven days	64.0	59.1	increased
33. Percentage of students who attended physical education (PE) class one or more days during an average school week	47.1	47.5	no change
34. Percentage of students who had ever been taught about AIDS or HIV infection in school	91.1	91.1	no change
35. Percentage of students who smoked cigarettes on 20 or more of the past 30 days	14.5	14.1	no change
36. Percentage of students who smoked more than 10 cigarettes per day on the days that they smoked during the past 30 days	3.8	5.2	no change
37. Percentage of students who attended physical education (PE) class daily	34.4	35.0	no change

* Change over time is statistically significant for $p < 0.05$.

Source: Centers for Disease Control and Prevention, Youth Risk Behavior Surveillance System, http://www.cdc.gov/nccdphp/dash/yrbs/index.htm

3.12 North Dakota, 1995 and 2001

(responses to the Youth Risk Behavior Surveillance System Survey questions, and direction of change at the 95 percent confidence level, North Dakota, 1995 and 2001)

		2001	1995	direction of change*
1.	Of students who rode a motorcycle during the past 12 months, the percentage who never or rarely wore a motorcycle helmet	52.0	56.1	no change
2.	Of students who rode a bicycle during the past 12 months, the percentage who never or rarely wore a bicycle helmet	95.5	98.2	decreased
3.	Percentage of students who during the past 30 days rode one or more times in a car or other vehicle driven by someone who had been drinking alcohol	43.5	48.7	decreased
4.	Percentage of students who during the past 30 days drove a car or other vehicle one or more times when they had been drinking alcohol	26.8	32.5	decreased
5.	Percentage of students who carried a weapon such as a gun, knife, or club on school property on one or more of the past 30 days	6.4	9.7	decreased
6.	Percentage of students who had been threatened or injured with a weapon on school property one or more times during the past 12 months	8.9	6.0	increased
7.	Percentage of students who were in a physical fight one or more times during the past 12 months	28.2	29.8	no change
8.	Percentage of students who were injured in a physical fight one or more times during the past 12 months and had to be treated by a doctor or nurse	2.8	3.3	no change
9.	Percentage of students who were in a physical fight on school property one or more times during the past 12 months	11.1	11.6	no change
10.	Percentage of students who seriously considered attempting suicide during the past 12 months	19.0	25.4	decreased
11.	Percentage of students who made a plan about how they would attempt suicide during the past 12 months	13.9	19.9	decreased
12.	Percentage of students who actually attempted suicide one or more times during the past 12 months	7.5	7.5	no change
13.	Percentage of students whose attempted suicide during the past 12 months resulted in an injury, poisoning, or overdose that had to be treated by a doctor or nurse	2.3	2.6	no change
14.	Percentage of students who smoked cigarettes on one or more of the past 30 days	35.3	39.6	no change
15.	Percentage of students who smoked two or more cigarettes per day on the days they smoked during the past 30 days	25.4	27.1	no change
16.	Percentage of students who smoked cigarettes on school property on one or more of the past 30 days	12.2	14.8	no change
17.	Percentage of students who used chewing tobacco or snuff on school property on one or more of the past 30 days	6.9	8.3	no change
18.	Percentage of students who had their first drink of alcohol other than a few sips before age 13	29.8	32.3	no change
19.	Percentage of students who had at least one drink of alcohol on one or more of the past 30 days	59.2	60.7	no change
20.	Percentage of students who had at least one drink of alcohol on school property on one or more of the past 30 days	6.4	8.6	no change
21.	Percentage of students who tried marijuana for the first time before age 13	6.9	5.3	no change
22.	Percentage of students who used marijuana one or more times during the past 30 days	22.0	14.9	increased
23.	Percentage of students who used marijuana on school property one or more times during the past 30 days	6.0	5.5	no change

(continued)

(continued from previous page)

	2001	1995	direction of change[*]
24. Percentage of students who used any form of cocaine, including powder, crack, or freebase one or more times during their life	9.3	5.2	increased
25. Percentage of students who took steroid pills or shots without a doctor's prescription one or more times during their life	4.3	4.7	no change
26. Percentage of students who used a needle to inject any illegal drug into their body one or more times during their life	2.4	3.7	decreased
27. Percentage of students who were offered, sold, or given an illegal drug on school property by someone during the past 12 months	27.3	27.6	no change
28. Percentage of students who had sexual intercourse for the first time before age 13	4.4	5.9	no change
29. Percentage of students who had sexual intercourse with four or more people during their life	12.1	12.3	no change
30. Percentage of students who had sexual intercourse with one or more people during the past three months	30.8	29.0	no change
31. Of students who had sexual intercourse during the past three months, the percentage who drank alcohol or used drugs before last sexual intercourse	33.5	31.9	no change
32. Of students who had sexual intercourse during the past three months, the percentage who used a condom during last sexual intercourse	59.1	48.5	increased
33. Percentage of students who described themselves as slightly or very overweight	31.9	34.6	no change
34. Percentage of students who were trying to lose weight	47.5	46.2	no change
35. Percentage of students who exercised to lose weight or to keep from gaining weight during the past 30 days	60.8	56.1	no change
36. Percentage of students who vomited or took laxatives to lose weight or to keep from gaining weight during the past 30 days	6.1	6.9	no change
37. Percentage of students who exercised or participated in physical activities for at least 20 minutes that made them sweat and breathe hard on three or more of the past seven days	60.4	59.7	no change
38. Percentage of students who attended physical education (PE) class one or more days during an average school week	48.0	52.6	no change
39. Percentage of students who had ever been taught about AIDS or HIV infection in school	89.4	87.5	no change
40. Percentage of students who smoked cigarettes on 20 or more of the past 30 days	18.7	19.8	no change
41. Percentage of students who smoked more than 10 cigarettes per day on the days that they smoked during the past 30 days	5.0	8.4	decreased
42. Percentage of students who have ever had sexual intercourse but have not had sexual intercourse during the past three months	26.7	26.7	no change
43. Percentage of students who attended physical education (PE) class daily	31.6	31.1	no change
44. Percentage of students who have never had sexual intercourse, who have had sexual intercourse but not during the past three months, or who used a condom the last time they had sexual intercourse during the past three months	87.6	85.2	no change

[*] Change over time is statistically significant for $p < 0.05$.
Source: Centers for Disease Control and Prevention, Youth Risk Behavior Surveillance System, http://www.cdc.gov/nccdphp/dash/yrbs/index.htm

3.13 South Dakota, 1991 and 2001

(responses to the Youth Risk Behavior Surveillance System Survey questions, and direction of change at the 95 percent confidence level. South Dakota, 1991 and 2001)

		2001	1991	direction of change[*]
1.	Of students who rode a bicycle during the past 12 months, the percentage who never or rarely wore a bicycle helmet	93.1	98.1	decreased
2.	Percentage of students who never or rarely wear a seat belt when riding in a car driven by someone else	27.4	54.1	decreased
3.	Percentage of students who during the past 30 days rode one or more times in a car or other vehicle driven by someone who had been drinking alcohol	38.1	49.9	decreased
4.	Percentage of students who during the past 30 days drove a car or other vehicle one or more times when they had been drinking alcohol	21.9	27.9	no change
5.	Percentage of students who were in a physical fight one or more times during the past 12 months	30.8	40.4	decreased
6.	Percentage of students who were injured in a physical fight one or more times during the past 12 months and had to be treated by a doctor or nurse	2.4	4.1	no change
7.	Percentage of students who seriously considered attempting suicide during the past 12 months	19.3	29.9	decreased
8.	Percentage of students who made a plan about how they would attempt suicide during the past 12 months	17.7	18.3	no change
9.	Percentage of students who actually attempted suicide one or more times during the past 12 months	13.1	8.2	increased
10.	Percentage of students who ever tried cigarette smoking, even one or two puffs	67.4	69.4	no change
11.	Percentage of students who smoked a whole cigarette for the first time before age 13	25.8	22.8	no change
12.	Percentage of students who smoked cigarettes on one or more of the past 30 days	33.1	30.9	no change
13.	Percentage of students who smoked two or more cigarettes per day on the days they smoked during the past 30 days	23.7	22.9	no change
14.	Percentage of students who had at least one drink of alcohol on one or more days during their life	81.5	83.8	no change
15.	Percentage of students who had their first drink of alcohol other than a few sips before age 13	31.6	33.6	no change
16.	Percentage of students who had at least one drink of alcohol on one or more of the past 30 days	50.2	57.9	no change
17.	Percentage of students who had five or more drinks of alcohol in a row, that is, within a couple of hours, on one or more of the past 30 days	36.5	41.0	no change
18.	Percentage of students who used marijuana one or more times during their life	36.3	21.5	increased
19.	Percentage of students who tried marijuana for the first time before age 13	8.8	6.8	no change
20.	Percentage of students who used marijuana one or more times during the past 30 days	18.4	9.6	increased
21.	Percentage of students who used any form of cocaine, including powder, crack, or freebase one or more times during their life	7.6	5.2	no change
22.	Percentage of students who used any form of cocaine, including powder, crack, or freebase one or more times during the past 30 days	3.1	1.8	no change
23.	Percentage of students who took steroid pills or shots without a doctor's prescription one or more times during their life	5.4	3.9	no change
24.	Percentage of students who had sexual intercourse	40.0	48.3	no change
25.	Percentage of students who had sexual intercourse for the first time before age 13	3.5	7.1	decreased

(continued)

(continued from previous page)

	2001	1991	direction of change[*]
26. Percentage of students who had sexual intercourse with four or more people during their life	11.5	16.0	no change
27. Percentage of students who had sexual intercourse with one or more people during the past three months	29.4	34.0	no change
28. Of students who had sexual intercourse during the past three months, the percentage who drank alcohol or used drugs before last sexual intercourse	28.5	37.1	decreased
29. Of students who had sexual intercourse during the past three months, the percentage who used a condom during last sexual intercourse	58.3	48.5	no change
30. Percentage of students who had been pregnant or gotten someone pregnant one or more times	3.8	6.0	no change
31. Percentage of students who described themselves as slightly or very overweight	30.9	35.2	decreased
32. Percentage of students who were trying to lose weight	46.3	45.8	no change
33. Percentage of students who did exercises to strengthen or tone their muscles on three or more of the past seven days	51.6	47.8	no change
34. Percentage of students who attended physical education (PE) class one or more days during an average school week	22.1	23.9	no change
35. Percentage of students who had ever been taught about AIDS or HIV infection in school	87.0	88.4	no change
36. Percentage of students who smoked cigarettes on 20 or more of the past 30 days	17.3	16.2	no change
37. Percentage of students who smoked more than 10 cigarettes per day on the days that they smoked during the past 30 days	3.6	3.8	no change
38. Percentage of students who have ever had sexual intercourse but have not had sexual intercourse during the past three months	27.0	29.7	no change
39. Percentage of students who attended physical education (PE) class daily	12.0	15.3	no change
40. Percentage of students who have never had sexual intercourse, who have had sexual intercourse but not during the past three months, or who used a condom the last time they had sexual intercourse during the past three months	87.9	82.7	no change

* Change over time is statistically significant for p< 0.05.
Source: Centers for Disease Control and Prevention, Youth Risk Behavior Surveillance System, http://www.cdc.gov/nccdphp/dash/yrbs/index.htm

3.14 Utah, 1991 and 2001

(responses to the Youth Risk Behavior Surveillance System Survey questions, and direction of change at the 95 percent confidence level. Utah, 1991 and 2001)

		2001	1991	direction of change*
1.	Of students who rode a motorcycle during the past 12 months, the percentage who never or rarely wore a motorcycle helmet	40.8	55.0	decreased
2.	Of students who rode a bicycle during the past 12 months, the percentage who never or rarely wore a bicycle helmet	84.5	93.8	decreased
3.	Percentage of students who never or rarely wear a seat belt when riding in a car driven by someone else	7.5	26.6	decreased
4.	Percentage of students who during the past 30 days rode one or more times in a car or other vehicle driven by someone who had been drinking alcohol	17.1	24.8	decreased
5.	Percentage of students who during the past 30 days drove a car or other vehicle one or more times when they had been drinking alcohol	6.4	8.9	no change
6.	Percentage of students who carried a weapon such as a gun, knife, or club on one or more of the past 30 days	16.8	24.3	decreased
7.	Percentage of students who were in a physical fight one or more times during the past 12 months	27.9	41.8	decreased
8.	Percentage of students who were injured in a physical fight one or more times during the past 12 months and had to be treated by a doctor or nurse	3.7	4.7	no change
9.	Percentage of students who seriously considered attempting suicide during the past 12 months	19.4	25.5	decreased
10.	Percentage of students who made a plan about how they would attempt suicide during the past 12 months	14.5	16.5	no change
11.	Percentage of students who actually attempted suicide one or more times during the past 12 months	9.2	7.1	increased
12.	Percentage of students whose attempted suicide during the past 12 months resulted in an injury, poisoning, or overdose that had to be treated by a doctor or nurse	3.9	2.2	no change
13.	Percentage of students who ever tried cigarette smoking, even one or two puffs	30.5	48.8	decreased
14.	Percentage of students who smoked a whole cigarette for the first time before age 13	12.2	18.6	decreased
15.	Percentage of students who smoked cigarettes on one or more of the past 30 days	8.3	16.8	decreased
16.	Percentage of students who smoked two or more cigarettes per day on the days they smoked during the past 30 days	5.1	11.5	decreased
17.	Percentage of students who had at least one drink of alcohol on one or more days during their life	40.6	50.3	decreased
18.	Percentage of students who had at least one drink of alcohol on one or more of the past 30 days	17.9	26.6	decreased
19.	Percentage of students who had five or more drinks of alcohol in a row, that is, within a couple of hours, on one or more of the past 30 days	10.9	16.6	decreased
20.	Percentage of students who used marijuana one or more times during their life	19.7	19.1	no change
21.	Percentage of students who tried marijuana for the first time before age 13	4.5	6.5	no change
22.	Percentage of students who used marijuana one or more times during the past 30 days	9.7	8.6	no change
23.	Percentage of students who used any form of cocaine, including powder, crack, or freebase one or more times during their life	4.1	5.2	no change
24.	Percentage of students who took steroid pills or shots without a doctor's prescription one or more times during their life	4.2	3.1	no change
25.	Percentage of students who described themselves as slightly or very overweight	28.7	30.0	no change

(continued)

(continued from previous page)

		2001	1991	direction of change[*]
26.	Percentage of students who were trying to lose weight	44.1	40.3	no change
27.	Percentage of students who did exercises to strengthen or tone their muscles on three or more of the past seven days	54.4	51.6	no change
28.	Percentage of students who attended physical education (PE) class one or more days during an average school week	59.0	60.6	no change
29.	Percentage of students who had ever been taught about AIDS or HIV infection in school	88.6	77.5	increased
30.	Percentage of students who smoked cigarettes on 20 or more of the past 30 days	4.2	8.3	decreased
31.	Percentage of students who smoked more than 10 cigarettes per day on the days that they smoked during the past 30 days	1.0	2.6	no change
32.	Percentage of students who attended physical education (PE) class daily	23.7	37.4	decreased

* Change over time is statistically significant for $p < 0.05$.
Source: Centers for Disease Control and Prevention, Youth Risk Behavior Surveillance System. http://www.cdc.gov/nccdphp/dash/ yrbs/index.htm

3.15 Vermont, 1993 and 2001

(responses to the Youth Risk Behavior Surveillance System Survey questions, and direction of change at the 95 percent confidence level, Vermont, 1993 and 2001)

	2001	1993	direction of change*
1. Of students who rode a bicycle during the past 12 months, the percentage who never or rarely wore a bicycle helmet	54.8	83.9	decreased
2. Percentage of students who never or rarely wear a seat belt when riding in a car driven by someone else	10.9	19.0	decreased
3. Percentage of students who did not go to school on one or more of the past 30 days because they felt unsafe at school or on their way to or from school	4.1	3.9	no change
4. Percentage of students who were injured in a physical fight one or more times during the past 12 months and had to be treated by a doctor or nurse	26.5	41.8	decreased
5. Percentage of students who were in a physical fight on school property one or more times during the past 12 months	3.3	4.8	decreased
6. Percentage of students who made a plan about how they would attempt suicide during the past 12 months	13.4	16.7	decreased
7. Percentage of students who actually attempted suicide one or more times during the past 12 months	6.8	8.6	decreased
8. Percentage of students whose attempted suicide during the past 12 months resulted in an injury, poisoning, or overdose that had to be treated by a doctor or nurse	2.3	2.0	no change
9. Percentage of students who smoked a whole cigarette for the first time before age 13	21.5	27.5	decreased
10. Percentage of students who smoked cigarettes on one or more of the past 30 days	23.7	33.5	decreased
11. Percentage of students who smoked two or more cigarettes per day on the days they smoked during the past 30 days	16.4	24.4	decreased
12. Percentage of students who had their first drink of alcohol other than a few sips before age 13	26.0	37.1	decreased
13. Percentage of students who had at least one drink of alcohol on one or more of the past 30 days	48.1	52.6	no change
14. Percentage of students who had five or more drinks of alcohol in a row, that is, within a couple of hours, on one or more of the past 30 days	29.0	31.4	no change
15. Percentage of students who tried marijuana for the first time before age 13	12.2	6.8	increased
16. Percentage of students who used marijuana one or more times during the past 30 days	30.3	19.2	increased
17. Percentage of students who used any form of cocaine, including powder, crack, or freebase one or more times during the past 30 days	4.1	2.0	increased
18. Percentage of students who had sexual intercourse for the first time before age 13	5.0	7.5	decreased
19. Percentage of students who had sexual intercourse with four or more people during their life	10.3	14.5	decreased
20. Percentage of students who had sexual intercourse with one or more people during the past three months	29.1	34.6	decreased
21. Of students who had sexual intercourse during the past three months, the percentage who drank alcohol or used drugs before last sexual intercourse	28.0	20.4	increased
22. Of students who had sexual intercourse during the past three months, the percentage who used a condom during last sexual intercourse	59.5	52.9	increased
23. Percentage of students who had been pregnant or gotten someone pregnant one or more times	2.9	4.2	no change
24. Percentage of students who described themselves as slightly or very overweight	30.0	34.4	decreased
25. Percentage of students who were trying to lose weight	41.1	42.1	no change

(continued)

(continued from previous page)

		2001	1993	direction of change[*]
26.	Percentage of students who exercised or participated in physical activities for at least 20 minutes that made them sweat and breathe hard on three or more of the past seven days	67.2	68.6	no change
27.	Percentage of students who attended physical education (PE) class one or more days during an average school week	49.1	53.4	no change
28.	Percentage of students who smoked cigarettes on 20 or more of the past 30 days	12.7	17.4	decreased
29.	Percentage of students who smoked more than 10 cigarettes per day on the days that they smoked during the past 30 days	3.7	6.6	decreased
30.	Percentage of students who have ever had sexual intercourse but have not had sexual intercourse during the past three months	25.4	31.7	decreased
31.	Percentage of students who attended physical education (PE) class daily	27.7	37.3	no change
32.	Percentage of students who have never had sexual intercourse, who have had sexual intercourse but not during the past three months, or who used a condom the last time they had sexual intercourse during the past three months	88.4	83.8	increased

* Change over time is statistically significant for $p < 0.05$.
Source: Centers for Disease Control and Prevention, Youth Risk Behavior Surveillance System, http://www.cdc.gov/nccdphp/dash/yrbs/index.htm

3.16 Wisconsin, 1993 and 2001

(responses to the Youth Risk Behavior Surveillance System Survey questions, and direction of change at the 95 percent confidence level, Wisconsin, 1993 and 2001)

		2001	1993	direction of change
1.	Of students who rode a bicycle during the past 12 months, the percentage who never or rarely wore a bicycle helmet	88.4	95.7	decreased
2.	Percentage of students who never or rarely wear a seat belt when riding in a car driven by someone else	20.9	29.1	decreased
3.	Percentage of students who during the past 30 days rode one or more times in a car or other vehicle driven by someone who had been drinking alcohol	36.3	38.7	no change
4.	Percentage of students who during the past 30 days drove a car or other vehicle one or more times when they had been drinking alcohol	17.0	14.7	no change
5.	Percentage of students who carried a weapon such as a gun, knife, or club on one or more of the past 30 days	13.3	18.9	decreased
6.	Percentage of students who carried a gun on one or more of the past 30 days	4.8	8.7	decreased
7.	Percentage of students who carried a weapon such as a gun, knife, or club on school property on one or more of the past 30 days	3.4	9.0	decreased
8.	Percentage of students who did not go to school on one or more of the past 30 days because they felt unsafe at school or on their way to or from school	6.0	5.6	no change
9.	Percentage of students who had been threatened or injured with a weapon on school property one or more times during the past 12 months	8.4	7.9	no change
10.	Percentage of students who were in a physical fight one or more times during the past 12 months	31.4	39.4	decreased
11.	Percentage of students who were in a physical fight on school property one or more times during the past 12 months	11.4	16.1	decreased
12.	Percentage of students who seriously considered attempting suicide during the past 12 months	19.9	27.4	decreased
13.	Percentage of students who actually attempted suicide one or more times during the past 12 months	8.6	9.6	no change
14.	Percentage of students whose attempted suicide during the past 12 months resulted in an injury, poisoning, or overdose that had to be treated by a doctor or nurse	2.5	2.8	no change
15.	Percentage of students who ever tried cigarette smoking, even one or two puffs	64.0	69.3	decreased
16.	Percentage of students who smoked a whole cigarette for the first time before age 13	22.2	26.9	decreased
17.	Percentage of students who smoked cigarettes on one or more of the past 30 days	32.6	31.8	no change
18.	Percentage of students who smoked two or more cigarettes per day on the days they smoked during the past 30 days	22.2	21.9	no change
19.	Percentage of students who smoked cigarettes on school property on one or more of the past 30 days	9.8	13.5	decreased
20.	Percentage of students who had their first drink of alcohol other than a few sips before age 13	28.2	36.8	decreased
21.	Percentage of students who had at least one drink of alcohol on one or more of the past 30 days	54.1	48.1	increased
22.	Percentage of students who had five or more drinks of alcohol in a row, that is, within a couple of hours, on one or more of the past 30 days	34.2	29.0	increased
23.	Percentage of students who tried marijuana for the first time before age 13	42.7	22.8	increased
24.	Percentage of students who used marijuana one or more times during their life	8.3	5.2	increased
25.	Percentage of students who tried marijuana for the first time before age 13	25.1	11.2	increased

(continued)

		2001	1993	direction of change*
26.	Percentage of students who used any form of cocaine, including powder, crack, or freebase one or more times during their life	8.1	4.6	increased
27.	Percentage of students who used any form of cocaine, including powder, crack, or freebase one or more times during the past 30 days	3.4	2.7	no change
28.	Percentage of students who were offered, sold, or given an illegal drug on school property by someone during the past 12 months	26.6	19.6	increased
29.	Percentage of students who had sexual intercourse	39.3	47.0	decreased
30.	Percentage of students who had sexual intercourse for the first time before age 13	4.0	7.3	decreased
31.	Percentage of students who had sexual intercourse with four or more people during their life	10.2	14.3	decreased
32.	Percentage of students who had sexual intercourse with one or more people during the past three months	29.1	32.5	no change
33.	Of students who had sexual intercourse during the past three months, the percentage who drank alcohol or used drugs before last sexual intercourse	25.7	21.7	no change
34.	Of students who had sexual intercourse during the past three months, the percentage who used a condom during last sexual intercourse	59.2	58.3	no change
35.	Percentage of students who had been pregnant or gotten someone pregnant one or more times	3.9	5.1	no change
36.	Percentage of students who described themselves as slightly or very overweight	32.4	35.5	no change
37.	Percentage of students who were trying to lose weight	43.3	43.6	no change
38.	Percentage of students who exercised or participated in physical activities for at least 20 minutes that made them sweat and breathe hard on three or more of the past seven days	64.9	64.3	no change
39.	Percentage of students who had ever been taught about AIDS or HIV infection in school	92.0	84.1	increased
40.	Percentage of students who smoked cigarettes on 20 or more of the past 30 days	16.4	15.8	no change
41.	Percentage of students who smoked more than 10 cigarettes per day on the days that they smoked during the past 30 days	4.0	5.0	no change
42.	Percentage of students who have ever had sexual intercourse but have not had sexual intercourse during the past three months	25.9	30.8	decreased
43.	Percentage of students who have never had sexual intercourse, who have had sexual intercourse but not during the past three months, or who used a condom the last time they had sexual intercourse during the past three months	88.2	86.7	no change

* Change over time is statistically significant for p< 0.05.
Source: Centers for Disease Control and Prevention, Youth Risk Behavior Surveillance System, http://www.cdc.gov/nccdphp/dash/yrbs/index.htm

3.17 Wyoming, 1995 and 2001

(responses to the Youth Risk Behavior Surveillance System Survey questions, and direction of change at the 95 percent confidence level. Wyoming, 1995 and 2001)

		2001	1995	direction of change*
1.	Of students who rode a motorcycle during the past 12 months, the percentage who never or rarely wore a motorcycle helmet	44.9	44.2	no change
2.	Of students who rode a bicycle during the past 12 months, the percentage who never or rarely wore a bicycle helmet	86.2	93.8	decreased
3.	Percentage of students who never or rarely wear a seat belt when riding in a car driven by someone else	20.0	33.4	decreased
4.	Percentage of students who during the past 30 days rode one or more times in a car or other vehicle driven by someone who had been drinking alcohol	35.9	42.3	decreased
5.	Percentage of students who during the past 30 days drove a car or other vehicle one or more times when they had been drinking alcohol	20.2	22.4	no change
6.	Percentage of students who carried a weapon such as a gun, knife, or club on one or more of the past 30 days	22.9	25.6	no change
7.	Percentage of students who carried a gun on one or more of the past 30 days	10.1	10.8	no change
8.	Percentage of students who carried a weapon such as a gun, knife, or club on school property on one or more of the past 30 days	8.4	14.1	decreased
9.	Percentage of students who did not go to school on one or more of the past 30 days because they felt unsafe at school or on their way to or from school	8.0	3.4	increased
10.	Percentage of students who had been threatened or injured with a weapon on school property one or more times during the past 12 months	9.4	7.3	increased
11.	Percentage of students who were in a physical fight one or more times during the past 12 months	31.4	35.6	decreased
12.	Percentage of students who were injured in a physical fight one or more times during the past 12 months and had to be treated by a doctor or nurse	2.9	4.8	decreased
13.	Percentage of students who were in a physical fight on school property one or more times during the past 12 months	13.5	16.8	decreased
14.	Percentage of students who seriously considered attempting suicide during the past 12 months	18.5	23.6	decreased
15.	Percentage of students who made a plan about how they would attempt suicide during the past 12 months	14.2	17.4	decreased
16.	Percentage of students who actually attempted suicide one or more times during the past 12 months	7.4	8.3	no change
17.	Percentage of students whose attempted suicide during the past 12 months resulted in an injury, poisoning, or overdose that had to be treated by a doctor or nurse	2.4	2.6	no change
18.	Percentage of students who ever tried cigarette smoking, even one or two puffs	64.6	73.0	decreased
19.	Percentage of students who smoked a whole cigarette for the first time before age 13	24.1	30.9	decreased
20.	Percentage of students who smoked cigarettes on one or more of the past 30 days	28.4	39.5	decreased
21.	Percentage of students who smoked two or more cigarettes per day on the days they smoked during the past 30 days	19.3	25.9	decreased
22.	Percentage of students who smoked cigarettes on school property on one or more of the past 30 days	10.7	17.2	decreased
23.	Percentage of students who used chewing tobacco or snuff on one or more of the past 30 days	18.1	25.1	decreased
24.	Percentage of students who used chewing tobacco or snuff on school property on one or more of the past 30 days	11.5	18.3	decreased

(continued)

(continued from previous page)

		2001	1995	direction of change*
25.	Percentage of students who had at least one drink of alcohol on one or more days during their life	82.3	81.1	no change
26.	Percentage of students who had their first drink of alcohol other than a few sips before age 13	33.9	42.0	decreased
27.	Percentage of students who had at least one drink of alcohol on one or more of the past 30 days	51.3	52.1	no change
28.	Percentage of students who had five or more drinks of alcohol in a row, that is, within a couple of hours, on one or more of the past 30 days	38.1	38.8	no change
29.	Percentage of students who had at least one drink of alcohol on school property on one or more of the past 30 days	6.1	7.3	no change
30.	Percentage of students who used marijuana one or more times during their life	41.0	38.1	no change
31.	Percentage of students who tried marijuana for the first time before age 13	9.8	8.3	no change
32.	Percentage of students who used marijuana one or more times during the past 30 days	20.4	21.9	no change
33.	Percentage of students who used marijuana on school property one or more times during the past 30 days	4.4	6.7	decreased
34.	Percentage of students who used any form of cocaine, including powder, crack, or freebase one or more times during their life	9.5	9.5	no change
35.	Percentage of students who used any form of cocaine, including powder, crack, or freebase one or more times during the past 30 days	4.3	4.7	no change
36.	Percentage of students who sniffed glue, breathed the contents of aerosol spray cans, or inhaled any paints or sprays to get high one or more times during their life	16.0	28.0	decreased
37.	Percentage of students who took steroid pills or shots without a doctor's prescription one or more times during their life	5.3	4.7	no change
38.	Percentage of students who used a needle to inject any illegal drug into their body one or more times during their life	2.6	2.8	no change
39.	Percentage of students who were offered, sold, or given an illegal drug on school property by someone during the past 12 months	18.9	24.3	decreased
40.	Percentage of students who had sexual intercourse	46.5	48.9	no change
41.	Percentage of students who had sexual intercourse for the first time before age 13	5.2	8.9	decreased
42.	Percentage of students who had sexual intercourse with four or more people during their life	13.8	16.4	no change
43.	Percentage of students who had sexual intercourse with one or more people during the past three months	32.9	32.0	no change
44.	Of students who had sexual intercourse during the past three months, the percentage who drank alcohol or used drugs before last sexual intercourse	30.2	30.1	no change
45.	Of students who had sexual intercourse during the past three months, the percentage who used a condom during last sexual intercourse	61.8	53.7	increased
46.	Percentage of students who had been pregnant or gotten someone pregnant one or more times	4.1	5.7	no change
47.	Percentage of students who described themselves as slightly or very overweight	27.5	26.9	no change
48.	Percentage of students who were trying to lose weight	41.7	40.3	no change
49.	Percentage of students who exercised to lose weight or to keep from gaining weight during the past 30 days	59.3	55.7	increased
50.	Percentage of students who vomited or took laxatives to lose weight or to keep from gaining weight during the past 30 days	4.8	6.0	no change
51.	Percentage of students who exercised or participated in physical activities for at least 20 minutes that made them sweat and breathe hard on three or more of the past seven days	69.0	68.1	no change

(continued)

(continued from previous page)

		2001	1995	direction of change[*]
52.	Percentage of students who did exercises to strengthen or tone their muscles on three or more of the past seven days	56.2	55.0	no change
53.	Percentage of students who attended physical education (PE) class one or more days during an average school week	58.2	58.0	no change
54.	Percentage of students who had ever been taught about AIDS or HIV infection in school	89.9	88.9	no change
55.	Percentage of students who smoked cigarettes on 20 or more of the past 30 days	13.6	19.4	decreased
56.	Percentage of students who smoked more than 10 cigarettes per day on the days that they smoked during the past 30 days	3.4	5.7	decreased
57.	Percentage of students who have ever had sexual intercourse but have not had sexual intercourse during the past three months	29.1	34.6	decreased
58.	Percentage of students who attended physical education (PE) class daily	30.9	36.4	no change
59.	Percentage of students who have never had sexual intercourse, who have had sexual intercourse but not during the past three months, or who used a condom the last time they had sexual intercourse during the past three months	87.5	85.2	no change

* Change over time is statistically significant for p< 0.05.
Source: Centers for Disease Control and Prevention, Youth Risk Behavior Surveillance System, http://www.cdc.gov/nccdphp/dash/ yrbs/index.htm

3.18 Boston, 1993 and 2001

(responses to the Youth Risk Behavior Surveillance System Survey questions, and direction of change at the 95 percent confidence level, Boston, 1993 and 2001)

		2001	1993	direction of change
1.	Of students who rode a motorcycle during the past 12 months, the percentage who never or rarely wore a motorcycle helmet	47.3	49.0	no change
2.	Of students who rode a bicycle during the past 12 months, the percentage who never or rarely wore a bicycle helmet	87.2	92.3	decreased
3.	Percentage of students who never or rarely wear a seat belt when riding in a car driven by someone else	30.3	57.0	decreased
4.	Percentage of students who during the past 30 days rode one or more times in a car or other vehicle driven by someone who had been drinking alcohol	25.2	31.1	decreased
5.	Percentage of students who during the past 30 days drove a car or other vehicle one or more times when they had been drinking alcohol	5.5	7.9	decreased
6.	Percentage of students who carried a weapon such as a gun, knife, or club on one or more of the past 30 days	16.4	27.5	decreased
7.	Percentage of students who carried a gun on one or more of the past 30 days	4.4	10.0	decreased
8.	Percentage of students who carried a weapon such as a gun, knife, or club on school property on one or more of the past 30 days	7.9	15.8	decreased
9.	Percentage of students who did not go to school on one or more of the past 30 days because they felt unsafe at school or on their way to or from school	9.8	14.4	decreased
10.	Percentage of students who had been threatened or injured with a weapon on school property one or more times during the past 12 months	8.8	12.0	decreased
11.	Percentage of students who were in a physical fight one or more times during the past 12 months	33.3	43.0	decreased
12.	Percentage of students who were injured in a physical fight one or more times during the past 12 months and had to be treated by a doctor or nurse	4.6	7.8	decreased
13.	Percentage of students who were in a physical fight on school property one or more times during the past 12 months	11.2	15.2	decreased
14.	Percentage of students who seriously considered attempting suicide during the past 12 months	16.1	23.7	decreased
15.	Percentage of students who made a plan about how they would attempt suicide during the past 12 months	12.9	19.7	decreased
16.	Percentage of students who actually attempted suicide one or more times during the past 12 months	11.5	13.5	no change
17.	Percentage of students whose attempted suicide during the past 12 months resulted in an injury, poisoning, or overdose that had to be treated by a doctor or nurse	5.0	4.3	no change
18.	Percentage of students who ever tried cigarette smoking, even one or two puffs	57.1	64.7	decreased
19.	Percentage of students who smoked a whole cigarette for the first time before age 13	13.5	21.0	decreased
20.	Percentage of students who smoked cigarettes on one or more of the past 30 days	15.4	20.9	decreased
21.	Percentage of students who smoked two or more cigarettes per day on the days they smoked during the past 30 days	8.3	12.6	decreased
22.	Percentage of students who smoked cigarettes on school property on one or more of the past 30 days	7.2	11.2	decreased
23.	Percentage of students who had at least one drink of alcohol on one or more days during their life	73.9	67.4	increased
24.	Percentage of students who had their first drink of alcohol other than a few sips before age 13	30.1	30.6	no change
25.	Percentage of students who had at least one drink of alcohol on one or more of the past 30 days	41.7	40.1	no change

(continued)

(continued from previous page)

		2001	1993	direction of change*
26.	Percentage of students who had five or more drinks of alcohol in a row, that is, within a couple of hours, on one or more of the past 30 days	18.1	20.3	no change
27.	Percentage of students who had at least one drink of alcohol on school property on one or more of the past 30 days	6.3	5.9	no change
28.	Percentage of students who used marijuana one or more times during their life	40.1	30.7	increased
29.	Percentage of students who tried marijuana for the first time before age 13	11.4	7.7	increased
30.	Percentage of students who used marijuana one or more times during the past 30 days	21.7	17.8	increased
31.	Percentage of students who used marijuana on school property one or more times during the past 30 days	6.0	6.5	no change
32.	Percentage of students who used any form of cocaine, including powder, crack, or freebase one or more times during their life	3.6	3.8	no change
33.	Percentage of students who took steroid pills or shots without a doctor's prescription one or more times during their life	3.1	3.8	no change
34.	Percentage of students who were offered, sold, or given an illegal drug on school property by someone during the past 12 months	31.0	21.7	increased
35.	Percentage of students who had sexual intercourse	51.6	60.6	decreased
36.	Percentage of students who had sexual intercourse for the first time before age 13	13.1	18.2	decreased
37.	Percentage of students who had sexual intercourse with four or more people during their life	21.0	25.9	decreased
38.	Percentage of students who had sexual intercourse with one or more people during the past three months	36.5	42.0	decreased
39.	Of students who had sexual intercourse during the past three months, the percentage who drank alcohol or used drugs before last sexual intercourse	17.4	18.4	no change
40.	Of students who had sexual intercourse during the past three months, the percentage who used a condom during last sexual intercourse	72.0	63.9	increased
41.	Percentage of students who had been pregnant or gotten someone pregnant one or more times	7.8	11.1	decreased
42.	Percentage of students who described themselves as slightly or very overweight	28.4	27.5	no change
43.	Percentage of students who were trying to lose weight	41.0	36.4	increased
44.	Percentage of students who exercised or participated in physical activities for at least 20 minutes that made them sweat and breathe hard on three or more of the past seven days	49.8	50.2	no change
45.	Percentage of students who did exercises to strengthen or tone their muscles on three or more of the past seven days	36.5	36.4	no change
46.	Percentage of students who attended physical education (PE) class one or more days during an average school week	56.5	62.7	no change
47.	Percentage of students who had ever been taught about AIDS or HIV infection in school	84.3	83.0	no change
48.	Percentage of students who smoked cigarettes on 20 or more of the past 30 days	4.9	8.3	decreased
49.	Percentage of students who smoked more than 10 cigarettes per day on the days that they smoked during the past 30 days	1.5	3.1	decreased
50.	Percentage of students who have ever had sexual intercourse but have not had sexual intercourse during the past three months	29.5	30.2	no change
51.	Percentage of students who attended physical education (PE) class daily	11.0	9.8	no change
52.	Percentage of students who have never had sexual intercourse, who have had sexual intercourse but not during the past three months, or who used a condom the last time they had sexual intercourse during the past three months	90.0	85.2	increased

* Change over time is statistically significant for p< 0.05.
Source: Centers for Disease Control and Prevention, Youth Risk Behavior Surveillance System, http://www.cdc.gov/nccdphp/dash/yrbs/index.htm

3.19 Chicago, 1991 and 2001

(responses to the Youth Risk Behavior Surveillance System Survey questions, and direction of change at the 95 percent confidence level, Chicago, 1991 and 2001)

		2001	1991	direction of change*
1.	Of students who rode a motorcycle during the past 12 months, the percentage who never or rarely wore a motorcycle helmet	67.6	73.8	no change
2.	Of students who rode a bicycle during the past 12 months, the percentage who never or rarely wore a bicycle helmet	92.6	95.9	decreased
3.	Percentage of students who never or rarely wear a seat belt when riding in a car driven by someone else	34.0	51.6	decreased
4.	Percentage of students who during the past 30 days rode one or more times in a car or other vehicle driven by someone who had been drinking alcohol	34.0	37.4	no change
5.	Percentage of students who during the past 30 days drove a car or other vehicle one or more times when they had been drinking alcohol	10.7	8.5	no change
6.	Percentage of students who carried a weapon such as a gun, knife, or club on one or more of the past 30 days	21.2	33.2	decreased
7.	Percentage of students who were in a physical fight one or more times during the past 12 months	40.8	51.3	decreased
8.	Percentage of students who were injured in a physical fight one or more times during the past 12 months and had to be treated by a doctor or nurse	5.7	8.0	no change
9.	Percentage of students who seriously considered attempting suicide during the past 12 months	17.3	25.0	decreased
10.	Percentage of students who made a plan about how they would attempt suicide during the past 12 months	15.3	17.6	no change
11.	Percentage of students who actually attempted suicide one or more times during the past 12 months	11.8	9.6	no change
12.	Percentage of students whose attempted suicide during the past 12 months resulted in an injury, poisoning, or overdose that had to be treated by a doctor or nurse	2.7	3.5	no change
13.	Percentage of students who ever tried cigarette smoking, even one or two puffs	64.5	72.4	decreased
14.	Percentage of students who smoked a whole cigarette for the first time before age 13	21.0	21.2	no change
15.	Percentage of students who smoked cigarettes on one or more of the past 30 days	24.7	16.3	increased
16.	Percentage of students who smoked two or more cigarettes per day on the days they smoked during the past 30 days	12.8	8.8	no change
17.	Percentage of students who had at least one drink of alcohol on one or more days during their life	74.5	75.3	no change
18.	Percentage of students who had their first drink of alcohol other than a few sips before age 13	32.4	30.9	no change
19.	Percentage of students who had at least one drink of alcohol on one or more of the past 30 days	42.3	42.1	no change
20.	Percentage of students who had five or more drinks of alcohol in a row, that is, within a couple of hours, on one or more of the past 30 days	21.4	18.9	no change
21.	Percentage of students who used marijuana one or more times during their life	49.3	26.7	increased
22.	Percentage of students who tried marijuana for the first time before age 13	15.6	9.4	increased
23.	Percentage of students who used marijuana one or more times during the past 30 days	28.7	11.8	increased
24.	Percentage of students who used any form of cocaine, including powder, crack, or freebase one or more times during their life	4.4	4.3	no change

(continued)

(continued from previous page)

	2001	1991	direction of change*
25. Percentage of students who used any form of cocaine, including powder, crack, or freebase one or more times during the past 30 days	2.6	2.5	no change
26. Percentage of students who took steroid pills or shots without a doctor's prescription one or more times during their life	5.2	4.1	no change
27. Percentage of students who had sexual intercourse	58.1	64.3	no change
28. Percentage of students who had sexual intercourse for the first time before age 13	17.2	24.2	decreased
29. Percentage of students who had sexual intercourse with four or more people during their life	22.5	29.8	no change
30. Percentage of students who had sexual intercourse with one or more people during the past three months	40.9	44.9	no change
31. Of students who had sexual intercourse during the past three months, the percentage who drank alcohol or used drugs before last sexual intercourse	23.7	16.5	no change
32. Of students who had sexual intercourse during the past three months, the percentage who used a condom during last sexual intercourse	70.0	50.3	increased
33. Percentage of students who had been pregnant or gotten someone pregnant one or more times	9.6	11.0	no change
34. Percentage of students who described themselves as slightly or very overweight	28.6	26.0	no change
35. Percentage of students who were trying to lose weight	43.6	35.3	increased
36. Percentage of students who did exercises to strengthen or tone their muscles on three or more of the past seven days	51.0	42.1	increased
37. Percentage of students who attended physical education (PE) class one or more days during an average school week	70.5	87.9	decreased
38. Percentage of students who had ever been taught about AIDS or HIV infection in school	86.9	75.7	increased
39. Percentage of students who smoked cigarettes on 20 or more of the past 30 days	7.6	5.7	no change
40. Percentage of students who smoked more than 10 cigarettes per day on the days that they smoked during the past 30 days	1.7	1.6	no change
41. Percentage of students who have ever had sexual intercourse but have not had sexual intercourse during the past three months	30.3	30.1	no change
42. Percentage of students who attended physical education (PE) class daily	57.1	73.9	decreased
43. Percentage of students who have never had sexual intercourse, who have had sexual intercourse but not during the past three months, or who used a condom the last time they had sexual intercourse during the past three months	87.9	78.2	increased

* Change over time is statistically significant for p< 0.05.
Source: Centers for Disease Control and Prevention, Youth Risk Behavior Surveillance System, http://www.cdc.gov/nccdphp/dash/yrbs/index.htm

3.20 Dallas, 1991 and 2001

(responses to the Youth Risk Behavior Surveillance System Survey questions, and direction of change at the 95 percent confidence level, Dallas, 1991 and 2001)

		2001	1991	direction of change*
1.	Of students who rode a motorcycle during the past 12 months, the percentage who never or rarely wore a motorcycle helmet	60.1	51.8	no change
2.	Of students who rode a bicycle during the past 12 months, the percentage who never or rarely wore a bicycle helmet	91.9	96.2	decreased
3.	Percentage of students who never or rarely wear a seat belt when riding in a car driven by someone else	8.5	13.7	decreased
4.	Percentage of students who during the past 30 days rode one or more times in a car or other vehicle driven by someone who had been drinking alcohol	39.6	44.8	decreased
5.	Percentage of students who during the past 30 days drove a car or other vehicle one or more times when they had been drinking alcohol	11.4	12.9	no change
6.	Percentage of students who carried a weapon such as a gun, knife, or club on one or more of the past 30 days	15.9	30.5	decreased
7.	Percentage of students who were in a physical fight one or more times during the past 12 months	41.0	46.9	decreased
8.	Percentage of students who were injured in a physical fight one or more times during the past 12 months and had to be treated by a doctor or nurse	3.9	6.2	decreased
9.	Percentage of students who seriously considered attempting suicide during the past 12 months	16.1	24.9	decreased
10.	Percentage of students who made a plan about how they would attempt suicide during the past 12 months	13.3	14.2	no change
11.	Percentage of students who actually attempted suicide one or more times during the past 12 months	11.0	6.6	increased
12.	Percentage of students whose attempted suicide during the past 12 months resulted in an injury, poisoning, or overdose that had to be treated by a doctor or nurse	3.0	2.6	no change
13.	Percentage of students who ever tried cigarette smoking, even one or two puffs	68.0	72.7	decreased
14.	Percentage of students who smoked a whole cigarette for the first time before age 13	19.4	23.4	decreased
15.	Percentage of students who smoked cigarettes on one or more of the past 30 days	17.8	13.9	increased
16.	Percentage of students who smoked two or more cigarettes per day on the days they smoked during the past 30 days	8.5	8.5	no change
17.	Percentage of students who had at least one drink of alcohol on one or more days during their life	81.1	78.6	no change
18.	Percentage of students who had their first drink of alcohol other than a few sips before age 13	34.3	33.2	no change
19.	Percentage of students who had at least one drink of alcohol on one or more of the past 30 days	44.0	44.4	no change
20.	Percentage of students who had five or more drinks of alcohol in a row, that is, within a couple of hours, on one or more of the past 30 days	20.7	22.9	no change
21.	Percentage of students who used marijuana one or more times during their life	43.5	29.0	increased
22.	Percentage of students who tried marijuana for the first time before age 13	13.7	10.0	increased
23.	Percentage of students who used marijuana one or more times during the past 30 days	20.4	10.6	increased
24.	Percentage of students who used any form of cocaine, including powder, crack, or freebase one or more times during their life	10.4	5.8	increased

(continued)

(continued from previous page)

	2001	1991	direction of change[*]
25. Percentage of students who used any form of cocaine, including powder, crack, or freebase one or more times during the past 30 days	5.2	1.8	increased
26. Percentage of students who took steroid pills or shots without a doctor's prescription one or more times during their life	3.9	3.6	no change
27. Percentage of students who had sexual intercourse	56.8	66.6	decreased
28. Percentage of students who had sexual intercourse for the first time before age 13	12.2	21.1	decreased
29. Percentage of students who had sexual intercourse with four or more people during their life	20.6	32.1	decreased
30. Percentage of students who had sexual intercourse with one or more people during the past three months	38.8	47.5	decreased
31. Of students who had sexual intercourse during the past three months, the percentage who drank alcohol or used drugs before last sexual intercourse	20.9	18.0	no change
32. Of students who had sexual intercourse during the past three months, the percentage who used a condom during last sexual intercourse	56.6	48.5	increased
33. Percentage of students who had been pregnant or gotten someone pregnant one or more times	8.0	11.2	decreased
34. Percentage of students who described themselves as slightly or very overweight	32.9	29.7	no change
35. Percentage of students who were trying to lose weight	47.2	36.8	increased
36. Percentage of students who did exercises to strengthen or tone their muscles on three or more of the past seven days	44.2	38.4	increased
37. Percentage of students who attended physical education (PE) class one or more days during an average school week	46.4	39.3	no change
38. Percentage of students who had ever been taught about AIDS or HIV infection in school	83.0	79.9	no change
39. Percentage of students who smoked cigarettes on 20 or more of the past 30 days	3.6	4.1	no change
40. Percentage of students who smoked more than 10 cigarettes per day on the days that they smoked during the past 30 days	0.7	1.0	no change
41. Percentage of students who have ever had sexual intercourse but have not had sexual intercourse during the past three months	31.6	28.5	no change
42. Percentage of students who attended physical education (PE) class daily	10.3	32.6	decreased
43. Percentage of students who have never had sexual intercourse, who have had sexual intercourse but not during the past three months, or who used a condom the last time they had sexual intercourse during the past three months	83.4	75.8	increased

* Change over time is statistically significant for $p < 0.05$.
Source: Centers for Disease Control and Prevention, Youth Risk Behavior Surveillance System, http://www.cdc.gov/nccdphp/dash/yrbs/index.htm

3.21 Ft. Lauderdale, 1991 and 2001

(responses to the Youth Risk Behavior Surveillance System Survey questions, and direction of change at the 95 percent confidence level, Ft. Lauderdale, 1991 and 2001)

		2001	1991	direction of change
1.	Of students who rode a motorcycle during the past 12 months, the percentage who never or rarely wore a motorcycle helmet	44.2	28.6	increased
2.	Of students who rode a bicycle during the past 12 months, the percentage who never or rarely wore a bicycle helmet	89.2	98.3	decreased
3.	Percentage of students who never or rarely wear a seat belt when riding in a car driven by someone else	10.3	21.4	decreased
4.	Percentage of students who during the past 30 days rode one or more times in a car or other vehicle driven by someone who had been drinking alcohol	27.5	31.8	no change
5.	Percentage of students who during the past 30 days drove a car or other vehicle one or more times when they had been drinking alcohol	10.8	10.9	no change
6.	Percentage of students who carried a weapon such as a gun, knife, or club on one or more of the past 30 days	10.9	16.3	decreased
7.	Percentage of students who were in a physical fight one or more times during the past 12 months	30.3	37.3	decreased
8.	Percentage of students who were injured in a physical fight one or more times during the past 12 months and had to be treated by a doctor or nurse	4.6	3.8	no change
9.	Percentage of students who seriously considered attempting suicide during the past 12 months	13.9	26.7	decreased
10.	Percentage of students who made a plan about how they would attempt suicide during the past 12 months	11.0	15.4	decreased
11.	Percentage of students who actually attempted suicide one or more times during the past 12 months	7.6	6.1	no change
12.	Percentage of students whose attempted suicide during the past 12 months resulted in an injury, poisoning, or overdose that had to be treated by a doctor or nurse	3.2	1.2	increased
13.	Percentage of students who ever tried cigarette smoking, even one or two puffs	54.6	65.0	decreased
14.	Percentage of students who smoked a whole cigarette for the first time before age 13	15.9	21.9	decreased
15.	Percentage of students who smoked cigarettes on one or more of the past 30 days	18.3	15.9	no change
16.	Percentage of students who smoked two or more cigarettes per day on the days they smoked during the past 30 days	12.3	11.6	no change
17.	Percentage of students who had at least one drink of alcohol on one or more days during their life	73.9	79.1	decreased
18.	Percentage of students who had their first drink of alcohol other than a few sips before age 13	27.6	30.2	no change
19.	Percentage of students who had at least one drink of alcohol on one or more of the past 30 days	43.9	47.9	no change
20.	Percentage of students who had five or more drinks of alcohol in a row, that is, within a couple of hours, on one or more of the past 30 days	21.1	22.0	no change
21.	Percentage of students who used marijuana one or more times during their life	40.8	27.3	increased
22.	Percentage of students who tried marijuana for the first time before age 13	8.9	6.9	no change
23.	Percentage of students who used marijuana one or more times during the past 30 days	21.8	13.5	increased
24.	Percentage of students who used any form of cocaine, including powder, crack, or freebase one or more times during their life	7.2	3.0	increased

(continued)

(continued from previous page)

	2001	1991	direction of change*
25. Percentage of students who used any form of cocaine, including powder, crack, or freebase one or more times during the past 30 days	2.6	0.8	increased
26. Percentage of students who took steroid pills or shots without a doctor's prescription one or more times during their life	4.5	2.6	increased
27. Percentage of students who had sexual intercourse	47.3	55.5	decreased
28. Percentage of students who had sexual intercourse for the first time before age 13	8.8	13.1	decreased
29. Percentage of students who had sexual intercourse with four or more people during their life	15.1	20.6	decreased
30. Percentage of students who had sexual intercourse with one or more people during the past three months	33.5	39.1	decreased
31. Of students who had sexual intercourse during the past three months, the percentage who drank alcohol or used drugs before last sexual intercourse	22.6	15.3	increased
32. Of students who had sexual intercourse during the past three months, the percentage who used a condom during last sexual intercourse	73.1	42.9	increased
33. Percentage of students who had been pregnant or gotten someone pregnant one or more times	4.0	5.5	no change
34. Percentage of students who described themselves as slightly or very overweight	26.2	32.3	decreased
35. Percentage of students who were trying to lose weight	41.1	42.8	no change
36. Percentage of students who did exercises to strengthen or tone their muscles on three or more of the past seven days	42.7	39.6	no change
37. Percentage of students who attended physical education (PE) class one or more days during an average school week	44.2	40.5	no change
38. Percentage of students who had ever been taught about AIDS or HIV infection in school	87.5	85.2	no change
39. Percentage of students who smoked cigarettes on 20 or more of the past 30 days	7.0	8.2	no change
40. Percentage of students who smoked more than 10 cigarettes per day on the days that they smoked during the past 30 days	2.2	2.1	no change
41. Percentage of students who have ever had sexual intercourse but have not had sexual intercourse during the past three months	29.0	29.9	no change
42. Percentage of students who attended physical education (PE) class daily	23.7	32.2	decreased
43. Percentage of students who have never had sexual intercourse, who have had sexual intercourse but not during the past three months, or who used a condom the last time they had sexual intercourse during the past three months	91.1	77.8	increased

* Change over time is statistically significant for p< 0.05.
Source: Centers for Disease Control and Prevention, Youth Risk Behavior Surveillance System, http://www.cdc.gov/nccdphp/dash/yrbs/index.htm

3.22 Houston, 1995 and 2001

(responses to the Youth Risk Behavior Surveillance System Survey questions, and direction of change at the 95 percent confidence level, Houston, 1995 and 2001)

		2001	1995	direction of change
1.	Of students who rode a motorcycle during the past 12 months, the percentage who never or rarely wore a motorcycle helmet	53.1	47.7	no change
2.	Of students who rode a bicycle during the past 12 months, the percentage who never or rarely wore a bicycle helmet	87.9	90.1	no change
3.	Percentage of students who never or rarely wear a seat belt when riding in a car driven by someone else	12.0	14.2	no change
4.	Percentage of students who during the past 30 days rode one or more times in a car or other vehicle driven by someone who had been drinking alcohol	38.6	43.8	decreased
5.	Percentage of students who during the past 30 days drove a car or other vehicle one or more times when they had been drinking alcohol	13.8	14.0	no change
6.	Percentage of students who carried a weapon such as a gun, knife, or club on one or more of the past 30 days	15.7	20.5	decreased
7.	Percentage of students who carried a gun on one or more of the past 30 days	6.1	10.7	decreased
8.	Percentage of students who carried a weapon such as a gun, knife, or club on school property on one or more of the past 30 days	5.8	9.3	decreased
9.	Percentage of students who did not go to school on one or more of the past 30 days because they felt unsafe at school or on their way to or from school	9.5	12.7	decreased
10.	Percentage of students who had been threatened or injured with a weapon on school property one or more times during the past 12 months	8.7	10.2	no change
11.	Percentage of students who were in a physical fight one or more times during the past 12 months	33.9	33.6	no change
12.	Percentage of students who were injured in a physical fight one or more times during the past 12 months and had to be treated by a doctor or nurse	4.8	5.0	no change
13.	Percentage of students who were in a physical fight on school property one or more times during the past 12 months	13.4	15.6	no change
14.	Percentage of students who seriously considered attempting suicide during the past 12 months	14.5	21.9	decreased
15.	Percentage of students who made a plan about how they would attempt suicide during the past 12 months	11.7	15.7	no change
16.	Percentage of students who actually attempted suicide one or more times during the past 12 months	10.2	11.8	no change
17.	Percentage of students whose attempted suicide during the past 12 months resulted in an injury, poisoning, or overdose that had to be treated by a doctor or nurse	2.8	4.8	no change
18.	Percentage of students who ever tried cigarette smoking, even one or two puffs	62.2	66.9	no change
19.	Percentage of students who smoked a whole cigarette for the first time before age 13	20.4	19.5	no change
20.	Percentage of students who smoked cigarettes on one or more of the past 30 days	21.8	26.9	decreased
21.	Percentage of students who smoked two or more cigarettes per day on the days they smoked during the past 30 days	10.8	16.1	decreased
22.	Percentage of students who smoked cigarettes on school property on one or more of the past 30 days	6.0	8.6	decreased
23.	Percentage of students who used chewing tobacco or snuff on one or more of the past 30 days	3.5	4.8	no change
24.	Percentage of students who used chewing tobacco or snuff on school property on one or more of the past 30 days	2.2	3.3	no change

(continued)

(continued from previous page)

	2001	1995	direction of change
25. Percentage of students who had at least one drink of alcohol on one or more days during their life	75.2	72.7	no change
26. Percentage of students who had their first drink of alcohol other than a few sips before age 13	31.0	34.8	no change
27. Percentage of students who had at least one drink of alcohol on one or more of the past 30 days	43.9	44.4	no change
28. Percentage of students who had five or more drinks of alcohol in a row, that is, within a couple of hours, on one or more of the past 30 days	25.4	23.0	no change
29. Percentage of students who had at least one drink of alcohol on school property on one or more of the past 30 days	6.8	6.1	no change
30. Percentage of students who used marijuana one or more times during their life	40.7	37.0	no change
31. Percentage of students who tried marijuana for the first time before age 13	12.9	9.7	increased
32. Percentage of students who used marijuana one or more times during the past 30 days	20.4	20.7	no change
33. Percentage of students who used marijuana on school property one or more times during the past 30 days	5.2	7.5	decreased
34. Percentage of students who used any form of cocaine, including powder, crack, or freebase one or more times during their life	8.9	7.6	no change
35. Percentage of students who used any form of cocaine, including powder, crack, or freebase one or more times during the past 30 days	4.3	3.6	no change
36. Percentage of students who sniffed glue, breathed the contents of aerosol spray cans, or inhaled any paints or sprays to get high one or more times during their life	8.7	16.2	decreased
37. Percentage of students who took steroid pills or shots without a doctor's prescription one or more times during their life	5.7	5.1	no change
38. Percentage of students who used a needle to inject any illegal drug into their body one or more times during their life	2.3	3.2	no change
39. Percentage of students who were offered, sold, or given an illegal drug on school property by someone during the past 12 months	31.4	29.8	no change
40. Percentage of students who had sexual intercourse	49.5	55.4	no change
41. Percentage of students who had sexual intercourse for the first time before age 13	9.8	16.7	decreased
42. Percentage of students who had sexual intercourse with four or more people during their life	16.2	22.5	decreased
43. Percentage of students who had sexual intercourse with one or more people during the past three months	35.9	37.1	no change
44. Of students who had sexual intercourse during the past three months, the percentage who drank alcohol or used drugs before last sexual intercourse	23.7	21.5	no change
45. Of students who had sexual intercourse during the past three months, the percentage who used a condom during last sexual intercourse	65.1	55.3	increased
46. Percentage of students who had been pregnant or gotten someone pregnant one or more times	6.3	9.9	decreased
47. Percentage of students who described themselves as slightly or very overweight	28.8	23.9	increased
48. Percentage of students who were trying to lose weight	45.7	37.0	increased
49. Percentage of students who exercised to lose weight or to keep from gaining weight during the past 30 days	58.1	49.0	increased
50. Percentage of students who vomited or took laxatives to lose weight or to keep from gaining weight during the past 30 days	4.6	6.0	no change
51. Percentage of students who exercised or participated in physical activities for at least 20 minutes that made them sweat and breathe hard on three or more of the past seven days	55.2	53.1	no change

(continued)

(continued from previous page)

		2001	1995	direction of change[*]
52.	Percentage of students who did exercises to strengthen or tone their muscles on three or more of the past seven days	50.7	44.5	increased
53.	Percentage of students who attended physical education (PE) class one or more days during an average school week	49.8	65.0	decreased
54.	Percentage of students who had ever been taught about AIDS or HIV infection in school	81.2	79.7	no change
55.	Percentage of students who smoked cigarettes on 20 or more of the past 30 days	4.6	8.4	decreased
56.	Percentage of students who smoked more than 10 cigarettes per day on the days that they smoked during the past 30 days	0.9	3.4	decreased
57.	Percentage of students who have ever had sexual intercourse but have not had sexual intercourse during the past three months	27.2	32.9	no change
58.	Percentage of students who attended physical education (PE) class daily	17.1	39.1	decreased
59.	Percentage of students who have never had sexual intercourse, who have had sexual intercourse but not during the past three months, or who used a condom the last time they had sexual intercourse during the past three months	87.6	83.6	increased

* Change over time is statistically significant for $p < 0.05$.
Source: Centers for Disease Control and Prevention, Youth Risk Behavior Surveillance System, http://www.cdc.gov/nccdphp/dash/yrbs/index.htm

3.23 Miami, 1991 and 2001

(responses to the Youth Risk Behavior Surveillance System Survey questions, and direction of change at the 95 percent confidence level, Miami, 1991 and 2001)

	2001	1991	direction of change*
1. Of students who rode a motorcycle during the past 12 months, the percentage who never or rarely wore a motorcycle helmet	49.5	37.8	increased
2. Of students who rode a bicycle during the past 12 months, the percentage who never or rarely wore a bicycle helmet	88.1	97.8	decreased
3. Percentage of students who never or rarely wear a seat belt when riding in a car driven by someone else	18.1	28.4	decreased
4. Percentage of students who during the past 30 days rode one or more times in a car or other vehicle driven by someone who had been drinking alcohol	26.7	29.1	no change
5. Percentage of students who during the past 30 days drove a car or other vehicle one or more times when they had been drinking alcohol	8.8	9.0	no change
6. Percentage of students who carried a weapon such as a gun, knife, or club on one or more of the past 30 days	11.3	24.4	decreased
7. Percentage of students who were in a physical fight one or more times during the past 12 months	32.7	41.4	decreased
8. Percentage of students who were injured in a physical fight one or more times during the past 12 months and had to be treated by a doctor or nurse	4.3	3.7	no change
9. Percentage of students who seriously considered attempting suicide during the past 12 months	11.9	25.8	decreased
10. Percentage of students who made a plan about how they would attempt suicide during the past 12 months	9.8	15.2	decreased
11. Percentage of students who actually attempted suicide one or more times during the past 12 months	8.1	6.8	no change
12. Percentage of students whose attempted suicide during the past 12 months resulted in an injury, poisoning, or overdose that had to be treated by a doctor or nurse	3.4	1.6	increased
13. Percentage of students who ever tried cigarette smoking, even one or two puffs	50.9	66.2	decreased
14. Percentage of students who smoked a whole cigarette for the first time before age 13	13.0	20.6	decreased
15. Percentage of students who smoked cigarettes on one or more of the past 30 days	16.9	14.7	no change
16. Percentage of students who smoked two or more cigarettes per day on the days they smoked during the past 30 days	9.5	9.0	no change
17. Percentage of students who had at least one drink of alcohol on one or more days during their life	69.4	76.8	decreased
18. Percentage of students who had their first drink of alcohol other than a few sips before age 13	29.8	35.1	decreased
19. Percentage of students who had at least one drink of alcohol on one or more of the past 30 days	39.9	42.8	no change
20. Percentage of students who had five or more drinks of alcohol in a row, that is, within a couple of hours, on one or more of the past 30 days	19.1	17.2	no change
21. Percentage of students who used marijuana one or more times during their life	31.9	21.6	increased
22. Percentage of students who tried marijuana for the first time before age 13	7.7	6.7	no change
23. Percentage of students who used marijuana one or more times during the past 30 days	17.0	9.7	increased
24. Percentage of students who used any form of cocaine, including powder, crack, or freebase one or more times during their life	8.1	5.8	no change

(continued)

(continued from previous page)

	2001	1991	direction of change*
25. Percentage of students who used any form of cocaine, including powder, crack, or freebase one or more times during the past 30 days	4.0	2.2	increased
26. Percentage of students who took steroid pills or shots without a doctor's prescription one or more times during their life	3.2	3.6	no change
27. Percentage of students who had sexual intercourse	50.8	54.8	no change
28. Percentage of students who had sexual intercourse for the first time before age 13	9.1	15.0	decreased
29. Percentage of students who had sexual intercourse with four or more people during their life	17.1	20.4	no change
30. Percentage of students who had sexual intercourse with one or more people during the past three months	35.3	35.0	no change
31. Of students who had sexual intercourse during the past three months, the percentage who drank alcohol or used drugs before last sexual intercourse	18.3	14.9	no change
32. Of students who had sexual intercourse during the past three months, the percentage who used a condom during last sexual intercourse	68.8	45.1	increased
33. Percentage of students who had been pregnant or gotten someone pregnant one or more times	7.0	6.7	no change
34. Percentage of students who described themselves as slightly or very overweight	26.7	27.6	no change
35. Percentage of students who were trying to lose weight	42.7	37.7	increased
36. Percentage of students who did exercises to strengthen or tone their muscles on three or more of the past seven days	43.7	42.0	no change
37. Percentage of students who attended physical education (PE) class one or more days during an average school week	41.3	51.3	no change
38. Percentage of students who had ever been taught about AIDS or HIV infection in school	83.1	82.4	no change
39. Percentage of students who smoked cigarettes on 20 or more of the past 30 days	5.4	5.8	no change
40. Percentage of students who smoked more than 10 cigarettes per day on the days that they smoked during the past 30 days	1.3	1.7	no change
41. Percentage of students who have ever had sexual intercourse but have not had sexual intercourse during the past three months	30.2	35.9	decreased
42. Percentage of students who attended physical education (PE) class daily	15.4	44.6	decreased
43. Percentage of students who have never had sexual intercourse, who have had sexual intercourse but not during the past three months, or who used a condom the last time they had sexual intercourse during the past three months	89.1	81.0	increased

*Change over time is statistically significant for $p < 0.05$.
Source: Centers for Disease Control and Prevention, Youth Risk Behavior Surveillance System, http://www.cdc.gov/nccdphp/dash/yrbs/index.htm

3.24 Philadelphia, 1991 and 2001

(responses to the Youth Risk Behavior Surveillance System Survey questions, and direction of change at the 95 percent confidence level, Philadelphia, 1991 and 2001)

		2001	1991	direction of change*
1.	Of students who rode a motorcycle during the past 12 months, the percentage who never or rarely wore a motorcycle helmet	55.5	41.7	increased
2.	Of students who rode a bicycle during the past 12 months, the percentage who never or rarely wore a bicycle helmet	90.9	96.3	decreased
3.	Percentage of students who never or rarely wear a seat belt when riding in a car driven by someone else	34.5	52.1	decreased
4.	Percentage of students who during the past 30 days rode one or more times in a car or other vehicle driven by someone who had been drinking alcohol	23.3	32.1	decreased
5.	Percentage of students who during the past 30 days drove a car or other vehicle one or more times when they had been drinking alcohol	4.9	6.7	no change
6.	Percentage of students who carried a weapon such as a gun, knife, or club on one or more of the past 30 days	12.7	36.2	decreased
7.	Percentage of students who were in a physical fight one or more times during the past 12 months	41.7	56.0	decreased
8.	Percentage of students who were injured in a physical fight one or more times during the past 12 months and had to be treated by a doctor or nurse	5.3	8.2	decreased
9.	Percentage of students who seriously considered attempting suicide during the past 12 months	16.6	26.1	decreased
10.	Percentage of students who made a plan about how they would attempt suicide during the past 12 months	15.3	15.5	no change
11.	Percentage of students who actually attempted suicide one or more times during the past 12 months	12.0	8.1	increased
12.	Percentage of students whose attempted suicide during the past 12 months resulted in an injury, poisoning, or overdose that had to be treated by a doctor or nurse	3.1	2.5	no change
13.	Percentage of students who ever tried cigarette smoking, even one or two puffs	62.6	76.4	decreased
14.	Percentage of students who smoked a whole cigarette for the first time before age 13	17.7	24.9	decreased
15.	Percentage of students who smoked cigarettes on one or more of the past 30 days	15.8	19.5	no change
16.	Percentage of students who smoked two or more cigarettes per day on the days they smoked during the past 30 days	9.4	12.9	no change
17.	Percentage of students who had at least one drink of alcohol on one or more days during their life	70.3	76.7	decreased
18.	Percentage of students who had their first drink of alcohol other than a few sips before age 13	32.4	37.0	no change
19.	Percentage of students who had at least one drink of alcohol on one or more of the past 30 days	31.6	44.1	decreased
20.	Percentage of students who had five or more drinks of alcohol in a row, that is, within a couple of hours, on one or more of the past 30 days	13.6	20.1	decreased
21.	Percentage of students who used marijuana one or more times during their life	42.7	37.3	no change
22.	Percentage of students who tried marijuana for the first time before age 13	10.6	12.9	no change
23.	Percentage of students who used marijuana one or more times during the past 30 days	21.4	16.2	increased
24.	Percentage of students who used any form of cocaine, including powder, crack, or freebase one or more times during their life	2.6	5.2	decreased

(continued)

(continued from previous page)

		2001	1991	direction of change[*]
25.	Percentage of students who used any form of cocaine, including powder, crack, or freebase one or more times during the past 30 days	1.3	1.5	no change
26.	Percentage of students who took steroid pills or shots without a doctor's prescription one or more times during their life	4.1	4.6	no change
27.	Percentage of students who had sexual intercourse	61.6	68.0	no change
28.	Percentage of students who had sexual intercourse for the first time before age 13	17.1	21.9	no change
29.	Percentage of students who had sexual intercourse with four or more people during their life	25.9	31.6	no change
30.	Percentage of students who had sexual intercourse with one or more people during the past three months	42.1	50.7	no change
31.	Of students who had sexual intercourse during the past three months, the percentage who drank alcohol or used drugs before last sexual intercourse	13.5	15.5	no change
32.	Of students who had sexual intercourse during the past three months, the percentage who used a condom during last sexual intercourse	64.3	47.6	increased
33.	Percentage of students who had been pregnant or gotten someone pregnant one or more times	10.1	14.5	no change
34.	Percentage of students who described themselves as slightly or very overweight	27.6	27.7	no change
35.	Percentage of students who were trying to lose weight	41.8	34.5	increased
36.	Percentage of students who did exercises to strengthen or tone their muscles on three or more of the past seven days	36.2	38.4	no change
37.	Percentage of students who attended physical education (PE) class one or more days during an average school week	52.6	71.7	decreased
38.	Percentage of students who had ever been taught about AIDS or HIV infection in school	89.2	83.1	increased
39.	Percentage of students who smoked cigarettes on 20 or more of the past 30 days	6.4	9.6	no change
40.	Percentage of students who smoked more than 10 cigarettes per day on the days that they smoked during the past 30 days	0.9	2.3	no change
41.	Percentage of students who have ever had sexual intercourse but have not had sexual intercourse during the past three months	31.2	25.6	no change
42.	Percentage of students who attended physical education (PE) class daily	23.8	41.1	decreased
43.	Percentage of students who have never had sexual intercourse, who have had sexual intercourse but not during the past three months, or who used a condom the last time they had sexual intercourse during the past three months	85.3	73.9	increased

* Change over time is statistically significant for p< 0.05.
Source: Centers for Disease Control and Prevention, Youth Risk Behavior Surveillance System, http://www.cdc.gov/nccdphp/dash/ yrbs/index.htm

3.25 San Diego, 1991 and 2001

(responses to the Youth Risk Behavior Surveillance System Survey questions, and direction of change at the 95 percent confidence level, San Diego, 1991 and 2001)

		2001	1991	direction of change˙
1.	Of students who rode a motorcycle during the past 12 months, the percentage who never or rarely wore a motorcycle helmet	34.9	46.0	decreased
2.	Of students who rode a bicycle during the past 12 months, the percentage who never or rarely wore a bicycle helmet	72.1	92.8	decreased
3.	Percentage of students who never or rarely wear a seat belt when riding in a car driven by someone else	7.4	14.9	decreased
4.	Percentage of students who during the past 30 days rode one or more times in a car or other vehicle driven by someone who had been drinking alcohol	28.0	30.5	no change
5.	Percentage of students who during the past 30 days drove a car or other vehicle one or more times when they had been drinking alcohol	8.5	11.2	no change
6.	Percentage of students who carried a weapon such as a gun, knife, or club on one or more of the past 30 days	12.3	22.8	decreased
7.	Percentage of students who were in a physical fight one or more times during the past 12 months	33.5	38.6	no change
8.	Percentage of students who were injured in a physical fight one or more times during the past 12 months and had to be treated by a doctor or nurse	4.5	3.6	no change
9.	Percentage of students who seriously considered attempting suicide during the past 12 months	21.0	28.2	decreased
10.	Percentage of students who made a plan about how they would attempt suicide during the past 12 months	16.9	16.7	no change
11.	Percentage of students who actually attempted suicide one or more times during the past 12 months	10.5	6.3	increased
12.	Percentage of students whose attempted suicide during the past 12 months resulted in an injury, poisoning, or overdose that had to be treated by a doctor or nurse	3.5	2.2	no change
13.	Percentage of students who ever tried cigarette smoking, even one or two puffs	61.8	67.6	no change
14.	Percentage of students who smoked a whole cigarette for the first time before age 13	16.7	21.8	decreased
15.	Percentage of students who smoked cigarettes on one or more of the past 30 days	17.1	17.9	no change
16.	Percentage of students who smoked two or more cigarettes per day on the days they smoked during the past 30 days	8.2	10.2	no change
17.	Percentage of students who had at least one drink of alcohol on one or more days during their life	76.5	73.8	no change
18.	Percentage of students who had their first drink of alcohol other than a few sips before age 13	30.1	30.5	no change
19.	Percentage of students who had at least one drink of alcohol on one or more of the past 30 days	41.0	44.8	no change
20.	Percentage of students who had five or more drinks of alcohol in a row, that is, within a couple of hours, on one or more of the past 30 days	24.3	25.5	no change
21.	Percentage of students who used marijuana one or more times during their life	41.8	35.9	no change
22.	Percentage of students who tried marijuana for the first time before age 13	13.5	10.6	no change
23.	Percentage of students who used marijuana one or more times during the past 30 days	22.5	18.1	no change
24.	Percentage of students who used any form of cocaine, including powder, crack, or freebase one or more times during their life	8.8	8.1	no change

(continued)

(continued from previous page)

	2001	1991	direction of change[*]
25. Percentage of students who used any form of cocaine, including powder, crack, or freebase one or more times during the past 30 days	3.8	2.6	no change
26. Percentage of students who took steroid pills or shots without a doctor's prescription one or more times during their life	5.2	2.2	increased
27. Percentage of students who had sexual intercourse	38.2	48.0	decreased
28. Percentage of students who had sexual intercourse for the first time before age 13	5.6	10.6	decreased
29. Percentage of students who had sexual intercourse with four or more people during their life	11.2	15.8	no change
30. Percentage of students who had sexual intercourse with one or more people during the past three months	26.6	30.3	no change
31. Of students who had sexual intercourse during the past three months, the percentage who drank alcohol or used drugs before last sexual intercourse	24.1	22.4	no change
32. Of students who had sexual intercourse during the past three months, the percentage who used a condom during last sexual intercourse	62.7	43.1	increased
33. Percentage of students who had been pregnant or gotten someone pregnant one or more times	4.7	6.2	no change
34. Percentage of students who described themselves as slightly or very overweight	29.3	29.8	no change
35. Percentage of students who were trying to lose weight	45.6	38.9	increased
36. Percentage of students who did exercises to strengthen or tone their muscles on three or more of the past seven days	52.4	51.9	no change
37. Percentage of students who attended physical education (PE) class one or more days during an average school week	63.7	67.2	no change
38. Percentage of students who had ever been taught about AIDS or HIV infection in school	89.4	96.4	decreased
39. Percentage of students who smoked cigarettes on 20 or more of the past 30 days	4.7	6.8	no change
40. Percentage of students who smoked more than 10 cigarettes per day on the days that they smoked during the past 30 days	0.9	1.0	no change
41. Percentage of students who have ever had sexual intercourse but have not had sexual intercourse during the past three months	29.9	36.8	no change
42. Percentage of students who attended physical education (PE) class daily	40.9	55.2	decreased
43. Percentage of students who have never had sexual intercourse, who have had sexual intercourse but not during the past three months, or who used a condom the last time they had sexual intercourse during the past three months	90.4	82.9	increased

* Change over time is statistically significant for p< 0.05.
Source: Centers for Disease Control and Prevention, Youth Risk Behavior Surveillance System, http://www.cdc.gov/nccdphp/dash/yrbs/index.htm

Index